CARDIOVASCULAR

DISEASE AND

DIABETES

Notice

Medicine is an ever-changing science. As new research and clinical experience broaden our knowledge, changes in treatment and drug therapy are required. The authors and the publisher of this work have checked with sources believed to be reliable in their efforts to provide information that is complete and generally in accord with the standards accepted at the time of publication. However, in view of the possibility of human error or changes in medical sciences, neither the authors nor the publisher nor any other party who has been involved in the preparation or publication of this work warrants that the information contained herein is in every respect accurate or complete, and they disclaim all responsibility for any errors or omissions or for the results obtained from use of the information contained in this work. Readers are encouraged to confirm the information contained herein with other sources. For example and in particular, readers are advised to check the product information sheet included in the package of each drug they plan to administer to be certain that the information contained in this work is accurate and that changes have not been made in the recommended dose or in the contraindications for administration. This recommendation is of particular importance in connection with new or infrequently used drugs.

CARDIOVASCULAR

DISEASE AND

DIABETES

Editor
Luther T. Clark, MD, FACC, FACP
Professor of Clinical Medicine
Chief, Division of Cardiovascular Medicine
State University of New York Downstate Medical Center
Chief of Cardiology, Kings County Hospital Center
Brooklyn, New York

Associate Editor
Samy I. McFarlane, MD, MPH, FACP
Professor of Medicine
Chief, Division of Endocrinology, Diabetes and Hypertension
State University of New York Downstate Medical Center &
Kings County Hospital Center
Brooklyn, New York

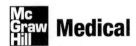 **Medical**

New York / Chicago / San Francisco / Lisbon / London / Madrid / Mexico City
Milan / New Delhi / San Juan / Seoul / Singapore / Sydney / Toronto

Cardiovascular Disease and Diabetes

Copyright © 2007 by The McGraw-Hill Companies, Inc. All rights reserved. Printed in the United States of America. Except as permitted under the United States Copyright Act of 1976, no part of this publication may be reproduced or distributed in any form or by any means, or stored in a database or retrieval system, without the prior written permission of the publisher.

1 2 3 4 5 6 7 8 9 0   FRG/FRG   0 9 8 7 6

ISBN-13: 9780-07-143681-6
ISBN-10: 0-07-143681-2

This book was set in Palatino by International Typesetting and Composition.
The editors were Hilarie Surrena, Karen G. Edmonson, and Peter J. Boyle.
The production supervisor was Sherri Souffrance.
Project management was provided by International Typesetting and Composition.
The indexer was Robert Swanson.
Quebecor World Fairfield was printer and binder.

This book is printed on acid-free paper.

Library of Congress Cataloging-in-Publication Data

Cardiovascular disease and diabetes / edited by Luther T.
  Clark; associate editor, Samy I. McFarlane.
      p. ; cm.
   Includes bibliographical references and index.
   ISBN 0-07-143681-2 (alk. paper)
   1. Diabetic angiopathies.   2. Cardiovascular system—Diseases—Etiology.   3.
Cardiovascular system—Diseases—Complications.   I. Clark, Luther T.   II. McFarlane,
Samy I.
   [DNLM: 1. Cardiovascular Diseases—complications.   2. Diabetes
Complications—therapy.   3. Cardiovascular Diseases—therapy.   4. Diabetes
Mellitus—therapy. WK 840 C267   2007]
   RC700.D5C3722   2007
   616.1′071—dc22   2006046614

CONTENTS

CONTRIBUTORS

Mary Ann Banerji, MD, FACP
Associate Professor of
    Medicine
State University of New York
    Downstate Medical Center
Brooklyn, New York
Chapter 15

Paramdeem Baweja, MD
Clinical Assistant Instructor of
    Medicine
Division of Cardiovascular
    Medicine
State University of New York
    Downstate Medical Center
Brooklyn, New York
Chapter 3

Clinton D. Brown, MD
Associate Professor of
    Medicine
Medical Director of Ambulatory
    Dialysis and Lipid Clinic
State University of New York
    Downstate Medical Center
Brooklyn, New York
Chapter 8

Ruth C. Browne, ScD
Director, Arthur Ashe Institute for
    Urban Health
State University of New York
    Downstate Medical Center
Brooklyn, New York
Chapter 20

Chard Bubb, MD
Clinical Assistant Instructor of
    Medicine
Division of Endocrinology,
    Diabetes and Hypertension
State University of New York
    Downstate Medical Center
Kings County Hospital Center
Brooklyn, New York
Chapter 2

Joshua Burack, MD, FACS
Clinical Associate Professor of
    Surgery
State University of New York
    Downstate Medical Center
Kings County Hospital Center
Brooklyn, New York
Chapter 12

Erdal Cavusoglu, MD
Assistant Professor of Medicine
Associate Director of the Cardiac
    Cath Lab
Division of Cardiovascular Medicine
State University of New York
    Downstate Medical Center
Brooklyn, New York
Chapter 17

Roseann Chesler, PhD
Research Assistant Professor
State University of New York
    Downstate Medical Center
Brooklyn, New York
Chapter 10

Luther T. Clark, MD, FACC, FACP
Professor of Clinical Medicine
Chief, Division of Cardiovascular
    Medicine
State University of New York
    Downstate Medical Center
Chief of Cardiology
Kings County Hospital Center
Brooklyn, New York
Chapters 1, 3, 5, 14, 19, 20, 21, 22

Karen Scott Collins, MD, MPH
Deputy Chief Medical Officer
Health Care Quality and Clinical
    Services
New York City Health and
    Hospitals Corporation
New York, New York
Chapter 21

Uzodinma R. Dim, MD
Clinical Instructor of
    Medicine
State University of New York
    Downstate Medical Center
Brooklyn, New York
Chapter 3

Luis Garcia, PA-C
New York Methodist Hospital
Brooklyn, New York
Chapter 5

Yohannes Gebreegziabher, MD
Clinical Instructor of
    Medicine
Division of Cardiovascular
    Medicine
State University of New York
    Downstate Medical Center
Brooklyn, New York
Chapter 2

Suzette Graham-Hill, MD
Assistant Professor of Medicine
Division of Cardiovascular
    Medicine
State University of New York
    Downstate Medical Center
Brooklyn, New York
Chapter 14

Amir Hayat, MD
Senior Research Specialist
Department of Medicine
State University of New York
    Downstate Medical Center
Brooklyn, New York
Chapter 13

Girardin Jean-Louis, PhD
Associate Professor, Psychiatry and
    Ophthalmology
Research Coordinator, Brooklyn
    Health Disparities Research Center
State University of New York
    Downstate Medical Center
Brooklyn, New York
Chapter 19

John Kassotis, MD, EngSciD, FACP
Visiting Associate Professor of
    Medicine
Director, Electrophysiology Section
State University of New York
    Downstate Medical Center
Brooklyn, New York
Chapters 5, 6, 19

Ronald Kokolis, MD
Clinical Instructor of Medicine
Division of Cardiovascular Medicine
State University of New York
    Downstate Medical Center
Brooklyn, New York
Chapter 20

Spyros Kokolis, MD
Clinical Instructor of Medicine
Division of Cardiovascular Medicine
State University of New York
   Downstate Medical Center
Brooklyn, New York
Chapters 5, 17

Manish Lakhani, MD
Clinical Instructor of Medicine
Division of Cardiovascular
   Medicine
State University of New York
   Downstate Medical Center
Brooklyn, New York
Chapter 17

John C. LaRosa, MD, FACP
Professor of Medicine
President and Chief Executive
   Officer
State University of New York
   Downstate Medical Center
Brooklyn, New York
Chapters 8, 18

Judie H. LaRosa, PhD, RN
Professor of Preventive Medicine
   and Community Health
Deputy Director, Master of Public
   Health Program
State University of New York
   Downstate Medical Center
Brooklyn, New York
Chapter 18

Jason M. Lazar, MD, FACC, FACCP
Visiting Associate Professor of
   Medicine
Director, Noninvasive Cardiology
State University of New York
   Downstate Medical Center
Brooklyn, New York
Chapter 11, 16

Robert C. Lowery, MD, FACS
Professor and Chief
Division of Cardiothoracic Surgery
State University of New York
   Downstate Medical Center
Brooklyn, New York
Chapter 12

Amgad N. Makaryus, MD
Clinical Instructor of Medicine
Division of Cardiology
North Shore University Hospital
New York University School of
   Medicine
Manhasset, New York
Chapter 2

Nagarathna Manjappa, MD
Clinical Instructor of Medicine
Department of Medicine
State University of New York
   Downstate Medical Center
Brooklyn, New York
Chapter 13

Jonathan D. Marmur, MD, FACC, FRCP(c)
Professor of Medicine
Director, Cardiac Catheterization
   and Interventional Cardiology
State University of New York
   Downstate Medical Center
Brooklyn, New York
Chapters 4, 17

Samy I. McFarlane, MD, MPH, FACP
Professor of Medicine
Chief, Division of Endocrinology,
   Diabetes and Hypertension
State University of New York
   Downstate Medical Center
Kings County Hospital Center
Brooklyn, New York
Chapters 2, 22

Judith Mitchell, MD, FACC
Associate Professor of Medicine
Director, Heart Failure Center
State University of New York
  Downstate Medical Center
Brooklyn, New York
Chapter 7

Cristina Mitre
Clinical Instructor of Medicine
Division of Cardiovascular
  Medicine
State University of New York
  Downstate Medical Center
Brooklyn, New York
Chapter 4

Susana R. Morales, MD
Associate Professor of Clinical
  Medicine
Associate Chair for Educational
  Affairs
Weill Medical College of
  Cornell University
New York, New York
Chapter 20

Hanan Morcos, MD
Clinical Instructor of Medicine
Division of Cardiovascular
  Medicine
State University of New York
  Downstate Medical Center
Brooklyn, New York
Chapter 6

Roman Royzman, MD
Clinical Instructor of Medicine
Division of Cardiovascular
  Medicine
State University of New York
  Downstate Medical Center
Brooklyn, New York
Chapter 22

Louis Salciccioli, MD, FACC, FACP
Assistant Professor of Medicine
Director, Advanced Cardiac
  Imaging
State University of New York
  Downstate Medical Center
Brooklyn, New York
Chapter 11, 16

Moro O. Salifu, MD, MPH, FACP
Associate Professor of Medicine
Director, Nephrology Fellowship
  Program
State University of New York
  Downstate Medical Center
Brooklyn, New York
Chapter 13

Gerald A. Soff, MD
Professor of Medicine
Chief, Division of
  Hematology/Oncology
State University of New York
  Downstate Medical Center
Brooklyn, New York
Chapter 17

Michael A. Weber, FACP, FACC
Professor of Medicine
State University of New York
  Downstate Medical Center
Brooklyn, New York
Chapter 9

Marilyn White, MD
Associate Director, Research and
  Training
Arthur Ashe Institute for Urban
  Health
State University of New York
  Downstate Medical Center
Brooklyn, New York
Chapter 20

Reba Williams, MD
Senior Director Healthcare Quality
  and Clinical Services
New York City Health and
  Hospitals Corporation
New York, New York
Chapter 21

Ferdinand Zizi, MBA
Program Manager, Brooklyn Health
  Disparities Research Center
State University of New York
  Downstate Medical Center
Brooklyn, New York
Chapter 19

To my mother, Princetta, who sacrificed so that I might succeed
and
To Mitchell and Timmy Karro, for their wisdom and guidance
and
To my wife, Camille, for her love, patience, support, and encouragement
and
To my children Jason Myles and Monica Marie, who give me
joy and inspiration

The burden of diabetes and diabetes-related cardiovascular disease is now, more than ever, a worldwide problem with enormous consequences in terms of human suffering and economic costs. In the United States, the number of people with diabetes was approximately 2 million in the 1960s. This increased to 15 million by the year 2000, 21 million in 2006, with projected estimates of 50 million (diagnosed and undiagnosed) by the year 2025. Worldwide, the prevalence of diabetes is projected to exceed 300 million cases by the year 2025. Despite accelerating advances in the understanding of diabetes and cardiovascular diseases, the rapidly increasing diabetes epidemic—largely a consequence of the obesity epidemic— may result in reversal of the declining cardiovascular disease mortality trends of the past three decades.

Both type 1 and type 2 diabetes are powerful and independent risk factors for cardiovascular disease. Atherosclerosis accounts for approximately 80% of all premature deaths and 75% of hospitalizations in patients with diabetes. Approximately three-fourths of these deaths result from coronary artery disease and the remaining from cerebrovascular or peripheral vascular diseases. Although optimal control and intensive management of risk factors can reduce cardiovascular disease by as much as 50%, the quality of care provided patients with diabetes remains far from optimal, with less than 30% of diabetics achieving currently recommended treatment goals. Recent accelerated advances in genetics and genomics, new therapies and treatment strategies, and new technologies all herald new opportunities for prevention, treatment, and stemming the tide of the diabetes-cardiovascular disease conundrum.

In *Cardiovascular Disease and Diabetes*, the authors provide a comprehensive assessment of the pathophysiology and clinical management of cardiovascular disease in patients with diabetes. In addition, this multidisciplinary team of contributors provides chapters on other important aspects of diabetes and cardiovascular diseases, including impact on health disparities and the chronic care model as a best practices strategy. Both primary care physicians and specialists who treat patients with diabetes and heart disease should find *Cardiovascular Disease and Diabetes* useful for improving their understanding of the cardiovascular complication of diabetes and for day-to-day clinical decision making and patient management. Dr. Luther Clark and collaborators, all expert clinicians and scientists from the State University of New York Downstate and Kings County Medical Centers, have to be congratulated for such a timely, comprehensive, well-integrated, and practical book.

Valentin Fuster, MD, PhD, FACC

As we approach the end of the first decade of the 21st century, diabetes mellitus and its complications remain among the greatest challenges to modern medicine. This is true despite the fact that diabetes is preventable and its major complications treatable. If the current epidemic of diabetes continues unabated in the United States and worldwide, the prevalence will exceed 330 million by the year 2025. This translates into a staggering toll of acute and chronic complications that will reverse the declining cardiovascular disease mortality trend that we have witnessed during the past several decades. A pandemic of obesity, an increasingly sedentary lifestyle, increased prevalence of other major cardiovascular risk factors (hypertension, dyslipidemia, etc), increased lifespan, and poor glycemic control in diabetics all contribute to this burgeoning health crisis.

Approximately 80% of all deaths and more than 75% of all hospitalizations in patients with diabetes are due to cardiovascular disease, primarily complications of coronary heart disease. Given the major clinical and public health implications of cardiovascular disease and diabetes, it is critically important that we take full advantage of recent advances in our knowledge of pathobiology and treatment to reduce cardiovascular risks and improve outcomes in patients with diabetes.

The purpose of *Cardiovascular Disease and Diabetes* is to provide a comprehensive state-of-the-art text on the epidemiology, pathophysiology, and recent advances in management of cardiovascular disease in patients with diabetes. Special emphasis is placed on recent and emerging concepts, and modern approaches to patient management. *Cardiovascular Disease and Diabetes* is intended for practicing clinicians. Both primary care physicians and specialists who treat patients with diabetes and cardiovascular disease will find this book to be a useful reference for understanding pathophysiologic concepts and a manual of the latest treatment recommendations. The special cardiovascular problems associated with diabetes are discussed in detail with specific evidence-based management recommendations.

Cardiovascular Disease and Diabetes is written by a panel of seasoned clinicians and expert scientists who comprehensively review both the clinical and scientific aspects of diabetic cardiovascular disease. The contributors provide new information on the mechanisms of diabetes-associated cardiovascular disease, associated risk factors, and acute and chronic cardiac syndromes. Chapters are devoted to epidemiology, mechanisms of diabetes-associated cardiovascular disease, associated coronary risk factors (hypertension, dyslipidemia, obesity, metabolic syndrome), specific cardiovascular syndromes that complicate diabetes (acute coronary syndromes, sudden cardiac death, heart failure, nephropathy), CHD risk assessment, hemostatic abnormalities, and the shifting paradigm of care for diabetes and cardiac disease from acute, life-threatening disorders to chronic, long-term conditions in an aging population. It is an essential guide for treatment, prevention, and unraveling of the diabetes conundrum.

Luther T. Clark, MD, FACC, FACP

ACKNOWLEDGMENTS

Many friends and colleagues have provided support and inspiration for the writing of this text. I am particularly indebted to my fellow clinicians and educators at the State University of New York Downstate Medical Center and Kings County Hospital Center whose commitment to improving the quality of medical care for patients with cardiovascular disease and diabetes and to educating future generations of clinicians inspired me to take on the challenge of editing and contributing to *Cardiovascular Disease and Diabetes*.

I would like to acknowledge and express my gratitude to all of the contributors who committed to writing chapters and followed through despite their busy and overextended schedules. The selfless donation of their time and expertise demonstrate their commitment to patient care and to education. I want to particularly thank them for their patience in responding to my persistence and urging as deadlines approached.

Grateful thanks are also due to Cassandra A. McCullough for her research assistance, Janet Goldson-McKenzie for coordinating the many logistics and schedules necessary for my involvement as editor/contributor, and Carlota Brown for her expertise in handling the final details and followups necessary to meet deadlines.

I want to acknowledge and thank the cardiology fellows, residents, and students whom I've worked with over the years for their inspiration and illumination of the need for putting this book together.

Finally, I wish to thank my strongest supporter, my wife, Camille, without whose support and encouragement, this would have been an impossible endeavor.

CARDIOVASCULAR DISEASES AND DIABETES: AN EPIDEMIOLOGIC OVERVIEW

Luther T. Clark

Cardiovascular disease (CVD) is the leading cause of mortality in the United States and a leading cause of death and disability throughout the world. Diabetes mellitus is a well-established independent risk factor for CVD in both men and women, and an important contributor to the increasing threat of CVD. Prevention of CVD and management of established CVD in patients with diabetes are among the greatest challenges facing clinicians, patients, and society. Although the two conditions are closely linked, they are usually managed separately by different teams of specialists. Improvement in the overall quality of care for diabetes and reduction of the disproportionate burden of CVD will require better strategies for coordinated, comprehensive, acute, and chronic care.

GLOBAL BURDEN OF CARDIOVASCULAR DISEASE AND DIABETES

Cardiovascular Disease

Worldwide, there are approximately 17 million deaths annually from CVD, 7.2 million due to ischemic heart disease, 5.5 million to cerebrovascular disease, and 4.0 million to hypertensive and other cardiac conditions.[1,2] In addition, there are at least 20 million annual survivors of heart attack and strokes. Approximately 80% of the worldwide CVD mortality occurs in developing countries (Fig. 1-1) and the number is increasing.[3] This is largely due to an

International Cardiovascular Disease Statistics

Death rates for total cardiovascular disease, coronary heart disease, stroke and total deaths in selected countries (most recent year available) (Revised 2005)

Men ages 35–74
Rate per 100,000 population

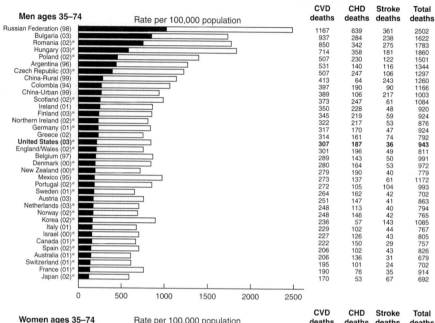

	CVD deaths	CHD deaths	Stroke deaths	Total deaths
Russian Federation (98)	1167	639	361	2502
Bulgaria (03)	937	284	238	1622
Romania (02)*	850	342	275	1783
Hungary (03)*	714	358	181	1860
Poland (02)*	507	230	122	1501
Argentina (96)	531	140	116	1344
Czech Republic (03)*	507	247	106	1297
China-Rural (99)	413	64	243	1260
Colombia (94)	397	190	90	1166
China-Urban (99)	389	106	217	1003
Scotland (02)*	373	247	61	1084
Ireland (01)	350	228	48	920
Finland (03)*	345	219	59	924
Northern Ireland (02)*	322	217	53	876
Germany (01)*	317	170	47	924
Greece (02)	314	161	74	792
United States (03)*	**307**	**187**	**36**	**943**
England/Wales (02)*	301	196	49	811
Belgium (97)	289	143	50	991
Denmark (00)*	280	164	53	972
New Zealand (00)*	279	190	40	779
Mexico (95)	273	137	61	1172
Portugal (02)*	272	105	104	993
Sweden (01)*	264	162	42	702
Austria (03)	251	147	41	863
Netherlands (03)*	248	113	40	794
Norway (02)*	248	146	42	765
Korea (02)*	236	57	143	1085
Italy (01)	229	102	44	767
Israel (00)*	227	126	43	805
Canada (01)*	222	150	29	757
Spain (02)*	206	102	43	826
Australia (01)*	206	136	31	679
Switzerland (01)*	195	101	24	702
France (01)*	190	76	35	914
Japan (02)*	170	53	67	692

Women ages 35–74
Rate per 100,000 population

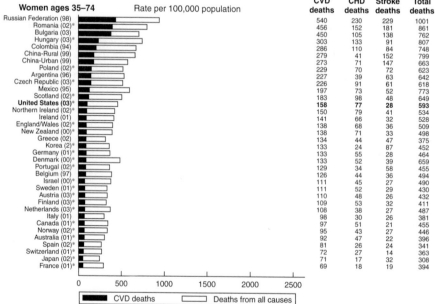

	CVD deaths	CHD deaths	Stroke deaths	Total deaths
Russian Federation (98)	540	230	229	1001
Romania (02)*	456	152	181	861
Bulgaria (03)	450	105	138	762
Hungary (03)*	303	133	91	807
Colombia (94)	286	110	84	748
China-Rural (99)	279	41	152	799
China-Urban (99)	273	71	147	663
Poland (02)*	229	70	72	623
Argentina (96)	227	39	63	642
Czech Republic (03)*	226	91	61	618
Mexico (95)	197	73	52	773
Scotland (02)*	183	98	48	649
United States (03)*	**158**	**77**	**28**	**593**
Northern Ireland (02)*	150	79	41	534
Ireland (01)	141	66	32	528
England/Wales (02)*	138	68	36	509
New Zealand (00)*	138	71	33	498
Greece (02)	134	44	47	375
Korea (2)*	133	24	87	452
Germany (01)*	133	55	28	464
Denmark (00)*	133	52	39	659
Portugal (02)*	129	34	58	455
Belgium (97)	126	44	36	494
Israel (00)*	111	45	27	490
Sweden (01)*	111	52	29	430
Austria (03)	110	48	26	432
Finland (03)*	109	53	32	411
Netherlands (03)*	108	38	27	487
Italy (01)	98	30	26	381
Canada (01)*	97	51	21	455
Norway (02)*	95	43	27	446
Australia (01)*	92	47	22	396
Spain (02)*	81	26	24	341
Switzerland (01)*	72	27	14	363
Japan (02)*	71	17	32	308
France (01)*	69	18	19	394

■ CVD deaths   □ Deaths from all causes

Note : Rates adjusted to the European Standard population. ICD/9 codes are 390–459 for cardiovascular disease; 410–414 for coronary heart disease; and 430–438 for stroke. Countries using ICD/10 are noted with.*
* ICD/10 codes are 100–199 for cardiovascular disease; 120–125 for coronary hear disease; and 160-169 for stroke.
Source : The World Heath Organization Web page, **who.int/whosis/, NCHS and NHLBI.**

Figure 1-1 **Death rates for total CVD, CHD, stroke, and total deaths in selected countries (revised in 2005). Note: Rates adjusted for the European Standard**

Table 1-1 **Worldwide Prevalence of Diabetes and Impaired Glucose Tolerance in 2003 and Projected for 2025**

All Diabetes and IGT	2003	2025
Total world population (billions)	6.3	8.0
Adult population (billions) (20–79 years)	3.8	5.3
Number of people with diabetes (millions) (20–79 years)	194	333
World diabetes prevalence (%) (20–79 years)	5.1	6.3
Number of people with IGT (millions) (20–79 years)	314	472
IGT prevalence (%) (20–79 years)	8.2	9.0

Source: Data from International Diabetes Federation. Diabetes Atlas, 2003: Available at: www.idf.org/e-atlas. Accessed March 20, 2006.

aging population and increased exposure to major CVD risk factors, including smoking, hypertension, hypercholesterolemia, physical inactivity, obesity, and diabetes. The growing epidemic of obesity and diabetes are of special concern.

Diabetes Mellitus

Globally, diabetes is one of the most common noncommunicable diseases, and is the fourth or fifth leading cause of death in most developed countries.[4,5] Its prevalence is increasing at a rate that is now epidemic in many developing and newly industrialized nations. In 2003, there were 194 million adults worldwide with diabetes and 314 million adults with impaired glucose tolerance (IGT; Table 1-1).[4] These numbers are projected to increase to 333 and 472 million, respectively, by the year 2025 (Table 1-1).

population. ICD/9 codes are 390–459 for CVD; 410–414 for CHD; and 430–438 for stroke. Countries using ICD/10 are noted with asterisk (*). ICD/10 codes are 100–199 for CVD; 120–125 for CHD; and 160–169 for stroke. (*Source: Adapted from Thom T, Haase N, Rosamond W, et al. Heart disease and stroke statistics— 2006 update. A report from the American Heart Association Statistics Committee and Stroke Statistics Subcommittee. Circulation 2006;113:e85–e151; The World Health Organization Web page: who.int/whosis/; NCHS and NHLBI.*)

In the United States, approximately 7.0% of the population (20.8 million people) has diabetes, 14.6 million diagnosed and 6.2 million undiagnosed.[6] Among U.S. adults 20 years of age or older, 20.6 million (9.6% of the adult population) have diabetes (10.9 million or 10.5% of men and 9.7 million or 8.8% of women ≥20 years old have diabetes). The prevalence of diabetes in the United States has tripled during the past three decades and the number of individuals affected continues to increase—at enormous human and economic costs.

CARDIOVASCULAR DISEASES IN THE UNITED STATES

Prevalence

More than 71 million Americans have one or more types of CVD (Fig. 1-2; Table 1-2),[3] including coronary heart disease (CHD; 6.5 million), heart failure (5.0 million), and stroke (5.5 million). CVD is responsible annually for more than 900,000 deaths and 6.4 million hospital discharges. The estimated total annual cost of CVD and stroke in the United States is $403.1 billion, including health care services, medications, and lost productivity.

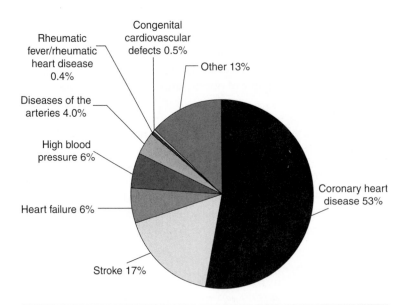

Figure 1-2 **Percentage breakdown of deaths from CVDs (United States: 2003 [preliminary]).** (*Source: Adapted from Thom T, Haase N, Rosamond W, et al. Heart disease and stroke statistics—2006 update. A report from the American Heart Association Statistics Committee and Stroke Statistics Subcommittee. Circulation 2006;113:e85–e151; CDC/NCHS and NHLBI.*)

Table 1-2 **CVD Prevalence, Mortality, Hospital Discharges, and Estimated 2006 Cause by Population Group**

Population Group	Prevalence 2003	Mortality 2003#*	Hospital Discharges 2003	Cost 2006
Total	71,300,000 (34.2%)	910,614	6,434,000	$403.1 billion
Total males	33,100,000 (34.4%)	426,772 (46.9%)[†]	3,239,000	—
Total females	38,200,000 (33.9%)	483, 842 (53.1%)[†]	3,196,000	—
NH white males	34.3%	368,182	—	—
NH white females	32.4%	419,248	—	—
NH black males	41.1%	49,032	—	—
NH black females	44.7%	55,803	—	—
Mexican American males	29.2%	—	—	—
Mexican American females	29.3%	—	—	—

Abbreviation: NH, non-Hispanic; (—), data not available.

*Hash (#) reperesents preliminary data.

[†]These percentages represent the portion of total CVD mortality that is for males vs. females.
Source: Prevalence: NHANES (1999–1992), CDC/NCHS, and NHLBI. Percentages for racial/ethnic groups are age-adjusted for Americans aged 20 and older. These data are based on self-reports. Estimates from NHANES 1999–2002 applied to 2003 population estimates. Mortality: CDC/NCHS: these data represent underlying cause of death only; data for white and black males and females include Hispanics; data include congenital CVD. Hospital discharges: National Hospital Discharge Survey, CDC/NCHS; data include people discharged alive and dead. Cost: NHLBI; data include estimated direct an indirect cost for 2006.

Mortality

Despite recent declines, mortality from CVD (heart disease and stroke) remains the leading cause of death in the United States for both men and women[3] (Fig. 1-3; Table 1-2), and for most ethnic groups. The decline in cardiovascular mortality during the past two decades has been less dramatic for women than men. In 2003, CVD accounted for 37.3% of all deaths in the United States and was an underlying or contributing cause of death in about 58% of cases.[3] The death rates (deaths/1000 population) were 364.2 for males and 262.5 for females. In contrast, cancer death rates were 232.3 for males and 160.2 for females. Death rates for females were 25.2 for breast cancer and 41.1 for lung

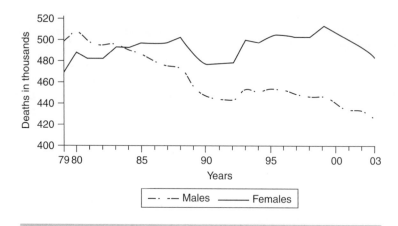

Figure 1-3 **CVD mortality trends for males and females (United States: 1979–2003 [preliminary]).** (*Source: Adapted from Thom T, Haase N, Rosamond W, et al. Heart disease and stroke statistics— 2006 update. A report from the American Heart Association Statistics Committee and Stroke Statistics Subcommittee. Circulation 2006;113: e85–e151; CDC/NCHS and NHLBI.*)

cancer. One in 30 females die from breast cancer while 1 in 2.6 die from CVD. Among the various ethnic groups in the United States, heart disease is the leading cause of death for American Indians and Alaska Natives, blacks (or African Americans), Hispanics, and whites. Cancer is the leading cause of death for Asians and Pacific Islanders, with heart disease a close second.[7]

African Americans have the highest overall mortality rate from CHD of any ethnic group (Fig. 1-4), particularly out-of-hospital deaths, and especially at younger ages.[8,9] Hispanics, on the other hand, and despite an excess of CHD risk factors similar to that in African Americans (Table 1-3)[10] have a lower CVD mortality rate than non-Hispanic blacks and non-Hispanic whites (see Fig. 1-4).[11–14] The lower CVD mortality rates in Hispanics despite a high burden of CVD risk factors has been referred to as the "Hispanic Paradox."[13] Blacks are the only ethnic group in the United States in which mortality rates continue to exceed the 2010 targets.

DIABETES MELLITUS AND OTHER CARDIOVASCULAR DISEASE RISK FACTORS

The major risk factors for CVD are cigarette smoking, hypertension, dyslipidemia, diabetes, and obesity. Although the prevalence of major CVD risk factors in the population in the United States has decreased during the past

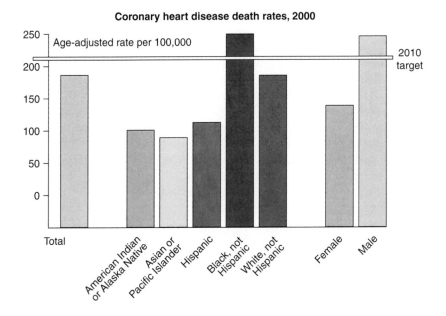

Figure 1-4 **CHD death rates by ethnicity and gender in reference to the 2010 Healthy People 2000 target.** (*Source: Adapted from http://www.cdc. gov/nchs/hphome.htm*)

Table 1-3 **CHD Risk Factors That Are More Prevalent in Non-Hispanic blacks and Hispanics Than in Non-Hispanic whites in the United States**

More prevalent in non-Hispanic blacks than non-hispanic whites	*More prevalent in Hispanics than non-hispanic whites*
Hypertension	Type 2 DM
Type 2 DM	Obesity
Obesity	Low HDL-C (females)
Metabolic syndrome (females)	Elevated TGs
Cigarette smoking	Metabolic syndrome
Physical inactivity	Physical inactivity

Source: Data from Refs. 8, 10, and 11.

several decades[3] (Fig. 1-5), obesity and diabetes are notable exceptions[3] (Figs. 1-6 and 1-7) with the increasing prevalence of obesity and type 2 diabetes in children and adolescents (Fig. 1-8) a particular concern. Most individuals with CHD have at least one major risk factor[3,15,16] and risk factors often cluster in individual patients. Data from the 2003 Behavioral Risk Factor Surveillance System (BRFSS) study of adults aged 18 and older showed that the prevalence of two or more risk factors for CVD increased among successive age groups.[3] The prevalence of having two or more risk factors was similar in women (36.4%) and men (37.8%), highest among blacks (48.7%) and American Indians/Alaska Natives (46.7%) and lowest among Asians (25.9%).[3,15] These findings portend the potential for an increased burden of CVD and further erosion of the mortality declines observed during the past several decades.

Diabetes Mellitus

PREVALENCE

Diabetes mellitus is a heterogeneous disease that has been classified as type 1 and type 2. More than 90% of diabetes is of the type 2 variety, and is

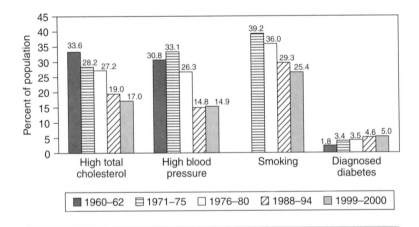

Figure 1-5 **Trends in cardiovascular risk factors in the U.S. population aged 20–74 (NHES: 1960–1962; NHANES: 1971–1975 to 1999–2000). In this study, high total cholesterol was defined as ≥240 mg/dL; high blood pressure was defined as ≥140/90 mmHg.** (*Source: Adapted from Thom T, Haase N, Rosamond W, et al. Heart disease and stroke statistics—2006 update. A report from the American Heart Association Statistics Committee and Stroke Statistics Subcommittee. Circulation 2006;113: e85–e151; Gregg EW, Narayan KMV. Type 2 diabetes and cognitive function: Are cognitive impairment and dementia complications of type 2 diabetes? Clin Geriatr 2000;8:57–72.*)

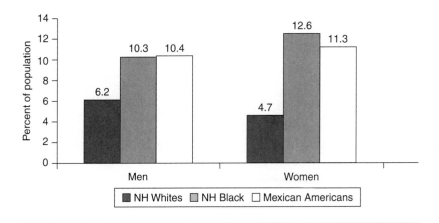

Figure 1-6 **Age-adjusted prevalence of physician-diagnosed diabetes in Americans aged 20 and older by race/ethnicity and sex (NHANES: 1999–2002). NH indicates non-Hispanics.** (*Source: Adapted from Thom T, Haase N, Rosamond W, et al. Heart disease and stroke statistics—2006 update. A report from the American Heart Association Statistics Committee and Stroke Statistics Subcommittee.* Circulation *2006;113:e85–e151; CDC/NCHS and NHLBI.*)

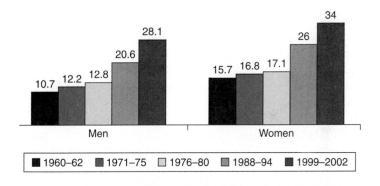

Figure 1-7 **Age-adjusted prevalence of obesity in Americans aged 20–74 by sex and survey (NHES 1960–1962; NHANES: 1971–1974, 1976–1980, 1988–1994, and 1999–2002). Note: Obesity is defined as BMI of 30.0 or higher.** (*Source: Adapted from Thom T, Haase N, Rosamond W, et al. Heart disease and stroke statistics—2006 update. A report from the American Heart Association Statistics Committee and Stroke Statistics Subcommittee.* Circulation *2006;113:e85–e151; Health, United States, 2004, CDC/NCHS.*)

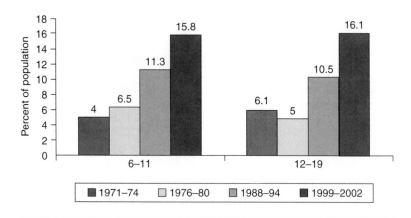

Figure 1-8 **Trends in the prevalence of overweight among U.S. children and adolescents by age and survey (NHANES: 1971–1974, 1976–1980, 1988–1994, and 1999–2002; NHANES: 1971–1974 to 1999–2002).** *(Source: Adapted from Thom T, Haase N, Rosamond W, et al. Heart disease and stroke statistics—2006 update. A report from the American Heart Association Statistics Committee and Stroke Statistics Subcommittee. Circulation 2006;113:e85–e151; Health, United States, 2004, CDC/NCHS.)*

primarily a disease of insulin resistance and hyperglycemia. Type 1 diabetes accounts for less than 10% of cases and is characterized by severe insulinopenia, hyperglycemia, and occasional bouts of ketoacidosis.

Worldwide, there are approximately 194 million adult cases of diabetes and this number is expected to increase to 333 million by 2025 (Table 1-1).[2,4] In the United States, approximately 7.0% of the population (20.8 million people) has diabetes mellitus, 14.6 million diagnosed and 6.2 million undiagnosed.[2] Among adults 20 years of age or older, 20.6 million (9.6% of the adult population) have diabetes (10.9 million or 10.5% of men and 9.7 million or 8.8% of women ≥20 years old have diabetes).

The impact of diabetes is not uniform across ethnic groups. Compared to whites, type 2 diabetes is 2 to 3 times more prevalent in African Americans, 2.5 times more prevalent in Hispanics (particularly those of Puerto Rican and Mexican origin), and 5 times more prevalent in Native Americans.[17] In the United States, approximately 8.7% (13.1 million) of all non-Hispanic whites ≥20 years and 13.3% (3.2 million) of all non-Hispanic blacks ≥20 years have diabetes. Mexican Americans, the largest Hispanic/Latino subgroup, are 1.7 times as likely to have diabetes as non-Hispanic whites. If the prevalence of diabetes among Mexican Americans is applied to the total

Hispanic/Latino population, about 2.5 million (9.5%) Hispanic/Latino Americans aged 20 years or older would have diabetes.

DIABETES AND CARDIOVASCULAR RISK

Both type 1 and type 2 diabetes are potent and independent risk factors for CHD, stroke, peripheral arterial disease, blindness, and nephropathy. In patients with diabetes mellitus, CVD is the major cause of morbidity and mortality.[18] Approximately 80% of all deaths and more than 75% of all hospitalizations in patients with diabetes are due to CVD—primarily complication of CHD.

The incidence and severity of microvascular disease (nephropathy, retinopathy, neuropathy, and peripheral small vessel disease) are directly related to the duration and severity of hyperglycemia in type 1 diabetes. However, macrovascular disease (coronary, cerebrovascular, and peripheral vascular) is multifactorial in origin with many contributing factors, some of which are interlinked and appear to be related to insulin resistance and hyperinsulinemia (i.e., hypertension, dyslipidemia, obesity, and coagulation abnormalities).[19–21]

Hypertension

Both systolic hypertension and diastolic hypertension are established risk factors for CVD.[22] Hypertension increases risk for CHD, heart failure, stroke, end-stage renal disease (ESRD), left ventricular hypertrophy, left ventricular dysfunction, heart failure, and overall mortality. Hypertension is approximately twice as common in diabetic as in nondiabetic patients, and about three of four adults with diabetes have blood pressure ≥130/80 mmHg or use prescription medications for hypertension. Patients with diabetic nephropathy are at particular risk since 75–85% of those with overt diabetic nephropathy will have hypertension.[23,24] Left ventricular dysfunction in hypertensive diabetics may be predominantly diastolic, systolic, or both. However, even in the absence of coexisting hypertension, diabetes may be associated with increased left ventricular mass and diastolic dysfunction.[25–27]

Obesity

An estimated 97 million adults in the United States are overweight or obese. *Obesity* is defined as a body mass index (weight in kg divided by the square of height in meters) ≥30 kg/m^2 and *overweight* as 25–29.9 kg/m^2.[28] Obesity increases risk for development of type 2 diabetes, CHD, stroke, hypertension, and is associated with insulin resistance in normoglycemic individuals as well as those with type 2 diabetes.[28–36] Abdominal (central), visceral, or predominantly upper-body distribution of body fat is a stronger risk factor for CVD than is obesity per se. The steady increase in diabetes in the United

States and worldwide is largely due to an increasing global epidemic of obesity. The linkage between obesity and diabetes is so strong that some experts have coined a new term to describe it, "diabesity."[37,38]

Atherogenic Dyslipidemia

Dyslipidemia is common in patients with diabetes. Diabetic dyslipidemia refers to atherogenic dyslipidemia occurring in persons with type 2 diabetes and is characterized by the triad of elevated triglyceride (TG) levels, reduced high-density lipoprotein cholesterol (HDL-C) levels, and a preponderance of small dense low-density lipoprotein cholesterol (LDL-C) particles. Often referred to as "atherogenic dyslipidemia,"[39,40] all of the three components of this atherogenic dyslipidemia triad are associated with atherogenesis and increased CHD risk.[41-44]

ELEVATED TRIGLYCERIDES

Elevated serum TG levels ($\geq$150 mg/dL) are an independent risk factor for CHD. Hypertriglyceridemia can be caused by diabetes mellitus, obesity, physical inactivity, a high-carbohydrate diet (>60% of calories), as well as certain drugs (estrogens, corticosteroids), excessive alcohol intake, and genetic disorders.

LOW HDL CHOLESTEROL

Low HDL-C is defined by the National Cholesterol Education Program Adult Treatment Panel III (NCEP ATP III) guidelines as <40 mg/dL in men and women.[39,40] However, for diagnosis of the metabolic syndrome, HDL <40 mg/dL in men or <50 mg/dL in women are considered abnormal and one of the diagnostic criteria. Low HDL-C is a strong and independent predictor of CHD.[39-44] Low HDL-C may be caused by factors associated with insulin resistance, such as elevated TGs, type 2 diabetes, excess weight, physical inactivity, high carbohydrate consumption, cigarette smoking, and certain drugs (beta-blockers, anabolic steroids, and progesterone). In individuals with low HDL-C levels, the primary therapeutic objective is to achieve the recommended LDL-C goal.[39,40] If the TG level is >200 mg/dL, reduction of non-HDL-C (total cholesterol minus HDL-C) is the secondary target. If the TG level is not elevated, specific therapies to increase HDL-C may be considered.

TOTAL AND LDL CHOLESTEROL

Total and LDL-C levels in persons with diabetes are similar to those of persons without diabetes. However, LDL particles in persons with type 2 diabetes are smaller and the number is usually greater. The NCEP ATP III recommends that in individuals with diabetes, as in others, LDL-C should be the primary target of lipid-modifying therapy.[39,40] Intensive treatment is recommended for very high-risk, high-risk, and moderately high-risk patients.

CIGARETTE SMOKING

Cigarette smoking is a powerful risk factor for atherosclerosis and CHD. The risk of CVD is doubled in patients with diabetes who smoke cigarettes and the benefits of modifying other risk factors are substantially attenuated.[45] Although the prevalence of cigarette smoking in diabetics is similar to that in nondiabetics, the imperative for smoking cessation is greater in diabetics.

CARDIOVASCULAR DISEASES AND DIABETES

Coronary Heart Disease

Approximately 30% of patients hospitalized with acute coronary syndromes have diabetes. Diabetics present with first myocardial infarction at younger ages than nondiabetics, experience greater mortality during the acute phase of myocardial infarction and during the postinfarction period,[46,47] often have complications (including arrhythmias, congestive heart failure, and recurrent ischemia/infarction), and more often have multivessel coronary artery disease on angiography. Myocardial infarction in diabetics may occur without chest pain and present as unexplained heart failure, malignant arrhythmias, or even with acutely uncontrolled blood sugars and diabetic ketoacidosis.

Although recent advances in treatment for acute myocardial infarction have dramatically improved survival in both nondiabetic and diabetic patients, diabetes still doubles the case fatality rate.[47] Diabetic women have particularly poor outcomes with mortality rates that are almost twofold greater than diabetic men. The excess in-hospital mortality and increased frequency of clinical heart failure occur despite similar residual left ventricular ejection fractions as in nondiabetics.

Silent Myocardial Ischemia

Diabetic patients have a higher frequency of silent ischemia or ischemia with atypical symptoms than their nondiabetic counterparts. In the Framingham Heart Study, 32–42% of diabetic patients with myocardial infarction had atypical symptoms (dyspnea, fatigue, confusion, nausea, and vomiting) compared to 6–15% of those patients without diabetes.[48,49] Although the increased frequency of silent ischemia in diabetics may be due to the associated cardiac autonomic neuropathy, silent myocardial ischemia is not uncommon in diabetic patients with CHD and no evidence of autonomic neuropathy. Optimal glycemic control may slow the development of cardiac autonomic neuropathy and lessen propensity for silent ischemic episodes.

Heart Failure and Cardiomyopathy

Diabetes increases the likelihood of development of heart failure from all causes. Congestive heart failure is twice as prevalent in diabetic men and five times as common in diabetic women as in their nondiabetic counterparts (see Chapters 2 and 7). Although this appears to be largely a consequence of the higher rates of CHD and hypertension, even after adjustments for coronary disease, age, blood pressure, weight, rheumatic heart disease, and serum cholesterol, diabetics are still at increased risk for developing heart failure.

Diabetic cardiomyopathy may be a distinct entity, resulting primarily from the interactions of hypertension and diabetes. It can also coexist with coronary artery disease, and may explain the higher prevalence of congestive heart failure in diabetic patients following myocardial infarction. Diabetic cardiomyopathy is characterized by myocardial hypertrophy, increased interstitial connective tissue, and microvascular pathology with systolic and diastolic ventricular dysfunction. The cardiomyopathy appears to be multifactorial in origin and may occur in the absence of coronary, valvular, or other known cardiac diseases. Clinically, these patients usually have a dilated congestive cardiomyopathy.

Cardiac Autonomic Neuropathy

Cardiac autonomic neuropathy is one of the long-term complications of diabetes. It is often present in patients with peripheral or autonomic neuropathy, and may be recognized by the presence of decreased heart rate variability with respiration and/or decreased rise in heart rate during standing. Impaired parasympathetic activity is more common, may be seen relatively early in diabetes, and is manifested as increased resting heart rate and decreased respiratory variation in heart rate. Postural hypotension is common in diabetic patients with autonomic neuropathy, particularly following bed rest or in patients taking antihypertensive medications. The increased risk of sudden cardiac death in diabetic patients with autonomic neuropathy may be in part related to the high incidence of QT prolongation (at rest and following exercise), which may be associated with increased risk for malignant ventricular arrhythmias.

CARDIORENAL DISEASE: DIABETIC NEPHROPATHY

Diabetes mellitus is the leading cause of renal failure worldwide with a prevalence greater than that of glomerulonephritis and hypertensive renal disease. Diabetic nephropathy is a clinical syndrome characterized by persistent albuminuria, elevated blood pressure, a relentless decline in glomerular filtration rate, and a high risk of cardiovascular morbidity and mortality.[17] According to the U.S. Renal Data System (USRDS), 45% of patients with ESRD in 2002 had diabetes as the primary cause.[50] In patients with ESRD, clinical and subclinical coronary artery diseases are common in both diabetics and nondiabetics at the time of initiation of ESRD therapy. Patients with chronic kidney disease have accelerated atherosclerosis and are at increased risk for cardiovascular events although direct evidence demonstrating a causal relationship is lacking.[51–53]

SUMMARY

As we near the end of the first decade of the twenty-first century, the burdens of CVDs and diabetes continue to increase, and are approaching epidemic proportions. This is a consequence of a multiplicity of factors, including an aging population, an increased exposure to cardiovascular risk factors, and in particular, the dramatic increase in the prevalence of overweight, obesity, and the metabolic syndrome. These risk factors predispose to the development of both diabetes and CVD, and pose great challenges to clinicians, public health practices, and patients. New and improved strategies are necessary if we are to stem the increasing tide of obesity, diabetes, and CVD. Otherwise, the mortality declines observed during the last several decades will not only cease, but will also be reversed.

REFERENCES

1. Smith SC Jr, Jackson R, Pearson TA, et al. Principles for National and Regional Guidelines on Cardiovascular Disease Prevention: A Scientific Statement from the World Heart and Stroke Forum. *Circulation* 2004;109:3112–3121.

2. Fleck F. Cardiovascular disease: a global health time bomb. *Bull World Health Organ* 2004;82(6):470–471. ISSN 0042-9686. Available at: http://www.earth.columbia.edu/news/2004/images/raceagainsttime_FINAL_051104.pdf

3. Thom T, Haase N, Rosamond W, et al. Heart disease and stroke statistics—2006 update. A report from the American Heart Association Statistics Committee and Stroke Statistics Subcommittee. *Circulation* 2006;113:e85–e151.

4. International Diabetes Federation. Diabetes Atlas, 2003. Available at: www.idf.org/e-atlas. Accessed March 20, 2006.

5. Wild S, Roglic G, Green A, et al. Global prevalence of diabetes. Estimates for the year 2000 and projections for 2030. *Diabetes Care* 2004;27:1047–1053.

6. CDC. National Diabetes Fact Sheet—United States, 2005. Available at: http://www.cdc.gov/diabetes/pubs/pdf/ndfs_2005.pdf Accessed 3/18/06

7. Arias E, Anderson RN, Kung HC, et al. Deaths: final data for 2001. *Natl Vital Stat Rep* 2003;52:1–115.

8. Clark LT. Issues in minority health: atherosclerosis and coronary heart disease in African Americans. *Med Clin North Am* 2005;89:977–1001.

9. Clark LT, Ferdinand KC, Flack JM, et al. Coronary heart disease in African Americans. *Heart Dis* 2001;3:97–108.

10. Liao Y, Cooper R, Cao G, et al. Mortality from coronary heart disease and cardiovascular disease among adult U.S. Hispanics. *J Am Coll Cardiol* 1997;30:1200–1205.

11. Ford ES, Giles WH, Dietz WH. Prevalence of the metabolic syndrome among US adults: findings from the Third National Health and Nutritional Examination Survey. *JAMA* 2002;287:356–359.

12. Hunt KJ, Williams K, Resendez RG, et al. All-cause and cardiovascular mortality among diabetic participants in the San Antonio Heart Study: evidence against the "Hispanic Paradox." *Diabetes Care* 2002;25(9):1557–1563.

13. Markides KS, Coreil J. The health of Hispanics in the southwestern United States: an epidemiologic paradox. *Public Health Rep* 1986;101:253–265.

14. Resnick HE, Jones K, Ruotolo G, et al. Insulin resistance, the metabolic syndrome, and risk of incident cardiovascular disease in nondiabetic American Indians. The Strong Heart Study. *Diabetes Care* 2003;26:861–867.

15. CDC. Declining prevalence of no known major risk factors for heart disease and stroke among adults—United States, 1991–2001. *MMWR* 2004;53:4–7.

16. Greenland P, Knoll MD, Stamler J, et al. Major risk factors as antecedents of fatal and nonfatal coronary heart disease events. *JAMA* 2003;290:891–897.

17. Jawa A, Kcomt J, Fonseca VA. Diabetic nephropathy and retinopathy. *Med Clin North Am* 2004;88:1001–1036.

18. Wingard DL, Barrett-Connor E. Heart disease and diabetes. In Harris M, ed., *Diabetes in America*, 2nd ed. National Institute of Health, National Institute of Diabetes and Digestive and Kidney Diseases. NIH Publication No. 95-1468, 1995:429–445.

19. Haffer SM, Meittinen H. Insulin resistance implications for type II diabetes mellitus and coronary heart disease. *Am J Med* 1997;103:152–162.

20. Koch M, Gradaus F, Schoebel F, et al. Relevance of conventional cardiovascular risk factors for the prediction of coronary disease in diabetic patients on renal replacement therapy. *Nephrol Dial Transplant* 1997;12:1187–1191.

21. Escalante DA, Kim DK, Garber AJ. Atherosclerotic cardiovascular disease. *Curr Ther Diab* 1998;176–190.

22. Chobanian AV, Bakris GL, Black HR, et al. The Seventh Report of the Joint National Committee on Prevention, Detection, Evaluation, and Treatment of High Blood Pressure: the JNC7 Report. *JAMA* 2003;289:2560–2571.

23. World Health Organization: definition, diagnosis and classification of diabetes mellitus and its complications: report of a WHO consultation. Part 1: diagnosis and classification of diabetes mellitus. Geneva: World Health Organization, 1999. Available at: *http://www.staff.ncl.ac.uk/philip.home/who_dmg.pdf.* Accessed March 7, 2006.

24. Vikram NK, Pandey RM, Misra A, et al. Non-obese (body mass index < 25 kg/m^2) Asian Indians with normal waist circumference have high cardiovascular risk. *Nutrition* 2003;19(6):503–509.

25. Epstein M, Sowers JR. Diabetes mellitus and hypertension. *Hypertension* 1992;19:403–418.

26. Weidmann P, Boehlen LM, deCourten M. Pathogenesis and treatment of hypertension associated with diabetes mellitus. *Am Heart J* 1993;125:1498–1513.

27. Galderisi M, Anderson K, Wilson P, et al. Echocardiographic evidence for the existence of a distinct diabetic cardiomyopathy (The Framingham Heart Study). *Am J Cardiol* 1991;68:85–89.

28. NHLBI Obesity Education Initiative Expert Panel. Clinical guidelines on the identification, evaluation, and treatment of overweight and obesity in adults: the evidence report. *Obes Res* 1998;6(Suppl 2):51S–209S.

29. Pi-Sunyer FX. Pathophysiology and long-term management of the metabolic syndrome. *Obes Res* 2004;12:174S–180S.

30. Despres JP. The insulin resistance–dyslipidemic syndrome of visceral obesity: effect on patient's risk. *Obes Res* 1998;6:8S–17S.

31. Bjorntorp P. Body fat distribution, insulin resistance, and metabolic diseases. *Nutrition* 1997;13:795–803.

32. Brunzell JD, Hokanson JE. Dyslipidemia of central obesity and insulin resistance. *Diabetes Care* 1999;22:C10–C13.

33. Bonow RO. Primary prevention of cardiovascular disease: a call to action. *Circulation* 2002;106:3140–3141.

34. Reilly MP, Rader DJ. The metabolic syndrome: more than the sum of its parts? *Circulation* 2003;108:1546–1551.

35. Lüscher TF, Creager MA, Beckman JA, et al. Diabetes and vascular disease: pathophysiology, clinical consequences, and medical therapy. Part II. *Circulation* 2003;108:1655–1661.

36. Klein S, Burke LE, Bray GA, et al. AHA Scientific Statement. Clinical implications of obesity with specific focus on cardiovascular disease. *Circulation* 2004;110:2952–2967.

37. From the NIH: successful diet and exercise therapy is conducted in Vermont for "diabesity." *JAMA* 1980;243:519–520.

38. Astrup A, Finer N. Redefining type 2 diabetes: "diabesity" or "obesity dependent diabetes mellitus?" (Review). *Obes Rev* 2000;1:57–59.

39. Third Report of the National Cholesterol Education Program (NCEP) Expert Panel on Detection, Evaluation, and Treatment of High Blood Cholesterol in Adults (Adult Treatment Panel III) Final Report. *Circulation* 2002;106:3146–3421.

40. Grundy SM, Cleeman JI, Bairey Merz CN, et al. Implications of recent clinical trials for the National Cholesterol Education Program Adult Treatment Panel III guidelines. *Circulation* 2004;110:227–239.

41. Gordon DJ, Probstfield JL, Garrison RJ, et al. High-density lipoprotein cholesterol and cardiovascular disease: four prospective American studies. *Circulation* 1989;79:8–15.

42. Assmann G, Schulte H. Relation of high-density lipoprotein cholesterol and triglycerides to incidence of atherosclerotic coronary artery disease (the PROCAM experience). *Am J Cardiol* 1992;70:733–737.

43. Austin MA. Plasma triglyceride as a risk factor for cardiovascular disease. *Can J Cardiol* 1998;14(Suppl B):14B–17B.

44. Boden WE. High-density lipoprotein cholesterol as an independent risk factor in cardiovascular disease: assessing the data from Framingham to the Veterans Affairs High-Density Lipoprotein Intervention Trial. *Am J Cardiol* 2000;86: 19L–22L.

45. Grundy SM, Benjamin IJ, Burke GL, et al. Diabetes and cardiovascular disease: a statement for healthcare professionals from the American Heart Association.

Circulation 1999;100:1134–1146. [Published erratum appears in *Circulation* 2000;101:1629–1631].

46. Jacoby R, Nesto R. Acute myocardial infarction in the diabetic patient: pathophysiology, clinical course and prognosis. *J Am Coll Cardiol* 1992;20:736–744.

47. Woodfield S, Lundergan C, Reiner J, et al. Angiographic findings and outcomes in diabetic patients treated with thrombolytic therapy for acute myocardial infarction: the GUSTO-I experience. *J Am Coll Cardiol* 1996;28:1661–1669.

48. Kannel WB. Lipids, diabetes and coronary heart disease: insights from the Framingham Study. *Am Heart J* 1985;110:1100–1107.

49. Tzivoni D, Benhorin J, Stern S. Significance and management of silent myocardial ischemia. *Adv Cardiol* 1990;37:312–319.

50. U.S. Renal Data System, USRDS 2005 Annual Data Report. Incidence and prevalence. Available at: http://www.usrds.org/2005/ref/B.pdf

51. Stack AG. Coronary artery disease and peripheral vascular disease in chronic kidney disease: an epidemiological perspective. *Cardiol Clin* 2005;23:285–298.

52. Lindner A, Charra B, Sherrard DJ, et al. Accelerated atherosclerosis in prolonged maintenance hemodialysis. *N Engl J Med* 1974;290:697–701.

53. Foley RN, Parfrey PS, Sarnak MJ. Clinical epidemiology of cardiovascular disease in chronic renal disease. *Am J Kidney Dis* 1998;32:S112–S119.

MECHANISMS OF CARDIOVASCULAR DISEASE IN DIABETES

Samy I. McFarlane
Yohannes Gebreegziabher
Chard Bubb
Amgad N. Makaryus

Cardiovascular disease (CVD) is the main cause of morbidity and mortality in patients with diabetes mellitus (DM). Major advances in understanding of the pathophysiology of CVD in DM have evolved in recent years. Such knowledge of basic biochemical, molecular, and cellular mechanisms is important for development of effective prevention and treatment strategies of this serious and common disorder. A combination of complex factors such as hyperglycemia, insulin resistance, dyslipidemia, hypertension, oxidative stress, endothelial dysfunction, inflammation, and hypercoagulability, contribute not only to the initiation and progression of atherosclerosis and thrombosis, but also to direct myocardial dysfunction in patients with DM. In this chapter, we discuss the complex mechanisms of CVD in patients with diabetes and insulin-resistant states highlighting the current therapeutic interventions to reduce the disease burden in this high-risk population.

INCREASED CARDIOVASCULAR DISEASE RISK IN DIABETES MELLITUS

Scope of the Problem

Diabetes mellitus poses a significant public health challenge in the United States. The prevalence of DM is increasing rapidly to pandemic proportions.

In 2002, an estimated 18.2 million people (6.3% of the population) had DM, and the direct and indirect health care costs associated with DM were $132 billion.[1] Almost 35 million Americans (20% of all people in the midadult years and 35% of the entire older population) have some degree of abnormal glucose tolerance.[2] Moreover, approximately 35% of DM remains undiagnosed.[3,4] The global prevalence of DM is predicted to increase to 300 million by 2025.[5] DM will continue to be a growing clinical and public health problem because of the increasing frequency of major underlying risk factors for the disease: obesity, westernized diet, and sedentary lifestyles.

CVD is the leading cause of morbidity and mortality in patients with DM. Overall, mortality related to heart disease is estimated to be two to three times higher in patients with DM compared with those without the disease.[6,7] The proportion of CVD attributable to DM or impaired glucose tolerance is as high as 80%.[8] In one of the largest cohort of 347,978 men who were screened for the Multiple Risk Factor Intervention Trial (MR-FIT) and followed for an average of 12 years, DM was significantly associated with increase risk of CVD death in all age groups studied.[9] Other major studies such as the Framingham study and the Nurses' Health Study have demonstrated an increased mortality from CVD in patients with DM.[6,10] In addition, mortality associated with conventional CVD risk factors other than DM, such as hypertension, dyslipidemia, family history, and cigarette smoking, was significantly higher in men with DM than in nondiabetic men.[9] These major CVD risk factors remain important determinants of CVD in patients with DM. In addition, other emerging risk factors (nontraditional), such as albuminuria and elevated fibrinogen level appear to disproportionately increase CVD risk in individuals with DM and insulin resistance.[11–14]

RISK QUANTIFICATION AND STRATIFICATION

Patients with DM are known to be at increased risk of CVD.[6,9,10] Moreover, patients with DM have an increased risk of cardiovascular events once the diagnosis of CVD has been established. Because of this increased risk, it has been suggested that DM may be considered a CVD or a "coronary risk equivalent" indicating that patients with DM belong in the same risk category as patients with known CVD.[15] The relationship between DM and increased CVD risk begins earlier in the progression from normal glucose tolerance to frank DM.[16] The risk of atherosclerotic CVD increases with increasing plasma glucose concentration.[17] For example, in the United Kingdom Prospective DM Study (UKPDS), each 1% increase in the HbA1c level was associated with a 14% increase in the incidence of fatal and nonfatal myocardial infarction.[15]

The coexistence of other cardiovascular risk factors, like hypertension and dyslipidemia, with DM increases the risk of developing CVD in DM. A cluster of several maladaptive cardiovascular risk factors, termed metabolic syndrome or "syndrome X," is defined as the presence of three or more of the following CVD risk factors: blood pressure >130/85 mmHg, abdominal obesity defined by waist circumference >40 in. in men and >35 in. in women, triglycerides >150 mg/dL, serum high-density lipoprotein (HDL) cholesterol <40 mg/dL in men and <50 mg/dL in women, and fasting glucose >110 mg/dL.[18] This metabolic syndrome increases CVD risk and is therefore, it is also called the cardiometabolic syndrome (CMS).[19] Early detection of CVD risk factors in patients with established DM and aggressive intervention should delay onset of CVD. There is evidence that early treatment of these comorbid conditions such as hypertension, obesity, and dyslipidemia reduces the magnitude of CVD in patients with DM.[20] For example, in the UKPDS, lowering systolic BP improved CVD risk in patients with type 2 DM.[21]

PATHOPHYSIOLOGIC MECHANISMS OF CARDIOVASCULAR DISEASE IN DIABETES MELLITUS

The pathophysiologic mechanisms by which DM increases CVD are complex and multifactorial. DM is associated with an increased risk for atherosclerosis independent of the diabetes-induced increase of the known risk factors such as hypertension, dyslipidemia, and insulin resistance. This increased atherosclerosis risk is likely related to the combination of hyperglycemia-induced oxidative stress, altered lipoproteins, increased advanced glycation products, endothelial dysfunction, and inflammation (Table 2-1). Both insulin resistance syndrome (IRS) and hyperglycemia seem to affect the risk of CVD in patients with DM.[22-24] DM is also associated with direct myocardial dysfunction, in addition to the increased risk of coronary atherosclerosis.[25] Macrovascular atherosclerotic CVD (coronary artery disease, cerebrovascular disease, and peripheral vascular disease) is responsible for the majority of morbidity and mortality associated with DM. Atherosclerosis, an arterial wall disease characterized by endothelial dysfunction, vascular smooth muscle growth, inflammation, remodeling, fibrosis, and thrombosis, occurs early and is a more progressive disease in patients with DM.[26] DM can also affect cardiac function independently of coronary artery atherosclerosis by causing endothelial dysfunction in the microcirculation, stimulating abnormal sympathetic tone, depressing cardiac myofilament calcium responsiveness, impairing calcium cycling, limiting myocardial glycolytic oxidative metabolism, and causing diastolic dysfunction by decreasing cardiac compliance.[27-30]

The pathogenesis of CVD in DM includes a constellation of multifactorial metabolic and hemodynamic abnormalities (Table 2-1). In addition to metabolic abnormalities, oxidative stress, inflammation, endothelial dysfunction, hypercoagulability, and myocardial fibrosis; the pathophysiology of CVD in DM involves the traditional cardiac risk factors (hypertension, dyslipidemia, cigarette smoking, genetic factors, hyperglycemia, insulin resistance, and hyperinsulinemia), which are increased in DM.

Table 2-1 **Metabolic and Hemodynamic Abnormalities in DM Associated with Increased Risk of CVD**

Atherosclerotic CVD

Metabolic and biochemical abnormalities
   Hyperglycemia, dyslipidemia (hypertriglyceridemia, reduced HDL-C, increased small dense LDL), hyperinsulinemia, insulin resistance, hyperhomocysteinemia, rennin-angiotensin activation
Increased oxidative stress
   Increased generation of AGEs, activation of polyol pathway and hexosamine pathway, lipid peroxidation, and protein kinase C activation
   Vascular smooth muscle hyperplasia and hypertrophy, intimal lipid accumulation
Endothelial dysfunction
   Decreased NO bioavailability, impaired endothelial vasorelaxation, impaired permeability of endothelial tight junction
   Increased sympathetic nervous system activity and sodium retention
Low-grade chronic inflammation and fibrosis
   Increased CRP, cytokines, TNF-α, ANG-II, vascular endothelial growth factor (VEGF), increased P-selectin, VCAM-1, ICAM-1
Prothrombotic state
   Increased PAI-1, increased platelet activation, increased fibrinogen

Cardiac dysfunction

Impaired myocardial glycolytic oxidative metabolism, microcirculatory endothelial dysfunction, abnormal sympathetic function, impaired calcium cycling, reduced cardiac compliance, and diastolic dysfunction

Associated risk factors

Hypertension and obesity

THE ROLE OF OXIDATIVE STRESS IN DIABETIC CARDIOVASCULAR DISEASE

Though there is lack of clinical evidence on the benefits of the use of antioxidants in DM, data on the pathophysiologic role of oxidative stress on diabetic CVD are quite convincing.[31,32] While reactive oxygen species (ROS) are normally generated under physiologic conditions and are involved as signaling molecules and defense mechanisms as in phagocytosis; excess generation of ROS resulting in oxidative stress has pathologic effects including damage to proteins, lipids, and DNA resulting in impaired cellular structure and function.[33,34]

Oxidative stress is a pathologic state in which excess ROS overwhelm endogenous antioxidant systems. Oxidative stress is the result of excess formation and/or insufficient removal of either ROS such as superoxide ($^{\cdot}O_2^-$), hydroxyl ($^{\cdot}OH$), peroxyl ($^{\cdot}RO_2$), hydro peroxyl ($^{\cdot}HRO_2^-$), hydrogen peroxide (H_2O_2), and hydrochlorous acid (HOCl) or reactive nitrogen species (RNS) like nitric oxide ($^{\cdot}NO$), nitrogen dioxide ($^{\cdot}NO_2^-$), peroxynitrite ($ONOO^-$), nitrous oxide (HNO_2), and alkyl peroxynitrates (RONOO). $^{\cdot}O_2^-$, $^{\cdot}NO$, and $ONOO^-$ are well-studied ROS and are believed to have important roles in diabetic cardiovascular complications.[35] These ROS and RNS are produced by several enzymatic and nonenzymatic processes such as oxidative phosphorylation, nicotinamide adenine dinucleotide phosphate (NADPH) oxidase, xanthine oxidase, the uncoupling of lipoxygenases, cytochrome P450 monooxygenases, and glucose autooxidation.

In addition to the increased production of ROS in DM, hyperglycemia and other reducing sugars in DM cause glycation and glycooxidation of molecules in the arterial wall generating advanced glycation end products (AGEs; Fig. 2-1).[36] Hyperglycemia accelerates formation of nonenzymatic AGEs which accumulate in vascular tissue, leading to increased endothelial dysfunction and increased ROS generation.[37] Moreover, hyperglycemia increases sorbitol formation reducing NADPH which is required for the antioxidant activity of glutathione reductase and normal function of many enzymes such as nitric oxide synthetase (NOS).[38]

$^{\cdot}O_2^-$ is one of the most important ROS in the vasculature. $^{\cdot}O_2^-$ activates several damaging pathways in DM including accelerated formation of AGEs, the polyol pathway, the hexosamine pathway, lipid peroxidation, and protein kinase C (see Fig. 2-1); all of which have been proven to be involved in both micro- and macrovascular complications.[36] $^{\cdot}O_2^-$ and H_2O_2 stimulate nuclear signaling mechanisms causing proliferation and migration of vascular smooth muscle cells (VSMCs), pathologic angiogenesis, and apoptosis.[39,40]

$^{\cdot}NO$, produced from L-arginine by endothelial NOS, mediates endothelium-dependent vasorelaxation in VSMC, and inhibits platelet and leukocyte adhesion to vascular endothelium (Table 2-2). However, $^{\cdot}NO$ easily reacts with $^{\cdot}O_2^-$, generating the highly reactive molecule $ONOO^-$, and triggering a cascade of harmful events.[41] $ONOO^-$ causes protein nitration and lipid peroxidation. ROS-induced membrane lipid peroxidation and protein nitration alters the structure and the fluidity of cell membranes, which ultimately affects normal cellular function resulting in endothelial dysfunction.[42,43] Moreover, oxygen-derived free radicals impair endothelium-dependent vasodilation through inactivation of NO.[44,45]

In DM, ROS production in vascular tissue is increased.[46] Glucose autooxidation and cellular oxidation of glucose lead to generation of excess ROS in mitochondria.[43,47] DM is associated with increased generation of

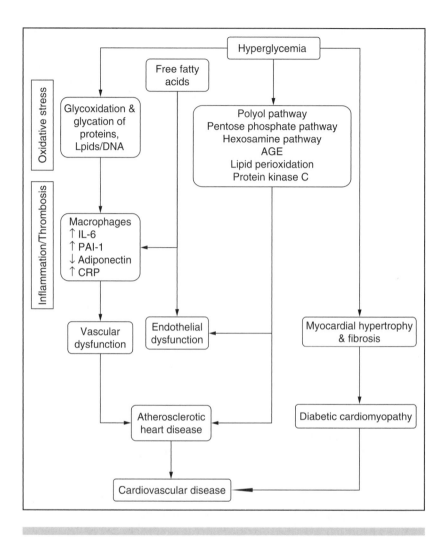

Figure 2-1 **The pathogenesis of CVD in DM. IL, interleukin; PAI-1, plasmin activator inhibitor-1; CRP, C-reactive protein; AGE, advanced glycosylated end products; ↑, increase; ↓, decrease.**

oxygen-derived free radicals by autooxidation by both glucose-dependent and glucose-independent mechanisms. There is also hyperglycemia-induced enhanced metabolism of glucose through the polyol (sorbitol) pathway (see Fig. 2-1), which result in increased production of $\cdot O_2^-$. The increased ROS in DM result in impaired vasorelaxation, vascular dysfunction, damage to membrane lipids, proteins, and nucleic acids, which will cause endothelial dysfunction and accelerated atherosclerosis. Moreover,

Table 2-2 **Alterations in Vascular Endothelium Associated with DM**

Abnormality	Significance
↓ Release of and responsiveness to NO	Impaired endothelial function and reactivity
↑ Expression, synthesis, and plasma levels of endothelin-1	Vasoconstriction and hypertension
↑ Adhesion-molecule expression (VCAM-1; ICAM-1)	Increased monocyte adhesion to vessel wall
↑ Adhesion of platelets and monocytes	Foam cell formation, thrombosis, and inflammation
↑ Procoagulant activity (PAI-1; fibrinogen)	Thrombosis
↑ Advanced glycosylated end products	Increased stiffness of arterial wall
Impaired fibrinolytic activity	Decreased clot breakdown

Abbreviations: ↑, increased; ↓, decreased; NO, nitric oxide; PAI-1, plasmin activator inhibitor; VCAM-1, vascular cell adhesion molecule-1; ICAM-1, intercellular adhesion molecule-1.

excess generation of mitochondrial ROS due to hyperglycemia initiates a vicious circle by activating signaling molecules such as nuclear factor-κB, polyol (sorbitol) and hexosamine pathways, protein kinase C, and AGEs. Enhanced production of AGEs, sorbitol, and proinflammatory cytokines exerts a positive feedback on ROS and RNS synthesis and potentiates protein kinase C-mediated vascular dysfunction by altering gene expression as well as vascular function and structure. All these complex interrelated pathologic modifications contribute to the pathogenesis of vascular dysfunction (see Fig. 2-1).

Increased formation of oxidized low-density lipoprotein (LDL) particles is another important mechanism by which oxidative stress contributes to CVD. Oxidized LDL particles are produced by ROS, vascular wall lipoxygenases, and myeloperoxidases.[48] Increased circulating levels of oxidized LDL have been found in both DM and prediabetic conditions.[49,50] Accumulation of oxidized LDL within the arterial wall stimulates monocyte infiltration, and VSMC migration and proliferation. Oxidized LDL is not recognized by the LDL receptor, and is taken up by scavenger receptors in macrophages and VSMCs leading to foam cell formation and atherosclerotic plaques.[51–53] DM further exacerbates the uptake of oxidized LDL by foam cells. Macrophage foam cells release inflammatory cytokines and growth factors, which further accelerate progression of endothelial dysfunction and atherosclerosis.

AGE AND RAGE IN DIABETIC CARDIOVASCULAR DISEASE

Biochemical interactions of glucose and proteins are being recognized as the underlying mechanism in the pathogenesis of DM-related cardiovascular complications. Chronic hyperglycemia is the main factor in the pathophysiologic mechanisms of diabetic micro- and macrovascular complications.[54-57] One of the mechanisms in the pathogenesis of accelerated atherosclerosis and cardiac dysfunction in DM is hyperglycemia-induced nonenzymatic glycation of proteins and lipids resulting in increased AGEs formation (see Fig. 2-1).[58]

AGE forms irreversible cross-links with many macromolecules like collagen and elastin, thereby resulting in stiff collagen. AGEs may also be involved in atherogenesis by oxidizing LDL. Moreover, AGE acts on AGE receptors (RAGE) on endothelial cells, macrophages, and epithelial cells which stimulate the release of cytokines and growth factors.[59] Through the RAGE-mediated signal transduction, AGE and non-AGE proinflammatory molecules activate several critical molecular pathways that promote angiogenesis, vascular stiffening, and extracellular matrix accumulation. AGEs accumulate slowly in the connective tissue throughout the body and contribute to myocardial stiffness, endothelial dysfunction, atherosclerotic plaque formation, and altered vascular injury responses.[60,61] Thus, AGE cross-links are increasingly felt to play a role in atherosclerosis, myocardial dysfunction, nephropathy, cataracts, retinopathy, and neuropathy.[58] AGEs also play a role in increased cardiovascular risk associated with aging.[62]

The nonenzymatic glycation of proteins occurs by covalent binding of aldehyde or ketone groups of reducing sugars to free N-terminal and lysyl side chain amino groups of proteins. This results in ketoamines called Amadori's products such as glycosylated hemoglobin and fructosamine. The Amadori's products have a reactive free carbonyl group and also degrade to highly reactive carbonyl compounds. These highly reactive carbonyl intermediates such as 3-deoxy-glucosone, glyoxal, and methyl-glyoxal can react again with free amino groups to form several other AGE products such as imidazolone, N—carboxy-methyl-lysine (CML), N—carboxy-ethyl-lysine (CEL), glyoxal-lysine dimer (GOLD), and methyl-glyoxal-lysine dimer (MOLD).[60,63]

Therapeutic agents to reduce formation and accumulation of AGEs in DM have gained interest as potentially cardioprotective. Interventions to reduce AGE-mediated injury by inhibition of AGE formation or prevention of new cross-link formation and breaking of preexisting AGE cross-link have shown good results in animal models of experimental DM.[64] A variety of agents have been developed which include aminoguanidine, ALT-946, pyridoxamine, benfotiamine, OPB-9195, alagebrium chloride, N-phenacylthiazolium bromide, and LR-90. However, the clinical utility of AGE inhibition in humans remains to be seen. Further studies are needed before these agents become part of the therapeutic armamentarium of DM.[65]

ENDOTHELIAL DYSFUNCTION IN DIABETES MELLITUS

Studies have shown that chronic hyperglycemia and insulin resistance cause endothelial dysfunction. Endothelial dysfunction contributes to the development of atherosclerosis, hypertension, microalbuminuria, and diabetic nephropathy.[66] Though atherosclerosis in patients with DM is multifactorial, current theories place endothelial dysfunction as the central initiating factor of the increased atherosclerosis (see Figure 2-2).

The endothelial cell serves as an interface between circulating blood and VSMCs, and therefore facilitates a complex array of functions in intimate interaction with the VSMC, as well as cells within the blood compartment such as monocytes. The normal endothelium mediates vasodilatation, suppresses thrombosis, and suppresses vascular inflammation and hypertrophy. Endothelial dysfunction, manifested as an impaired response to vasodilators, and increased thrombosis, inflammation, and VSMC growth and hypertrophy, is well documented in DM (see Table 2-2).[67,68] Factors associated with endothelial dysfunction in DM include hyperglycemia, increased free fatty acids (FFAs), altered lipoproteins, oxidative stress, overexpression of growth factors and cytokines, increased derivatives of glycation, and activation of protein kinase C.

The endothelial cell and VSMC functions are integrated by complex chemical mediators. The endothelial cells produce NO by the enzyme NOS. NO diffuses into the VSMC and activates the enzyme guanylate cyclase, which produces cyclic guanosine monophosphate (cGMP) which in turn induces smooth muscle relaxation and vasodilation. The continual vasodilation produced by basal NO production has a role in regulation of blood pressure. In type 2 DM, NO-dependent vasodilation is impaired due to an imbalance in production and inactivation. Reduction of NO may also occur in hypertension associated with DM by way of increased plasma asymmetric dimethylarginine (ADMA) levels, an endogenous competitive inhibitor of NOS, or suppression of free scavenger superoxide dismutase (SOD).[69–71]

The endothelial cells also produce mediators that induce vasoconstriction, including endothelin, prostaglandins, and angiotensin-II; thereby regulating vascular tone by maintaining a balance between vasodilation and constriction. The key enzyme that regulates the local generation of angiotensin-II is angiotensin-converting enzyme (ACE). ACE is synthesized by the Endothelial cell (EC), expressed in the surface of the EC, and exerts activity on the bloodborne angiotensin-I. Angiotensin-I is produced by cleavage of a precursor macromolecule (angiotensinogen). Angiotensin-II binds to and regulates VSMC tone via specific angiotensin (ANG) receptors. Depending on the specific receptor activated, angiotensin-II can exert regulatory effects on several VSMC functional activities including vasoconstriction, growth, proliferation, and differentiation. Overall, the actions of angiotensin-II oppose those of NO. Angiotensin-II causes vascular and end-organ dysfunction independent of its vasoconstrictive effects by promoting oxidative stress and endothelial dysfunction.[72] Acting through its type I receptor (AT_1), angiotensin-II also mediates ROS production through NADPH oxidase activation.[73]

Other important markers of endothelial dysfunction, which are expressed in DM, include E-selectin, and intercellular adhesion molecule 1 (ICAM-1), vascular cellular adhesion molecule 1 (VCAM-1), and monocyte chemoattractant protein 1 (MCP-1).[74–78] These markers bind to leukocyte glycoproteins and increase leukocyte adhesion and migration to endothelial cells. Increased leukocyte infiltration to endothelial cells results in release of inflammatory cytokines, matrix metalloproteinases, growth factors, and procoagulants. These processes increase initiation and progression of atherosclerosis and thrombosis.

Increased oxidative stress associated with DM results in endothelial dysfunction. The pathophysiologic alterations that cause endothelial dysfunction, atherosclerosis, and hypertension in DM, also occur in the renal mesangial cells resulting in diabetic glomerulosclerosis and proteinuria. The relationship among vascular endothelial dysfunction, microalbuminuria, and chronic kidney disease is increasingly recognized through epidemiologic and clinical trials.[79] Endothelial dysfunction may be induced by hyperglycemia-stimulated increases in tissue growth factors causing renal mesangial hypertrophy, and enhanced vasomotor tone and vascular/glomerular permeability via vasoconstrictive arachidonic acid metabolites.[80–82] Studies have revealed that albuminuria and chronic kidney disease are strong independent predictors of CVD in DM.[83,84]

Endothelial cell dysfunction has been defined by blunting of the NO-dependent vasodilation response to acetylcholine or a paradoxical vaso-constrictive response to acetylcholine or similar pharmacologic agents like methacholine. Endothelial dysfunction involves either an increase or a decrease in any of the endothelial cell-related messengers and/or by alterations in any of the functional changes such as alterations in regulation of the vessel lumen, increased permeation of macromolecules, increased or decreased production of vasoactive factors producing abnormal vasoconstriction or vasodilation, and increased prothrombotic and or procoagulant activity. Since endothelial functions cannot be measured directly, several indirect methods have been developed to estimate these functions. These include the assessment of plasma concentrations of endothelial-cell-derived proteins, including von Willebrand factor (vWF), VCAM-1, and ICAM-1, as well as the more complicated measurement of NO-dependent vasodilatation or flow-mediated dilatation (FMD) of the brachial artery by noninvasive ultrasound.[85] Increased plasma concentrations of vWF, VCAM-1, and ICAM-1, and a decreased FMD have been associated with an increased risk of CVD.[86,87]

METABOLIC DERANGEMENTS CONTRIBUTING TO CARDIOVASCULAR DISEASE IN DIABETES MELLITUS

Several studies indicate that postprandial metabolic derangements associated with DM are important CVD risk factors.[88] Epidemiologic studies have also shown an association between 2-hour glucose concentrations after a 75 g glucose load and the occurrence of CVD in the general population.[89,90] Metabolic derangements associated with DM and metabolic syndrome or IRS include hyperglycemia, AGEs, increased levels of FFAs, lipoprotein abnormalities (increased very low-density lipoprotein [VLDL] and decreased HDL and small dense lipoproteins), and hyperinsulinemia.

Hyperglycemia and hypertriglyceridemia associated with DM induce oxidative stress, endothelial dysfunction, inflammation, and VSMC hypertrophy and fibrosis.[26]

Hyperglycemia results in increasing oxidative stress, diminishing NO, and enhanced AGE formation, thus increasing glycation of circulating lipoproteins. Intracellular hyperglycemia causes overproduction of superoxide by the mitochondrial electron transport chain, which results in increased polyol pathway influx; increased advanced glycation end-product formation; activation of protein kinase C isoforms, and increased hexosamine pathway flux. These end products result in hyperglycemia-induced vascular damage.[91] This hyperglycemia-induced oxidative stress also results in modification of intracellular proteins resulting in altered cellular function, DNA damage, activation of the transcription factor nuclear factor-κB, which results in abnormal changes in gene expression, decreased production of NO, and increased expression of cytokines, growth factors, as well as procoagulant and proinflammatory molecules.[78] In addition, hyperglycemia alters lipid metabolism, activation of protein kinase C, insulin signaling, and increases adhesion molecule gene expression and inflammatory cytokines.

Fasting hypertriglyceridemia has been shown to be an independent risk factor for CVD.[92] High levels of FFAs can lead to increased oxidative stress and diminished NO synthesis. DM is associated with high triglyceride-rich lipoproteins like smaller VLDL and low HDL. In addition, LDL particles are smaller, denser, and more atherogenic in patients with DM. These DM-associated lipid abnormalities increase the risk of atherosclerosis and directly alter myocardial metabolism of FFAs and glucose.[93]

Postprandial hyperglycemia and increased FFAs are associated with several alterations of the coagulation system.[94,95] Increased FFAs have been shown to be associated with a prothrombotic change characterized by increased plasminogen activator inhibitor-1 (PAI-1) activity. In addition, postprandial hyperglycemia increases circulating cytokine concentrations (interleukin-6 [IL-6] and tumor necrosis factor [TNF]).[96] Postprandial hyperglycemia may have a cytotoxic effect on endothelial cells by inducing increased levels of apoptosis.[97–99] Thus, postprandial hyperglycemia increases atherosclerosis risk by inducing an inflammatory state of increased fibrosis and hypercoagulability. Although postprandial hyperglycemia may not be an independent CVD risk factor, it is likely a risk marker suggestive of underlying metabolic disturbances such as insulin resistance and dyslipidemia, which may have an even greater impact on CVD risk.

LOW-GRADE INFLAMMATION, COAGULATION, AND THROMBOSIS IN DIABETES MELLITUS

Low-grade chronic inflammation and coagulation are two important processes involved in the development of atherosclerosis, which is the underlying mechanism for CVD.[100] Recent advances in basic science have established a fundamental role for inflammation in mediating CVD through the initiation, progression, and thrombotic complications of atherosclerosis. Subclinical elevations of inflammatory markers including C-reactive protein (CRP), IL-6, fibrinogen, andPAI-1 are observed in insulin resistance and type 2 DM.[101–103] Elevated levels of CRP have been related to CVD risk.[104] CRP levels are elevated in type 1 and 2 diabetes, increased insulin resistance, and the metabolic syndrome.[105–107]

DM is associated with excessive amount of adipose tissue. Visceral obesity contributes to the clustering of multiple risk factors for CVD. Increased visceral fat store is associated with macrophage infiltration that secrete proinflammatory molecules such as TNF-α, IL-6, and IL-1β.[108] These cytokines augment inflammation and decrease insulin sensitivity.[106] Cytokines from adipocytes may also contribute to insulin resistance by increasing TNF-α and IL-6 or decreasing adiponectin.[109] Adiponectin is an insulin-sensitizing adipocytokine that is decreased with obesity, CMS, and DM.[110] Indices of oxidative stress are significantly correlated with body mass index and inversely related to plasma adiponectin.[111]

Moreover, inflammatory adipocytokines give rise to E-selectin and ICAM-1 in the endothelium, which participates in the migration of inflammatory cells to the subendothelial space, promoting the development of foam cells and unstable atherosclerotic plaque.[112]

Cytokines may play crucial roles in the initiation and progression of atherosclerotic lesions. Cytokines contribute to increased oxidative stress and generation of growth factors, which are important for the proliferation and migration of smooth muscle cells. These cytokines may also induce platelet aggregation, increase the synthesis of platelet activating factor, stimulate lipolysis as well as the expression of adhesion molecules, and upregulate the synthesis and cell surface expression of procoagulant activity in endothelial cells. The increased oxidation and glycooxidation of proteins and lipids in DM may result in increased cytokine release from macrophage activation. AGE-mediated cytokine release is associated with overproduction of multiple growth factors, including platelet-dependent growth factor, insulin-like growth factor-1 (IGF-1), granulocyte/monocyte colony stimulating factor, and transforming growth factor-β.

An additional pathogenic phenomenon is increased formation of immune complexes that contain modified lipoproteins. High levels of soluble immune complexes containing modified LDL predict the development of macrovascular complications in type 1 DM and are associated with the presence of CVD in type 2 DM. These immune complexes induce the release of large amounts of cytokines and stimulate the expression and release of matrix metalloproteinase-1. Activation of macrophages by immune complexes leads to the release of TNF, which has been shown to upregulate the synthesis of CRP. High levels of high-sensitivity assayable CRP have been demonstrated in patients with insulin resistance. Thus, the increase in immune complexes in DM may lead to the initiation and progression of atherosclerosis and may also contribute to plaque rupture, thrombosis, and cardiovascular events.

Increased macrophage content has been shown in the atherosclerotic lesions of persons with DM. This is likely a consequence of an increase in recruitment of macrophages into the vessel wall by the higher levels of cytokines and adhesion molecules present in DM. T cells have been reported to respond to AGEs by releasing interferon-γ. T-cell activation can inhibit SMC proliferation and collagen biosynthesis, thereby leading to the formation of vulnerable plaques and acute cardiovascular events.

DM is also considered to be a prothrombotic state. The most important regulator of tissue plasminogen activator (t-PA) is PAI. PAI-1 overexpression may be attributable to direct effects of insulin and proinsulin. Increases in tissue factor, fibrinogen, factor VII activity, and PAI-1 in both plasma and the atherosclerotic plaque; decreases in urokinase in the plaque; and increases in platelet aggregation, have all been described in DM. Tissue factor, the main activator of the extrinsic coagulation pathway, is increased in animal models of DM and obesity.[113,114] t-PA has a critical role in the dissolution of clots and maintenance of vessel lumen.

The prothrombotic state in DM appears to contribute to both the pathogenesis of progressive atherosclerosis, thrombosis, and acute cardiovascular events in DM. Increased plasma and plaque PAI-1 decrease VSMC migration and are also associated with decreased expression of urokinase within the vessel wall and plaque. T cell and macrophage activation in the setting of a thin fibrous cap may precipitate plaque rupture and induce acute coronary syndromes. DM may also be associated with an increased frequency of atherosclerotic plaque rupture.[115] DM has also been shown to increase the rate of restenosis after percutaneous transluminal coronary angioplasty (PTCA)[116–118] and coronary artery bypass grafting (CABG).[119]

DIABETIC CARDIOMYOPATHY

Diastolic Dysfunction

Diabetes mellitus is a major risk factor for development of impaired left ventricular (LV) function and clinical heart failure. Existence of diabetic cardiomyopathy, independent of associated hypertension and atherosclerotic coronary artery disease, is supported by several epidemiologic and clinical observations.[120,121] LV dysfunction in DM is primarily a diastolic abnormality. Diastolic dysfunction is observed in diabetic patients without evidence of other heart disease.[122–124] Diastolic dysfunction characterized by reduced early peak mitral velocity, increased late peak mitral velocity, and prolonged deceleration time and isovolumic relaxation time is common in both type 1 and type 2 DM.[125] Moreover, DM may also be associated with systolic dysfunction as several studies have shown a significant association between DM and idiopathic dilated cardiomyopathy.[126–129]

MECHANISMS OF DIABETIC CARDIOMYOPATHY

The mechanism of diabetic cardiomyopathy is likely to be a combination of abnormalities, including metabolic disturbances, oxidative stress, microvascular disease, myocardial remodeling, fibrosis, autonomic dysfunction, and insulin resistance. Impaired cardiac myocyte glucose supply and glycolysis may be the initial mechanism of diabetic cardiomyopathy.[130–133] Hyperglycemia increases levels of FFA, oxidative stress, and growth factors and causes abnormalities in substrate supply and utilization, calcium homeostasis, and lipid metabolism. In DM, there is reduced myocardial glucose uptake probably due to the cellular depletion of glucose transporters and inhibitory effect of increased fatty acid oxidation through the pyruvate dehydrogenase complex.[134–136] Moreover, high FFA may lead to abnormally high oxygen requirements during FFA metabolism and the intracellular accumulation of potentially toxic intermediates of FFA.[137,138] Oxidative stress-induced abnormalities of calcium handling can also contribute to diabetic cardiomyopathy. Diminished calcium sensitivity, reduction of sarcoplasmic reticulum Ca^{2+}-ATPase, and decreased sarcoplasmic reticulum calcium pump protein have been documented in DM and may result in impaired LV function.[139,140] In addition, alterations in the expression of myosin isoenzymes, regulatory proteins, and myosin phosphorylation may contribute to the development of myofibrillar remodeling in the diabetic heart.[141]

Local renin-angiotensin system upregulation in DM may enhance oxidative damage inducing cardiac cell apoptosis and necrosis.[142–144] Angiotensin-II increases collagen production.[145] Alterations of endothelin-1 and its receptors are also associated with increased focal fibrous scarring with apoptotic cardiomyocytes.[146] Hypertrophy and interstitial fibrosis of myocardium are observed in DM.[147] Angiotensin-II and endothelin-1-induced myocardial microvascular changes, myocardial cell injury, and interstitial fibrosis may contribute to the development of diabetic cardiomyopathy. Patients with DM are noticed to have a significantly greater thickening of the capillary basement membrane, accumulation of toluidine blue-positive materials, and interstitial fibrosis.[148] In addition, abnormalities in coronary small vessel function and impaired endothelium-dependent coronary vasodilation occur in DM and dilated cardiomyopathy.[149–152]

Cardiac autonomic neuropathy also plays a role. Sympathetic denervation is an important feature of cardiac autonomic neuropathy in DM.[153] Cardiac sympathetic denervation is present in newly diagnosed type 1 diabetes patients without evidence of localized myocardial perfusion defects.[154] However, regional sympathetic damage is relatively common in type 2 diabetes.[155] Cardiac autonomic neuropathy is associated with altered myocardial blood flow; with regions of persistent sympathetic innervation exhibiting the greatest deficits of vasodilator reserve resulting LV regional dysfunction.[156]

Diabetic cardiomyopathy is initiated by hyperglycemia at an early stage and characterized by metabolic disturbances such as depletion of GLUT4, increased FFAs, carnitine deficiency, calcium homeostasis changes, and insulin resistance. Cellular changes such as defects in calcium transport and fatty acid metabolism may lead to increases in myocyte apoptosis and necrosis, angiotensin-II, and cardiac autonomic neuropathy resulting in myocyte injury, loss, and myocardial fibrosis. This stage of diabetic cardiomyopathy is mainly characterized by myocellular hypertrophy and myocardial fibrosis. The further changes in metabolism and development of myocardial fibrosis result in myocardial microvascular changes, which are characterized by both myocardial microvascular structural and functional changes probably accompanying recurrent microvascular spasm.

INTERVENTIONS TO REDUCE CARDIOVASCULAR DISEASE IN DIABETES MELLITUS

Risk Factor Focus

Increasing evidence indicates that controlling both major CVD risk factors (cigarette smoking, hypertension, elevated LDL cholesterol (LDL-C) and diabetic dyslipidemia, and hyperglycemia) and underlying risk factors (obesity, physical inactivity, and adverse nutrition) will reduce onset of CVD and its complications in patients with DM.[157] Emphasis should be given to modification of all of these CVD risk factors in a patient with DM. The mechanisms of metabolic disturbances, myocardial fibrosis, microvascular disease, cardiac autonomic neuropathy, and insulin resistance imply that various treatments might be effective for preventing or delaying the development of

CVD in DM. Steps to reduce atherogenesis consist of the basic treatment for vascular disease and should be started at the early stage of diabetic cardiomyopathy. Management of the traditional risk factors and lifestyle modification programs should be instituted as early as possible.

Lifestyle Modification

Dietary counseling with regular physical activity and health weight maintenance is essential in patients with DM. Exercise improves glucose homeostasis by reducing blood glucose and increasing insulin sensitivity. Exercise training improves cardiac output and reverses negative remodeling on the contractile properties of the heart thereby improving myocardial function. Exercise increases the skeletal muscle GLUT4 gene and protein expression. In skeletal muscle, exercise has been demonstrated to recruit a separate pool of GLUT4 to that activated by insulin. This leads to an additive effect of insulin and exercise on glucose uptake and therefore improves blood glucose levels. When regular physical activity is not contraindicated, the usual prescription of 30 minutes of moderate-intensity exercise daily should be recommended. Cigarette smoking is a major risk factor for CVD, and patients with DM who smoke cigarettes should be assisted to stop smoking.[158]

Hypertension

The prevalence of hypertension is increased in patients with DM and the American diabetes association (ADA) recommends a goal of <130/80 mmHg. Recommendations on thresholds for intervention for blood pressure in diabetics vary across the guidelines. In the UKPDS, beneficial effects on complications, in particular stroke, were achieved at 144/82 mmHg in the tighter control group[159,160] consistent with results from the hypertension optimal treatment (HOT) study.[160] However, analysis of the UKPDS population suggested that increased benefit was derived at levels below this cutoff. These findings led to the more stringent recommended target of <130/80 mmHg for people with type 2 diabetes uncomplicated by nephropathy.

The International Diabetes Foundation Task Force[161] recommends initiating medication for lowering blood pressure in diabetes not complicated by raised albumin excretion rate, using any agent except for α-adrenergic blockers. Avoidance of α-adrenergic blockers as first-line therapy is based on evidence from the antihypertensive and lipid-lowering treatment to prevent heart attack (ALLHAT) trial.[163] ACE inhibitors and angiotensin-II receptor blockers may offer some advantages over other agents in patients' kidney damage and albuminuria. They further recommend initiating therapy with β-adrenergic blockers in people with angina, β-adrenergic blockers or ACE inhibitors in people with previous myocardial infarction, ACE inhibitors or diuretics in those with heart failure. They recommend caution with combined thiazide and β-adrenergic blockers because of the risk of deterioration in metabolic control.[162]

Dyslipidemia

DM is associated with elevated triglycerides, small LDL particles, and low levels of HDL cholesterol, all of which contribute to atherogenesis and coronary plaque rupture. The recently updated clinical guidelines of the National Cholesterol Education Program support the inclusion of patients with diabetes in the high-risk category and confirm the benefits of LDL-lowering therapy in these patients to LDL-C goal <100 mg/dL. In patients with an even more increased risk, an LDL-C goal of <70 mg/dL is a therapeutic option.[164]

The International Diabetes Foundation Task Force[162] recommends initiating a statin at standard dose for all type 2 diabetics >40 years old or in all with manifested CVD; a statin at standard dose for all type 2 diabetics >20 years old with microalbuminuria or assessed as being at particularly high risk; in addition to statin, fenofibrate where serum triglycerides are >2.3 mmol/L (>200 mg/dL), once LDL-C is as optimally controlled as possible. Consideration of other lipid-lowering drugs (ezetimibe, nicotinic acid, and concentrated omega-3 fatty acids) in those failing to reach lipid-lowering targets or intolerant of conventional drugs is also recommended.[162]

These recommendations are backed by recently published large multi-center trials. The Heart Protection Study (utilizing simvastatin) recruited people with diabetes even if they had no history of cardiovascular risk, and the results showed a strong benefit.[165] The CARDS trial similarly studied people with diabetes who had no overt evidence of CVD, and showed marked benefit with atorvastatin.[166] These studies suggest that statin treatment for all people with type 2 diabetes if they are over 40 years of age regardless of their other risk factors.

Control of Hyperglycemia

Control of hyperglycemia is important for the prevention of microvascular disease. The primary goal for glycemic therapy is to achieve a near-normal fasting glucose level and a HbA1c level <7%. Glipizide has been shown to reduce the degree of insulin resistance in the myocardium and improves cardiac function in diabetes. Insulin and IGF-1 share multiple intracellular signaling pathways, and both receptors mediate antiapoptotic effects. Improvements in the signaling of these molecules may have an effect to preserve cardiomyocyte number. Metformin and the thiazolidinediones are used to treat insulin resistance. Metformin reduces FFA efflux from fat cells, thereby suppressing hepatic glucose production, and indirectly improving peripheral insulin sensitivity and endothelial function. In contrast, thiazolidinediones improve peripheral insulin sensitivity by reducing circulating FFAs but also by increasing production of adiponectin, which improves insulin sensitivity. Thiazolidinediones also improve endothelial function and may prevent or delay the onset of diabetes.

Aspirin

Patients with DM and insulin resistance have a prothrombotic state as described earlier. Low-dose aspirin therapy is indicated for secondary prevention of CVD. Aspirin is probably useful for patients with DM without manifested CVD because of increased risk for acute coronary syndromes. Aspirin 75–100 mg daily is recommended for people with evidence of CVD or at high risk for CVD. The use of clopidogrel may be considered in patients with aspirin intolerance.[162]

Antioxidants

Despite the evidence for the role of oxidative stress in the progression of CVD, randomized clinical trials examining antioxidant vitamins including vitamin E and beta-carotene have resulted in negative results. Drugs used for the reduction of CVD risk factors, such as ACE inhibitors, AT_1 receptor blockers, calcium channel blocker, and statins possess antioxidant activity which may be useful in prevention and improvement of insulin resistance, DM, and CVD in DM through pleiotropic effects.

SUMMARY

Atherosclerosis and myocardial dysfunction are increased in patients with DM. Hyperglycemia, increased FFAs, AGEs, lipoprotein abnormalities, oxidative stress, and glycosylation contribute to atherosclerosis, myocardial dysfunction, and increased cardiovascular complications of DM. Endothelial dysfunction with low-grade inflammatory processes and procoagulant states contribute to both initiation and progression of atherosclerosis, plaque rupture, and thrombosis in patients with DM. New insights into these complex pathophysiologic mechanisms of diabetic CVD may lead to novel therapeutic interventions. Interventions directed to risk factor reduction and early inhibition of the pathophysiologic mechanisms should be developed and implemented.

REFERENCES

1. National Center for Chronic Disease Prevention and Health Promotion. National Diabetes Fact Sheet: general information and national estimates on diabetes in the United States, 2003. Available at: www.cdc.gov/diabetes/pubs/estimates. htm. Accessed September 30, 2005.

2. Grundy SM, Howard B, Smith S Jr, et al. Prevention Conference VI: diabetes and cardiovascular disease: executive summary: conference proceeding for healthcare professionals from a special writing group of the American Heart Association. *Circulation* 2002;105(18):2231–2239.

3. Mokdad AH, Ford ES, Bowman BA, et al. Diabetes trends in the U.S.: 1990-1998. *Diabetes Care* 2000;23(9):1278–1283.

4. Mokdad AH, Ford ES, Bowman BA, et al. The continuing increase of diabetes in the US. *Diabetes Care* 2001;24(2):412.

5. King H, Aubert RE, Herman WH. Global burden of diabetes, 1995-2025: prevalence, numerical estimates, and projections. *Diabetes Care* 1998;21:1414–1431.

6. Kannel WB, McGee DL. Diabetes and cardiovascular disease. The Framingham study. *JAMA* 1979;241(19):2035–2038.

7. Sowers JR, Stump CS. Insights into the biology of diabetic vascular disease: what's new? *Am J Hypertens* 2004;17(11 Pt 2):2S–6S; quiz A2-4.

8. Haffner SM, Lehto S, Ronnemma T, et al. Mortality from coronary heart disease in subjects with type 2 diabetes and in nondiabetic subjects with and without myocardial infarction. *N Engl J Med* 1998;339:229–234.

9. Stamler J, Vaccaro O, Neaton JD, et al. Diabetes, other risk factors, and 12-yr cardiovascular mortality for men screened in the Multiple Risk Factor Intervention Trial. *Diabetes Care* 1993;16(2):434–444.

10. Hu FB, Stampfer MJ, Solomon CG, et al. The impact of diabetes mellitus on mortality from all causes and coronary heart disease in women: 20 years of follow-up. *Arch Intern Med* 2001;161(14):1717–1723.

11. McFarlane SI, Banerji M, Sowers JR. Insulin resistance and cardiovascular disease. *J Clin Endocrinol Metab* 2001;86(2):713–718.

12. Deckert T, Yokoyama H, Mathiesen E, et al. Cohort study of predictive value of urinary albumin excretion for atherosclerotic vascular disease in patients with insulin dependent diabetes. *BMJ* 1996;312:871–874.

13. Mogensen CE. Microalbuminuria predicts clinical proteinuria and early mortality in maturity-onset diabetes. *N Engl J Med* 1984;310:356–360.

14. Heinrich J, Balleisen L, Schulte HGA, et al. Fibrinogen and factor VII in the prediction of coronary risk: results from the PROCAM study in healthy men. *Arterioscler Thromb* 1994;14:54–59.

15. Expert Panel on Detection, Evaluation, and Treatment of High Blood Cholesterol in Adults (Adult Treatment Panel III). Executive Summary of The Third Report of The National Cholesterol Education Program (NCEP). *JAMA* 2001;285(19):2486–2497.

16. Stratton IM, Adler AI, Neil HA, et al. Association of glycaemia with macrovascular and microvascular complications of type 2 diabetes (UKPDS 35): prospective observational study. *BMJ* 2000;321(7258):405–412.

17. Hu FB, Stampfer MJ, Haffner SM, et al. Elevated risk of cardiovascular disease prior to clinical diagnosis of type 2 diabetes. *Diabetes Care* 2002;25(7):1129–1134.

18. Grundy SM, Brewer HB Jr, Cleeman JI, et al. American Heart Association; National Heart, Lung, and Blood Institute. Definition of metabolic syndrome: Report of the National Heart, Lung, and Blood Institute/American Heart Association conference on scientific issues related to definition. *Circulation* 2004;109(3):433–438.

19. Castro JP, El-Atat FA, McFarlane SI, et al. Cardiometabolic syndrome: pathophysiology and treatment. *Curr Hypertens Rep* 2003;5(5):393–401.

20. Sowers JR. Treatment of hypertension in patients with diabetes. *Arch Intern Med* 2004;164(17):1850–1857.

21. UK Prospective Diabetes Study Group. Tight blood pressure control and risk of macrovascular and microvascular complications in type 2 diabetes: UKPDS 38. *BMJ* 1998;317(7160):703–713. [Erratum in: *BMJ* 1999;318(7175):29].

22. Orchard TJ, Olson JC, Erbey JR, et al. Insulin resistance-related factors, but not glycemia, predict coronary artery disease in type 1 diabetes: 10-year follow-up data from the Pittsburgh Epidemiology of Diabetes Complications Study. *Diabetes Care* 2003;26(5):1374–1379.

23. Haffner SM, Miettinen H. Insulin resistance implications for type II diabetes mellitus and coronary heart disease. *Am J Med* 1997;103(2):152–162.

24. Lehto S, Ronnemaa T, Pyorala K, et al. Poor glycemic control predicts coronary heart disease events in patients with type 1 diabetes without nephropathy. *Arterioscler Thromb Vasc Biol* 1999;19:1014–1019.

25. Eckel RH, Wassef M, Chait A, et al. Prevention Conference VI: Diabetes and Cardiovascular Disease: Writing Group II: pathogenesis of atherosclerosis in diabetes. *Circulation* 2002;105(18):e138–e143.

26. Moreno PR, Murcia AM, Palacios IF, et al. Coronary composition and macrophage infiltration in atherectomy specimens from patients with diabetes mellitus. *Circulation* 2000;102(18):2180–2184.

27. Jweied EE, McKinney RD, Walker LA, et al. Depressed cardiac myofilament function in human diabetes mellitus. *Am J Physiol Heart Circ Physiol* 2005; [Epub ahead of print]. Accessed October 8, 2005.

28. Clark RJ, McDonough PM, Swanson E, et al. Diabetes and the accompanying hyperglycemia impairs cardiomyocyte calcium cycling through increased nuclear O-GlcNAcylation. *J Biol Chem* 2003;278(45):44230–44237.

29. Mahgoub MA, Abd-Elfattah AS. Diabetes mellitus and cardiac function. *Mol Cell Biochem* 1998;180(1/2):59–64.

30. Marwick TH. Diabetic heart disease. *Heart* 2005; [Epub ahead of print]. Accessed September 20, 2005.

31. Kris-Etherton PM, Lichtenstein AH, Howard BV, et al. Nutrition Committee of the American Heart Association Council on Nutrition, Physical Activity, and Metabolism. Antioxidant vitamin supplements and cardiovascular disease. *Circulation* 2004;110(5):637–641.

32. Baynes JW, Thorpe SR. Role of oxidative stress in diabetic complications: a new perspective on an old paradigm. *Diabetes* 1999;48(1):1–9.

33. Yorek MA. The role of oxidative stress in diabetic vascular and neural disease. *Free Radic Res* 2003;37(5):471–480.

34. Niedowicz DM, Daleke DL. The role of oxidative stress in diabetic complications. *Cell Biochem Biophys* 2005;43(2):289–330.

35. Johansen JS, Harris AK, Rychly DJ, et al. Oxidative stress and the use of antioxidants in diabetes: linking basic science to clinical practice. *Cardiovasc Diabetol* 2005;4(1):5.

36. Schmidt AM, Hori O, Brett J, et al. Cellular receptors for advanced glycation end products. Implications for induction of oxidant stress and cellular dysfunction in the pathogenesis of vascular lesions. *Arterioscler Thromb* 1994;14(10):1521–1528.

37. Vlassara H. Recent progress on the biologic and clinical significance of advanced glycosylation end products. *J Lab Clin Med* 1994;124(1):19–30.

38. Ido Y, Kilo C, Williamson JR. Interactions between the sorbitol pathway, non-enzymatic glycation, and diabetic vascular dysfunction. *Nephrol Dial Transplant* 1996;11(Suppl 5):72–75.

39. Rao GN, Berk BC. Active oxygen species stimulate vascular smooth muscle cell growth and proto-oncogene expression. *Circ Res* 1992;70:593–599.

40. Dimmeler S, Zeiher AM. Reactive oxygen species and vascular cell apoptosis in response to angiotensin II and pro-atherosclerotic factors. *Regul Pept* 2000; 90:19–25.

41. Turko IV, Marcondes S, Murad F. Diabetes-associated nitration of tyrosine and inactivation of succinyl-CoA:3-oxoacid CoA-transferase. *Am J Physiol Heart Circ Physiol* 2001;281(6):H2289–H2294.

42. Griendling KK, FitzGerald GA. Oxidative stress and cardiovascular injury: Part II: animal and human studies. *Circulation* 2003;108(17):2034–2040.

43. Griendling KK, FitzGerald GA. Oxidative stress and cardiovascular injury: Part I: basic mechanisms and in vivo monitoring of ROS. *Circulation* 2003;108(16): 1912–1916.

44. De Vriese AS, Verbeuren TJ, Van de Voorde J, et al. Endothelial dysfunction in diabetes. *Br J Pharmacol* 2000;130(5):963–974.

45. McFarlane SI, Sowers JR. Cardiovascular endocrinology 1: aldosterone function in diabetes mellitus: effects on cardiovascular and renal disease. *J Clin Endocrinol Metab* 2003;88(2):516–523.

46. Sowers JR. Insulin resistance and hypertension. *Am J Physiol Heart Circ Physiol* 2004;286(5):H1597–H1602.

47. Nishikawa T, Edelstein D, Du XL, et al. Normalizing mitochondrial superoxide production blocks three pathways of hyperglycaemic damage. *Nature* 2000;404(6779):787–790.

48. Mertens A, Holvoet P. Oxidized LDL and HDL: antagonists in atherothrombosis. *FASEB J* 2001;15(12):2073–2084.

49. Toshima S, Hasegawa A, Kurabayashi M, et al. Circulating oxidized low density lipoprotein levels. A biochemical risk marker for coronary heart disease. *Arterioscler Thromb Vasc Biol* 2000;20(10):2243–2247.

50. Kopprasch S, Pietzsch J, Kuhlisch E, et al. In vivo evidence for increased oxidation of circulating LDL in impaired glucose tolerance. *Diabetes* 2002;51(10): 3102–3106.

51. Boullier A, Bird DA, Chang MK, et al. Scavenger receptors, oxidized LDL, and atherosclerosis. *Ann N Y Acad Sci* 2001;47:214–222; discussion 222–223.

52. Gough PJ, Greaves DR, Suzuki H, et al. Analysis of macrophage scavenger receptor (SR-A) expression in human aortic atherosclerotic lesions. *Arterioscler Thromb Vasc Biol* 1999;19(3):461–471.

53. Hirano K, Yamashita S, Nakagawa Y, et al. Expression of human scavenger receptor class B type I in cultured human monocyte-derived macrophages and atherosclerotic lesions. *Circ Res* 1999;85(1):108–116.

54. The Diabetes Control and Complications Trial Research Group. The effect of intensive treatment of diabetes on the development and progression of long-term complications in insulin-dependent diabetes mellitus. *N Engl J Med* 1993;329: 977–986.

55. The Diabetes Control and Complications Trial/Epidemiology of Diabetes Interventions and Complications Research Group, Retinopathy and nephropathy in patients with type 1 diabetes four years after a trial of intensive therapy. *N Engl J Med* 2000;342:381–389.

56. Kuusisto J, Mykkanen L, Pyorala K, et al. Non-insulin-dependent diabetes and its metabolic control are important predictors of stroke in elderly subjects. *Stroke* 1994;25:1157–1164.

57. Colwell JA. Multifactorial aspects of the treatment of the type II diabetic patient. *Metabolism* 1997;46:1–4.

58. Cooper ME. Importance of advanced glycation end products in diabetes-associated cardiovascular and renal disease. *Am J Hypertens* 2004;17:31S–38S.

59. Brett J, Schmidt AM, Yan SD, et al. Survey of the distribution of a newly characterized receptor for advanced glycation end products in tissues. *Am J Pathol* 1993;143(6):1699–1712.

60. Basta G, Schmidt AM, De Caterina R. Advanced glycation end products and vascular inflammation: implications for accelerated atherosclerosis in diabetes. *Cardiovasc Res* 2004;63(4):582–592.

61. Twigg SM, Chen MM, Joly AH, et al. Advanced glycosylation end products up-regulate connective tissue growth factor (insulin-like growth factor-binding protein-related protein 2) in human fibroblasts: a potential mechanism for expansion of extracellular matrix in diabetes mellitus. *Endocrinology* 2001;142(5): 1760–1769.

62. Li SY, Du M, Dolence EK, et al. Aging induces cardiac diastolic dysfunction, oxidative stress, accumulation of advanced glycation end products and protein modification. *Aging Cell* 2005;4(2):57–64.

63. Thornalley PJ, Langborg A, Minhas HS. Formation of glyoxal, methylglyoxal and 3-deoxyglucosone in the glycation of proteins by glucose. *Biochem J* 1999;344: 109–116.

64. Huijberts MS, Wolffenbuttel BH, Boudier HA, et al. Aminoguanidine treatment increases elasticity and decreases fluid filtration of large arteries from diabetic rats. *J Clin Invest* 1993;92(3):1407–1411.

65. Bolton WK, Cattran DC, Williams ME, et al. ACTION I Investigator Group. Randomized trial of an inhibitor of formation of advanced glycation end products in diabetic nephropathy. *Am J Nephrol* 2004;24(1):32–40. [Epub 2003, Dec 17].

66. Sowers JR. Insulin resistance and hypertension. *Mol Cell Endocrinol* 1990;74(2): C87–C89.

67. Calles-Escandon J, Cipolla M. Diabetes and endothelial dysfunction: a clinical perspective. *Endocr Rev* 2001;22(1):36–52.

68. Feener EP, King GL. Endothelial dysfunction in diabetes mellitus: role in cardiovascular disease. *Heart Fail Monit* 2001;1(3):74–82.

69. Takiuchi S, Fujii H, Kamide K, et al. Plasma asymmetric dimethylarginine and coronary and peripheral endothelial dysfunction in hypertensive patients. *Am J Hypertens* 2004;17(9):802–808.

70. Williams SB, Cusco JA, Roddy MA, et al. Impaired nitric oxide-mediated vasodilation in patients with non-insulin-dependent diabetes mellitus. *J Am Coll Cardiol* 1996;27(3):567–574.

71. Fukai T, Folz RJ, Landmesser U, et al. Extracellular superoxide dismutase and cardiovascular disease. *Cardiovasc Res* 2002;55(2):239–249.

72. Sowers JR, Haffner S. Treatment of cardiovascular and renal risk factors in the diabetic hypertensive. *Hypertension* 2002;40(6):781–788.

73. Dzau VJ. Theodore Cooper Lecture: tissue angiotensin and pathobiology of vascular disease: a unifying hypothesis. *Hypertension* 2001;37(4):1047–1052.

74. Meigs JB, Hu FB, Rifai N, et al. Biomarkers of endothelial dysfunction and risk of type 2 diabetes mellitus. *JAMA* 2004;291(16):1978–1986.

75. Kim JA, Berliner JA, Natarajan RD, et al. Evidence that glucose increases monocyte binding to human aortic endothelial cells. *Diabetes* 1994;43(9):1103–1107.

76. Manduteanu I, Voinea M, Serban G, et al. High glucose induces enhanced monocyte adhesion to valvular endothelial cells via a mechanism involving ICAM-1, VCAM-1 and CD18. *Endothelium* 1999;6(4):315–324.

77. Takahara N, Kashiwagi A, Nishio Y, et al. Oxidized lipoproteins found in patients with NIDDM stimulate radical-induced monocyte chemoattractant protein-1 mRNA expression in cultured human endothelial cells. *Diabetologia* 1997;40(6): 662–670.

78. Cushing SD, Berliner JA, Valente AJ, et al. Minimally modified low density lipoprotein induces monocyte chemotactic protein 1 in human endothelial cells and smooth muscle cells. *Proc Natl Acad Sci U S A* 1990;87(13):5134–5138.

79. Sowers JR, Epstein M, Frohlich ED. Diabetes, hypertension, and cardiovascular disease: an update. *Hypertension* 2001;37(4):1053–1059. [Review. Erratum in: *Hypertension* 200137(5):1350].

80. Abdel-Wahab N, Weston BS, Roberts T, et al. Connective tissue growth factor and regulation of the mesangial cell cycle: role in cellular hypertrophy. *J Am Soc Nephrol* 2002;(10):2437–2445.

81. Fernandez-Real JM, Ricart W. Insulin resistance and chronic cardiovascular inflammatory syndrome. *Endocr Rev* 2003;24(3):278–301.

82. Sowers JR, Epstein M. Diabetes mellitus and associated hypertension, vascular disease, and nephropathy. An update. *Hypertension* 1995;26(6 Pt 1):869–879.

83. Borch-Johnsen K, Kreiner S. Proteinuria: value as predictor of cardiovascular mortality in insulin dependent diabetes mellitus. *Br Med J (Clin Res Ed)* 1987;294(6588):1651–1654.

84. Parving HH, Gall MA, Nielsen FS. Dyslipidaemia and cardiovascular disease in non-insulin-dependent diabetic patient with and without diabetic nephropathy. *J Intern Med Suppl* 1994;736:89–94.

85. Widlansky ME, Gokce N, Keaney JF Jr, et al. The clinical implications of endothelial dysfunction. *J Am Coll Cardiol* 2003;42:1149–1160.

86. Widlansky ME, Gokce N, Keaney JF Jr, et al. The clinical implications of endothelial dysfunction. *J Am Coll Cardiol* 2003;42:1149–1160.

87. Corretti MC, Anderson TJ, Benjamin EJ, et al. Guidelines for the ultrasound assessment of endothelial-dependent flow-mediated vasodilation of the brachial artery: a report of the International Brachial Artery Reactivity Task Force. *J Am Coll Cardiol* 2002;39:257–265.

87. Lefebvre PJ, Scheen AJ. The postprandial state and risk of cardiovascular disease. *Diabet Med* 1998;15(Suppl 4):S63–S68.

89. Coutinho M, Gerstein HC, Wang Y, et al. The relationship between glucose and incident cardiovascular events. A metaregression analysis of published data from 20 studies of 95,783 individuals followed for 12.4 years. *Diabetes Care* 1999;22:233–240.

90. DECODE Study Group. Glucose tolerance and mortality: comparison of WHO and American Diabetes Association diagnostic criteria. European Diabetes Epidemiology Group, Diabetes Epidemiology: collaborative analysis of diagnostic criteria in Europe. *Lancet* 1999;354:617–621.

91. Brownlee M. Biochemistry and molecular cell biology of diabetic complications. *Nature* 2001;414:813–820.

92. Hokanson JE, Austin MA. Plasma triglyceride level is a risk factor for cardiovascular disease independent of high-density lipoprotein cholesterol level: a meta-analysis of population-based prospective studies. *J Cardiovasc Risk* 1996;3:213–219.

93. Teno S, Uto Y, Nagashima H, et al. Association of postprandial hypertriglyceridemia and carotid intima-media thickness in patients with type 2 diabetes. *Diabetes Care* 2000;23(9):1401–1406.

94. Ceriello A. Coagulation activation in diabetes mellitus: the role of hyperglycaemia and therapeutic prospects. *Diabetologia* 1993;36:1119–1125.

95. Ceriello A, Giacomello R, Stel G, et al. Hyperglycemia-induced thrombin formation in diabetes. The possible role of oxidative stress. *Diabetes* 1995;44:924–928.

96. Esposito K, Nappo F, Marfella R, et al. Inflammatory cytokine concentrations are acutely increased by hyperglycemia in humans. *Circulation* 2002;106:2067–2072.

97. Shizukuda Y, Reyland ME, Buttrick PM. Protein kinase C-delta modulates apoptosis induced by hyperglycemia in adult ventricular myocytes. *Am J Physiol Heart Circ Physiol* 2002;282:H1625–H1634.

98. Brownlee M. Biochemistry and molecular cell biology of diabetic complications. *Nature* 2001;414:813–820.

99. Risso A, Mercuri F, Quagliaro L, et al. Intermittent high glucose enhances apoptosis in human umbilical vein endothelial cells in culture. *Am J Physiol Endocrinol Metab* 2001;281:E924–E930.

100. Lusis A. Atherosclerosis. *Nature* 2000;407:233–241.

101. Duncan BB, Schmidt MI, Pankow JS, et al. Atherosclerosis risk in communities study. Low-grade systemic inflammation and the development of type 2 diabetes: the atherosclerosis risk in communities study. *Diabetes* 2003;52(7):1799–1805.

102. Spranger J, Kroke A, Mohlig M, et al. Inflammatory cytokines and the risk to develop type 2 diabetes: results of the prospective population-based European

Prospective Investigation into Cancer and Nutrition (EPIC)-Potsdam Study. *Diabetes* 2003;52(3):812–817.

103. Festa A, D'Agostino R Jr, Tracy RP, et al. Insulin Resistance Atherosclerosis Study. Elevated levels of acute-phase proteins and plasminogen activator inhibitor-1 predict the development of type 2 diabetes: the insulin resistance atherosclerosis study. *Diabetes* 2002;51(4):1131–1137.

104. Libby P, Ridker PM, Maseri A. Inflammation and atherosclerosis. *Circulation* 2002;105:1135–1143.

105. Ford ES. Body mass index, diabetes, and C-reactive protein among US adults. *Diabetes Care* 1999;22:1971–1977.

106. Gomes MB, Piccirillo LJ, Nogueira VG, et al. Acute-phase proteins among patients with type 1 diabetes. *Diabet Metab* 2003;29:405–411.

107. Festa A, D'Agostino R, Howard G, et al. Chronic subclinical inflammation as part of the insulin resistance syndrome. *Circulation* 2000;102:42–47.

108. Teno S, Uto Y, Nagashima H, et al. Association of postprandial hypertriglyceridemia and carotid intima-media thickness in patients with type 2 diabetes. *Diabetes Care* 2000;23(9):1401–1406.

109. Duncan BB, Schmidt MI, Pankow JS, et al. Adiponectin and the development of type 2 diabetes: the atherosclerosis risk in communities study. *Diabetes* 2004;53(9):2473–2478.

110. Havel PJ. Update on adipocyte hormones: regulation of energy balance and carbohydrate/lipid metabolism. *Diabetes* 2004;53(Suppl 1):S143–S151.

111. Furukawa S, Fujita T, Shimabukuro M, et al. Increased oxidative stress in obesity and its impact on metabolic syndrome. *J Clin Invest* 2004;114(12):1752–1761.

112. Libby P. Changing concepts of atherogenesis. *J Intern Med* 2000;247(3):349–358.

113. Samad F, Pandey M, Loskutoff DJ. Tissue factor gene expression in the adipose tissues of obese mice. *Proc Natl Acad Sci USA* 1998;95(13):7591–7596.

114. Kislinger T, Tanji N, Wendt T, et al. Receptor for advanced glycation end products mediates inflammation and enhanced expression of tissue factor in vasculature of diabetic apolipoprotein E-null mice. *Arterioscler Thromb Vasc Biol* 2001;21(6):905–910.

115. Burke AP, Kolodgie FD, Farb A, et al. Healed plaque ruptures and sudden coronary death: evidence that subclinical rupture has a role in plaque progression. *Circulation* 2001;103(7):934–940.

116. Kornowski R, Mintz GS, Kent KM, et al. Increased restenosis in diabetes mellitus after coronary interventions is due to exaggerated intimal hyperplasia. A serial intravascular ultrasound study. *Circulation* 1997;95(6):1366–1369.

117. Moreno PR, Fallon JT, Murcia AM, et al. Tissue characteristics of restenosis after percutaneous transluminal coronary angioplasty in diabetic patients. *J Am Coll Cardiol* 1999;34(4):1045–1049.

118. Carter AJ, Bailey L, Devries J, et al. The effects of uncontrolled hyperglycemia on thrombosis and formation of neointima after coronary stent placement in a novel diabetic porcine model of restenosis. *Coron Artery Dis* 2000;11:473–479.

119. Ahmed JM, Hong MK, Mehran R, et al. Influence of diabetes mellitus on early and late clinical outcomes in saphenous vein graft stenting. *J Am Coll Cardiol* 2000;36(4):1186–1193.

120. Regan TJ, Lyons MM, Ahmed SS, et al. Evidence for cardiomyopathy in familial diabetes mellitus. *J Clin Invest* 1977;60:884–899.

121. Fang ZY, Prins JB, Marwick TH. Diabetic cardiomyopathy: evidence, mechanisms, and therapeutic implications. *Endocr Rev* 2004;25(4):543–567.

122. Zarich SW, Arbuckle BE, Cohen LR, et al. Diastolic abnormalities in young asymptomatic diabetic patients assessed by pulsed Doppler echocardiography. *J Am Coll Cardiol* 1988;12:114–120.

123. Airaksinen J, Ikaheimo M, Kaila J, et al. Impaired left ventricular filling in young female diabetics. An echocardiographic study. *Acta Med Scand* 1984;216:509–516.

124. Ruddy TD, Shumak SL, Liu PP, et al. The relationship of cardiac diastolic dysfunction to concurrent hormonal and metabolic status in type I diabetes mellitus. *J Clin Endocrinol Metab* 1988;66:113–118.

125. Poirier P, Bogaty P, Garneau C, et al. Diastolic dysfunction in normotensive men with well-controlled type 2 diabetes: importance of maneuvers in echocardiographic screening for preclinical diabetic cardiomyopathy. *Diabetes Care* 2001;24:5–10.

126. Hamby RI, Zoneraich S, Sherman L. Diabetic cardiomyopathy. *JAMA* 1974; 229:1749–1754.

127. Coughlin SS, Pearle DL, Baughman KL, et al. Diabetes mellitus and risk of idiopathic dilated cardiomyopathy. The Washington, DC Dilated Cardiomyopathy Study. *Ann Epidemiol* 1994;4:67–74.

128. Fang ZY, Yuda S, Anderson V, et al. Echocardiographic detection of early diabetic myocardial disease. *J Am Coll Cardiol* 2003;41:611–617.

129. Kannel WB, Hjortland M, Castelli WP. Role of diabetes in congestive heart failure: the Framingham study. *Am J Cardiol* 1974;34:29–34.

130. Rodrigues B, Cam MC, McNeill JH. Metabolic disturbances in diabetic cardiomyopathy. *Mol Cell Biochem* 1998;180:53–57.

131. Ohtake T, Yokoyama I, Watanabe T, et al. Myocardial glucose metabolism in noninsulin-dependent diabetes mellitus patients evaluated by FDG-PET. *J Nucl Med* 1995;36:456–463.

132. Chen V, Ianuzzo CD, Fong BC, et al. The effects of acute and chronic diabetes on myocardial metabolism in rats. *Diabetes* 1984;33:1078–1084.

133. Belke DD, Larsen TS, Gibbs EM, et al. Altered metabolism causes cardiac dysfunction in perfused hearts from diabetic (db/db) mice. *Am J Physiol Endocrinol Metab* 2000;279:E1104–E1113.

134. Garvey WT, Hardin D, Juhaszova M, et al. Effects of diabetes on myocardial glucose transport system in rats: implications for diabetic cardiomyopathy. *Am J Physiol* 1993;264:H837–H844.

135. Eckel J, Reinauer H. Insulin action on glucose transport in isolated cardiac myocytes: signalling pathways and diabetes induced alterations. *Biochem Soc Trans* 1990;18:1125–1127.

136. Liedtke AJ, DeMaison L, Eggleston AM, et al. Changes in substrate metabolism and effects of excess fatty acids in reperfused myocardium. *Circ Res* 1988;62: 535–542.

137. Rodrigues B, Cam MC, McNeill JH. Metabolic disturbances in diabetic cardiomyopathy. *Mol Cell Biochem* 1998;180:53–57.

138. Yazaki Y, Isobe M, Takahashi W, et al. Assessment of myocardial fatty acid abnormalities in patients with idiopathic dilated cardiomyopathy using I123 BMIPP SPECT: correlation with clinicopathological findings and clinical course. *Heart* 1999;81:153–159.

139. Takeda N, Nakamura I, Hatanaka T, et al. Myocardial mechanical and myosin isoenzyme alterations in streptozotocin-diabetic rats. *Jpn Heart J* 1988;29: 455–463.

140. Abe T, Ohga Y, Tabayashi N, et al. Left ventricular diastolic dysfunction in type 2 diabetes mellitus model rats. *Am J Physiol Heart Circ Physiol* 2002;282: H138–H148.

141. Dhalla NS, Liu X, Panagia V, et al. Subcellular remodeling and heart dysfunction in chronic diabetes. *Cardiovasc Res* 1988;40:239–247.

142. Sechi LA, Griffin CA, Schambelan M. The cardiac renin-angiotensin system in STZ-induced diabetes. *Diabetes* 1994;43:1180–1184.

143. Bojestig M, Nystrom FH, Arnqvist HJ, et al. The renin-angiotensin-aldosterone system is suppressed in adults with type 1 diabetes. *J Renin Angiotensin Aldosterone Syst* 2001;1:353–356.

144. Frustaci A, Kajstura J, Chimenti C, et al. Myocardial cell death in human diabetes. *Circ Res* 2000;87:1123–1132.

145. Lijnen PJ, Petrov VV, Fagard RH. Induction of cardiac fibrosis by angiotensin II. Methods. *Find Exp Clin Pharmacol* 2000;22:709–723.

146. Chen S, Evans T, Mukherjee K, et al. Diabetes-induced myocardial structural changes: role of endothelin-1 and its receptors. *J Mol Cell Cardiol* 2000;32:1621–1629.

147. Nunoda S, Genda A, Sugihara N, et al. Quantitative approach to the histopathology of the biopsied right ventricular myocardium in patients with diabetes mellitus. *Heart Vessels* 1985;1:43–47.

148. Kawaguchi M, Techigawara M, Ishihata T, et al. A comparison of ultrastructural changes on endomyocardial biopsy specimens obtained from patients with diabetes mellitus with and without hypertension. *Heart Vessels* 1997;12:267–274.

149. Nitenberg A, Foult JM, Blanchet F, et al. Multifactorial determinants of reduced coronary flow reserve after dipyridamole in dilated cardiomyopathy. *Am J Cardiol* 1985;55:748–754.

150. Treasure CB, Vita JA, Cox DA, et al. Endothelium-dependent dilation of the coronary microvasculature is impaired in dilated cardiomyopathy. *Circulation* 1990;81:772–779.

151. Itenberg A, Valensi P, Sachs R, et al. Impairment of coronary vascular reserve and ACh-induced coronary vasodilation in diabetic patients with angiographically normal coronary arteries and normal left ventricular systolic function. *Diabetes* 1993;42:1017–1025.

152. Strauer BE, Motz W, Vogt M, et al. Impaired coronary flow reserve in NIDDM: a possible role for diabetic cardiopathy in humans. *Diabetes* 1997;46(Suppl 2): S119–S124.

153. Miyanaga H, Yoneyama S, Kamitani T, et al. Clinical usefulness of 123I-metaiodobenzylguanidine myocardial scintigraphy in diabetic patients with cardiac sympathetic nerve dysfunction. *Jpn Circ J* 1995;59:599–607.

154. Schnell O, Muhr D, Weiss M, e al. Reduced myocardial 123I-metaiodobenzylguanidine uptake in newly diagnosed IDDM patients. *Diabetes* 1996;45:801–805.

155. Turpeinen AK, Vanninen E, Kuikka JT, et al. Demonstration of regional sympathetic denervation of the heart in diabetes. Comparison between patients with NIDDM and IDDM. *Diabetes Care* 1996;19:1083–1090.

156. Stevens MJ, Dayanikli F, Raffel DM, et al. Scintigraphic assessment of regionalized defects in myocardial sympathetic innervation and blood flow regulation in diabetic patients with autonomic neuropathy. *J Am Coll Cardiol* 1998;31:1575–1584.

157. Grundy SM, Benjamin IJ, Burke GL, et al. Diabetes and cardiovascular disease: a statement for healthcare professionals from the American Heart Association. *Circulation* 1999;100:1134–1146.

158. American Diabetes Association. Smoking and diabetes: Clinical Practice Guideline 2001. *Diabetes Care* 2001;24(Suppl 1):S64–S65.

159. UK Prospective Diabetes Study Group. Tight blood pressure control and risk of macrovascular and microvascular complications in type 2 diabetes: UKPDS 38. *BMJ* 1998;317:703–713.

160. Hansson L, Zanchetti A, Carruthers SG, et al. Effects of intensive blood pressure lowering and low-dose aspirin in patients with hypertension: principal results of the Hypertension Optimal Treatment (HOT) randomised trial. *Lancet* 1998;351:1755–1762.

161. IDF Clinical Guidelines Task Force. *Global Guideline for Type 2 Diabetes*. Brussels: International Diabetes Federation, 2005.

162. American Diabetes Association. Aspirin therapy in diabetes: Clinical Practice Recommendations. *Diabetes Care* 2001;24(Suppl 1):S62–S63.

163. Major outcomes in high-risk hypertensive patients randomized to angiotensin-converting enzyme inhibitor or calcium channel blocker vs diuretic: The Antihypertensive and Lipid-Lowering Treatment to Prevent Heart Attack Trial (ALLHAT). *JAMA* Dec. 18 2002;288(23):2981–2997.

164. Grundy SM, Cleeman JI, Merz CN, et al. Implications of recent clinical trials for the National Cholesterol Education Program Adult Treatment Panel III Guidelines. *Circulation* 2004;110:227–239.

165. Heart Protection Study Collaborative Group. MRC/BHF Heart Protection Study of cholesterol-lowering with simvastatin in 5963 people with diabetes: a randomized placebo-controlled trial. *Lancet* 2003;361:2005–2016.

166. Colhoun HM, Betteridge DJ, Durrington PN, et al. on behalf of the CARDS investigators. Primary prevention of cardiovascular disease with atorvastatin in type 2 diabetes in the Collaborative Atorvastatin Diabetes Study (CARDS): a multicentre randomized controlled trial. *Lancet* 2004;364:685–696.

TYPE 2 DIABETES, CORONARY RISK EQUIVALENCE, AND ASYMPTOMATIC CORONARY ARTERY DISEASE

Luther T. Clark
Paramdeep Baweja
Uzodinma R. Dim

Cardiovascular disease (CVD) is a leading cause of death in persons with diabetes, accounting for almost 80% of mortality in diabetic patients in the United States.[1,2] Diabetes increases risk for atherosclerotic vascular disease approximately two- to four-fold, in particular, coronary atherosclerosis, but also cerebral and peripheral arterial diseases (PADs).[3-5] The prevalence of diabetes mellitus has increased dramatically during the past several decades, with approximately 200 million people currently affected worldwide. Furthermore, it is estimated that the prevalence of diabetes will continue to increase and worldwide will exceed 360 million patients in the year 2030. Type 2 diabetes is the most prevalent form, accounting for almost 90% of all diabetes.[6,7] The increasing number of patients with diabetes and the onset of diabetes at younger ages have many consequences, including: (1) requirement for more years of medical attention and therapy for individuals with diabetes, its complications, and associated risk factors; (2) increased coronary and noncoronary atherosclerosis; and (3) increased frequency of other associated coronary heart disease (CHD) risk factors, including hypertension, dyslipidemia, and obesity.

DIABETES AND CORONARY RISK EQUIVALENCE

A guiding principle of CHD risk-modifying therapy is that the intensity of treatment should be individually tailored and based on the overall risk burden.[8–10] The Second Report of the National Cholesterol Education Program (NCEP) Expert Panel on Detection, Evaluation, and Treatment of High Blood Cholesterol in Adults (ATP II) in 1993[9] recommended using CHD risk status as a guide to the intensity of lipid-modifying therapy. This report divided the population at risk for CHD into three groups, based on known CHD, multiple CHD risk factors, or isolated hypercholesterolemia without other risk factors.

The term "CHD risk equivalent" was introduced[8,9] to identify those individuals without established CHD who have a risk for future major CHD events the same as that for individuals with established CHD. The NCEP lists diabetes as a CHD risk equivalent. However, some investigators have recently questioned the appropriateness of such categorization for all patients with diabetes.[11] The first half of this chapter reviews the concept of CHD risk equivalence and examines the appropriateness of classifying diabetes as a CHD equivalent. The second half of the chapter addresses the problem of asymptomatic coronary artery disease (CAD) in type 2 diabetes and provides the latest recommendations for evaluation and treatment.

Definition of CHD Risk Equivalent

The third NCEP report (ATP III) in 1993, in setting its treatment goals, adopted the same strategy as that used in ATP II to risk stratify patients into low-, moderate-, and high-risk categories. Patients with established CHD remained the prototype for the "high-risk" category, which was further defined as risk for a hard CHD event (myocardial infarction [MI] or fatal CHD) >20% over a 10-year period.[8–10] This risk of >20% over 10 years was based on that observed in patients with stable angina and those who have had coronary revascularization.[8,10]

The NCEP ATP III guidelines defined a *CHD risk equivalent* as risk for a major coronary event (MI or coronary death) equal to that of persons with established CHD >20% over 10 years.[8] The NCEP identified three population groups as CHD risk equivalents: (1) those with diabetes; (2) those with other forms of clinical atherosclerotic disease (PAD, abdominal aortic aneurysm, and carotid artery disease; transient ischemic attack [TIA] or stroke of carotid origin or >50% obstruction of a carotid artery); and (3) those without clinical atherosclerotic disease or diabetes but have multiple risk factors that convey an absolute 10-year risk for a major coronary event of >20%.

Risk of Recurrent Events in Established CHD

Although mortality rates from CHD have declined during the past several decades, persons with CHD remain at significant risk for recurrent events and subsequent mortality. Evidence of coronary disease in the absence of clinical MI carries the same risk for future CHD events as does a clinical MI. The recurrent rate of major coronary events in individuals with any clinical evidence of CHD is >20% over 10 years.[8] Extrapolation from the placebo groups in several recent secondary prevention trials demonstrates recurrent CHD risks that range from about 26% over 10 years in those with "average" cholesterol levels[12,13] to 56% in those with high cholesterol levels.[14] In women with existing CHD, rates were similar to men, and older persons had higher rates than younger persons.[15] In several recent studies in which diabetic patients were followed for at least 10 years, the high mortality risk was affirmed with 10-year mortality rates that ranged from 17 to 33%[11,16–20] (Table 3-1). It is possible that the observed event rates in these studies may be lower than that of the general population of diabetics due to the well-known healthy volunteer effect of clinical trial participants.

Diabetes Mellitus and CHD Risk Equivalence

TYPE 2 DIABETES MELLITUS

Diabetes mellitus is the most common CHD risk equivalent. Both type 1 and type 2 diabetes increase risk for CHD. Women with diabetes have greater relative risk (but not absolute risk) than men with diabetes.[21–23] The increased CHD risk in diabetics can be attributed to the hyperglycemia and insulin

Table 3-1 **Mortality Rates in Diabetic Patients Without Baseline CHD**

Author	Year	Subject (n)	Follow-up Duration (Year)	Mortality Rate (%)
Howard et al.[11]	2006	1910	10	10 (nonfatal MI 13%)
Whiteley et al.[16]	2005	3015	25	26
Hu et al.[17]	2003	3705	25	24
Eberly et al.[18]	2003	1122	18	17
Cho et al.[19]	2002	1285	10	24
Muggeo et al.[20]	2000	1409	10	33

resistance, major risk factors, as well as other metabolic abnormalities.[24,25] The NCEP classified type 2 diabetes as a CHD risk equivalent[1] because: (1) individuals with type 2 diabetes have a 10-year risk for major coronary events (MI and CHD death) that approximates that of individuals with CHD but without diabetes[3,26,27]; and (2) patients with type 2 diabetes have high mortality rates at time of acute MI and a poor prognosis for long-term survival following MI.[19,21,28,29] Thus, individuals with type 2 diabetes should be managed with the same intensity of risk reduction as those with established CHD.

The Finnish cohort study in 1998 by Haffner et al.[3] is perhaps the most frequently cited study demonstrating type 2 diabetes as a CHD equivalent. This study demonstrated that the 7-year incidence of MI (fatal and nonfatal) among 1378 nondiabetic subjects (ages 45–65 years) with and without prior MI at baseline was 18.8 and 3.5%, respectively ($P < 0.001$). In 1059 type 2 diabetic subjects, the incidence rates of MI in those without and with prior MI at baseline were 20.2 and 45.0%, respectively ($P < 0.001$). Thus, in this Finnish population, persons with type 2 diabetes without prior CHD had a risk for a MI as high as persons without diabetes with previous MI (Fig. 3-1).

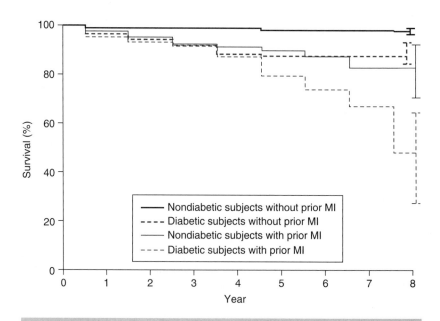

Figure 3-1   **CHD mortality in diabetic and nondiabetic subjects with and without previous MI. Kaplan-Meier estimates of the probability of death from CHD in 1059 subjects with type 2 diabetes and 1378 nondiabetic subjects with and without prior MI. MI denotes myocardial infarction. Vertical bars indicate 95% confidence intervals.**

In another trial, the Organization to Assess Strategies for Ischemic Syndromes (OASIS) study,[26] which evaluated the 2-year prognosis of 8013 (1718 diabetic) diabetic and nondiabetic patients hospitalized with unstable angina or non-Q-wave MI, the investigators also found that diabetic patients without prior CVD had the same event rates for all adverse outcomes as nondiabetic patients with previous history of vascular disease. The findings of this study supported the concept of diabetes as a CHD risk equivalent. The concept is further supported by a series of observational studies in which diabetics and nondiabetics were followed for periods of at least 10 years. In these studies (Table 3-1), the mortality rates of patients with diabetes without CHD had 10-year mortality rates of 17–33%.[11,16–20]

TYPE 1 DIABETES MELLITUS

Although type 1 diabetes increases risk for CHD, some persons with type 1 diabetes (i.e., young individuals without other risk factors) have a 10-year risk for CHD <15–20%. These patients nevertheless have a high long-term risk and the intensity of low-density lipoprotein (LDL) lowering and other risk-modifying therapy should be based on clinical judgment. In recent-onset type 1 diabetes in the absence of other risk factors, reduction of LDL cholesterol to <130 mg/dL may be sufficient. However, as the duration of disease increases, the lower LDL goal (<100 mg/dL) should be considered. In patients with CVD and type 1 or type 2 diabetes, the reasonable LDL goal of <70 mg/dL and intensive treatment of other risk factors are recommended.

Noncoronary Clinical Atherosclerotic Disease and CHD Equivalence

Noncoronary clinical atherosclerotic disease is a powerful predictor of CHD risk. PAD, symptomatic carotid artery disease, asymptomatic carotid artery stenosis, and abdominal aortic aneurysm put patients at high risk for major coronary events and so can also be considered CHD risk equivalents.

PERIPHERAL ARTERIAL DISEASE

Peripheral arterial disease refers to atherosclerotic involvement of a limb artery that is flow limiting. More than 8 million persons in the United States have PAD, a disorder that occurs most frequently in persons ≥60 years of age. The prevalence of PAD (defined as intermittent claudication) increases with age with a prevalence of <3% below age 60 and >20% at ages ≥75.[30,31] Persons with PAD are at increased risk for subsequent CVD morbidity and mortality. The risk factors for PAD are the same as those for CHD, although some risk factors (diabetes mellitus, cigarette smoking, and the metabolic syndrome) appear to be especially important. Patients with PAD frequently have coexisting CVD. The prevalence of CVD in persons with PAD has been variably reported depending on the assessment instrument for CVD. However, in one angiographic study,[32] 90% of patients with PAD undergoing reconstructive surgery had CAD. Approximately 50% of deaths in patients with PAD are due to CAD, 15% due to stroke, and 10% due to abdominal vascular disease.[30–33]

DIABETES AND PERIPHERAL ARTERIAL DISEASE

Diabetes increases the risk of developing PAD by more than fourfold.[34] When compared to nondiabetics, diabetic patients more often have distal PAD in the profunda femoris and arteries below the knee, a lower incidence of aorto-iliac disease, and a similar incidence of occlusive disease in the superficial femoral artery. Blood glucose control, cessation of cigarette smoking, control of elevated blood pressure, control of dyslipidemia, and control of other risk factors are the cornerstones of treatment. Prevention of lower extremity ischemia and distal arterial reconstruction are the most effective defenses against limb amputation. Diabetes is a contributing factor to approximately half of non-trauma-related limb amputations—largely due to the associated severe PAD and more rapid progression of PAD to critical limb ischemia. Diabetics have a 40-fold greater likelihood of limb amputation than nondiabetics, the major contributory factors being PAD, infection, and neuropathy.

High-Risk Persons with Multiple Risk Factors

Some individuals with multiple risk factors are at intermediate risk for major CHD events and others are at high risk. The Framingham risk algorithm provides a tool for calculating absolute risk in males and females (Figs. 3-2 and 3-3) with multiple risk factors.[8] Global risk can be determined and those individuals at high risk identified. Those individuals in whom the risk exceeds 20% over 10 years can be considered to have a CHD risk equivalent.

ASYMPTOMATIC CORONARY ARTERY DISEASE IN TYPE 2 DIABETES

Asymptomatic Myocardial Ischemia

Diabetics have a high rate of asymptomatic coronary disease, silent ischemia, and unrecognized MI.[35,36] The lack of warning symptoms during infarction and ischemia in patients with diabetes has been attributed to autonomic neuropathy involving sympathetic fibers, which are a key component of angina perception.[37] In support of this hypothesis is the observation that the uptake of metaiodobenzylguanidine (MIBG), a norepinephrine analog, is reduced in diabetic patients with silent ischemia.[38] This finding suggests sympathetic denervation, which has also been observed with positron emission tomography (PET).[39,40] Recent evidence from the Detection of Ischemia in Asymptomatic Diabetics (DIAD) study suggests that more than 22% of asymptomatic patients with type 2 diabetes show evidence of ischemia on stress myocardial perfusion imaging.[36] Some investigators have reported higher prevalences of occult CAD

Estimate of 10-year risk for men (Framingham point scores)

Age	Points	Total cholesterol	Points at ages 20–39	Points at ages 40–49	Points at ages 50–59	Points at ages 60–69	Points at ages 70–79
20–34	–9						
35–39	–4	<160	0	0	0	0	0
40–44	0	160–199	4	3	2	1	0
45–49	3	200–239	7	5	3	1	0
50–54	6	240–279	9	6	4	2	1
55–59	8	≥280	11	8	5	3	1
60–64	10						
65–69	11		Points at ages 20–39	Points at ages 40–49	Points at ages 50–59	Points at ages 60–69	Points at ages 70–79
70–74	12						
75–79	13	Non smoker	0	0	0	0	0
		Smoker	8	5	3	1	1

HDL	Points	Systolic BP	If untreated	If treated
≥60	–1	<120	0	0
50–59	0	120–129	0	1
40–49	1	130–139	1	2
<40	2	140–159	1	2
		≥160	2	3

Point total	10-year risk	Point total	10-year risk
<0	<1%	11	8%
0	1%	12	10%
1	1%	13	12%
2	1%	14	16%
3	1%	15	20%
4	1%	16	25%
5	2%	≥17	≥30%
6	2%		
7	3%		
8	4%		
9	5%		
10	6%		

Figure 3-2 **Framingham risk algorithm for calculating risk of major CHD events (MI or fatal CHD) in men.** *(Source: Adapted from Third Report of the National Cholesterol Education Program (NCEP) Expert Panel on Detection, Evaluation, and Treatment of High Blood Cholesterol in Adults (Adult Treatment Panel III) Final Report. Circulation 2002;106:3146–3421.)*

and inducible ischemia among asymptomatic diabetics. In a study of 1427 asymptomatic diabetics without prior MI or revascularization undergoing nuclear stress testing, Rajagopalan et al.[41] reported that 826 patients (58%) had an abnormal stress single-photon emission computed tomography (SPECT) scan. In another study of 1737 diabetics, investigators in the Cedars-Sinai group[42] recently reported an overall 42% abnormal SPECT rate with no differences between asymptomatic patients and those with angina. These observed differences in the prevalence of silent CAD in these studies may reflect differences in participant selection and study designs.

10-year risk estimates for Women (Framingham point scores)

Age	Point	Total cholesterol	Points at ages 20–39	Points at ages 40–49	Points at ages 50–59	Points at ages 60–69	Points at ages 70–79
20–34	–7						
35–39	–3	<160	0	0	0	0	0
40–44	0	160–199	4	3	2	1	1
45–49	3	200–239	8	6	4	2	1
50–54	6	240–279	11	8	5	3	2
55–59	8	≥280	13	10	7	4	2
60–64	10						
65–69	12		Points at ages 20–39	Points at ages 40–49	Points at ages 50–59	Points at ages 60–69	Points at ages 70–79
70–74	14						
75–79	16	Non smoker	0	0	0	0	0
		Smoker	9	7	4	2	1

HDL	Points	Systolic BP	If untreated	If treated
≥60	–1	<120	0	0
50–59	0	120–129	1	3
40–49	1	130–139	2	4
<40	2	140–159	3	5
		≥160	4	6

Point total	10-year risk	Point total	10-year risk
<9	<1%	20	11%
9	1%	21	14%
10	1%	22	17%
11	1%	23	22%
12	1%	24	27%
13	2%	≥25	≥30%
14	2%		
15	3%		
16	4%		
17	5%		
18	6%		
19	8%		

Figure 3-3 **Framingham risk algorithm for calculating risk of major CHD events (MI or fatal CHD) in women.** *(Source: Adapted from Third Report of the National Cholesterol Education Program (NCEP) Expert Panel on Detection, Evaluation, and Treatment of High Blood Cholesterol in Adults (Adult Treatment Panel III) Final Report.* Circulation *2002;106:3146–3421.)*

Cardiac Testing for Asymptomatic Ischemia in Diabetes

In 1998, the American Diabetes Association (ADA) issued guidelines for diagnostic testing for detection of coronary disease in patients with type 2 diabetes[43,44] (Table 3-2). A variety of noninvasive techniques are available for detecting asymptomatic ischemia, including exercise-electrocardiography, nuclear imaging, and stress echocardiography (see Chap. 17 for a more detailed discussion of imaging techniques and their roles in evaluating diabetic

Table 3-2 **Indication for Cardiac Testing in Diabetic Patients**

Testing for CAD is warranted in patients with the following:
  Typical or atypical cardiac symptoms
  Resting electrocardiograph suggestive of ischemia or infarction
  Peripheral or carotid occlusive arterial disease
  Sedentary lifestyle, age ≥35 years, and plans to begin a vigorous exercise program
Two or more of the risk factors listed below (a–e) in addition to diabetes:
a. Total cholesterol ≥240 mg/dL, LDL cholesterol ≥160 mg/dL, or HDL cholesterol <35 mg/dL
b. Blood pressure >140/90 mmHg
c. Smoking
d. Family history of premature CAD
e. Positive micro/macroalbuminuria test

Source: Adapted from Ref. 43.

patients). An important consideration when requesting exercise testing is that diabetic patients are less likely to be able to satisfactorily perform on a standard treadmill test than are nondiabetics. Figures 3-4 and 3-5 provide algorithms for evaluation of symptomatic and asymptomatic patients with diabetes.

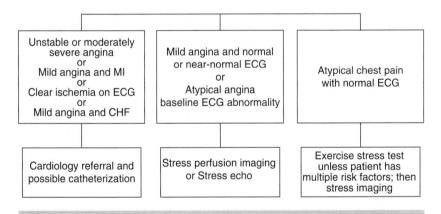

Figure 3-4 **Cardiac testing of the symptomatic diabetic patient. In patients with diabetes and symptoms that are either clearly related to ischemia or atypical in nature but suspected to be of cardiac origin, testing can be undertaken using the algorithm in Fig. 3-3.*A multiple risk factor patient is defined as an individual with two or more risk factors (see Table 3-1).** *(Adapted from American Diabetes Association. Consensus development conference on the diagnosis of coronary heart disease in people with diabetes.* Diabetes Care *1998;21:1551–1559.)*

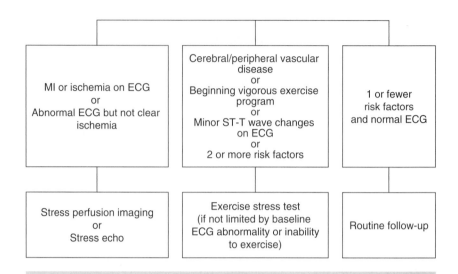

Figure 3-5 **Cardiac testing of the asymptomatic diabetic patient. Patients with two or more risk factors or those beginning a vigorous exercise program should have an exercise stress test. In patients with clear suggestive evidence of ischemia or infarction on ECG, stress perfusion imaging or stress echo should be used. If expertise with both modalities is available, perfusion imaging would be preferred.** *(Adapted from American Diabetes Association. Consensus development conference on the diagnosis of coronary heart disease in people with diabetes.* Diabetes Care *1998;21:1551–1559.)*

Exercise stress testing with only electrocardiography has limited value for assessing ischemia in diabetic patients both because of the low predictive value of the test and the limited ability of many patients with diabetes to exercise prespecified target levels. Stress testing combined with imaging studies provides greater and more reliable diagnostic value and is preferred for assessment of myocardial ischemia.

Imaging studies afford several advantages as they permit visualization of perfusion (using nuclear imaging) or systolic wall motion (mainly echocardiography, but magnetic resonance imaging can also be used) abnormalities, both sensitive markers of ischemia. In addition, the imaging studies can be performed in combination with pharmacologic stress rather than physical exercise when necessary. Both nuclear myocardial perfusion imaging and stress echocardiography have been demonstrated to have a high accuracy for the detection of CAD in patients with type 2 diabetes. In diabetic patients, the validity period of a normal study is different than for nondiabetics. This can be limited to 2–3 years, indicating a quicker progression of CAD in these patients. Elhendy et al.[45] demonstrated that the event rate in diabetic patients with a normal exercise echocardiogram increased from 0% in the first year to 1.8% at 3-year and 7.6% at 5-year follow-up.

For asymptomatic diabetic patients, the ADA guidelines recommend that those patients with an abnormal resting ECG, evidence of peripheral vascular disease, or two or more risk factors should be evaluated for occult CAD. The follow-up recommendations for a positive test are described in Fig. 3-6. Asymptomatic diabetic patients with a "mildly" positive stress test, for example, modest (1–1.5 mm) ST depression at a moderate- to high exercise level (Bruce stage 3 or greater), are considered to be a low-risk group and further workup with an imaging test is recommended. In asymptomatic diabetic patients who have "moderately" positive electrocardiographic stress tests, further noninvasive stratification with perfusion imaging is also warranted. In asymptomatic diabetic patients with a "markedly" positive stress test, indicated by features including hypotension during exercise; a positive test with a heart rate <120, or exercise capacity <6 minutes (stage 1 or 2 of a Bruce protocol or 5 metabolic equivalents (METS) or resting oxygen consumption of 3.5 mL/kG/min of other protocols); ST depression involving 5 or more leads; or >2-mm maximum ST depression are recommended for direct evaluation with coronary angiography.

Pre-test risk	ETT results			
	Normal	Mildly positive	Moderately positive	Markedly positive
High 4–5 risk factors**	√√	√√√	√√√√	√√√√
Moderate 2–3 risk factors	√	√√√	√√√	√√√√
Low 0–1 risk factors	√	√√√	√√√	√√√√

√	Routine follow-up
√√	Close follow-up
√√√	Imaging
√√√√	Cardiology referral/possible catheterization

Figure 3-6 **Appropriate follow-up after screening exercise treadmill test (ETT). When initial exercise stress testing is done in asymptomatic diabetic patients, the type of follow-up depends on the pretest risk and the degree of abnormality on the stress test. Normal follow-up indicates annual revaluation of symptoms and signs of CHD and ECG. A repeat ETT should be considered in 3–5 years if clinical status is unchanged. Close follow-up means shorter intervals between evaluation and follow-up ETT (i.e., 1–2 years). Pretext risk is assigned based on the presence of other vascular disease and risk factors (see Table 3-1).** (Adapted from American Diabetes Association. Consensus development conference on the diagnosis of coronary heart disease in people with diabetes. Diabetes Care 1998;21:1551–1559.)

The ADA guidelines also indicate that coronary artery calcification (CAC) detected by electron beam computed tomography (EBCT) is recognized as being related to pathologic plaque area and the severity of coronary artery stenoses. However, significant coronary stenoses can exist in the absence of detectable calcification.

Detection of Silent Myocardial Ischemia in Asymptomatic Diabetics Study

The detection of silent myocardial ischemia in asymptomatic diabetics (DIAD) study is a prospective study designed to assess the prevalence of silent myocardial ischemia in asymptomatic diabetics.[36] The Rose Questionnaire was employed to insure that patients with angina symptoms were excluded. The study enrolled 1123 patients with type 2 diabetes, aged 50–75 years, with no known or suspected CAD, at 14 centers in the United States and Canada between July 2000 and August 2002. Participants will be followed for up to 5 years (until September 2007) for occurrence of cardiac events. In the DIAD study, patients were randomly assigned to either stress testing and 5-year clinical follow-up ($n = 522$) or to follow-up only. The prevalence of ischemia in 522 patients randomized to stress testing was assessed by adenosine technetium-99m sestamibi SPECT myocardial perfusion imaging. Pharmacologic testing eliminated the problem of inadequate exercise capacity anticipated in some diabetics. Within the group of patients that underwent stress testing, 113 patients (22%) had abnormal studies. Regional perfusion abnormalities were present in 16% (of the 113 patients). Markedly abnormal perfusion images occurred in 6% (of the 113 patients). Despite normal myocardial perfusion, 30 additional patients (6%) had other significant test abnormalities such as transient ST-segment depression during adenosine infusion, left ventricular dysfunction, or transient ischemic left ventricular dilation. Categorization of the DIAD population according to the presence or absence of criteria for screening as defined in the ADA consensus screening guidelines revealed that in the group of 306 patients with two or more risk factors, 66 (22%) had abnormal test results, whereas in the 204 patients with less than two risk factors, 45 (22%) also had abnormal test results. Hence, abnormal myocardial perfusion results were equally distributed among patients with two or more and less than two risk factors indicating an inability to stratify patients solely based on their number of risk factors. These preliminary results suggest that it is clinically appropriate and cost-effective to screen for silent myocardial ischemia in asymptomatic diabetics.

Exercise-Electrocardiography

Conventional ST-segment analysis during exercise-electrocardiography is moderately sensitive for detecting CHD. However, ST-segment analysis alone has low specificity and a high rate (10–35%) of false positive responses, particularly in asymptomatic persons and in women.[46] As a result, the diagnosis of myocardial ischemia by exercise-electrocardiography should be confirmed by further imaging techniques before the subject is labeled as having silent ischemia.[47]

Ambulatory ECG Recordings (Holter Monitoring)

Holter monitoring has the advantage of providing long-term ECG recordings of ischemic and arrhythmic events while patients are engaged in routine daily activities.[48] However, a limitation to the use of outpatient Holter monitoring, especially for the evaluation of therapeutic interventions, is the marked day-to-day variability in the frequency and duration of ST depression and ischemic episodes.[49]

Myocardial Contrast Echocardiography

The recent work by Scognamiglio et al. showed significant results in favor of myocardial contrast echocardiography.[50] The study involved 1900 asymptomatic patients with type 2 diabetes (age ≤60 years, mean 52 years), 60% of whom had ≥2 CHD risk factors (dyslipidemia, hypertension, smoking, a positive family history of premature coronary disease, or the presence of microalbuminuria or macroalbuminuria). All patients underwent stress testing with dipyridamole myocardial contrast echocardiography, and coronary angiography was performed in those with myocardial perfusion defects. The investigators found the two risk groups (≥2 vs. 0 or 1 risk factors) had equivalent rates of abnormal stress tests (60%) and of significant coronary disease on angiography (65%). This finding suggests that merely stratifying patients based on the presence or absence of multiple risk factors—as in the ADA 1998 guidelines—will result in missing significant CAD in a large percentage of patients. However, the study did demonstrate that patients with multiple risk factors had more severe coronary disease with significantly higher rates of three-vessel disease (33% vs. 8%), diffuse disease (55% vs. 18%), and vessel occlusion (31% vs. 4%); they had a lower rate of single-vessel disease (29% vs. 54%). Hence patients with ≤1 risk factor, have more favorable angiographic anatomy. As discussed earlier in this chapter, diabetic patients without previous MI have a risk for MI as high as the risk of reinfarction in a nondiabetic individual with previous MI. Since regular and routine stress testing is recommended for risk assessment in patients with previous MI, one can argue that patients with type 2 diabetes—CHD risk equivalents—should also routinely have exercise stress evaluations. However, even though these patients are at increased risk, given the extremely large numbers of type 2 diabetics, carrying out a recommendation for more routine diagnostic testing of asymptomatic diabetics would be a formidable and expensive undertaking.

Myocardial Perfusion Single-Photon Emission Computed Tomography

As previously discussed, evidence from the DIAD study found that 22% asymptomatic patients with type 2 diabetes show evidence of ischemia on stress myocardial perfusion imaging.[45] In a study of 1427 asymptomatic diabetics without prior MI or revascularization undergoing nuclear stress testing, Rajagopalan et al.[41] reported that 826 patients (58%) had an abnormal stress SPECT scan. A study from the Cedars-Sinai group[42] examining 1737 diabetics reported an overall 42% abnormal SPECT rate for asymptomatic patients. Both of these studies demonstrated that CAD prevalence in asymptomatic diabetics was independent of the number of risk factors. In another study, Kang et al.[51] reported similar sensitivities and specificities of myocardial perfusion SPECT for detecting angiographic CAD in diabetic and nondiabetic patients. Thus, a number of studies have confirmed that stress SPECT provides incremental prognostic value and can be used for risk stratification in diabetics.[52–54] Despite the evidence of usefulness of stress SPECT scanning for diagnostic evaluation, caution must be exercised since a relatively common finding in patients with diabetes is that the extent and severity of perfusion abnormalities on SPECT imaging suggest more extensive and severe ischemia than that found at coronary angiography. In a study conducted by Mayo Clinic investigators, 51 of 127 patients (40%) with high-risk nuclear scans (reflecting extensive and severe ischemia and/or scar) undergoing coronary angiography showed relatively mild angiographic CAD. These findings could be false positives or they may indicate underlying microvascular dysfunction.[55] A normal stress SPECT study is generally associated with a low risk (<1% annual risk of cardiac death or MI),[56] but the risk is higher in diabetics even with a normal SPECT.[42,53,57]

In summary, it appears that although current recommendations for stress testing in asymptomatic diabetics with multiple risk factors are appropriate, the recommendation to not evaluate further those asymptomatic diabetics without multiple risk factors may result in failure to diagnose significant ischemia in a substantial number of patients. In this group of patients, two alternative approaches were suggested by Di Carli et al.[58] The first approach is the suggestion for development of an aggregate score that incorporates and weighs risk factors. Although there is currently no generally accepted scoring system to do this, several studies have demonstrated that incorporating a clinical score into a testing strategy can enhance diagnostic yield and improve cost-effectiveness.[59,60] A second suggested approach is to utilize a test of atherosclerosis burden to identify asymptomatic diabetics with a higher likelihood of occult CAD. For example, previous studies have shown that the use of a calcium score threshold (e.g., 400) may identify those individuals with intermediate likelihood of SPECT abnormality.[61,62]

Electron Beam Computed Tomography and Coronary Artery Calcification

Coronary artery calcium on EBCT, as determined by a calcium score, can identify subclinical atherosclerosis in asymptomatic patients who may be at high risk for CHD. This imaging technique allows visualization of atherosclerosis (coronary artery calcium) rather than ischemia, and may thus permit identification of CAD prior to the onset of ischemia. Anand et al.[63] evaluated 510 asymptomatic patients with type 2 diabetes using EBCT and performed nuclear myocardial perfusion imaging in patients with a calcium score >100. For comparison, 53 randomly selected patients with a calcium score ≤100 also underwent SPECT. None of the patients with calcium score (10 had abnormalities on SPECT. The incidence of abnormal SPECT studies increased in parallel to the calcium score, from 18.4% in patients with calcium score between 11 and 100 to 71.4% in patients with a calcium score >1000. During a mean follow-up of 18 ± 5 months, no events occurred in the patients with a calcium score (10, whereas the majority (82%) of events occurred in patients with a calcium score >400. These observations suggest that sequential use of EBCT and SPECT may improve risk assessment and identification of high-risk asymptomatic diabetic patients.

Combined Pet and CT for CAD Detection

The combination of PET and multidetector computed tomography (CT) (PET-CT) is currently being evaluated for detection of significant CAD.[64,65] The combined PET-CT approach provides the potential for delineation of the anatomic extent and physiologic severity of coronary atherosclerosis and obstructive disease in a single setting. Individually employed, PET and CT have limitations that would be overcome with the combined approach. The integration of CT technology with PET technology provides the potential to evaluate for the presence of significant subclinical coronary atherosclerosis in patients with normal perfusion.

SUMMARY AND CONCLUSIONS

Patients with diabetes are at high risk for symptomatic and asymptomatic ischemic events. Despite the large number of studies conducted to date, the optimal approach to evaluation and detection of asymptomatic ischemia in patients with diabetes remains undefined and a topic of debate. The DIAD study may prove especially important in this regard. In the initial phase of the DIAD study, significant silent ischemia was determined to be present in 22% of asymptomatic individuals with diabetes. The ultimate significance of this finding and the relative risks of this group compared to those without silent ischemia await completion of the 5-year follow-up phase of the study—anticipated to be in 2007. Although it is clear that patients with diabetes (symptomatic and asymptomatic) are at high risk for the development of CHD events, any recommendation for widespread diagnostic testing of asymptomatic diabetics should be evidence-based and have a high likelihood of impacting therapy. At present, routine exercise testing and evaluations for subclinical ischemia in asymptomatic diabetics without other CHD risk factors are not recommended. However, type 2 diabetes is a CHD risk equivalent, and these patients should receive intensive management of their diabetes, vigorous control of all CHD risk factors, and appropriate use of recommended cardioprotective therapies (aspirin, beta-blockers, angiotensin-converting enzyme inhibitors, and statins) to reduce their risks of clinical events and mortality.

In addition to the above, practitioners should always keep a high index of suspicion for myocardial ischemia in patients with diabetes. It is well known that diabetics often have defective angina warning systems, and atypical clinical presentations such as diaphoresis and weakness may be due to ischemia as well as due to hypo- or hyperglycemia. The ADA recommends that diabetic patients with an abnormal resting ECG, evidence of peripheral vascular disease, or multiple CHD risk factors should be evaluated for occult CAD.[43] While the debate will continue regarding whether or not all asymptomatic diabetic patients should be evaluated for subclinical atherosclerosis,[58] it is clear that the detection of silent myocardial ischemia should be treated as vigorously as symptomatic ischemia with prompt initiation of appropriate anti-ischemic drug therapy,[66] appropriate cardioprotective therapies, and consideration of additional evaluation.

REFERENCES

1. American Diabetes Association. Consensus statement: role of cardiovascular risk factors in prevention and treatment of macrovascular disease in diabetes. *Diabetes Care* 1993;(Suppl 2):72–78.

2. Aronson D, Rayfield EJ, Chesebro JH. Mechanisms determining course and outcome of diabetic patients who have had acute myocardial infarction. *Ann Intern Med* 1997;126(4):296–306.

3. Haffner SM, Lehto S, Rönemaa T, et al. Mortality from coronary heart disease in subjects with type 2 diabetes and in nondiabetic subjects with and without prior myocardial infarction. *N Engl J Med* 1998;339(4):229–234.

4. Kannel WB, McGee DL. Diabetes and glucose tolerance as risk factors for cardiovascular disease: the Framingham study. *Diabetes Care* 1979;2(2):120–126.

5. Stamler J, Vaccaro O, Neaton JD, et al. Diabetes, other risk factors, and 12-yr cardiovascular mortality for men screened in the Multiple Risk Factor Intervention Trial. *Diabetes Care* 1993;16(2):434–444.

6. King H, Aubert RE, Herman WH. Global burden of diabetes, 1995-2025: prevalence, numerical estimates, and projections. *Diabetes Care* 1998;21(9):1414–1431.

7. Boyle JP, Honeycutt AA, Narayan KM, et al. Projection of diabetes burden through 2050: impact of changing demography and disease prevalence in the U.S. *Diabetes Care* 2001;24(11):1936–1940.

8. Third Report of the National Cholesterol Education Program (NCEP) Expert Panel on Detection, Evaluation, and Treatment of High Blood Cholesterol in Adults (Adult Treatment Panel III) Final Report. *Circulation* 2002;106:3146–3421.

9. Summary of the Second Report of the National Cholesterol Education Program (NCEP) Expert Panel on Detection, Evaluation, and Treatment of High Blood Cholesterol in Adults (Adult Treatment Panel II). *JAMA* 1993;269:3015–3023.

10. Grundy SM. Diabetes and coronary risk equivalency: what does it mean? *Diabetes Care* 2006;29:457–460.

11. Howard BV, Best LG, Galloway JM, et al. Coronary heart disease risk equivalence in diabetes depends on concomitant risk factors. *Diabetes Care* 2002;29:391–397.

12. Sacks FM, Pfeffer MA, Moye LA, et al. The effect of pravastatin on coronary events after myocardial infarction in patients with average cholesterol levels: Cholesterol and Recurrent Events Trial investigators. *N Engl J Med* 1996;335: 1001–1009.

13. The Long-Term Intervention with Pravastatin in Ischaemic Disease (LIPID) Study Group. Prevention of cardiovascular events and death with pravastatin in patients with coronary heart disease and a broad range of initial cholesterol levels. *N Engl J Med* 1998;339:1349–1357.

14. Randomised trial of cholesterol lowering in 4444 patients with coronary heart disease: the Scandinavian Simvastatin Survival Study (4S). *Lancet* 1994;344: 1383–1389.

15. LaRosa JC, He J, Vuppurti S. Effect of statins on risk of coronary disease: a meta analysis of randomized controlled trials. *JAMA* 1999;282:2340–2346.

16. Whiteley L, Padmanabhan S, Hole D, et al. Should diabetes be considered a coronary heart disease risk equivalent? Results from 25 years of follow-up in the Renfrew and Paisley survey. *Diabetes Care* 2005;28(7):1588–1593.

17. Hu FB, Stampfer MJ, Solomon CG, et al. The impact of diabetes mellitus on mortality from all causes and coronary heart disease in women: 20 years of follow-up. *Arch Intern Med* 2001;161(14):1717–1723.

18. Eberly LE, Cohen JD, Prineas R, et al. and Intervention Trial Research Group. Impact of incident diabetes and incident nonfatal cardiovascular disease on 18-year mortality: the multiple risk factor intervention trial experience. *Diabetes Care* 2003;26(3):848–854.

19. Cho E, Rimm EB, Stampfer MJ, et al. The impact of diabetes mellitus and prior myocardial infarction on mortality from all causes and from coronary heart disease in men. *J Am Coll Cardiol* 2002;40(5):954–960.

20. Muggeo M, Zoppini G, Bonora E, et al. Fasting plasma glucose variability predicts 10-year survival of type 2 diabetic patients: the Verona Diabetes Study. *Diabetes Care* 2000;23(1):45–50.

21. Abbott RD, Donahue RP, Kannel WB, et al. The impact of diabetes on survival following myocardial infarction in men vs women. The Framingham Study. *JAMA* 1988;260(23):3456–3460.

22. Barrett-Connor E, Wingard DL. Sex differential in ischemic heart disease mortality in diabetics: a prospective population-based study. *Am J Epidemiol* 1983; 118(4):489–496.

23. Lee WL, Cheung AM, Cape D, et al. Impact of diabetes on coronary artery disease in women and men: a meta-analysis of prospective studies. *Diabetes Care* 2000; 23(7):962–968.

24. Rosengren A, Welin L, Tsipogianni A, et al. Impact of cardiovascular risk factors on coronary heart disease and mortality among middle aged diabetic men: a general population study. *BMJ* 1989;299(6708):1127–1131.

25. Siegel RD, Cupples A, Schaefer EJ, et al. Lipoproteins, apolipoproteins, and low-density lipoprotein size among diabetics in the Framingham offspring study. *Metabolism* 1996;45(10):1267–1272.

26. Malmberg K, Yusuf S, Gerstein HC, et al. Impact of diabetes on long-term prognosis in patients with unstable angina and non-Q-wave myocardial infarction: results of the OASIS (Organization to Assess Strategies for Ischemic Syndromes) Registry. *Circulation* 2000;29;102:1014–1019.

27. Lotufo PA, Gaziano JM, Chae CU, et al. Diabetes and all-cause and coronary heart disease mortality among US male physicians. *Arch Intern Med* 2001;161(2): 242–247.

28. Behar S, Boyko V, Reicher-Reiss H, et al. Ten-year survival after acute myocardial infarction: comparison of patients with and without diabetes. SPRINT Study Group. Secondary Prevention Reinfarction Israeli Nifedipine Trial. *Am Heart J* 1997;133(3):290–296.

29. Chun BY, Dobson AJ, Heller RF. The impact of diabetes on survival among patients with first myocardial infarction. *Diabetes Care* 1997;20(5):704–708.

30. Criqui MH, Denenberg JO, Langer RD, et al. The epidemiology of peripheral arterial disease: importance of identifying the population at risk. *Vasc Med* 1997;3:221–226.

31. Aronow WS, Ahn C. Prevalence of coexistence of coronary artery disease, peripheral arterial disease, and atherothrombotic brain infarction in men and women ≥ 62 years of age. *Am J Cardiol* 1994;74:64–65.

32. Hertzer NR, Beven EG, Young JR, et al. Coronary artery disease in peripheral vascular patients. A classification of 1000 coronary angiograms and results of surgical management. *Ann Surg* 1984:199;223–233.

33. Dormandy J, Mahir M, Ascada G, et al. Fate of the patient with chronic leg ischaemia. *J Cardiovasc Surg* 1989;30:50–57.

34. Kazmier FJ, Bowie EJW, O'Fallon WM, et al. A prospective study of peripheral occlusive arterial disease in diabetes. IV. Platelet and plasma functions. *Mayo Clin Proc* 1981;56:243–253.

35. Nesto RW, Phillips RT, Kett KG, et al. Angina and exertional myocardial ischemia in diabetic and nondiabetic patients: assessment by exercise thallium scintigraphy. *Ann Intern Med* 1988;108:170–175.

36. Wackers FJ, Young LH, Inzucchi SE, et al. Detection of silent myocardial ischemia in asymptomatic diabetic subjects: the DIAD study. *Diabetes Care* 2004;27: 1954–1961.

37. Niakan E, Harati Y, Rolak LA, et al. Silent myocardial infarction and diabetic cardiovascular autonomic neuropathy. *Arch Intern Med* 1986;146:2229–2230.

38. Langer A, Freeman MR, Josse R, et al. Metaiodobenzylguanidine imaging in diabetes mellitus: assessment of cardiac sympathetic denervation and its relation to autonomic dysfunction and silent myocardial ischemia. *J Am Coll Cardiol* 1995;25: 610–618.

39. Di Carli MF, Bianco-Battles D, Landa ME, et al. Effects of autonomic neuropathy on coronary blood flow in patients with diabetes mellitus. *Circulation* 1999;100:813–819.

40. Stevens MJ, Raffel DM, Allman KC, et al. Cardiac sympathetic dysinnervation in diabetes: implications for enhanced cardiovascular risk. *Circulation* 1998;98: 961–968.

41. Rajagopalan N, Miller TD, Hodge DO, et al. Identifying high-risk asymptomatic diabetic patients who are candidates for screening stress single-photon emission computed tomography imaging. *J Am Coll Cardiol* 2005;45:43–49.

42. Zellweger MJ, Hachamovitch R, Kang X, et al. Prognostic relevance of symptoms versus objective evidence of coronary artery disease in diabetic patients *Eur Heart J* 2004;25:543–550.

43. American Diabetes Association. Consensus development conference on the diagnosis of coronary heart disease in people with diabetes: 10-11 February 1998. Miami, FL. *Diabetes Care* 1998;21:1551–1559.

44. Redberg RF, Greenland P, Fuster V, et al. Prevention Conference VI: Diabetes and Cardiovascular Disease: Writing Group III: risk assessment in persons with diabetes. *Circulation* 2002;105:e144–e152.

45. Elhendy A, Arruda AM, Mahoney DM, et al. Prognostic stratification of diabetic patients by exercise echocardiography. *J Am Coll Cardiol* 2001;37:1551–1557.

46. Yeung AC, Vekshtein VI, Krantz DS, et al. The effect of atherosclerosis on the vasomotor response of coronary arteries to mental stress. *N Engl J Med* 1991;325: 1551–1556.

47. Deedwania PC. Should asymptomatic subjects with silent ischemia undergo further evaluation and follow-up? *Int J Cardiol* 1994;44:101–103.

48. Deedwania PC. The need for a cost-effective strategy to detect ambulatory silent ischemia. *Am J Cardiol* 1994;74:1061–1062.

49. Patel DJ, Norrie MJ, Clarke D, et al. Natural variability of transient myocardial ischaemia during daily life: an obstacle when assessing efficacy of anti-ischaemic agents? *Heart* 1996;76:477–482.

50. Scognamiglio R, Negut C, Ramondo A, et al. Detection of coronary artery disease in asymptomatic patients with type 2 diabetes mellitus. *J Am Coll Cardiol* 2006; 47:65–71.

51. Kang X, Berman DS, Lewin H, et al. Comparative ability of myocardial perfusion single-photon emission computed tomography to detect coronary artery disease in patients with and without diabetes mellitus. *Am Heart J* 1999;137:949–957.

52. Berman DS, Kang X, Hayes SW, et al. Adenosine myocardial perfusion single-photon emission computed tomography in women compared with men: impact of diabetes mellitus on incremental prognostic value and effect on patient management. *J Am Coll Cardiol* 2003;41:1125–1133.

53. Giri S, Shaw LJ, Murthy DR, et al. Impact of diabetes on the risk stratification using stress single-photon emission computed tomography myocardial perfusion imaging in patients with symptoms suggestive of coronary artery disease. *Circulation* 2002;105:32–40.

54. Kang X, Berman DS, Lewin HC, et al. Incremental prognostic value of myocardial perfusion single photon emission computed tomography in patients with diabetes mellitus. *Am Heart J* 1999;138:1025–1032.

55. Campisi R, Di Carli MF. Assessment of coronary flow reserve and microcirculation: a clinical perspective. *J Nucl Cardiol* 2004;11:3–11.

56. Klocke FJ, Baird MG, Bateman TM, et al. ACC/AHA/ASNC guidelines for the clinical use of cardiac radionuclide imaging: a report of the American 1995 guidelines for the clinical use of radionuclide imaging. *J Am Coll Cardiol* 2003;42: 1318–1333.

57. Hachamovitch R, Hayes S, Friedman JD, et al. Determinants of risk and its temporal variation in patients with normal stress myocardial perfusion scans: what is the warranty period of a normal scan? *J Am Coll Cardiol* 2003;41:1329–1340.

58. Di Carli MF, Hachamovitch R. Should we screen for occult coronary artery disease among asymptomatic patients with diabetes? *J Am Coll Cardiol* 2005;45(1): 50–53.

59. Poornima IG, Miller TD, Christian TF, et al. Utility of myocardial perfusion imaging in patients with low-risk treadmill scores. *J Am Coll Cardiol* 2004;43:194–199.

60. Berman DS, Hachamovitch R, Kiat H, et al. Incremental value of prognostic testing in patients with known or suspected ischemic heart disease: a basis for optimal utilization of exercise technetium-99m sestamibi myocardial perfusion single-photon emission computed tomography (published erratum appears in *J Am Coll Cardiol* 1996;27:756). *J Am Coll Cardiol* 1995;26:639–647.

61. Berman DS, Wong ND, Gransar H, et al. Relationship between stress-induced myocardial ischemia and atherosclerosis measured by coronary calcium tomography. *J Am Coll Cardiol* 2004;44:923–930.

62. He ZX, Hedrick TD, Pratt CM, et al. Severity of coronary artery calcification by electron beam computed tomography predicts silent myocardial ischemia. *Circulation* 2000;101:244–251.

63. Anand DV, Lim ETS, Hopkins D, et al. Risk stratification in uncomplicated type 2 diabetes: prospective evaluation of the combined use of coronary artery calcium imaging and selective myocardial perfusion scintigraphy. *Eur Heart J* 2006;27: 713–721.

64. Di Carli MF, Dorbala S, Hachamovitch R. Integrated cardiac PET-CT for the diagnosis and management of CAD. *J Nucl Cardiol* 2006;13(2):139–144.

65. Namdar M, Hany TF, Koepfli P, et al. Integrated PET/CT for the assessment of coronary artery disease: a feasibility study. *J Nucl Med* 2005;46(6):930–935.

66. Rogers WJ, Bourassa MG, Andrews TC, et al. Asymptomatic Cardiac Ischemia Pilot (ACIP) study: outcome at 1 year for patients with asymptomatic cardiac ischemia randomized to medical therapy or revascularization. The ACIP Investigators. *J Am Coll Cardiol* 1995;26:594–605.

MANAGEMENT OF ACUTE CORONARY SYNDROMES IN DIABETIC PATIENTS

Cristina Mitre
Jonathan D. Marmur

Important factors in the pathogenesis of acute coronary syndromes (ACS) are vascular inflammation, rupture of vulnerable plaque, with increased thrombosis and distal microembolization. Diabetic patients, however, have hyperreactive platelets with exaggerated adhesion, aggregation, and thrombin generation, associated with more severe ischemic disease and adverse outcome.[1-4] Therefore, the treatment of ACS should address these factors, reducing inflammation, stabilizing the ruptured plaque, and preventing further microvascular damage.

The objectives of initial evaluation and management of patients with diabetes mellitus presenting with symptoms compatible with ACS are to identify immediate life-threatening signs and to ensure the most appropriate level of care based on diagnostic criteria and risk stratification. All patients with ACS should be admitted to an inpatient unit with continuous rhythm, blood pressure monitoring, careful observation for recurrent ischemic events, and frequent assessment.

Treatment algorithms, based on clinical risk stratification, are used to triage patients to early angiography to define the coronary anatomy with subsequent revascularization when appropriate.

MEDICAL THERAPY

The treatment of patients with diabetes mellitus and ACS is often similar to that in nondiabetic patients. Immediate measures, such as bed rest with continuous ECG monitoring, supplemental oxygen to maintain SaO_2 >90%, nitrates sublingual or spray followed by IV administration, and morphine IV to relieve pain and anxiety, are all common in patients with or without diabetes.[5]

Also, the initial medical therapy in diabetic patients presenting with ACS should be particularly directed toward tight glycemic control, regardless of any revascularization procedure.

Glycemic Control

Oral hypoglycemic agents and insulin should be used to achieve tight glycemic control, with target of a glycosylated hemoglobin (HbA1c) value of <7.0% (considered standard of care).[6] In patients with type 2 diabetes, insulin resistance represents the main defect, often in the setting of obesity. The newer agents, thiazolidinediones (rosiglitazone, pioglitazone), by selective binding at the peroxisome proliferator-activated receptor gamma (PPARγ) found in adipose tissue, skeletal muscle, and liver, act primarily by decreasing insulin resistance. Also, thiazolidinediones have shown to have favorable effects on endothelial function, reducing intimal hyperplasia after coronary stenting as assessed by intravascular ultrasound (IVUS).[7] In the United Kingdom Prospective Diabetes Study (UKPDS), there were significantly fewer microvascular complications with intensive glycemic control compared with conventional treatment of type 2 diabetes ($P = 0.009$).[8] Also, the UKPDS substudy in obese patients treated with metformin showed a statistically significant reduction (39%) in the incidence of myocardial infarction (MI) compared to the conventional arm ($P = 0.01$).[9] It is not yet clear whether achieving tight glycemic control by reducing insulin resistance offers better outcome compared to providing exogenous insulin or drugs stimulating endogenous insulin release in patients with type 2 diabetes and coronary artery disease (CAD). One major study designed to answer this question is the Bypass Angioplasty Revascularization Investigation 2 Diabetes (BARI 2D) trial.[10,11]

Another important aspect of treatment in diabetic patients with acute myocardial infarction (AMI) is the beneficial effect on survival of a regimen of glucose, insulin, and potassium (GIK). A meta-analysis of all randomized placebo-controlled studies of GIK therapy in AMI showed a statistical significant reduction in hospital mortality in the GIK group ($P = 0.004$).[12] The Diabetes Mellitus Insulin-Glucose Infusion in Acute Myocardial Infarction (DIGAMI) study also revealed a survival benefit obtained with insulin-glucose infusion compared to conventional therapy, with the most important predictors of outcome being the glucose level and HbA1c at the time of AMI.[13]

Antiplatelet and Anticoagulant Therapy

ASPIRIN

Although the role of aspirin (ASA) in ACS and especially in MI is well documented, limited data directly address ASA treatment in diabetes. The dose of ASA may be critical in diabetic subjects, with conflicting reports supporting this, demonstrating no benefit from 160 mg of ASA daily in diabetics (Second International Study of Infarct Survival [ISIS-2]).[14] Due to increased platelet turnover, a dose of 325 mg of ASA may be necessary to effectively suppress the thromboxane A_2. The Antiplatelet Trialists' Collaboration[15,16] performed a meta-analysis of secondary prevention studies and showed that diabetic and nondiabetic subjects benefited from ASA to the same degree. However, the Israeli Bezafibrate Infarction Prevention Study showed a greater benefit of ASA in diabetic patients with CAD reflected in 5% absolute reduction (10.9% vs. 15.9%) in cardiac mortality at 5-year follow-up compared to 2% in nondiabetic patients.[17]

Diabetic or nondiabetic patients presenting with suspected ACS, if not already receiving ASA, should be given the first dose in ED, chewed to rapidly establish a high blood level. Treatment should be continued if they were already receiving ASA. Subsequent doses should be given daily. The protective effect of ASA has been proven at 1–2 years follow-up in clinical trials and, although there are no longer-term studies conducted only in diabetic patients, the treatment should be continued indefinitely unless a contraindication develops.

THIENOPYRIDINES

Initially clopidogrel and ticlopidine were used in CAD patients as an alternative to ASA when there was intolerance or a contraindication to ASA use.[5] Clopidogrel became the preferred drug due to less side effects and better and more rapid platelet inhibition. Comparing results from six trials with thienopyridines, Bhatt et al. showed less major adverse cardiac events (e.g., death, MI, and target vessel revascularization [TVR]) with clopidogrel compared to ticlopidine.[18] Recent trials enrolling patients with ACS or referred for planned percutaneous coronary intervention (PCI) revealed improved outcome with clopidogrel and ASA therapy continued for 9 months to 1 year.[19,20] In CURE (clopidogrel in unstable angina to prevent recurrent events) and CREDO (Clopidogrel for the Reduction of Events During Observation) trials, the benefit was also observed in diabetic patients. However, there are no randomized studies with thienopyridines enrolling only diabetic patients with ACS. The major concern with clopidogrel treatment is the risk of bleeding in case surgery is needed, but stopping treatment at least 5–7 days prior to a surgical procedure seems to be a safe approach.[19] A particular aspect in diabetic patients presenting with ACS, considering the higher rate of multivessel disease and therefore the higher need for coronary artery bypass grafting (CABG), should be the initiation of clopidogrel after defining the anatomy of coronary arteries and deciding that surgery is not an option.

Glycoprotein IIb/IIIa Inhibitors

Recent meta-analyses of the major randomized trials with IV glycoprotein (GP) IIb/IIIa inhibitors demonstrated a survival benefit of these drugs in patients with ACS, especially in those undergoing PCI.[21-23] In patients who do not have a coronary intervention, trials with GP IIb/IIIa inhibitors showed a modest reduction in major adverse cardiac events and in some no benefit. A better outcome is noted in high-risk patients, such as those with increased baseline troponins, continuing ischemia, or comorbid conditions, especially in diabetic patients. In a meta-analysis of six major placebo-controlled trials with GP IIb/IIIa inhibitors, Roffi et al. found a significant reduction in 30-day mortality among diabetics (from 6.2 to 4.6%; $P = 0.007$; Fig. 4-1), whereas there was no effect among nondiabetics (Fig. 4-2).[24] Furthermore, the benefit was even more marked in diabetics undergoing PCI (Fig. 4-3). However, there was a lack of consistent reduction in all six trials and the authors performed only a univariate analysis. GP IIb/IIIa inhibitors in diabetic patients undergoing PCI were also found beneficial in a previous meta-analysis.[25] Whether the benefit is truly related to diabetes and whether it correlates with fasting glucose, HbA1c, or endogenous insulin levels, are questions that still have to be answered.

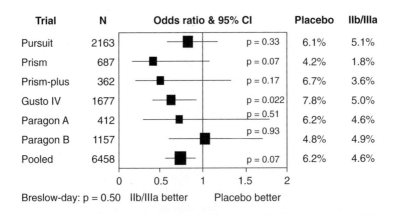

Figure 4-1 **Effect of GP IIb/IIIa inhibitor treatment on 30-day mortality in diabetic patients with ACS.** *(Source: Adapted from Roffi M, Chew DP, Mukherjee D, et al. Platelet glycoprotein IIb/IIIa inhibitors reduce mortality in diabetic patients with non-ST-segment elevation acute coronary syndromes. Circulation 2001;104:2767–2771.)*

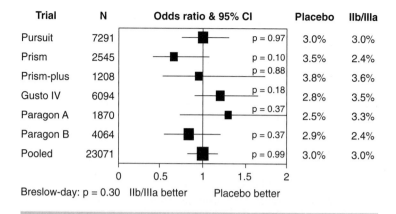

Figure 4-2 **Effect of GP IIb/IIIa inhibitor treatment on 30-day mortality in nondiabetic patients.** *(Source: Adapted from Roffi M, Chew DP, Mukherjee D, et al. Platelet glycoprotein IIb/IIIa inhibitors reduce mortality in diabetic patients with non-ST-segment elevation acute coronary syndromes.* Circulation *2001;104:2767–2771.)*

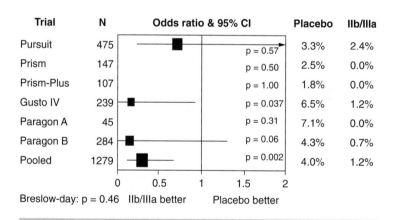

Figure 4-3 **Effect of GP IIb/IIIa inhibitor treatment on 30-day mortality in diabetic patients with ACS undergoing PCI.** *(Source: Adapted from Roffi M, Chew DP, Mukherjee D, et al. Platelet glycoprotein IIb/IIIa inhibitors reduce mortality in diabetic patients with non-ST-segment elevation acute coronary syndromes.* Circulation *2001;104: 2767–2771.)*

UNFRACTIONATED HEPARIN (UFH), LOW-MOLECULAR WEIGHT HEPARIN (LMWH), AND DIRECT THROMBIN INHIBITORS

Initial meta-analysis of randomized studies comparing UFH and LMWH did not reveal any significant difference in efficacy and safety between these two agents.[26] However, more recent publications suggest that LMWH represents a better choice not only in non-ST-elevation ACS, but also in AMI coupled with thrombolytic treatment.[27,28] The preference for LMWH is explained not only by obtaining a more predictable and stable anticoagulant effect, and lower incidence of heparin-induced thrombocytopenia, but also due to easier administration and cost-effectiveness. However, there are no randomized trials of LMWH versus UFH conducted only in diabetic patients with ACS, and therefore their benefit in this high-risk group is assumed based on results in the general population and subgroup analysis.

The newer direct thrombin inhibitors were proven to be superior to heparin for the prevention of death and MI in patients with ACS, primarily by reducing the MI rate, with a slight increase in bleeding complications.[29,30] No data are available for diabetic patients with only ACS.

Anti-Ischemic, Anti-Inflammatory Therapy

BETA-BLOCKERS

Controlled trials have demonstrated the beneficial effects of beta-blockers in patients with AMI. The use of beta-blockers in diabetes has been questioned because of their modulating effect on hypoglycemic symptoms and potential interference with insulin release. However, there are no randomized trials with beta-blockers conducted in diabetic patients with ACS. Malmberg et al.[31] reported improved outcome in diabetics with AMI after treatment with metoprolol compared to placebo in a retrospective analysis of two large studies: in the Göteborg Metoprolol trial mortality at 3 months was reduced by metoprolol from 17.9 to 7.5% and late infarction was reduced from 16.4 to 3.8%, and in the MIAMI (Metoprolol in AMI) trial mortality was decreased by metoprolol from 11.3 to 5.7% and late infarction from 4.5 to 3.1% during 15-day follow-up. In a large multicenter cohort of 2024 patients, including 340 diabetics, Kjekshus et al. reported in diabetic patients discharged on beta-blockers a 1-year mortality of only 10%, compared with 23% for diabetics not on beta-blockers.[32] More recently, Chen et al.[33] also reported a lower 1-year mortality rate for elderly diabetic patients with AMI receiving beta-blockers, insulin-treated (12.5% vs. 17.8%, $P < 0.001$), and non-insulin-treated (8.9% vs. 15.2%, $P < 0.001$) diabetics, to a similar extent as for nondiabetics, without increased risk of readmission for diabetic complications. In non-ST-elevation MI there are conflicting results, with studies reporting no benefit in reducing the cardiac event rate with propranolol, as in a subgroup analysis of BHAT (Beta-Blocker Heart Attack) trial.[34] However, Gottlieb et al.[35] report a reduction in mortality with beta-blockers in a study of 201,752 patients with MI from the Cooperative Cardiovascular Project, even in high-risk patients such as those with heart failure, pulmonary disease, and older age, or in those with nontransmural infarction, and a lower mortality reduction in diabetics or patients with very low left ventricular ejection fraction (LVEF <20%). Overall, there is compelling evidence that beta-blockers are effective in diabetic subjects with CAD and their use should be actively encouraged especially in post-MI secondary prevention. However, controlled randomized trials are needed to offer a better response regarding the benefit of beta-blockers in diabetic patients presenting with ACS.

ACE Inhibitors

The survival benefit obtained with angiotensin-converting enzyme (ACE) inhibitors in patients with AMI, especially in those with left ventricular dysfunction, was proven in previous studies. Subgroup analysis of Gruppo Italiano per lo Studio della Soprawivenza nell's Infarcto Miocardico (GISSI)[36] demonstrated that treatment with lisinopril was associated with a decreased 6-week mortality in diabetic patients (8.7% vs. 12.4%; odds ratio [OR], 0.68; 95% confidence interval [CI], 0.53–0.86), an effect that was significantly ($P < 0.025$) higher than that observed in nondiabetic patients. Furthermore, the survival benefit in diabetics was maintained at 6 months despite withdrawal from treatment at 6 weeks (12.9% vs. 16.1%; OR, 0.77; 95% CI, 0.62–0.95). A retrospective analysis using data from the Trandolapril Cardiac Evaluation (TRACE) study, which was a randomized, double-blind, placebo-controlled trial of trandolapril in 1749 patients with AMI and ejection fraction ≤35% showed a relative risk (RR) of death from any cause of 0.64 (95% CI, 0.45–0.91) for the diabetic group versus 0.82 (95% CI, 0.69–0.97) for the nondiabetic group.[37] Also, in diabetics, trandolapril markedly reduced the risk of progression to severe heart failure, while no significant reduction of this endpoint was noted in the nondiabetic group. In another subgroup analysis of diabetic patients with nonthrombolyzed anterior AMI who were enrolled in the Survival of Myocardial Infarction Long-Term Evaluation (SMILE) trial,[38] the newer agent zofenopril significantly reduced the incidence of the primary endpoint of death and severe congestive heart failure (8.6% vs. 18.3%; $P = 0.019$) at 6 weeks and the effect was greater than that observed in nondiabetic patients. However, the reduction in 1-year mortality did not reach statistical significance (13.7% vs. 16.5%; $P = 0.52$), suggesting that long-term treatment is probably needed to maintain the benefits of the early ACE inhibition in patients with diabetes. The benefit of long-term treatment with ACE inhibitors in diabetic patients with AMI was noticed by Gottlieb et al. in a retrospective survey,[39] with lower 1-year mortality rates than in diabetics not treated with ACE inhibitors (16.2% vs. 18.8%). The impact of ACE inhibition is less studied with non-ST-elevation ACS especially in diabetics.

Coexisting Risk Factors

Treatment of coexisting risk factors like hypertension, hyperlipidemia, obesity, and smoking should be an important aspect of ACS treatment in diabetic patients, irrespective of the mode of revascularization or no revascularization.

Clinical trials demonstrated consistent benefit of statins by decreasing low-density lipoprotein cholesterol (LDL-C) values and resulting in significant reduction in cardiac events and mortality. A recent meta-analysis[40] of five major randomized, placebo-controlled, double-blinded trials showed a reduction of 31% in major coronary events and 21% in all-cause mortality. Three major studies of secondary prevention in the post-MI period have demonstrated significant benefits in diabetic patient subgroups. A post hoc subgroup analysis on data from 202 diabetics out of a total 4444 subjects with previous MI or angina, included in the Scandinavian Simvastatin Survival Study (4S), demonstrated that cholesterol-lowering therapy following MI was highly effective in reducing total mortality, major cardiovascular events, and any atherosclerotic events.[41] These benefits may be more marked in diabetic than with nondiabetic subjects with coronary heart disease (CHD), because diabetics have higher absolute risk of recurrent events. Similar results were reported by the Cholesterol And Recurrent Events (CARE) trial, which included 586 diabetic subjects post-MI.[42] The reduction in mortality was comparable in both diabetic and nondiabetic subjects (25% vs. 23%, respectively). In a combined analysis of two secondary prevention trials with pravastatin, Sacks et al. also showed that pravastatin reduced the CHD event rate in diabetics with low LDL-C (<125 mg/dL) from 34 to 22% ($P = 0.004$), comparable to that of nondiabetics.[43] Another more recent trial, the Heart Protection Study, enrolled 5963 diabetics with and without cardiovascular disease and randomized them to 40 mg daily simvastatin or matching placebo.[44] The important contributions of this study are the definite benefit observed in the simvastatin group by 22% ($P < 0.0001$) reduction in cardiovascular events rate, and moreover a 27% reduction (95% CI, 13–40, $P = 0.0007$) among diabetics with pretreatment LDL-C concentration below 116 mg/dL. The findings of this study are in agreement with the recommendations made by the National Cholesterol Education Program Adult Treatment Panel III, which considered diabetes as a "CHD risk equivalent" with a target LDL-C of <100 mg/dL.[45] In summary, there appears to be strong evidence for the use of statin therapy in diabetic patients regardless of their baseline LDL-C level and presentation with or without CHD/ACS. Furthermore, statin therapy has been recently attributed anti-inflammatory and anticoagulant effects, reflected in reduction of C-reactive protein (CRP) and other inflammation markers, which may play an important role in reducing cardiovascular events especially in the diabetic population.[46–49]

REVASCULARIZATION

Thrombolytic Therapy

Thrombolytic agents lower the mortality of patients with AMI, including those with diabetes, who are usually older, have had a previous MI, have more comorbid conditions, hypertension and hyperlipidemia, and more severe CAD and worse LVEF.[50,51] Although there seem to be no major outcome differences among various thrombolytic strategies, in GUSTO-I (Global Utilization of Streptokinase and TPA for Occluded Coronary Arteries) trial there was improved survival of diabetics receiving accelerated tissue plasminogen activator (t-PA).[50] However, the 30-day and 1-year mortality remains high in AMI patients with diabetes receiving thrombolytics, at least 40–60% higher than in nondiabetics (Fig. 4-4), despite similar rates of vessel patency.[50-52] Diabetes mellitus is an important predictor of short- and long-term mortality after AMI, independent of the infarct size and other risk factors.

Thrombolytic Therapy versus PCI

There are multiple trials comparing the efficacy of thrombolytic regimens with primary PCI in patients presenting with ST-segment elevation AMI and several meta-analyses concur that PCI is associated with improved clinical outcomes.[53-56] During the last few years, technical advances and changes in patient care resulted in lower time to treatment for patients with ACS. However, only 8% of patients with AMI undergo primary PCI within 2 hours of symptom onset.[57] The time to reperfusion seems to be extremely important,

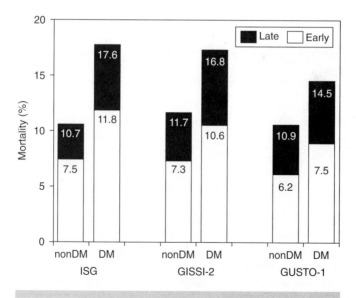

Figure 4-4 **Early (30–35 days) and late (6–12 months) mortality in AMI patients with and without diabetes receiving thrombolytics.** (Source: Adapted from Mak KH, Moliterno DJ, Granger CB, et al. for the GUSTO-I Investigators. Influence of diabetes mellitus on clinical outcome in the thrombolytic era of acute myocardial infarction. J Am Coll Cardiol 1997;30:171–179.)

as there are some differences in outcome after PCI or thrombolytics considering the time of intervention.[58] The recent DANAMI-2 (the Second Danish Acute Myocardial Infarction) trial showed benefit in favor of PCI for patients with AMI, even in those who were transferred to a PCI center, but the transport time was <3 hours.[59] The CAPTIM (Comparison of Angioplasty and Prehospital Thrombolysis in Acute Myocardial Infarction) trial, however, showed a strong trend toward lower 30-day mortality with prehospital thrombolysis compared to primary PCI if patients received treatment in <2 hours of symptom onset (2.2% vs. 5.7%, $P = 0.058$), while there was no difference after the first 2 hours (5.9% vs. 3.7%, $P = 0.47$).[60]

Most of these trials included patients with diabetes anywhere from 6 to 25%, but there are no studies conducted only in diabetics. Furthermore, diabetic patients are less likely to receive adequate treatment on time, thrombolytic or PCI, due to silent ischemia, late or atypical presentation, and comorbid conditions.[50] Also, due to multivessel disease, PCI was not the type of invasive revascularization most often used in patients with diabetes, as CABG had previously reported better survival results.

Invasive Revascularization

In most published reports of coronary revascularization, PCI or CABG, patients with diabetes have greater risk for complications and worse long-term prognosis than patients without diabetes.

PERCUTANEOUS TRANSLUMINAL CORONARY ANGIOPLASTY

The initial studies of revascularization in diabetics including only balloon angioplasty (percutaneous transluminal coronary angioplasty [PTCA]) had controversial short-term outcomes. In the 1985–1986 National Heart, Lung, and Blood Institute (NHLBI) registry of balloon angioplasty,[61] there were no differences in the rates of procedural success and complications of revascularization in 281 patients with diabetes as compared to 1833 patients without diabetes. However, diabetic (female) patients experienced more in-hospital death and MI (10% vs. 4.8%, $P = 0.02$) and were predictive of adverse outcome in the multivariate model. In contrast, 1133 diabetic patients had no increased risk of death, MI, or CABG compared with 9300 nondiabetic patients undergoing elective PTCA from 1980 to 1989 at Emory University, despite more frequent adverse baseline characteristics in diabetic patients.[62]

The long-term outcome after PTCA in diabetic patients has consistently been shown to be inferior to results in nondiabetics, as opposed to data for periprocedural in-hospital results. In the Emory University report at 5-year follow-up, the survival rates were 88 and 93% for patients with and without diabetes, respectively; with divergence of the survival curves evident within the first 1.5 years. Also, diabetic patients experienced more MI and more often required additional surgical and percutaneous revascularization procedures. Similarly, mortality in diabetics in the NHLBI registry was double that of to nondiabetics over a 9-year period (36% vs. 18%), with greater rate of MI and repeat revascularization.

In the PTCA and abciximab trials (Evaluation of 7E3 for the Prevention of Ischemic Complications [EPIC] and Evaluation of PTCA to Improve Long-Term Outcome with Abciximab GP IIb/IIIa Receptor Blockade [EPILOG]),[63] abciximab compared to placebo resulted in similar reduction in death, MI, or urgent revascularization at 30 days, 6 months, and 1-year in diabetic patients compared to nondiabetics, but there was no benefit on restenosis subsets.

The early divergence of ischemic event rates between diabetic and nondiabetic patients after PTCA corresponds to the period of highest risk for restenosis. In the first NHLBI PTCA registry, restenosis rate was 47% in diabetic versus 32% in nondiabetic patients ($P < 0.01$). Other reports have confirmed that diabetes mellitus is independently associated with a greater incidence of restenosis over a 6- to 9-month period after PTCA. The greater restenotic response to PTCA in diabetics was attributed to various pathophysiologic mechanisms, in particular exuberant neointimal hyperplasia and adverse arterial geometric remodeling. Another mechanism contributing to increased restenosis is the small vessel size/diameter in diabetic patients. Therefore, a similar degree of intimal hyperplasia or geometric remodeling will result in significant luminal obstruction in a small diameter vessel as compared to larger vessels in nondiabetics.

PERCUTANEOUS CORONARY INTERVENTION—STENTING

Coronary stenting,[64] by eliminating the geometric remodeling component of the restenosis process and decreasing the acute complication rates, has become the mainstay of PCI in a wide variety of patient groups and coronary lesion types. Coronary stents have been shown to decrease acute complications and restenosis even in high-risk patients such as diabetics, by providing a predictable large lumen (acute gain), preventing elastic recoil, decreasing acute/subacute closure in combination with antiplatelet therapy, and almost abolishing the geometric remodeling ("vessel shrinkage"). However, in diabetic patients the restenosis rate remains high, anywhere from 25 to 50% in most studies, with greater luminal loss due to neointimal hyperplasia, even without significant differences in acute complications compared to nondiabetic patients.[65–68] Diabetes mellitus was established as an independent predictor of restenosis and target lesion revascularization (TLR). Abizaid et al.[69] compared the acute results and restenosis rates in 789 consecutive patients undergoing stenting, in whom 112 were treated with oral hypoglycemics and 8% were insulin requiring. There was no difference in the acute procedural and clinical complications, angiographic success rates, but restenosis and TLR were increased in nondiabetics compared to diabetics using oral hypoglycemics to insulin dependent diabetes mellitus (IDDM). In the multivariate model, IDDM was an independent predictor of TLR and any late cardiac event.

More recent publications revealed the synergistic effect of stenting with abciximab, as in the EPISTENT (Evaluation of Platelet IIb/IIIa Inhibitor for Stenting) trial, with ischemic complications and 1-year mortality substantially improved, and the TVR reduced in diabetic patients to a rate comparable to nondiabetics.[70] The 6-month TVR rate was significantly reduced: 16.6% in stent-placebo, 18.4% in PTCA-abciximab versus 8.1% in stent-abciximab group ($P = 0.021$). This beneficial effect of extremely low TVR rate of 8.1%, comparable to 8.4% in nondiabetic stent cohort of the EPISTENT trial, was mediated by lower late loss index (0.40 in stent-abciximab vs. 0.60 in stent-placebo group; $P = 0.06$), implying decreased intimal hyperplasia volume and higher net gain. Abciximab was also reported to improve 30-day mortality (0.6% vs. 3.0%; $P = 0.03$) and repeat intervention (0% vs. 1.1%, $P = 0.03$) in diabetic patients undergoing PCI for non-AMI in Mayo Clinic Registry, even though there was no significant benefit at 1 year.[71]

Surgical Revascularization (CABG)

Diabetes mellitus is a potential risk factor for complications and adverse long-term outcome after surgical revascularization. In the early postoperative period, there is increased risk of mortality, stroke, wound infections, renal failure, and reoperation after CABG compared to nondiabetic patients. A study from Duke University[72] reported a poor long-term survival after CABG in diabetic versus nondiabetic patients (74% vs. 86%, $P = 0.02$). Limited data are available for the appropriate mode of revascularization in patients with diabetes mellitus after prior CABG. A report from Germany,[73] involving 489 CABG patients (99 diabetics), revealed a lower 3-year mortality after PTCA (7.2%) versus after redo-CABG (37.4%; $P < 0.006$), identifying diabetes as a risk factor for death with 1.43 RR in all patients.

Randomized Trials of PTCA Versus CABG

Recent analyses[74,75] of randomized trials of PTCA versus CABG in patients with multivessel disease have shown a lower mortality at long-term follow-up (1–8 years) in diabetics undergoing surgical revascularization (Fig. 4-5).[76–79] PTCA patients also required higher repeat intervention and had more frequent angina compared to patients who underwent CABG. There is no prospective randomized trial of PTCA versus CABG in diabetic patients only. In the BARI trial, diabetes mellitus was added as a subgroup analysis after TIMI II (The Thrombolysis in Myocardial Infarction II) trial report of increased mortality in

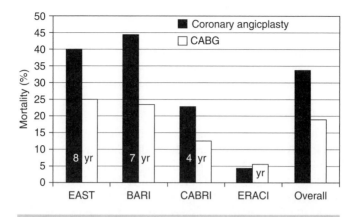

Figure 4-5 **Mortality rates in randomized trials of patients with diabetes mellitus undergoing CABG and coronary angioplasty.** *(Source: Adapted from Mak KH, Faxon DP. Clinical studies on coronary revascularization in patients with type 2 diabetes. Eur Heart J 2003;24:1087–1103.)*

diabetic patients after MI. Treated diabetics represented 19% of the BARI study population ($n = 353$), with a 5-year mortality of 19.4% in the CABG group, compared to 34.5% in the PTCA group ($P = 0.002$).[80] The cardiac mortality was 23.4% in PTCA versus 8.2% in the CABG group ($P = 0.0002$). This striking difference observed only in the diabetic subgroup, and not in any other subgroup of the BARI trial, lead to NHLBI alert[81] indicating that CABG should be the preferred treatment for patients with treated diabetes mellitus who have multivessel disease undergoing first revascularization. The benefit of CABG in diabetic patients in the BARI trial was mainly seen in those who received one or two internal mammary artery grafts.[82]

A plausible explanation for BARI results was suggested by Rozenman et al., after quantitative analysis of serial follow-up angiogram in diabetic ($n = 55$) versus nondiabetic patients ($n = 193$),[83] suggesting that mechanical trauma of PTCA promoted disease progression and new lesion formation. Another reasonable explanation could be the impact of rupture of vulnerable plaques, which tend to occur in proximal and midcoronary arteries and were likely to cause serious cardiovascular events in the PTCA versus CABG group, where the distal vascular bed is protected by the bypass conduit.

In the BARI observational registry,[84] patients who met eligibility criteria for the randomized trial, but were not randomized and underwent PTCA or CABG by choice, there was no significant difference in cardiac mortality (7.5% for PTCA vs. 6.0% for CABG; $P = 0.73$) or all cause mortality (14.4% for PTCA vs. 14.9% for CABG group; $P = 0.83$) at 5-year follow-up. Even after adjustment for the difference in clinical and angiographic factors, the RR in predicted mortality increased slightly, but not statistically different for PTCA versus CABG (RR increased from 1.07 to 1.35). Possible explanations for the disparity between randomized versus registry results are higher education level, more physical activity, less smoking, and better quality of life of the registry patients, which all may translate to better diabetic control.

Stent Versus CABG Trials

Stents have been shown to decrease acute complications and late restenosis compared to PTCA and have become the mainstay of treatment. Randomized trials using stent versus CABG in patients with CAD have conflicting results: in the Arterial Revascularization Therapy Study (ARTS), 1-year mortality was comparable between stenting (2.5%) and CABG (2.8%), while in the Stent or Surgery Study (SoS) mortality at mean 2 years follow-up was higher in the PCI group (4.5%) versus CABG (1.6%; $P = 0.01$), and in the Argentinian randomzed trial of coronory angioplasty with stenting versus coronary bypass surgery in patients with multiple vessel disease (ERACH II) study mortality at >1 year was higher in the surgery group (7.6% vs. 5.4%; $P = 0.017$).[85-87] The differences between results may be partially explained by patient selection, procedural technique and experience, and use of adjunctive medical therapies, such as abciximab. In the ARTS trial, diabetic patients had increased mortality when treated with stents (6.3% vs. 1.6%; $P = 0.013$).[88] Also, patients with diabetes receiving stents were more likely to experience adverse cardiovascular events and to undergo repeat revascularization.

Drug-Eluting Stents Trials

A major advance in the treatment of diabetic patients with CAD, presenting or not as ACS, has been achieved by using the new drug-eluting stents (DES). In CAD patients undergoing PCI with sirolimus- or paclitaxel-coated stents, there are supporting data of very low angiographic restenosis, cardiac adverse events, and TLR.[89-95] In diabetic patients enrolled in the sirolimus-eluting stent in de novo native coronary lesions (SIRIUS) trial, the TLR at 270 days was 6.9% in DES group versus 22.3% in bare-metal stent (BMS) group, and at 1-year follow-up 8.4% versus 26.4% ($P = 0.0002$).[90,91] Even in the highest-risk group of patients enrolled in the sirolimus-eluting stent in de novo native coronary lesions (SIRIUS) trial, with diabetes mellitus, reference-vessel diameter <2.5 mm and lesion length >15 mm, there was a relative reduction of 71% in clinical restenosis rate at 12 months.[91] In the randomized study with the sirolimus-eluting velocity balloon expandable stent in the treatment of patients with de novo coronary artery lesions (RAVEL) trial, the reported angiographic restenosis rate at 6 months was 0% in the DES group, similar to nondiabetic patients, while in diabetics receiving bare-metal stents it was 42% ($P = 0.001$). There were no TLR at 1 year in diabetics with DES compared with 36% rate in diabetics with standard stents ($P = 0.007$).[92] In the one year clinical results with the slow results Plymer-based, Paclitaxel-eluting TAXUS stent IV trial, similar results were again reported in nondiabetic and diabetic patients randomized to the paclitaxel-coated stent arm. The angiographic restenosis at 9 months in the DES group was 8.5% in nondiabetics (vs. 24.4% with bare-metal stent; $P < 0.001$), 5.8% in diabetics requiring oral medications (vs. 29.7%; $P = 0.003$), and 7.7% in diabetics requiring insulin (vs. 42.9%; $P = 0.007$).[94] Although not all the DES trials reported separate subanalyses in diabetic patients, from available data it can be concluded that restenosis rate after PCI with DES in these high-risk patients has decreased to values between 0 and 8%, for the first time similar to rates in nondiabetic patients.

Other Revascularization Procedures

Some diabetic patients with extensive diffuse small vessel disease or refractory recurrent restenosis or vein graft closure may be appropriate for other modes of revascularization like percutaneous or transmyocardial revascularization (TMR or PTMR), enhanced external counterpulsation (EECP), and angiogenic therapy.

CONCLUSIONS AND FUTURE DIRECTIONS

The best revascularization strategy, PCI using DES versus CABG, in patients with diabetes mellitus presenting with or without ACS, is currently being evaluated. The FREEDOM (Future Revascularization Evaluation in Patients with Diabetes Mellitus: Optimal Management of Multivessel Disease) study is a prospective multicenter trial comparing DES with CABG in diabetic patients. Also, the ARTS-2 trial will compare patients with multivessel disease undergoing PCI with DES (sirolimus) versus CABG. Aggressive risk factor reduction, especially glycemic control and lipid-lowering therapy, has to be combined with either of the revascularization strategies. One important study that will determine the optimal revascularization approach for diabetic patients is the BARI-2D randomized trial, which evaluates revascularization (CABG or PCI) along with routine versus strict glycemic control by a factorial 2×2 design in diabetic patients, with total mortality as primary endpoint.[11] Also, the role of abciximab during PCI with DES must be clarified, considering the cost versus effectiveness factors. In the RAVEL trial, only one diabetic patient in DES arm received GP IIb/IIIa inhibitor.

REFERENCES

1. Butler R, MacDonald TM, Struthers AD, et al. Clinical implications of diabetic heart disease. *Eur Heart J* 1998;19:1617–1627.
2. Schneider DJ, Nordt TK, Sobel BE. Attenuated fibrinolysis and accelerated atherogenesis in type II diabetic patients. *Diabetes* 1993;42:1–7.
3. Keating FK, Sobel BE, Schneider DJ. Effects of increased concentrations of glucose on platelet reactivity in healthy subjects and in patients with and without diabetes. *Am J Cardiol* 2003;92:1362–1365.

4. Davi G, Catalano I, Averna M, et al. Thromboxane biosynthesis and platelet function in type II diabetes mellitus. *N Engl J Med* 1990;322:1769–1774.

5. Braunwald E, Antman EM, Beasley JM, et al. ACC/AHA guideline update for the management of patients with unstable angina and non-ST-segment elevation myocardial infarction: a report of the American College of Cardiology/American Heart Association Task Force on Practice Guidelines. *J Am Coll Cardiol* 2002;40: 1366–1374. Available at: www.acc.org and www.americanheart.org

6. American Diabetes Association. Standards of medical care for patients with diabetes mellitus. *Diabetes Care* 2003;26(Suppl):S33–S50.

7. Takagi T, Akasaka T, Yamamuro A, et al. Troglitazone reduces neointimal proliferation after coronary stent implantation in patients with non insulin dependent diabetes mellitus: a serial intravascular ultrasound study. *J Am Coll Cardiol* 2000; 36:1529–1535.

8. UK Prospective Diabetes Study (UKPDS) Group. Intensive blood-glucose control with sulphonylureas or insulin compared with conventional treatment and risk of complications in patients with type 2 diabetes (UKPDS 33). *Lancet* 1998;352:837–853.

9. UK Prospective Diabetes Study (UKPDS) Group. Effect of intensive blood-glucose control with metformin on complications in overweight patients with type 2 diabetes (UKPDS 34). *Lancet* 1998;352:854–865.

10. Sobel BE, Frye R, Detre KM. Burgeoning dilemmas in the management of diabetes and cardiovascular disease. Rationale for the BARI 2D Trial. *Circulation* 2003;107:636–642.

11. Frye RL. Optimal care of patients with type 2 diabetes mellitus and coronary artery disease. *Am J Med* 2003;115(8A):93S–98S.

12. Fath-Ordoubadi F, Beatt KJ. Glucose-insulin-potassium therapy for treatment of acute myocardial infarction: an overview of randomized placebo-controlled trials. *Circulation* 1997;96:1152–1156.

13. Malmberg K, Norhammar A, Wedel H, et al. Glycometabolic state at admission: important risk marker of mortality in conventionally treated patients with diabetes mellitus and acute myocardial infarction: long-term results from the DIGAMI Study. *Circulation* 1999;99:2626–2632.

14. ISIS-2 Collaborative Group. Randomised trial of intravenous streptokinase, oral aspirin, both, or neither among 17,187 cases of suspected acute myocardial infarction: ISIS-2 (Second International Study of Infarct Survival). *Lancet* 1988;2:349–360.

15. Antiplatelet Trialists' Collaboration. Collaborative overview of randomized trials of antiplatelet therapy. *Br Med J* 1994;308:81–106.

16. Antithrombotic Trialists' Collaboration. Collaborative meta-analysis of randomized trials of antiplatelet therapy for prevention of death, myocardial infarction, and stroke in high-risk patients. *Br Med J* 2002;324:71–77.

17. Harpaz D, Gottlieb S, Graff E, et al. Effects of aspirin treatment on survival in non-insulin-dependent diabetic patients with coronary artery disease. Israeli Bezafibrate Infarction Prevention Study Group. *Am J Med* 1998;105:494–499.

18. Bhatt DL, Bertrand ME, Berger PB, et al. Meta-analysis of randomized and registry comparison of ticlopidine with clopidogrel after stenting. *J Am Coll Cardiol* 2002;39:9–14.

19. The clopidogrel in unstable angina to prevent recurrent events (CURE) trial investigators. Effects of clopidogrel in addition to aspirin in patients with acute coronary syndromes without ST-segment elevation. *N Engl J Med* 2001;345:494–502.

20. Steinhubl SR, Berger PB, Tift Mann III, for the CREDO Investigators. Early and sustained dual oral antiplatelet therapy following percutaneous coronary intervention. *JAMA* 2002;288:2411–2420.

21. Boersma E, Harrington RA, Moliterno DJ, et al. Platelet glycoprotein IIb/IIIa inhibitors in acute coronary syndromes: a meta-analysis of all major randomized clinical trials. *Lancet* 2002;359:189–198.

22. Roffi M, Chew DP, Mukherjee D, et al. Platelet glycoprotein IIb/IIIa inhibitors in acute coronary syndromes: gradient of benefit related to the revascularization strategy. *Eur Heart J* 2002;23:1441–1448.

23. Karvouni E, Katritsis DG, Ioannidis J. Intravenous glycoprotein IIb/IIIa receptor antagonists reduce mortality after percutaneous coronary interventions. *J Am Coll Cardiol* 2003;41:26–32.

24. Roffi M, Chew DP, Mukherjee D, et al. Platelet glycoprotein IIb/IIIa inhibitors reduce mortality in diabetic patients with non-ST-segment elevation acute coronary syndromes. *Circulation* 2001;104:2767–2771.

25. Bhatt DL, Marso SP, Lincoff AM, et al. Abciximab reduces mortality in diabetics following percutaneous coronary intervention. *J Am Coll Cardiol* 2000;35:922–928.

26. Eikelboom JW, Anand S, Malmberg K, et al. Unfractioned heparin and low-molecular-weight heparin in acute coronary syndromes without ST elevation: a meta-analysis. *Lancet* 2000;355:1936–1942.

27. Cohen M. The role of low-molecular-weight heparin in the management of acute coronary syndromes. *J Am Coll Cardiol* 2003;41:55S–61S.

28. Theroux P, Welsh RC. Meta-analysis of randomized trials comparing enoxaparin versus unfractioned heparin as adjunctive therapy to fibrinolysis in ST-elevation acute myocardial infarction. *Am J Cardiol* 2003;91:860–864.

29. The Direct Thrombin Inhibitor Trialists' Collaborative Group. Direct thrombin inhibitors in acute coronary syndromes: principal results of a meta-analysis based on individual patients' data. *Lancet* 2002;359:294–302.

30. Eikelboom J, White H, Yusuf H. The evolving role of direct thrombin inhibitors in acute coronary syndromes. *J Am Coll Cardiol* 2003;41:70S–78S.

31. Malmberg K, Herlitz J, Hjalmarson A, et al. Effects of metoprolol on mortality and late infarction in diabetics with suspected acute myocardial infarction. *Eur Heart J* 1989;10:423–428.

32. Kjekshus J, Gilpin E, Cali G, et al. Diabetic patients and beta-blockers after acute myocardial infarction. *Eur Heart J* 1990;11:43–50.

33. Chen J, Marciniak TA, Radford MJ, et al. Beta-blocker therapy for secondary prevention of myocardial infarction in elderly diabetic patients. Results from the National Cooperative Cardiovascular Project. *J Am Coll Cardiol* 1999;34:1388–1394.

34. Beta-blocker heart attack trial (BHAT). *JAMA* 1982;247:1707–1714.

35. Gottlieb SS, McCarter RJ, Vogel RA. Effect of beta-blockade on mortality among high-risk and low-risk patients after myocardial infarction. *N Engl J Med* 1998; 339(8):489–497.

36. Zuanetti G, Latini R, Maggioni AP, et al. Effect of the ACE inhibitor lisinopril on mortality in diabetic patients with acute myocardial infarction: data from the GISSI-3 study. *Circulation* 1997;96:4239–4245.

37. Gustafsson I, Torp-Pedersen C, Kober L, et al. Effect of the angiotensin-converting enzyme inhibitor trandolapril on mortality and morbidity in diabetic patients with left ventricular dysfunction after acute myocardial infarction. Trace Study Group. *J Am Coll Cardiol* 1999;34:83–89.

38. Borghi C, Bacchelli S, Esposti DD, et al. SMILE Study. Effects of the early ACE inhibition in diabetic nonthrombolyzed patients with anterior acute myocardial infarction. *Diabetes Care* 2003;26:1862–1868.

39. Gottlieb S, Leor J, Shotan A, et al. Comparison of effectiveness of angiotensin-converting enzyme inhibitors after acute myocardial infarction in diabetic versus nondiabetic patients. *Am J Cardiol* 2003;92:1020–1025.

40. LaRosa JC, He J, Vupputuri S. Effect of statins on risk of coronary disease. A meta-analysis of randomized controlled trials. *JAMA* 1999;282:2340–2346.

41. Pyorala K, Pedersen TR, Kjekshus J, et al. Cholesterol lowering with simvastatin improves prognosis of diabetic patients with coronary heart disease. A subgroup analysis of the Scandinavian Simvastatin Survival Study (4S). *Diabetes Care* 1997;20:614–620.

42. Goldberg RB, Mellies MJ, Sacks FM, et al for the CARE Investigators. Cardiovascular events and their reduction with pravastatin in diabetic and glucose-intolerant myocardial infarction survivors with average cholesterol levels. Subgroup analysis in the CARE trials. *Circulation* 1998;98:2513–2519.

43. Sacks FM, Tonkin AM, Craven T, et al. Coronary heart disease in patients with low LDL-cholesterol. Benefit of pravastatin in diabetics and enhanced role for HDL-cholesterol and triglycerides as risk factors. *Circulation* 2002;105:1424–1428.

44. Heart Protection Study Collaborative Group. MRC/BHF Heart Protection Study of cholesterol-lowering with simvastatin in 5963 people with diabetes: a randomized placebo-controlled trial. *Lancet* 2003;361:2005–2016.

45. Executive summary of the third report of the National Cholesterol Education Program (NCEP) expert panel on detection, evaluation, and treatment of high blood cholesterol in adults (adult treatment panel III). *JAMA* 2001;19:2486–2497.

46. Plenge JK, Hernandez TL, Weil KM, et al. Simvastatin lowers C-reactive protein within 14 days: an effect independent of low-density lipoprotein cholesterol reduction. *Circulation* 2002;106:1447–1452.

47. Sommeijer DW, MacGillavry MR, Meijers J, et al. Anti-inflammatory and anticoagulant effects of pravastatin in patients with type 2 diabetes. *Diabetes Care* 2004;27:468–473.

48. Lee SJ, Sacks FM. Effect of pravastatin on intermediate-density and low-density lipoproteins containing apolipoprotein CIII in patients with diabetes mellitus. *Am J Cardiol* 2003;92:121–124.

49. Kereiakes DJ. Adjunctive pharmacotherapy before percutaneous coronary intervention in non-ST-elevation acute coronary syndromes: the role of modulating inflammation. *Circulation* 2003;108:III22–III27.

50. Mak KH, Moliterno DJ, Granger CB, et al. for the GUSTO-I Investigators. Influence of diabetes mellitus on clinical outcome in the thrombolytic era of acute myocardial infarction. *J Am Coll Cardiol* 1997;30:171–179.

51. Granger CB, Califf RM, Young S, et al. Outcome of patients with diabetes mellitus and acute myocardial infarction treated with thrombolytic agents. The Thrombolysis and angioplasty in myocardial infarction (TAMI) study group. *J Am Coll Cardiol* 1993;21:920–925.

52. Woodfield SL, Lundergan CF, Reiner JS, et al. Angiographic findings and outcome in diabetic patients treated with thrombolytic therapy for acute myocardial infarction: the GUSTO-I experience. *J Am Coll Cardiol* 1996;28:1661–1669.

53. Michels KB, Yusuf S. Does PTCA in acute myocardial infarction affect mortality and reinfarction rates? A quantitative overview (meta-analysis) of the randomized clinical trials. *Circulation* 1995;91:476–485.

54. Weaver WD, Simes RJ, Betriu A, et al. Comparison of primary coronary angioplasty and intravenous thrombolytic therapy for acute myocardial infarction: a quantitative review. *JAMA* 1997;278:2093–2098.

55. Keeley EC, Boura JA, Grines CL. Primary angioplasty versus intravenous thrombolytic therapy for acute myocardial infarction: a quantitative review of 23 randomised trials. *Lancet* 2003;361:13–20.

56. Dalby M, Bouzamondo A, Lechat P, et al. Transfer for primary angioplasty versus immediate thrombolysis in acute myocardial infarction: a meta-analysis. *Circulation* 2003;108:1809–1814.

57. Cannon CP, Gibson CM, Lambrew CT, et al. Relationship of symptom-onset-to-balloon time and door-to-balloon time with mortality in patients undergoing angioplasty for acute myocardial infarction. *JAMA* 2000;283:2941–2947.

58. Giugliano RP, Braunwald E. Selecting the best reperfusion strategy in ST-elevation myocardial infarction. It's all a matter of time. *Circulation* 2003;108:2828–2830.

59. Andersen HR, Nielsen TT, Rasmussen K, et al. for the DANAMI-2 Investigators. A comparison of coronary angioplasty with fibrinolytic therapy in acute myocardial infarction. *N Engl J Med* 2003;349:733–742.

60. Steg PG, Bonnefoy E, Chabaud S, et al. for the CAPTIM Investigators. Impact of time to treatment on mortality after prehospital fibrinolysis or primary angioplasty: data from the CAPTIM randomized clinical trial. *Circulation* 2003;108:2851–2856.

61. Kip KE, Faxon DP, Detre KM, et al. Coronary angioplasty in diabetic patients: the NHLBI PTCA registry. *Circulation* 1996;94:1818–1825.

62. Weintraub WS, Stein B, Kosinski A, et al. Outcome of coronary bypass surgery versus coronary angioplasty in diabetic patients with multivessel coronary artery disease. *J Am Coll Cardiol* 1998;31:10–19.

63. Kleiman NS, Lincoff AM, Kereiakes DJ, et al. EPILOG Investigators. Diabetes mellitus, glycoprotein IIb/IIIa blockade, and heparin. *Circulation* 1998;97:1912–1920.

64. Lincoff AM. Does stenting prevent diabetic arterial shrinkage after percutaneous coronary revascularization? *Circulation* 1997;96:1374–1377.

65. Carroza JP, Kuntz RE, Fishman RF, et al. Restenosis after arterial injury caused by coronary stenting in patients with diabetes mellitus. *Ann Intern Med* 1993;118: 344–349.

66. Kornowski R, Mintz GS, Leon MB, et al. Increased restenosis in diabetes mellitus after coronary interventions is due to exaggerated intimal hyperplasia. *Circulation* 1997;95:1366–1369.

67. Elezi S, Kastrati A, Pache J, et al. Diabetes mellitus and the clinical and angiographic outcome after coronary stent placement. *J Am Coll Cardiol* 1998;32: 1866–1873.

68. Yokoi H, Nosaka T, Kimura T, et al. Coronary stenting in diabetic patients: early and follow-up results. *J Am Coll Cardiol* 1997;29:455A.

69. Abizaid A, Kornowski R, Mintz G, et al. The influence of diabetes mellitus on acute and late clinical outcomes following coronary stent implantation. *J Am Coll Cardiol* 1998;32:584–589.

70. Marso SP, Lincoff AM, Ellis SG, et al. Optimizing the percutaneous interventional outcomes for patients with diabetes mellitus: results of the EPISTENT (evaluation of platelet IIb/IIIa inhibitor for stenting trial) diabetic substudy. *Circulation* 1999;100:2477–2484.

71. Velianou JL, Mathew V, Wilson SH, et al. Effect of abciximab on late adverse events in patients with diabetes mellitus undergoing stent implantation. *Am J Cardiol* 2000;86:1063–1068.

72. Barsness GW, Peterson ED, Ohman EM, et al. Relationship between diabetes mellitus and long-term survival after coronary bypass and angioplasty. *Circulation* 1997;96:2551–2556.

73. Frantz E, Pfautsch P, Moddel S, Fleck E. No excess mortality after coronary angioplasty in diabetic patients with multivessel disease after prior bypass surgery. *J Am Coll Cardiol* 1997;29:455A.

74. Mak KH, Faxon DP. Clinical studies on coronary revascularization in patients with type 2 diabetes. *Eur Heart J* 2003;24:1087–1103.

75. Hoffman SN, TenBrook JA, Wolf MP, et al. A meta-analysis of randomized controlled trials comparing coronary artery bypass graft with percutaneous transluminal coronary angioplasty: one- to eight-year outcomes. *J Am Coll Cardiol* 2003;41:1293–1304.

76. King III SB, Kosinski AS, Guyton RA, et al. for the EAST Investigators. Eight-year mortality in the Emory Angioplasty vs. Surgery Trial (EAST). *J Am Coll Cardiol* 2000;35:1116–1121.

77. BARI investigators. Seven-year outcome in the Bypass Angioplasty Revascularization Investigation (BARI) by treatment and diabetic status. *J Am Coll Cardiol* 2000;35: 1122–1129.

78. Kurbaan AS, Bowker TJ, Ilsley CD, et al. on behalf of CABRI Investigators. Difference in mortality of the ACBRI diabetic and nondiabetic populations and its relation to coronary artery disease and the revascularization mode. *Am J Cardiol* 2001;87:947–950.

79. Pereira CF, Bernardi V, Martinez J, et al. Diabetic patients with multivessel disease treated with percutaneous coronary revascularization had similar outcome

than those treated with surgery: one year follow up results from two Argentine randomized studies (ERACI–ERACI II) (abstract). *J Am Coll Cardiol* 2000;35:3A.

80. The BARI investigators. Influence of diabetes on 5-year mortality and morbidity in a randomized trial comparing CABG and PTCA in patients with multivessel disease. The Bypass Angioplasty Revascularization Investigation (BARI). *Circulation* 1997;96:1761–1769.

81. Ferguson JJ. NHLBI BARI clinical alert on diabetics treated with angioplasty. *Circulation* 1995;92:3371.

82. Morris JJ, Smith LR, Jones RH, et al. Influence of diabetes and mammary artery grafting on survival after coronary bypass. *Circulation* 1991;84:275–284.

83. Rozenman Y, Saposnikov D, Mosseri M, et al. Long-term angiographic follow-up of coronary balloon angioplasty patients with diabetes mellitus: a clue to the explanation of the results of the BARI study. *J Am Coll Cardiol* 1997;30:1420–1425.

84. Detre KM, Guo P, Holubkov R, et al. Coronary revascularization in diabetic patients: a comparison of the randomized and observational components of the Bypass Angioplasty Revascularization Investigation (BARI). *Circulation* 1999;99: 633–640.

85. Serruys PW, Unger F, Sousa JE, et al. Comparison of coronary artery bypass surgery and stenting for the treatment of multivessel disease. *N Engl J Med* 2001;344:1117–1124.

86. The SoS Investigators. Coronary artery bypass surgery versus percutaneous coronary intervention with stent implantation in patients with multivessel coronary artery disease (the Stent or Surgery trial): a randomised controlled trial. *Lancet* 2002;360:965–970.

87. Rodriguez A, Bernardi V, Navia J, et al. Argentine randomized study: coronary angioplasty with stenting versus coronary artery bypass surgery in patients with multivessel disease (ERACI II): 30-day and one-year follow-up results. *J Am Coll Cardiol* 2001;37:51–58.

88. Abizaid A, Costa MA, Centemero M, et al. Clinical and economic impact of diabetes mellitus on percutaneous and surgical treatment of multivessel coronary disease patients. Insights from the Arterial Revascularization Therapy Study (ARTS) Trial. *Circulation* 2001;104:533–538.

89. Sousa JE, Costa MA, Abizaid AC, et al. for the SIRIUS Investigators. Sustained suppression of neointimal proliferation by sirolimus-eluting stents. One-year angiographic and intravascular ultrasound follow-up. *Circulation* 2001;104:2007–2011.

90. Moses JW, Leon MB, Popma JJ, et al. Sirolimus-eluting stents versus standard stents in patients with stenosis in a native coronary artery. *N Engl J Med* 2003; 349:1315–1323.

91. Holmes DR, Leon MB, Moses JW, et al. Analysis of 1-year clinical outcomes in the SIRIUS trial. A randomized trial of sirolimus-eluting stent versus a standard stent in patients at high risk for coronary restenosis. *Circulation* 2004;109:634–640.

92. Abizaid A, Costa MA, Blanchard D, et al. for the RAVEL Investigators. Sirolimus-eluting stents inhibit neointimal hyperplasia in diabetic patients. Insights from the RAVEL trial. *Eur Heart J* 2004;25:107–112.

93. Colombo A, Drzewiecki J, Banning A, et al. randomized study to assess the effectiveness of slow and moderate release polymer based paclitaxel-eluting stents for coronary artery lesions. *Circulation* 2003;108:788–794.

94. Stone GW, Ellis SG, Cox DA, et al. for the TAXUS-IV Investigators. A polymer-based, paclitaxel-eluting stent in patients with coronary artery disease. *N Engl J Med* 2004;350:221–231.

95. Gershlick A, De Scheerder I, Chevalier B, et al. Inhibition of restenosis with a paclitaxel-eluting, polymer-free coronary stent. The European evaluation of paclitaxel eluting stent (ELUTES) trial. *Circulation* 2004;109:487–493.

96. Sarembock IJ. Stent restenosis and the use of drug-eluting stents in patients with diabetes mellitus. *Curr Diab Rep* 2004;4:13–19.

SUDDEN CARDIAC DEATH
IN THE DIABETIC PATIENT

Spyros Kokolis
Luther T. Clark
Luis Garcia
John Kassotis

INTRODUCTION

Ventricular arrhythmias remain one of the most formidable tasks faced by the medical community. Their diagnosis and management affect the morbidity and mortality in patients that are predisposed to diseases that propagate ventricular arrhythmias. Sudden cardiac death (SCD) caused by ventricular arrhythmias can result in death within minutes of the onset of symptoms. Diabetes is a major contributor to this growing epidemic and it is becoming clear that diabetic patients remain at an increased risk.[1] Different studies have shown that the diabetic myocardium exhibits abnormalities in cellular ion transport, which may increase susceptibility to reperfusion-induced arrhythmia.[2]

SCD is characterized by a sudden loss of consciousness caused by cardiac arrest and cessation of cardiac function. Ventricular tachycardia (VT), and ventricular fibrillation (VF) are the most common causes of out-of-hospital cardiac arrest, accounting for approximately three-quarters of cases.[3,4] The results of clinical trials have shed light on various groups of patients at risk for SCD. These trials will assist the clinician in determining which patients are at an increased risk and who would benefit from an implantable cardioverter-defibrillator (ICD) insertion. It is important to recognize ventricular tachyarrhythmias, identify patients at risk, establish an appropriate workup, and determine therapy. This is a challenging task, and continues to evolve as data from clinical studies alter the management of VT and VF.

More than 90% of patients who experience cardiac arrest have demonstrable coronary artery disease (CAD).[4] Patients are at an elevated risk for developing ventricular arrhythmias after a myocardial infarction (MI) due to a significant reduction in left ventricular (LV) systolic function. The scar-related ventricular tachyarrhythmias are reentrant rhythm disturbances that propagate around areas of infarction and the bordering myocardium (see Fig. 5-1).[5] Nonsustained VT (NSVT) and sustained monomorphic and polymorphic VT comprise the remainder of the spectrum (Fig. 5-2). Ventricular premature complexes are morphologically abnormal and widened QRS complexes, which occur earlier than the previous sinus-driven complex.

Morphology is an important distinguishing characteristic. Monomorphic VT exhibits a constant QRS morphology, while polymorphic VT manifests various QRS morphologies, which vary from beat-to-beat measurement. Polymorphic VT has multiple random sites of reentry, in contrast to monomorphic VT which is characterized by a single reentrant loop with a particular exit site.

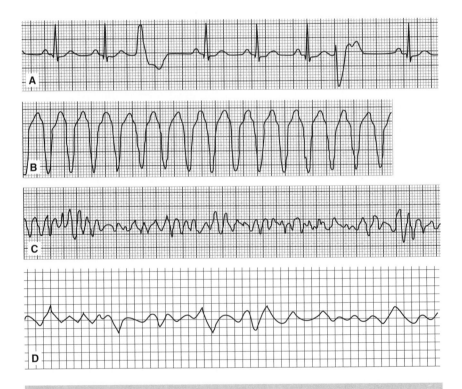

Figure 5-1 *(A) Normal sinus rhythm with PVCs. (B) Monomorphic VT. (C) Polymorphic VT. (D) Ventricular fibrillation.* (Source: Adapted from Garcia TB, Holtz N. 12-Lead ECG: The Art of Interpretation. Bartlett Publication, 2001.)

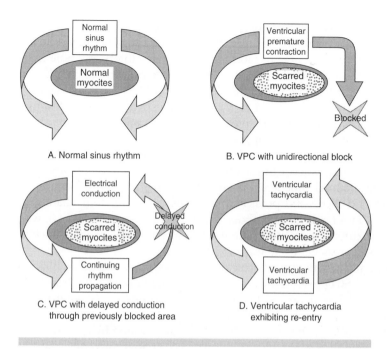

Figure 5-2 **Mechanism of reentrant VT.**

The morphology (right bundle branch block [RBBB] or left bundle branch block [LBBB]) is determined by the exit site (LV or right ventricle [RV]) and the axis. When the patient presents with a wide complex tachycardia, criteria have been established which assist the clinician in making a diagnosis of VT.

Duration is another important aspect in the description and classification of VT, NSVT, and sustained VT, which comprise these categories. VT <30 seconds in duration is classified as NSVT, and VT ≥30 seconds is classified as sustained VT. VT can be hemodynamically stable or unstable. Electrocardiographically, VF is visualized as irregular activation with no distinct P wave, QRS, ST segments, or T waves. VF is always associated with a hemodynamic collapse.

Various regression models have been used by investigators, analyzing the surface electrocardiogram (ECG), to localize the critical zone of reentry in VT. Such an analysis has proven useful in identifying the critical zone of reentry. Strategically placed radiofrequency lesions can disrupt the circuit and prevent recurrence of arrhythmias.[6]

The transmission of impulse conduction is facilitated by cardiac intercellular gap junctions. Gap junctions enhance conduction in the longitudinal direction. In the post-MI setting, gap junctions in the myocardial border zone (the intermediate zone between the infarct and normal myocardium) are disrupted and reorganized, establishing a potential substrate for reentrant VT.[7]

Reentrant VT is thought to originate from a premature impulse that encounters myocardium (refractory to stimulation) bordering the infarct. The impulse travels around the area of block, and then encounters excitable tissue in the region from the opposite side to complete the circuit (Fig. 5-2).[8,9] This mechanism of reentry established the electrophysiologic substrate required for the initiation and propagation of VT, and investigators began testing various antiarrhythmic agents, capable of disrupting various limbs of the reentrant model, in an attempt to suppress these arrhythmias.

The Vaughan Williams classification system categorized these antiarrhythmic agents according to their major site of action. Class I agents are sodium channel blockers, while class II, III, and IV agents act on beta-adrenergic receptors, potassium channels, and calcium channels, respectively. Class I agents are subdivided into subsets (A, B, and C), with the IC agents exhibiting the most potent sodium channel blockade, which can effectively suppress ventricular ectopy (Table 5-1).[10]

Initially, frequent ventricular ectopy was presumed to be a marker of an increased SCD risk. The Cardiac Arrhythmia Suppression Trial (CAST) was performed based on the belief that the suppression of ventricular ectopy would improve mortality.[11] Patients with a decreased left ventricular ejection fraction (LVEF), a history of MI, and documentation by electrocardiographic monitoring of greater than or equal to six premature ventricular complexes (PVCs) per hour were randomized to either a class IC agent (encainide, flecainide, or moricizine) or placebo. CAST was terminated prematurely on the discovery of a significantly higher mortality, in the treatment arm. It was subsequently shown, in an experimental canine postinfarction model, that flecainide converted NSVT to sustained VT, and flecainide-induced sustained VT was difficult to successfully terminate. Flecainide slowed conduction within the myocardium bordering the infarct, which was thought to facilitate the formation of incessant reentrant VT and may have resulted in the higher incidence of SCD in the treatment group. Based on these findings, the presence of structural heart disease (e.g., post-MI) is an absolute contraindication to the use of class IC agents. The Cardiac Arrhythmia Suppression Trial II (CAST II) was a double-blind placebo-controlled randomized trial that compared the survival effects of moricizine to placebo in post-MI arrhythmia patients. Similar to the antiarrhythmic agents used in CAST, the use of moricizine in CAST II to suppress PVCs proved lethal within the first 2 weeks. Following the initial 2-week initiation period with moricizine, there was no significant increase in mortality and morbidity compared to control.[12]

METHODOLOGY

This chapter attempts to outline the diagnosis and treatment options and establish an algorithm for the appropriate risk stratification of those patients at risk

Table 5-1 **ACC/AHA/NASPE 2002 Updated Guidelines for Implantation of**
Cardiac Pacemakers and Antiarrhythmia Devices*

Class I indications for ICD

Patients with cardiac arrest due to VF or VT and not due to a transient or
reversible cause. If the patient has spontaneous sustained VT in association
with structural heart disease or syncope of undetermined origin with hemodynamically significant sustained VT or VF induced with an EP study when drug
therapy is ineffective is also considered a class I indication for ICD implantation.
If patients have prior CAD, MI, LV dysfunction, inducible VF, NSVT, or sustained
VT at EP study that is not suppressible by a class I antiarrhythmic drug, they also
need a device implantation.

Class IIa indications for ICD

Patients with LVEF of ≤30% at least 1 month post-MI and 3 months postcoronary artery revascularization surgery (level of evidence: B)

Class IIb indications for ICD

Patients with cardiac arrest presumed to be due to VF when EP testing is pre-
cluded by other medical conditions, severe symptoms (e.g., syncope)
attributable to sustained ventricular tachyarrhythmias while awaiting cardiac
transplantation or familial or inherited conditions with a high risk for life-threatening
ventricular tachyarrhythmias such as long QT syndrome or hypertrophic
CMP are considered a class IIb indication for a device implantation.

Class III indications for ICD

Patients with syncope of undetermined cause without inducible ventricular tachyarrhythmias and without structural heart disease, or diseases that are amenable
to surgical or catheter ablation; for example, atrial arrhythmias associated with
Wolfe-Parkinson-White syndrome, RV outflow tract VT, idiopathic left ventricular
tachycardia, or fascicular VT or transient or reversible disorders (e.g., AMI, electrolyte imbalance, drugs, or trauma) are considered class II indications for defibrillator implantation. Patients who have significant psychiatric illnesses that may be
aggravated by device implantation or terminal illnesses with projected life
expectancy <6 months or NYHA class IV drug-refractory CHF in patients who are
not candidates for cardiac transplantation are also considered class III indications
for ICD implantation.

*In 2002, the American College of Cardiology, the American Heart Association, and Heart Rhythm Society
or HRS jointly issued guidelines for implantation of cardiac pacemakers and antiarrhythmia devices in
2002. Those collaborating organizations are now in the process of updating those guidelines to include
the new information now available from SCD-HeFT.
Source: Data from Ref. 10.

for SCD. It is important for the clinician to elicit a medical history of sustained VT, NSVT, and/or frequent ventricular ectopy, to properly risk-stratify patients for SCD following an MI. A complete physical examination and certain diagnostic tests including the evaluation of systolic and diastolic functions are imperative (e.g., LVEF). If there is a history of an ischemic cardiomyopathy (CMP), the clinician has to determine if the patient is actively ischemic. Patients who are actively ischemic require coronary revascularization (e.g., percutaneous coronary intervention [PCI] or coronary artery bypass grafting [CABG]).

Labs, Stress Testing, ECG, and Angiography

During the initial evaluation of patients with suspected ventricular arrhythmias, the standard 12-lead ECG is critical. From the ECG, one can identify abnormalities (e.g., Q waves suggesting previous MI, frequent PVCs, and conduction system abnormalities) that suggest structural heart disease capable of sustaining a potentially fatal ventricular arrhythmia. In addition, the ECG may identify patients with a genetic predisposition for SCD (e.g., Brugada syndrome, RV dysplasia, and long QT syndrome).

Following the evaluation of the ECG, lab testing to identify electrolyte abnormalities (e.g., potassium, magnesium, and calcium levels) that can precipitate VT/VF is imperative. Prescription and over-the-counter medications should be reviewed, and patients should be questioned about illicit drug use, cocaine in particular.

If the patient's ECG exhibits Q waves or ST-T wave changes suggestive of CAD, stress testing and coronary angiography are two important tests in determining the presence of ischemia and significant CAD.

ECG stress testing used with nuclear imaging can localize areas of ischemia and infarction and quantify both the patient's ischemic burden and exercise tolerance. The stress test is a functional study that identifies the ischemic burden caused by coronary artery lesions. Stress testing is an important adjunct to the coronary angiogram. A coronary angiogram identifies areas of relative occlusion. Angiographic findings are used as the basis for selection of revascularization therapy (e.g., PCI vs. CABG).

Signal-Averaged Electrocardiography

Signal-averaged electrocardiography (SAECG) is a noninvasive means of determining the presence of electrical late potentials in the ventricle. Signal averaging uses filtering and noise-reduction techniques to detect low-amplitude electrical potentials.[13] SAECG records myocardial activation that occurs after the QRS complex. These very low-amplitude delayed signals are not detected by a routine ECG and correspond to delayed and fragmented areas of slow conduction in the ventricle, which predispose to the development of VT.[13] SAECG has an excellent negative predictive value (approaching 95%) of future arrhythmic events; however, the positive predictive value is 14–29%. Thus, a positive SAECG is not helpful in determining which therapy is required. As a consequence, the SAECG alone has not been established as an accurate predictor of mortality, SCD, or arrhythmia recurrence. The results of the SAECG are used as an adjunct to other invasive or noninvasive diagnostic modalities in the evaluation of SCD and arrhythmia occurrence.

Holter Monitoring

Holter monitoring is most useful in patients with frequent symptoms (e.g., daily). The yield of Holter monitoring is poor in patients with occasional or rare symptoms. Holter monitoring is a noninvasive ambulatory ECG recording system capable of storing a record of electrical activity for extended periods, usually 24–48 hours. This method of testing allows the clinician to document arrhythmias that may correlate with the patient's symptoms.

The Electrophysiologic Study Versus Electrocardiographic Monitoring (ESVEM) trial established Holter monitoring as an important noninvasive diagnostic modality in the treatment of ventricular arrhythmias.[14] The ESVEM trial concluded that Holter monitoring and invasive electrophysiologic study (EPS) were equally effective in predicting the efficacy of drug therapy over an extended follow-up period. Holter monitoring is less useful in detecting the etiology of a patient's palpitations or syncope when the symptoms are sporadic. The positive predictive value of Holter monitoring in the detection of sustained VT/VF is low (<20%).[4] Therefore, Holter monitoring, not unlike the SAECG, is most useful in combination with other diagnostic modalities.

Various studies have revealed a significant increase in diagnostic yield with cardiac loop ECG recorder that is worn for 30 days or longer in order to improve the diagnosis of symptoms related to cardiac arrhythmias. Advancements in the portable monitoring systems have resulted in systems with expanded memory, which are smaller, easier to wear, and easier to tolerate. Longer memory loop recording capacity allows monitoring for a longer duration, typically 30 days. The data can be transmitted to the responsible physician via the telephone or Internet.

Currently, surgically implantable loop recording devices are available which can monitor a patient's rhythm and determine the etiology of their symptoms, which have been extremely elusive by more conventional diagnostic techniques. Such devices have significantly enhanced diagnostic yield and are capable of monitoring rhythm disturbances for over a year.

Electrical Programmed Stimulation

The invasive EPS uses programmed electrical stimulation to determine whether a patient is predisposed to experiencing a reentrant ventricular or supraventricular arrhythmia. EPS involves placing specially designed pacing and recording catheters into strategic locations within the heart by way of the peripheral venous or arterial system (e.g., femoral vein, femoral artery, and internal jugular). EPS is used to determine the exact source of a patient's rhythm disturbance.

EPS is most effective in eliciting those arrhythmias, which are reentrant in nature. Regarding the initiation of scar-related VT post-MI, the sensitivity and specificity is estimated at 58 and 95%, respectively. The positive and negative predictive values are 30 and 98%, respectively.[4] Unfortunately, the low sensitivity of EPS allows a number of patients who are predisposed to life-threatening ventricular arrhythmias to go undetected. The sensitivity of EPS is especially poor in patients with nonischemic depressions in LVEF.

However, in certain patient subsets, a positive EPS can help stratify one's risk for developing SCD. The Multicenter Automatic Defibrillator Implantation Trial (MADIT) study showed that patients post-MI with an LVEF ≤35%, documented NSVT and inducible VT, which failed procainamide suppression, had a risk of death that was 4.24 times greater than in patients without inducible VT.[15] In addition, patients treated with antiarrhythmic therapy who remain inducible are at increased risk for SCD.[4]

The MADIT II study has reorganized where EPS lies in the workup of certain patients at risk for SCD. In the past, patients with a LVEF ≤35% and a history of MI in the presence of NSVT required a positive EPS to warrant ICD implantation. MADIT II reveals that the empiric implantation of an ICD, in those patients with an EF <30%, resulted in a 31% reduction in mortality.[16]

Important subsets of patients excluded from the MADIT II study are patients with an MI and those who have an EF between 30 and 40%. These patients are at an increased risk of SCD, but need further workup to assess the need for ICD implantation.

Assessment of Left Ventricular Systolic Function

A significant reduction of LVEF is the single most powerful independent predictor of SCD in patients with ischemic heart disease.[17] LVEF is an independent risk factor for SCD, cardiovascular mortality, and overall mortality.[4] Patients with an LVEF of <40% require an extensive workup to determine SCD risk. The MADIT II determined that patients with an LVEF ≤30% and a history of MI are at an extremely high risk of SCD and need an ICD to improve survival.[16]

Severe reductions in EF are most commonly related to an MI, which establishes the substrate for reentrant ventricular arrhythmias. In the Antiarrhythmics Versus Implantable Defibrillators (AVID) trial, patients with an LVEF >40% had a 5% risk of developing a malignant ventricular tachyarrhythmia.[18] For every 5% reduction of EF below 40%, the risk of cardiac arrest or arrhythmic death increased by 15%.[4] The LVEF is most commonly quantified by two-dimensional echocardiography, which is pivotal in excluding structural heart disease; other means of quantifying LVEF are by left ventriculography and multiple-gated acquisition scans.

Risk Stratification of Patients Post-MI with NSVT

The management of patients with structural heart disease and NSVT differs from that of patients who have experienced sustained VT/VF. Post-MI patients with NSVT were evaluated in the Basel Antiarrhythmic Study of Infarct Survival (BASIS)[19] trial and the Canadian Amiodarone Myocardial Infarction Arrhythmia Trial (CAMIAT).[20] Patients were found to have an incidence of SCD of 10–14% in a 12- to 20-month follow-up.[4] NSVT in patients who have had a previous MI and have LV dysfunction have a 2-year mortality rate in the range of 30%.[21]

The importance of NSVT in patients with an ischemic CMP has been established in the Grupo de Estudio de la Sobrevida en la Insuficiencia Cardiaca en Argentina (GESICA) trial as an independent marker of increased mortality due to SCD, with a sensitivity of 89% and a specificity of 42%.[22] The importance of NSVT has also been established in the Multicenter Unsustained Tachycardia Trial (MUSTT)[23] and the MADIT.[21] Both trials enrolled patients with documented NSVT, decreased LVEF, and history of MI, and both found that patients who did not receive an ICD experienced mortality rates >50%.[15]

Based on the results of these clinical trials, NSVT in the context of depressed LVEF and ischemic heart disease has proven to increase patients' mortality risk. Patients without a previous MI or evidence of structural heart disease with electrocardiographic evidence of NSVT are at lower risk for adverse clinical outcomes (Fig. 5-3).[4,24]

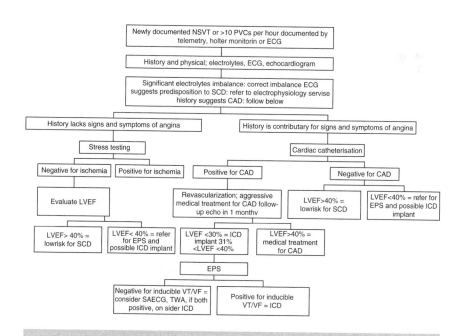

Figure 5-3 **Managing NSVT.** *(Source: Adapted from Garcia L, Kassotis J. Ventricular tachyarrhythmias.* Adv Phys Ass *2004;12(5–6):30–39.)*

Post-MI Complicated with VT and VF

Patients who have experienced a hemodynamically compromising VT or have experienced cardiac arrest secondary to VF in the absence of an acute MI have been the focus of the AVID and CASCADE (Cardiac Arrest in Seattle: Conventional Versus Amiodarone Drug Evaluation) clinical trials.[25] Both studies concluded that antiarrhythmic therapy with or without an ICD decreased mortality compared with placebo. Cardiac arrest survivors are at high risk of recurrence and SCD. Most of the patients studied in these clinical trials had a previous MI and a resultant LVEF of <35%, placing them at a high risk for both SCD and non-SCD. However, antiarrhythmic therapy alone was inferior to the implantation of an ICD in prevention of SCD (Fig. 5-4 and Table 5-2).[16,21,24,26–30]

NEWER MODALITIES

The following discussion describes newer diagnostic modalities designed to risk-stratify patients with an elevated risk of developing VT and SCD.

Microvolt T-wave Alternans

Microvolt T-wave alternans (TWA) is a beat-to-beat measurement of the amplitude and morphology of the ECG measurement of repolarization in the ST segment and T wave.[31] In order to perform a TWA, ECG leads are placed in the standard positions with three leads placed in an orthogonal position. The test can be performed during exercise stress testing, during ergometry, or by programmed electrical stimulation during an EPS. Patients are asked to exercise to a target heart rate ranging from 105 to 115 beats per minute for approximately 5 minutes.

The amplitude of QRS alterations is measured in microvolts using spectral analysis. Recent studies estimated the sensitivity and specificity of TWA as 77–86% and 72–75%, respectively, and the negative and positive predictive powers as 92 and 42%, respectively.[31,32] These statistics were determined by comparing TWA with invasive EPS.

When comparing SAECG with TWA, TWA had a higher sensitivity and a more accurate negative and positive predictive value when both tests were compared with EPS alone, in determining which patients would have inducible or spontaneous ventricular arrhythmias.[31,32] Most importantly, TWA has been established as an independent predictor of VT, VF, and SCD.

TWA has supplanted the SAECG as a noninvasive modality of risk-stratifying patients at risk for SCD and has emerged as a useful diagnostic tool, especially in patients with conduction system disease where SAECG is of limited utility (e.g., LBBB and RBBB). The combination of TWA and SAECG is superior to either modality alone in predicting a patient's risk of SCD from VT/VF.[32] Further studies are needed comparing the combination of TWA, SAECG, and EPS in predicting the risk of SCD.

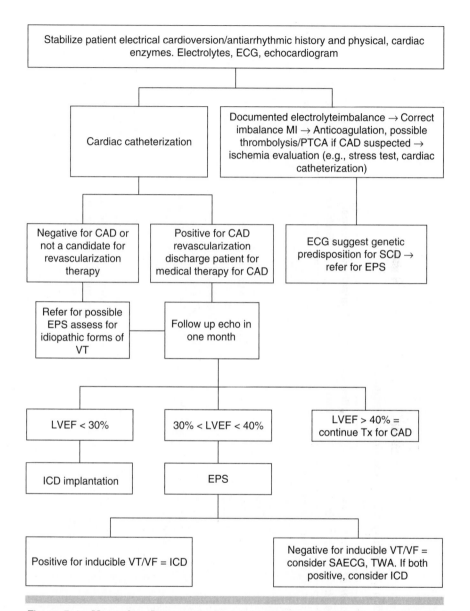

Figure 5-4 **Managing documented sustained VT and/or VF.** *(Source: Adapted from Garcia L, Kassotis J. Ventricular tachyarrhythmias.* Adv Phys Ass *2004; 12(5–6):30–39.)*

Table 5-2 *Clinical Trials Comparing ICD versus Drug Therapy*

Study	Number of Patients	Inclusion Criteria	Follow-up Time	Randomization	Primary Endpoint	Main Results
MADIT I[21]	196	Previous MI NSVT on monitoring LVEF <30% Inducible VT in EP lab	27 months	Pharmacologic treatment vs. ICD	Total mortality	54% relative risk reduction in total mortality in the ICD group
MADIT II[16]	1232	MI>30 days LVEF ≤30%	20 months	Conventional medical treatment vs.ICD	Death from all causes	31% relative risk reduction in total mortality
CABG-PATCH[26]	900	Severe CAD for CABG LVEF <60% NSVT or syncope	32 months	Control vs. ICD	Total mortality	Reduction in arrhythmic death with no effect on total mortality in the ICD group
MUSTT[27]	704	History of prior MI Asymptomatic NSVT LVEF ≤40% Inducible sustained VT	39 months	No therapy vs. EPS-guided antiarrhythmic therapy and ICD if at least one antiarrhythmic failed	Cardiac arrest or death from arrhythmia	Significant reduction in primary endpoint in the AA group receiving ICD and no difference between AA and no therapy groups

Study	N	Inclusion criteria	Follow-up	Comparison	Endpoint	Results
DINAMIT[28]	674	MI within 4–40 days LVEF ≤35% Reduced HR variability or basic HR ≥80 bpm	Up to 4 years	Conventional therapy vs. ICD	Total mortality	No difference in annual all-cause mortality
SCD-HeFT[29]	2521	LVEF ≤35% NYHA II or III Ischemic or nonischemic CMP	30 months	ICD vs. amiodarone vs. placebo	All-causes mortality reduction	Significant mortality reduction in ICD group at 5 years with no beneficial effect of amiodarone. Both ischemic and nonischemic CMP group benefited from ICD
COMPANION[30]	1520	LVEF ≤35% NYHA III or IV Heart failure Hospitalization within the last year	1 year	Optimal medical treatment vs. CRT alone vs. CRT + ICD	Occurrence of death or hospitalization from any cause	Reduction in the combined endpoint of all-cause mortality and all-cause hospitalization

Heart Rate Variability

Heart rate variability (HRV) is used to evaluate vagal and sympathetic influences on the heart and to identify patients at risk for cardiovascular disease.[13] The role of HRV is being studied as an independent marker of SCD. Once established, HRV can be used to risk-stratify patients for VT/VF and SCD. The loss of variability between R-R segments on the ECG reflects desensitization of the heart in response to the changes in the parasympathetic and sympathetic innervation. This loss in HRV is thought to reflect a predisposition for ventricular arrhythmias and SCD.

THERAPEUTIC MODALITIES

Our management of ventricular arrhythmias has changed after significant refinements in ICD technology. Antiarrhythmic drugs have proven unreliable in the prevention of SCD. Therefore, antiarrhythmic medications have taken on a secondary role as adjuvant therapy, primarily to minimize ICD discharges.

Among the available drug therapies, beta-blockers have emerged as the foundation of therapy in the prevention of SCD following an acute MI. The mortality benefit conferred by this class of agents occurs on immediate initiation of therapy following an acute event and at any point within the 2 years following an MI. Despite the benefits conferred by beta-blockers, SCD rates are still unacceptably high; therefore, beta-blockers are not viewed as primary therapy for the reduction of SCD secondary to ventricular arrhythmias.

Sotalol

Sotalol, a class III antiarrhythmic agent with beta-blocker (class II) properties, has shown promise in the prevention of SCD. However, the use of this drug is contraindicated in patients with bronchospastic pulmonary disease and impaired LV systolic function. The primary antiarrhythmic action is to prolong the action potential duration and thus the QT interval. Sotalol is a potassium channel blocker with nonselective beta-adrenergic receptor blocking properties.[13] Excessive prolongation of the QT interval results in a 2–8% risk of torsades de pointes (TdP). The negative inotropic properties of sotalol prevent its use in patients with a reduced LV systolic function, specifically in the presence of congestive heart failure (CHF). With one exception, no clinical trial has established a mortality benefit with the use of sotalol in patients following an MI. In fact, the use of D-sotalol was shown in the Survival With Oral D-Sotalol (SWORD) trial to increase mortality when administered to patients following an acute MI.[33] Sotalol use in patients with depressed LVEF increases the risk of developing TdP.

The ESVEM trial compared seven commonly used antiarrhythmic agents.[14] The majority of patients had a decreased LVEF, history of MI, and/or documented sustained VT/VF. Patients demonstrated the presence of inducible VT/VF during EPS and >10 PVCs per hour on Holter monitoring. Among the antiarrhythmic agents tested, patients treated with sotalol exhibited a trend toward a reduced mortality; however, this did not achieve statistical significance. Of the seven agents tested, sotalol exhibited the highest rates of suppression of inducible VT/VF during follow-up EPS.

Dofetilide

Dofetilide is a class III antiarrhythmic agent, which produces its antiarrhythmic actions by blocking a particular potassium channel (IK_r) in the myocardium. The effect of this potassium current blockade is to make the heart less susceptible to arrhythmias such as atrial fibrillation and atrial flutter. The EMERALD (European and Australian Multicenter Evaluation Research on Atrial Fibrillation and Dofetilide) and the SAFIRE (Symptomatic Atrial Fibrillation Investigation and Randomized Evaluation of Dofetilide) trials demonstrated dofetilide's effectiveness in converting patients with atrial fibrillation or flutter to normal sinus rhythm compared to placebo and may also have a role in increasing the electrical threshold for inducible VT or VF.[34] The principle risk associated with dofetilide use is an increased predisposition to the formation of TdP, in approximately 2% of patients taking the drug.

Radiofrequency ablation (RFA) of ischemic VT is an advancing treatment for patients experiencing an excessive number of ICD discharges in the setting of failed antiarrhythmic drug therapy. At present, hemodynamically stable VT capable of being mapped in the electrophysiology (EP) laboratory is amenable to RFA. Advanced imaging systems capable of identifying the origin and propagation of a single beat of reentrant VT, allow the ablation of a hemodynamically unstable VT.

Beta-Blockers

Beta-blockers decrease heart rate, blood pressure, and oxygen consumption and mute the deleterious effects of catecholamines, especially in CHF. It is believed that the combination of these physiologic actions prevents the occurrence and severity of ischemic events. The ability of these agents to enhance vagal tone and decrease sympathetic stimulation may result in a reduction of the number of VT/VF episodes.[35] By reducing the ischemic burden and preventing future coronary events, beta-blocker therapy can reduce the occurrence of VF and polymorphic VT, and if an ICD is present, the time to initial discharge.[36,37] The Norwegian Multicenter Study concluded that timolol, when given to patients 7 to 28 days post-MI over a 33-month period, achieved a 44.6% reduction of SCD.[36] However, beta-blockers are not effective in preventing scar-related reentrant monomorphic VT. In one study, esmolol did not alter the inducibility of VT in a canine post-MI model.[38]

Amiodarone

Amiodarone (a class III agent) has emerged as the single most important antiarrhythmic agent for the treatment of acute VT and VF. Intravenous amiodarone has replaced bretylium in the Advanced Cardiac Life Support protocol. In patients with frequent VT, amiodarone has been proven to decrease arrhythmia. Nevertheless, amiodarone has failed to exhibit a significant mortality benefit when compared with placebo in several high-risk subgroups.

Amiodarone is effective in the treatment of a variety of atrial and ventricular arrhythmias. Amiodarone's electrophysiologic properties include the ability to block sodium, calcium, and potassium channels; as well as antagonize alpha- and beta-receptors.[13] The electrophysiologic effects of amiodarone are to prolong the action potential duration and effective refractory periods. Amiodarone is a peripheral and coronary vasodilator and blocks the conversion of thyroxine (T4) to triiodothyronine (T3), which is thought to account for some of its electrophysiologic properties.[13] Amiodarone reduces the LV contractile force, heart rate, and systemic vascular resistance.

Amiodarone exhibits a variety of cardiac and noncardiac side effects. The most serious and potentially fatal side effect of amiodarone is pulmonary toxicity. The mechanism of pulmonary toxicity is thought to be a hypersensitivity reaction that can occur at any point during treatment. Immediate cessation of amiodarone is paramount if pulmonary toxicity is suspected. The likelihood of developing side effects is a function of the duration of therapy and dosage.

Amiodarone must be discontinued when liver enzymes exceed two to three times the normal range. The incidence of thyroid dysfunction during long-term use averages between 14 and 18%.[39] Hypothyroidism can be treated with levothyroxine without cessation of therapy. Hyperthyroidism may be treated with thionamides, potassium perchlorate, and/or glucocorticoids, and discontinuation of amiodarone therapy in rare instances. Patients may need a thyroidectomy to continue the administration of amiodarone.[39] The most common (70–100%) ocular side effect is corneal deposits.[40] Amiodarone rarely causes optic neuritis or a decrease in visual acuity.

Amiodarone has been shown to provide a mortality benefit in certain patients following an acute MI (Fig. 5-5).[24] In the European Myocardial Infarct Amiodarone Trial (EMIAT), patients with a history of MI and a LVEF <40% were randomized to either amiodarone or placebo.[17] Patients in the amiodarone group were found to have a decrease in arrhythmic mortality of 35% but no change in all-cause mortality. CAMIAT investigators compared patients with recent MI and >10 PVCs per hour or NSVT. They found a significant reduction in arrhythmic death among patients with asymptomatic NSVT who continued amiodarone treatment for at least 2 years.[20]

The CASCADE trial evaluated patients with a history of VF and an average LVEF of 35%.[2] Patients were randomized to either amiodarone therapy or placebo. Patients treated with amiodarone exhibited a lower cardiac mortality and fewer episodes of VF. To date, very few clinical trials have compared the efficacy of amiodarone with other antiarrhythmic drugs (e.g., sotalol).

Trials demonstrating a benefit of amiodarone treatment vs. placebo and vs. other antiarrhythmic.		
CAMIAT	**CASCADE**	**EMIAT**
• History of MI • History of NSVT or more than 10 PVCs/hour	• History of VF without reversible cause • History of more than 10 PVCs per hour or VT induced EPS • Avg. LVEF 35%	• History of MI and LVEF <40%
Patients treated with amiodarone vs. placebo	Patients treated with amiodarone vs. other antiarrhythmics	Patients treated with amiodarone vs. placebo
Relative risk reduction of 48.5% of arrhythmic death in amiodarone group	Survival free of cardiac death and sustained VT greater in amiodarone group	35% risk reduction of arrhythmic death in amiodarone group

Figure 5-5 **Amiodarone and other antiarrhythmics.** *(Source: Adapted from Garcia L, Kassotis J. Ventricular tachyarrhythmias.* Adv Phys Ass *2004;12(5–6):30–39.)*

Implantable Cardioverter-Defibrillators

The ICD has emerged as the cornerstone of therapy for patients at high risk for SCD. The ICD is most commonly placed in a prepectoral position with a lead positioned in the RV. ICDs are either single- or dual-chamber. The function of an ICD is to accurately identify and successfully terminate dangerous ventricular arrhythmias.

The newest generation of ICDs has the ability to terminate VT by either antitachycardia pacing (ATP) or by defibrillation. ATP therapy is activated when the ICD detects the presence of monomorphic VT above a preset rate (beats per minute), preprogrammed in the detection algorithm of the device. ATP attempts to overdrive and pace terminate the VT at a rate faster than the arrhythmia. If ATP fails to terminate the VT, the ICD will attempt to cardiovert the tachycardia by delivering an electrical shock (defibrillation; Fig. 5-4).[5] The advantage of ATP therapy is the cessation of the arrhythmia without patient discomfort, referred to as painless therapy.

In the prospective randomized multicenter trial of empirical ATP versus shocks for spontaneous rapid VT, pacing fast ventricular tachycardia reduces shock therapies (PainFREE Rx II), patients with ICDs had successful ATP which terminated their VT. This occurred without any need for painful shocks in these patients with implanted ICDs. This trial demonstrated the efficacy, safety, and improved patient quality of life by not shocking the patient out of the VT but by terminating the VT via anti-tachycardic pacing programmed in the ICD. In addition, this study revealed that pain-free therapy was successful, even with very rapid VT, which is traditionally thought to be resistant to overdrive pace termination.[3]

Over the last 10 years, many clinical trials have been conducted to determine, in a prospective randomized fashion, which subgroups of patients would benefit from ICD implantation (Table 5-2). The purpose of such clinical trials is to identify a survival benefit, increased efficacy, while minimizing the cost of device implantation. ICD therapy provides a survival benefit in patients with CAD who have suffered an MI and a resultant decrease in LVEF (<40%), documented NSVT, and inducible VT. Therefore, proper interpretation of the results from such well-designed clinical trials is necessary in the appropriate selection of patients who will benefit from such devices. Although ICD implantation has become as simple as the permanent pacemaker implantation, surgical risks, as well as, cost concerns make it imperative that the devices are implanted in the appropriate patient population.

PRIMARY AND SECONDARY PREVENTION TRIALS

Primary prevention trials of cardiac arrest or sustained VT/VF have attempted to identify patients who would benefit from ICD implantation. The CABG-PATCH trial enrolled patients who needed coronary artery bypass surgery, had documented LVEF ≤36%, and a positive SAECG.[26] Patients were randomized to placebo therapy or ICD implantation after revascularization. Results revealed no significant difference in survival between the groups tested. The results of the CABG-PATCH trial confirmed that not all patients with severe CAD require ICDs. The investigators determined that no statistical difference existed in survival between the two groups, suggesting other important causes of mortality. The LVEF may increase with revascularization, which reduces patient mortality. Most importantly, the CABG-PATCH trial highlighted the benefits of revascularization in the reduction of SCD in patients with ischemic heart disease and VT.

The MADIT trial enrolled patients who had an LVEF (35%, a history of MI, and documented NSVT. Patients with inducible VT, which was not suppressible during EPS after the infusion of procainamide, benefited from the implantation of an ICD. In the majority of patients, conventional therapy consisted of amiodarone. ICDs were found to reduce the overall mortality by 54%, and patients randomized to ICDs achieved a higher rate of survival compared with patients treated with amiodarone, demonstrating the importance of device implantation in this patient population.[21]

The MUSTT trial found that patients with an LVEF of ≤40%, with a history of MI, and a history of NSVT with inducible VT/VF during an invasive EPS, benefited from the implantation of an ICD compared with conventional antiarrhythmic therapy. In contrast to MADIT, MUSTT was a larger trial, a control group was instituted, and beta-blocker usage was greater in the control group, favoring antiarrhythmic therapy as a treatment modality. These important differences in the MUSTT trial helped to further confirm the results of MADIT by discovering a decrease in total mortality of 51% in the patients treated with ICDs. This was comparable with the 54% decrease in the MADIT ICD group.[15] Patients who received an ICD exhibited a significant reduction in overall mortality and arrhythmic death.

The AVID trial recruited patients if they had experienced a hemodynamically compromising VT/VF and had a LVEF of <35%. Patients were randomized to receive either an ICD or conventional antiarrhythmic therapy (amiodarone or sotalol). The efficacy of drug therapy was assessed by serial invasive EP evaluations. Patients who received an ICD, had an increased survival rate compared with conventional therapy at the 1-, 2-, and 3-year follow-ups.[18] These studies have both confirmed and further helped to identify those patients at high risk of developing a potentially lethal ventricular arrhythmia and SCD.

MADIT II

Patients with an LVEF ≤30% and history of MI >1 month prior to entry, became enrolled in the MADIT II study. Patients were randomized to either ICD or conventional therapy. A history of NSVT was not required, and EPS was not performed before enrollment. The study was terminated early when there was a 31% reduction in mortality in the ICD group.[16] This trial revealed the importance of ICD therapy as primary prevention in post-MI patients with reduced LVEF even in the absence of NSVT.

Patients who have a documented LVEF between 30 and 40% will continue to need electrophysiologic testing to determine the need for ICD implantation even though MADIT II revealed the benefit of prophylactic ICD therapy in patients with LVEF ≤30%.

The Sudden Cardiac Death in Heart Failure Trial (SCD-HeFT)

The Sudden Cardiac Death in Heart Failure Trial (SCD-HeFT) compared the efficacy of ICD, amiodarone, and placebo in treating 2521 patients with mild to moderate HF, with an EF ≤35%.

When compared to placebo, ICD therapy reduced all-cause mortality by 23%. The mortality benefit was observed in patients who were already optimally managed on drug therapy. In this study, amiodarone had no significant effect on all-cause mortality. SCD-HeFT demonstrated a greater benefit in the compensated groups of CHF class mortality (New York Heart Association [NYHA] class II > III and IV).

Radiofrequency Ablation

A well-established therapeutic modality for the treatment of a variety of supraventricular arrhythmias has been radiofrequency ablation (RFA).

Recently, with the evolution of refined imaging systems, RFA is emerging as an effective means in the elimination of a variety of ventricular arrhythmias. RFA has been previously shown to be effective in the treatment of idiopathic VT, originating from the LV and RV, and bundle branch reentry arrhythmias.

When placing catheters capable of mapping and pacing into strategic locations in the heart, RFA is performed, thus allowing one to map the origin and sites of propagation of abnormal electrical signals. Since most ventricular arrhythmias are reentrant, it is important to locate the critical site of slow conduction used in the reentrant arrhythmia. By delivering energy in the form of radiofrequency waves, heat is generated, destroying the tissue responsible for the propagation of such arrhythmic disturbances.

RFA remains an arduous and time-consuming task when attempted in patients with a scar-related VT, despite refinements in imaging and mapping techniques. RFA of scar-related VT is reserved for patients who have an ICD implanted and continue to receive electrical discharges despite antiarrhythmic therapy. In a group of patients who experienced multiple ICD discharges refractory to medical therapy, RFA was attempted and achieved a success rate of 75% and a reduction of 99.8% of discharges in appropriate defibrillator therapies.[42] Only hemodynamically stable monomorphic VT was ablated owing to the risk of rapid patient decompensation with hemodynamically unstable VT.

It is extremely difficult to locate by programmed electrical stimulation a hemodynamically unstable VT. Investigators using the Biosense CARTO system for three-dimensional mapping of the LV in 19 patients, who received frequent shocks by ICDs despite medical therapy were able to successfully locate the hemodynamically unstable VT.[43] Locations that correspond with the VT and electroanatomic mapping were subsequently ablated. Findings of the study included a 66% reduction in ICD shocks over an 18- to 48-week period and a decrease in the number of medications used before and after ablation. The study showed a promising role of RFA in the isolation and termination of hemodynamically unstable VT. Future studies on the benefits of VT ablation are needed to assess effects on morbidity and mortality, reduction in the use of antiarrhythmic agents, and the number of ICD discharges. Major complications associated with this type of RFA range from 8 to 11%, with death, MI, cerebrovascular accident, and cardiac tamponade being the most significant.[7,44]

In conclusion, even though RFA is a very effective therapy in certain kinds of VTs, such as the bundle branch reentrant tachycardia and idiopathic VT, its use and effectiveness in the scar-related VT are not as successful and it is currently used as an adjunct to ICD.

Antiarrhythmic Therapy after ICD

In patients with multiple ICD discharges, the first line of therapy is an antiarrhythmic drug. Questions such as the choice of the appropriate antiarrhythmic drug and the duration of treatment are difficult to generalize and are patient-specific. Considerations include comorbid disease and the degree of LV dysfunction.

The AVID investigators followed their patients who received ICDs prospectively and assessed the need for antiarrhythmic drug therapy intervention. The arrhythmia event rate was 90% in 64% of patients who experienced multiple ICD discharges in 1-year postimplantation.[45] Patients with an LVEF averaging 28%, a history of syncope, female gender, and recent smoker status were at highest risk for ICD therapy requiring pharmacologic intervention. After 1 year of antiarrhythmic therapy, the arrhythmia event rate decreased to 64%. Amiodarone was the most common drug used (42%).

The CASCADE investigators randomized their patients with history of VF and LVEF of 35% to amiodarone versus multiple antiarrhythmic agents in patients with an ICD. Amiodarone was found to decrease the incidence of shocks and decrease the incidence of syncope postshock.[2]

ICDs have been shown to drastically reduce the incidence of SCD in specific patient populations. At present, patients who have a severely reduced LVEF (≤30%) and a history of MI are at an extremely high risk for SCD and require an ICD. Patients with risk factors such as a LVEF between 30 and 40% and a history of MI continue to require inducible ventricular arrhythmias to warrant the insertion of an ICD, which have a proven mortality benefit (Fig. 5-6).

Using antiarrhythmic medications in patients who already have an ICD is a double-edged sword, on the one hand, they often slow the rate of VT making it more responsive to ATP and therefore sparing the patient the discomfort associated with the shock delivery, however, it can slow the VT rate below the detection limits of the ICD, thus the ICD will not intervene. On occasion, the VT slows into the normal heart rate range making management more difficult.

DAVID Trial and AVID Trial

The AVID trial revealed an improved survival with ICD therapy compared to conventional antiarrhythmic drug therapy. In the Dual-Chamber and VVI Implantable Defibrillator (DAVID) trial, VVI pacing at 40 beats per minute in patients with ICDs decreased the combined endpoint of death and hospitalization for CHF compared with dual-chamber rate adaptive pacemaker (DDDR) at 70 beats per minute.

The mortality in both the AVID and DAVID trial patients treated with VVI-40 ICDs and the time to rehospitalization for CHF was similar. Therefore, the composite endpoint did not differ between the two trials and there was no difference in mortality.

When comparing the AVID antiarrhythmic drug-treated patients with the DAVID DDDR-70 ICD patients, the trial showed that these groups had similar outcomes. The time to death was also similar in both of these VVI-40

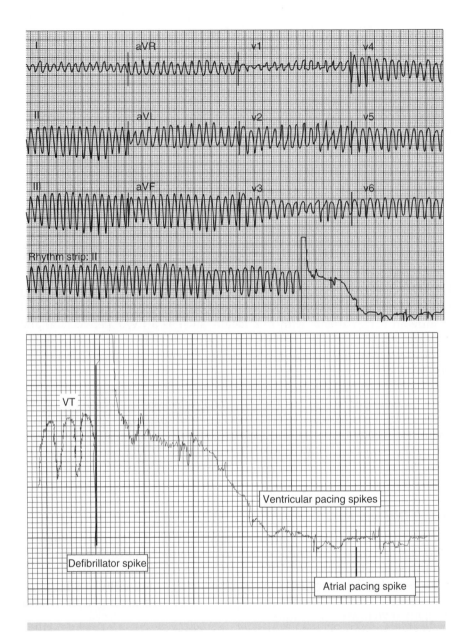

Figure 5-6 **Ventricular fibrillation converted to sinus rhythm by implantable cardioverter-defibrillator (ICD).** *(Source: ECG by Example. Second edition. Richard Dean Jenkins and Stephen John Gerred. Elsevier Publishing Company 2005: page 118–119)*

populations, despite an increased amount of coronary interventions, bypass surgery, and the higher use of beta-blockers in the DAVID trial.[46]

A significant percentage of patients with CHF have a resultant LBBB. The width of the QRS correlates inversely with a reduction in systolic function. From these studies, one concludes that an iatrogenic LBBB, secondary to RV pacing, has a deleterious outcome. Currently, devices are programmed with the intent of minimizing unnecessary RV pacing.

ICD versus CRT

Cardiac resynchronization therapy (CRT) has emerged recently as an essential treatment for the patient with refractory symptoms of CHF, on an optimal medical regimen. The rationale behind this therapy is that patients with CHF, who have a wide QRS >120 milliseconds with a LBBB, often have a ventricular dyssynchrony. Most recently, it has been shown that such patients experience both intra- and interventricular dyssynchrony. Pacing both ventricles simultaneously with a certain critical time delay can restore ventricular synchrony during cardiac systole with a resultant improvement in cardiac output and a clinical improvement in congestive symptoms.

The efficacy of CRT in patients with CHF has been evaluated in several studies. This discussion will focus on the results of the COMPANION (Comparison of Medical Therapy, Pacing, and Defibrillation in Heart Failure) and the CARE-HF (Cardiac Resynchronization in Heart Failure) clinical trials.

In the CARE-HF trial, patients with NYHA class III and IV CHF, LVEF (35%, and a QRS duration ≥120 milliseconds were randomized to receive either medical therapy with CRT or medical therapy alone. Patients with a QRS duration of <150 milliseconds were required to exhibit ventricular dyssynchrony, by two-dimensional echocardiography, prior to enrollment. The primary endpoint of the study was the time to death. After a mean follow-up time of 29 months, there was a reduction of the primary endpoint in the CRT group, independent of the age, sex, NYHA class, and QRS duration. This study revealed a decreased mortality in the CRT group attributed to the reduction in CHF exacerbations, improvement of the LVEF, and a reduction in the level of B-type natriuretic peptide (BNP) coupled with signs of reverse ventricular remodeling.

In the COMPANION trial patients were eligible for enrollment if they had a history of CHF, NYHA class III and IV, EF ≤35%, QRS duration >120 milliseconds, and a recent hospitalization for a CHF exacerbation, within the last year. Patients were randomized to either: CRT with ICD, CRT alone, or optimal medical therapy alone. The primary endpoint of this study was the composite endpoint of all-cause mortality and all-cause hospitalization. After a mean follow-up of 12 months, there was a significant reduction in the primary endpoint in both CRT arms.

Analyzing the data from both the COMPANION and CARE-HF trials revealed a similar reduction in mortality from the CRT and CRT with ICD arms. In this patient population, determining the necessity of ICD therapy becomes important. A randomized prospective trial designed to compare the two treatment modalities is necessary to reach a definitive conclusion. The majority of patients who are candidates for CRT are usually candidates for the insertion of an ICD.

Current Recommendations for ICD Insertion

Patients with a history of CHF who have a moderate to severely depressed LV systolic function (<40%) need aggressive risk stratification for SCD. At the present time, patients post-MI, whose resultant EF is <30% a month following the MI are candidates for ICD implantation. Patients following coronary intervention (e.g., PCI and CABG) need to be evaluated 3 months following revascularization. Patients with an EF that remains at or lower than 30% meet MADIT II criteria for the insertion of an ICD. In patients who have long-standing CHF with a depressed LVEF <35% in class III–IV CHF with a nonischemic dilated CMP warrants an ICD insertion. In the above referenced categories, those patients with a QRS duration of >120 milliseconds with either a left bundle or left bundle like interventricular conduction delay are candidates for CRT therapy. Currently, patients who have ischemic CMP and an EF >30% with significant ventricular ectopy should have an EPS study performed to assess their risk of developing a sustained ventricular arrhythmia. Also, any patient with a sustained ventricular arrhythmia or a known genetic predisposition for SCD is a candidate for device therapy.

SUMMARY

Following an assessment of LVEF and the presence of ischemia, the evaluation of a patient at risk for ventricular arrhythmias and CAD begins with a thorough medical history and a standard ECG. In order to assist the clinician in risk stratification for VT, VF, and SCD, the SAECG, HRV, microvolt TWA, and invasive EPS should be used in particular subgroups of patients. In terms of reducing the recurrence of VT/VF and subsequent ICD shocks, amiodarone is the superior antiarrhythmic agent. In addition, amiodarone has been shown to reduce arrhythmic death but has fallen short in reducing total mortality. Patients with a severely reduced LVEF (30% or below) with a history of MI are at extremely high risk for SCD and require an ICD. In order to reduce the incidence of SCD, aggressive risk stratification of patients is crucial. It is fundamental to know and understand the role of pharmacotherapy in conjunction with device therapy for the effective treatment of these patients to decrease future arrhythmic events and death.

CONCLUSION

In the United States, SCD is a major cause of death. Diabetes is a disease that propagates the destruction of the myocardial, vascular, and electrical environments in the cardiac cells. Diabetes needs to be quickly diagnosed and treated in order to decrease the deleterious effects that it has on the cardiovascular system. Widespread public awareness will increase knowledge and access to the diagnosis and treatment of patients with diabetes. This will allow for a decreased propagation or lower cardiovascular disease event rates in diabetic patients. Great progress has been made in determining patients who are candidates for ICD insertion. By controlling the epidemic and treatment of diabetes, fewer patients will necessitate ICD insertion. However, it is very important to facilitate a better understanding both amongst medical doctors and patients alike as to who would benefit from aggressive SCD risk stratification in the diabetic population. This is a treatment that has shown to provide a mortality benefit in patients that suffer cardiovascular disease that was initiated and propagated by diabetes.

REFERENCES

1. Eckel RH, Grundy SM, Zimmet PZ. The metabolic syndrome. *Lancet* 2005;365(9468): 1415–1428.

2. Kusama Y, Hearse DJ, Avkiran M. Diabetes and susceptibility to reperfusion-induced ventricular arrhythmias. *J Mol Cell Cardiol* 1992;24(4):411–421.

3. Myerburg RJ, Castellanos A. Cardiac arrest and sudden cardiac death. In: Braunwald E, Zipes DP, Lippy P, eds., *Heart Disease: A Textbook of Cardiovascular Medicine*, 6th ed. Philadelphia, PA: WB Saunders, 2001:890–931.

4. Camm AJ, Katritsis DG. Risk stratification of patients with ventricular arrhythmias. In: Zipes DP, Jalife J, eds., *Cardiac Electrophysiology: From Cell to Bedside*, 3rd ed. Philadelphia, PA: WB Saunders, 2000:808–817.

5. Garcia TB, Holtz N. *12-Lead ECG: The Art of Interpretation*. Bartlett Publication, 2001.

6. Ciaccio EJ, Coromilas J, Costeas CA, et al. Sinus rhythm electrogram shape measurements are predictive of the origins and characteristics of multiple reentrant ventricular tachycardia morphologies. *J Cardiovasc Electrophysiol* 2004;15(11): 1293–1301.

7. Peters NS, Wit AL. Myocardial architecture and ventricular arrhythmogenesis. *Circulation* 1998;97:1746–1754.

8. Delacretaz E, Stevenson WG. Catheter ablation of ventricular tachycardia in patients with coronary heart disease: part I: mapping. *Pacing Clin Electrophysiol* 2001;24:1261–1277.

9. Coromilas J, Saltman AE, Waldecker B, et al. Electrophysiological effects of flecainide on anisotropic conduction and reentry in infarcted canine hearts. *Circulation* 1995;91:2245–2263.

10. Gregoratos G, Abrams J, Epstein AE, et al. ACC/AHA/NASPE 2002 guideline update for implantation of cardiac pacemakers and antiarrhythmia devices: summary article. *Circulation* 2002;106:2145–2161.

11. Echt DS, Liebson PR, Mitchell LB, et al. Mortality and morbidity in patients receiving encainide, flecainide, or placebo. The Cardiac Arrhythmia Suppression Trial. *N Engl J Med* 1991;324:781–788.

12. Effect of the antiarrhythmic agent moricizine on survival after myocardial infarction. The Cardiac Arrhythmia Suppression Trial II Investigators. *N Engl J Med* 1992;327(4):227–233.

13. Miller JM, Zipes DP. Management of the patient with cardiac arrhythmias. In: Braunwald E, Zipes DP, Lippy P, eds., *Heart Disease: A Textbook of Cardiovascular Medicine*, 6th ed. Philadelphia, PA: WB Saunders, 2001:700–766.

14. Mason JW. A comparison of electrophysiologic testing with Holter monitoring to predict antiarrhythmic-drug efficacy for ventricular tachyarrhythmias. Electrophysiologic Study versus Electrocardiographic Monitoring Investigators. *N Engl J Med* 1993;329:445–451.

15. Prystowsky EN, Nisam S. Prophylactic implantable cardioverter defibrillator trials: MUSTT, MADIT, and beyond. *Am J Cardiol* 2000;86:1214–1215.

16. Moss AJ, Zareba W, Hall WJ, et al. Prophylactic implantation of a defibrillator in patients with myocardial infarction and reduced ejection fraction. *N Engl J Med* 2002;346:877–883.

17. Julian DG, Camm AJ, Frangin G, et al. Randomised trial of effect of Amiodarone on mortality in patients with left-ventricular dysfunction after recent myocardial infarction: EMIAT. *Lancet* 1997;349:667–674.

18. A comparison of antiarrhythmic-drug therapy with implantable defibrillators in patients resuscitated from near-fatal ventricular arrhythmias. The Antiarrhythmics versus Implantable Defibrillators (AVID) Investigators. *N Engl J Med* 1997;337:1576–1583.

19. Burkart F, Pfisterer M, Kiowski W, et al. Effect of antiarrhythmic therapy on mortality in survivors of myocardial infarction with asymptomatic complex ventricular arrhythmias: Basel Antiarrhythmic Study of Infarct Survival (BASIS). *J Am Coll Cardiol* 1990;16:1711–1718.

20. Cairns JA, Connolly SJ, Roberts R, et al. Randomised trial of outcome after myocardial infarction in patients with frequent or repetitive ventricular premature depolarisations: CAMIAT. Canadian Amiodarone Myocardial Infarction Arrhythmia Trial Investigators. *Lancet* 1997;349:675–682.

21. Moss AJ, Hall WJ, Cannom DS, et al. Improved survival with an implanted defibrillator in patients with coronary disease at high risk for ventricular arrhythmia. Multicenter Automatic Defibrillator Implantation Trial Investigators. *N Engl J Med* 1996;335:1933–1940.

22. Doval HC, Nul DR, Grancelli HO, et al. Randomised trial of low-dose Amiodarone in severe congestive heart failure. Grupo de Estudio de la Sobrevida en la Insuficiencia Cardiaca en Argentina (GESICA). *Lancet* 1994;344:493–498.

23. Buxton AE, Fisher JD, Josephson ME, et al. Prevention of sudden death in patients with coronary artery disease: the Multicenter Unsustained Tachycardia Trial (MUSTT). *Prog Cardiovasc Dis* 1993;36:215–226.

24. Garcia L, Kassotis J. Ventricular tachyarrhythmias. *Adv Phys Ass* 2004;12(5–6): 30–39.

25. Greene HL. The CASCADE Study: randomized antiarrhythmic drug therapy in survivors of cardiac arrest in Seattle. CASCADE Investigators. *Am J Cardiol* 1993;72:70F–74F.

26. Bigger JT Jr. Prophylactic use of implanted cardiac defibrillators in patients at high risk for ventricular arrhythmias after coronary-artery bypass graft surgery. Coronary Artery Bypass Graft (CABG) Patch Trial Investigators. *N Engl J Med* 1997;337:1569–1575.

27. Buxton AE, Lee KL, Fisher JD, et al. A randomized study of the prevention of sudden death in patients with coronary artery disease. Multicenter Unsustained Tachycardia Trial Investigators. *N Engl J Med* 1999;341(25):1882–1890.

28. Hohnloser SH, Kuck KH, Dorian P, et al. Prophylactic use of an implantable cardioverter-defibrillator after acute myocardial infarction. *N Engl J Med* 2004;351(24):2481–2488.

29. Bardy GH, Lee KL, Mark DB, et al. Amiodarone or an implantable cardioverter-defibrillator for congestive heart failure. *N Engl J Med* 2005;352:225–237.

30. Bristow MR, Saxon LA, Boehmer J, et al. Cardiac-resynchronization therapy with or without an implantable defibrillator in advanced chronic heart failure. *N Engl J Med* 2004;350:2140–2150.

31. Estes NA III, Michaud G, Zipes DP, et al. Electrical alternans during rest and exercise as predictors of vulnerability to ventricular arrhythmias. *Am J Cardiol* 1997;80:1314–1318.

32. Gold MR, Bloomfield DM, Anderson KP, et al. A comparison of T-wave alternans, signal averaged electrocardiography and programmed ventricular stimulation for arrhythmia risk stratification. *J Am Coll Cardiol* 2000;36:2247–2253.

33. Waldo AL, Camm AJ, deRuyter H, et al. Effect of d-sotalol on mortality in patients with left ventricular dysfunction after recent and remote myocardial infarction. The SWORD Investigators. Survival With Oral d-Sotalol. *Lancet* 1996;348:7–12.

34. Singh BN, Wadhani N. Antiarrhythmic and proarrhythmic properties of QT-prolonging antianginal drugs. *J Cardiovasc Pharmacol Ther* 2004;9(Suppl 1): S85–S97.

35. Reiter MJ, Reiffel JA. Importance of beta blockade in the therapy of serious ventricular arrhythmias. *Am J Cardiol* 1998;82:9I–19I.

36. Timolol-induced reduction in mortality and reinfarction in patients surviving acute myocardial infarction. *N Engl J Med* 1981;304:801–807.

37. Levine JH, Mellits ED, Baumgardner RA, et al. Predictors of first discharge and subsequent survival in patients with automatic implantable cardioverter-defibrillators. *Circulation* 1991;84:558–566.

38. Kassotis J, Sauberman RB, Cabo C, et al. Beta receptor blockade potentiates the antiarrhythmic actions of d-sotalol on reentrant ventricular tachycardia in a canine model of myocardial infarction. *J Cardiovasc Electrophysiol* 2003;14(11): 1233–1244.

39. Bogazzi F, Bartalena L, Gasperi M, et al. The various effects of Amiodarone on thyroid function. *Thyroid* 2001;11:511–519.

40. Mantyjarvi M, Tuppurainen K, Ikaheimo K. Ocular side effects of Amiodarone. *Surv Ophthalmol* 1998;42:360–366.

41. Wathen MS, DeGroot PJ, Sweeney MO, et al. Prospective Randomized Multicenter Trial of Empirical Antitachycardia Pacing Versus Shocks for Spontaneous Rapid Ventricular Tachycardia in Patients With Implantable Cardioverter-Defibrillators: Pacing Fast Ventricular Tachycardia Reduces Shock Therapies (PainFREE Rx II) Trial Results. *Circulation* 2004;110(17): 2591–2596.

42. Strickberger SA, Man KC, Daoud EG, et al. A prospective evaluation of catheter ablation of ventricular tachycardia as adjuvant therapy in patients with coronary artery disease and an implantable cardioverter-defibrillator. *Circulation* 1997;96:1525–1531.

43. Sra J, Bhatia A, Dhala A, et al. Electroanatomically guided catheter ablation of ventricular tachycardias causing multiple defibrillator shocks. *Pacing Clin Electrophysiol* 2001;24:1645–1652.

44. Calkins H, Epstein A, Packer D, et al. Catheter ablation of ventricular tachycardia in patients with structural heart disease using cooled radiofrequency energy: results of a prospective multicenter study. Cooled RF Multi Center Investigators Group. *J Am Coll Cardiol* 2000;35:1905–1914.

45. Steinberg JS, Martins J, Sadanandan S, et al. Antiarrhythmic drug use in the implantable defibrillator arm of the Antiarrhythmics Versus Implantable Defibrillators (AVID) Study. *Am Heart J* 2001;142:520–529.

46. Sharma A, Epstein AE, Herre JM, et al. A comparison of the AVID and DAVID trials of implantable defibrillators. *Am J Cardiol* 2005;95(12);1431–1435.

SYNCOPE IN THE DIABETIC PATIENT

Hanan Morcos
John Kassotis

INTRODUCTION

Syncope is a sudden and brief loss of consciousness associated with a loss of postural tone, characterized by spontaneous recovery. The loss of consciousness, which is a characteristic of syncope, is attributed to a reduction in cerebral blood flow. A distinguishing feature of syncope is the rapid recovery of mental status, with no postevent residual. Syncope is a common presenting symptom to the emergency department (ED), accounting for as much as 3% of all ED visits and up to 6% of hospital admissions per year.[1] Syncope is a common clinical problem characterized by a significant morbidity and mortality. Syncope may be the only warning sign before sudden cardiac death (SCD).

Elderly persons have a 6% annual incidence of syncope.[2] Surveys of young adults have revealed that up to 50% report a prior episode of loss of consciousness; most of these episodes are isolated events that never come to medical attention. Patients who experience recurrent unexplained "blackouts" experience significant anxiety, which makes the diagnosis even more difficult. Patients with this disorder report a poor quality of life. The prognosis of patients with syncope varies greatly with the underlying cause. In general, those patients with syncope have an increased mortality compared with participants without syncope.[3] When comparing the various etiologies accounting for syncope, the highest mortality was found in patients with structural heart disease.[3] Patients with neurocardiogenic syncope did not exhibit a significant increase in mortality.

Emotional stress, pain, lower extremity blood pooling, postural changes, heat prostration, dehydration, heavy sweating, exhaustion, micturition, coitus, coughing, and blood loss have all been implicated as causes of syncope. Medications are commonly at the root cause of syncope and near-syncope. Syncope occurring during exercise, associated with palpitations, or in those with family history of recurrent syncope or sudden death may suggest a cardiac etiology.

Poorly controlled diabetes can result in significant morbidity and mortality. Diabetic patients are at risk for the development of renal dysfunction, coronary and peripheral vascular disease, associated hypertension, and accelerated atherosclerosis. Diabetics may develop peripheral neuropathies and dysautonomia. Not uncommonly, the diabetic patient will present with syncope. The following discussion will focus on the patient who presents with syncope and will attempt to highlight the important diagnostic and therapeutic modalities available to the practitioner who encounters patients with this disorder.

CLINICAL EVALUATION/PRESENTATION

The history and physical examination are the most important components in the evaluation of a patient presenting with syncope. When approached systematically, the history is invaluable in the differential diagnosis of syncope. Initial evaluation should aim at distinguishing between true syncope from other etiologic causes of a loss of consciousness. Both the patient and any witnesses should be interviewed at the time of presentation. During the interview, important issues that need to be addressed include presence of a prodrome; character and duration of prodrome; postrecovery residual change in mental status; prior history of similar episodes; medication history; presence of structural heart disease; family history of SCD; precipitating factors; and other associated symptoms.

In the evaluation of the patients with syncope it is important to distinguish true syncope from other syndromes. Dizziness, presyncope, and vertigo do not result in a loss of consciousness or postural tone. Vertigo is associated with an abnormal sensorium of motion. "Drop attacks" lead to falls without a loss of consciousness. Those patients who require defibrillation to regain consciousness are defined as cardiac arrest survivors. Distinguishing syncope from seizure can be difficult, since both can have a common presentation. However, there are certain features that help decipher the two. It is important to look for the precipitants of the episode, the premonitory or prodromal symptoms, the symptoms that accompany the episode, and the events that follow it. A loss of consciousness that is precipitated by pain, exercise, micturition, defecation, or a stressful event is usually syncope rather than a seizure. Symptoms such as sweating and nausea that occur before or during the episode are associated with syncope, whereas "aura" is typical of seizures.

Characteristics which are uncommon in cardiogenic syncope include disorientation following the event; slow recovery of mentation; and unconsciousness lasting more than 5 minutes. Not uncommonly, patients complain of fatigue and diaphoresis during the recovery phase of syncope and are often noted to have pallor and bradycardia.

In the absence of trauma retrograde amnesia is an uncommon characteristic of syncope. When rhythmic movements (such as clonic or myoclonic jerks) are reported, seizure is the usual diagnosis, but syncope can also cause similar movements. Sometimes, the only way to distinguish the two is through direct observations in the laboratory (with the use of tilt testing) or by finding evidence of a seizure through electroencephalographic (EEG) studies. In patients with atypical presentations, tilt-table tests are performed with simultaneous EEG monitoring.

During the physical examination, attention should be given to the blood pressure in the supine, sitting, and standing positions. Blood pressure measurements should be taken on both arms. Careful attention should be given to the dermatologic examination for signs of collagen vascular disease, vasculitis, and the stigmata of long-standing diabetes. A funduscopic evaluation should be performed to detect a possible embolic event and the chronic changes seen with diabetes and hypertension. Auscultation of the carotids should be performed to detect a carotid bruit with careful observation of the carotid upstroke. A thorough neurologic examination should be performed looking for subtle neurologic deficits. The cardiac examination should focus on murmurs, extra heart sounds, and peripheral pulses to exclude structural heart disease, peripheral vascular disease, and the subclavian steal syndrome.

ETIOLOGY AND PATHOPHYSIOLOGY

Neurally mediated syncope (also known as vasovagal or neurocardiogenic syncope) comprises the largest group of disorders causing syncope, accounting for 24–32% (Fig. 6-1) of syncopal episodes.[4] Neurocardiogenic syncope results from reflex-mediated changes in vascular tone or heart rate. Although the mechanism is poorly understood, neurocardiogenic syncope is believed to occur in persons predisposed to the condition as a result of excessive peripheral venous pooling. This excessive venous pooling causes a sudden drop in peripheral venous return, resulting in a cardiac

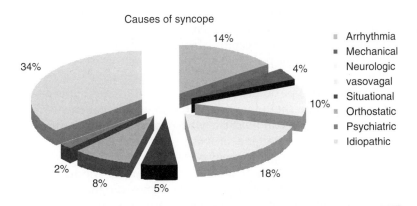

Causes of syncope

- Arrhythmia
- Mechanical
- Neurologic
- vasovagal
- Situational
- Orthostatic
- Psychiatric
- Idiopathic

Figure 6-1   **Prevalence of the causes of syncope.**

"hypercontractile" state, which, in turn, activates mechanoreceptors that normally respond only to stretch. Activation of these mechanoreceptors results in an increase in afferent neuronal discharge, mimicking a hypertensive state, and resulting in paradoxical vagal discharge decreasing the blood pressure and causing bradycardia. These mechanoreceptors are present throughout the body (including the bladder, rectum, esophagus, and lungs). A sudden activation of a large number of these receptors may also result in an increase of afferent signals to the brain prompting a neurocardiogenic response. This may explain why predisposed individuals may experience syncope prompted by a vigorous cough, micturition, and constipation.

Neurocardiogenic syncope is subdivided, on the basis of head-up tilt-table testing (TTT), into three types: type 1 (mixed vasovagal syncope); type 2 (cardioinhibitory syncope); and type 3 (pure vasodepressor syncope). Orthostatic syncope occurs as a result of orthostatic hypotension. When normal subjects stand, the systolic blood pressure drops only 5–15 mmHg and the diastolic blood pressure will rise slightly. In orthostatic syncope, the drop in systolic blood pressure on assuming the upright position is >20 mmHg, or decreases below 90 mmHg while the diastolic blood pressure decreases by 10 mmHg within 3 minutes of assuming the upright position.

Dysautonomia results from a failure of the autonomic nervous system to compensate for the acute decrease in venous return that occurs with upright posture. This compensatory failure is attributed to a failure of the baroreceptors to detect the drop in blood pressure or a derangement in the afferent limb of the autonomic nervous system to respond to the decrease in blood pressure. Alternatively or concomitantly, the failure of the peripheral circulation to respond to a drop in blood pressure is attributed to a reduction in end-organ responsiveness to circulating vasoconstrictors. Severe dysautonomia results in a dramatic drop in blood pressure and frank syncope.

Postural-orthostatic tachycardia syndrome (POTS) results from marked changes in heart rate (an increase of >30 beats per minute or an ambient heart rate of >120 beats per minute), which occurs during the first few minutes following resumption of the upright posture. The rapid heart rate may be associated with only mild orthostatic hypotension, however, many patients with POTS develop syncope. Beta-receptor hypersensitivity, decreased plasma volume, inappropriate venous pooling, and dysautonomia have been proposed as a potential mechanism of POTS.

Carotid sinus syncope occurs secondary to carotid sinus hypersensitivity. Carotid sinus syncope should be considered in elderly patients with recurrent syncope and in those individuals whose symptoms occur during shaving, turning the head, swimming, or while wearing a tight collar.

Cardiac causes of syncope account for 10–20% of syncopal episodes and can be subdivided into mechanical and electrical causes. Mechanical causes include hypertrophic cardiomyopathy; aortic stenosis; right ventricular outflow obstruction; myocardial infarction; pulmonary embolism; and cardiac tamponade. Electrical causes can be attributed to either tachyarrhythmias or bradyarrhythmias. Ventricular tachycardia, including torsades de pointes, is the most common tachyarrhythmia causing syncope. Other causes include the various supraventricular tachycardias including the Wolff-Parkinson-White syndrome. Patients with these various dysrhythmias may also experience a prodrome prior to passing out. Complaints may include chest pain, lightheadedness, dyspnea, or palpitations. Symptomatic bradycardia secondary to either sick sinus syndrome, AV nodal disease, or His-Purkinje disease resulting in heart block may cause syncope. Therefore, in the evaluation of patients with syncope, medications, which prolong the QT interval or suppress the SA or AV node should be excluded. Medications, which can cause syncope, include antihypertensive, antiarrhythmic, hypoglycemic, psychotropic agents; and illegal drugs (e.g., cocaine). Patients who had either a pacemaker or an implantable cardioverter-defibrillator (ICD) inserted should have the devices evaluated to either exclude malfunction or uncover a possible arrhythmic cause of the syncope.

Noncardiovascular causes of syncope comprise a small percentage (<15%). Included in this category are neurologic, metabolic, and psychogenic causes. Patients who experience syncope or near-syncope secondary to a neurologic cause usually will have associated physical findings. Potential neurologic causes include migraines, seizures, transient ischemic attacks, vertebro-basilar strokes, Arnold-Chiari malformations, and normal pressure hydrocephalus. Metabolic causes are rare, accounting for <5% of syncopal episodes. The most common metabolic causes include hypoglycemia, hypoxia, hypokalemia, and hyperventilation. Psychogenic causes of syncope include hysteria, anxiety/panic disorder, somatization disorder, conversion disorder, and depression. Cranial CT scanning and MRI have a very low yield in the work-up of patients who present with syncope in the absence of a focal neurologic deficit. Table 6-1 lists the common etiologies of syncope and their mean prevalence.

Table 6-1 **Causes of Syncope**

Causes	Mean Prevalence (%)
Neurocardiogenic	18
Situational	5
Carotid sinus	1
Orthostatic hypotension	8
Medications	3
Psychiatric	2
Neurologic	10
Structural heart disease	4
Arrhythmias	14
Unknown	34

WHICH TESTS ARE INDICATED IN THE WORK-UP OF SYNCOPE?

Routine Blood Testing

The routine use of blood tests such as cardiac enzymes, complete blood count, basic metabolic panel are of low diagnostic yield, with the exception of glucose testing in the diabetic patient. In patients with long-standing diabetes, an HbA1C may be useful to establish the degree of glycemic control.

Diagnostic Imaging

As previously mentioned, cranial CT scanning and MRI, in the absence of a history of syncope with a neurologic deficit are of low diagnostic yield, and have no role in the initial assessment of syncope.

12-Lead Electrocardiogram

The 12-lead electrocardiogram is an integral component of the work-up for syncope. The baseline ECG establishes the diagnosis in up to 5% of patients with syncope.[4] The ECG can demonstrate Wolff-Parkinson-White syndrome (short PR interval), long QT syndromes (prolonged QT interval), and Brugada syndrome (right bundle block pattern with ST elevations in V1, and V2). The ECG may reveal evidence of acute myocardial injury or evidence of infarction, conduction system abnormalities, ventricular ectopy, and arrhythmogenic right ventricular dysplasia (T-wave inversions in the right precordial leads).

Echocardiography

In the absence of physical findings suggestive of structural heart disease, the two-dimensional echocardiogram is of low diagnostic yield. Among the etiologies of syncope that are confirmed by echocardiography are aortic stenosis, hypertrophic cardiomyopathy, and atrial myxomas.

Holter Monitoring

Continuous ECG monitoring or Holter monitoring is indicated in patients suspected of having an arrhythmic cause of syncope on the basis of clinical history, physical examination, abnormal ECG, or structural heart disease. Overall, Holter monitoring is of low (about 4%)[5] diagnostic yield in the evaluation of patients with syncope, unless the arrhythmia occurs during an episode of syncope or presyncope. Detection of syncope or presyncope in the absence of an arrhythmia is also useful, although this does not exclude arrhythmia as the etiology of the symptoms.

Event Recording Devices

Event monitors are indicated in the evaluation of infrequent but recurrent episodes of presyncope or syncope. There are two forms of loop recorders:

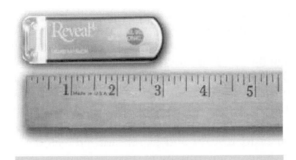

Figure 6-2 **Medtronic's Reveal implantable loop recorder.**

those worn or carried by the patient for weeks to months and those that are implanted for extended recording periods (from 18 to 24 months). The patient can activate both during and after an episode of presyncope or syncope. When activated, these devices are programmed to record the previous 4–5 minutes and the ensuing 1 minute. The implantable event monitor (Medtronic's Reveal) (Figs. 6-2 and 6-3) is meant for those patients who have extremely infrequent episodes of syncope (once or twice a year). This small leadless device, which incorporates two leads in its can, is implanted in the subcutaneous tissue of the chest, and can be triggered by the patient or automatically on the basis of programmed criteria. The diagnostic yield is 43–88% when used in selected population of patients, where there is a high probability of an arrhythmic etiology of the syncope.[6–8]

Signal-Averaged Electrocardiography

Signal-averaged electrocardiography (SAECG) is not recommended as part of the evaluation of syncope and presyncope. This is a noninvasive technique where 100–300 single QRS complexes are amplified, filtered for noise, and averaged to determine the low-amplitude, high-frequency signals in the

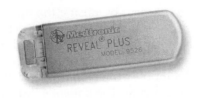

Figure 6-3 **Magnified Medtronic's Reveal plus implantable loop recorder.**

terminal portion of the QRS complex (late potentials). These late potentials are substrates for ventricular arrhythmias. Criteria for late potentials include total QRS duration >114 milliseconds, <20 Micro-V of root-mean-square signal amplitude in the last 40 milliseconds of the QRS complex, or duration of the terminal QRS complex remains longer than 38 milliseconds. SAECG cannot be used in patients with a bundle branch block or nonspecific intraventricular conduction delay as it is impossible to distinguish between late activation due to the conduction defect and the reentrant substrate. Patients with structural heart disease and significant left ventricular dysfunction with high probability of an arrhythmic etiology for their symptoms are more likely to benefit from an invasive electrophysiologic (EP) study. The SAECG has an excellent negative predictive value and is best used in the evaluation of certain high-risk patients (e.g., patients with possible arrhythmogenic right ventricular dysplasia and infiltrative cardiomyopathy).

Invasive Electrophysiologic Evaluation

Electrophysiologic testing is generally indicated in the patient with underlying structural heart disease and nonsustained ventricular tachycardia; documented supraventricular or ventricular arrhythmias amenable to radiofrequency ablative therapy; unexplained syncope; and those with syncope and evidence on ECG of SA nodal or AV nodal disease. The EP study can establish a diagnosis of sick sinus syndrome, carotid sinus hypersensitivity, conduction defects, supraventricular tachycardia, or ventricular tachycardia. However, role of EP testing in the evaluation of the patient with no structural heart disease and a negative head-up tilt-table test remains controversial.

TILT-Table Test

The tilt-table test has emerged as a valuable tool in not only determining the cause of syncope in patients who are susceptible to neurocardiogenic syncope, but also in shedding light as to the exact mechanism. TTT is not the initial procedure of choice in patients with structural heart disease; however, TTT should be considered early in the work-up of patients with no evidence of cardiac disease.

There is a great deal of variation in the protocols used in TTT. However, most protocols test the patient by raising the tilt to an angle varying from 60–80° (Fig. 6-4), for 30–45 minutes. In addition to the standard head-up tilt-table test, pharmacologic provocation is used to enhance sensitivity. Pharmacologic provocation is accomplished with either nitroglycerin or isoproterenol. The endpoint of this test is termination of the protocol or once syncope or presyncope occurs. The patient's heart rate and blood pressure are constantly monitored throughout the protocol.

There are several different hemodynamic responses to TTT and it is important to distinguish the hemodynamic pattern of neurocardiogenic

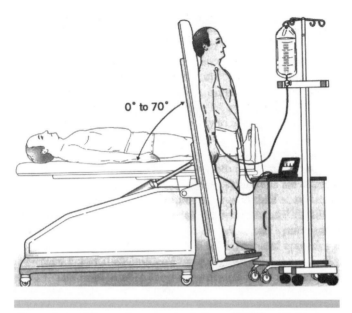

Figure 6-4 **Schematic representation of a tilt-table test.**

syncope from dysautonomic response. TTT can also distinguish the vagal response from that elicited in patients with POTS. Table 6-2 summarizes the various responses possible during upright TTT. It should be noted that although TTT is effective in the diagnosis of these disorders, once identified, TTT is not useful in monitoring therapeutic efficacy.

There are three types of responses that are characteristic of neurocardiogenic syncope, and one characterized as pure orthostasis.

1. *Mixed response (type 1)*: Immediately after head-up tilt, the heart rate increases appropriately and the blood pressure also increases slightly. The blood pressure remains stable and the heart rate increases slightly during the head-up tilt period. With the onset of syncope or presyncope, there is a collapse in blood pressure that occurs prior to a mild reduction or no change in the heart rate. In this type of response, the heart rate does not fall below 40 beats per minute for >10 seconds. Figure 6-5 is an example of this type of response.
2. *Cardioinhibitory response (type 2)*: Cardioinhibitory syncope is characterized by a decrease in heart rate to a ventricular rate of <40 beats per minute for >10 seconds or with an asystolic pause >3 seconds. The blood pressure clearly decreases after the decrease in heart rate. Restoration of heart rate occurs after the patient resumes the recumbent position. Figure 6-6 is an example of this hemodynamic response.

Table 6-2 **Hemodynamic Responses to TTT**

Syndrome	Immediate Response	During TTT	Syncopal Crisis
Mixed vasovagal syncope (type 1)	HR increases and BP increases slightly	BP remains stable and HR increases slightly	Collapse in BP precedes mild decline in HR
Cardioinhibitory syncope (type 2)	HR increases moderately and BP somewhat unstable	BP is somewhat unstable	Collapse in BP occurs during or before significant bradycardia lasting >10 seconds or asystolic pause lasting >3 seconds
Pure vasodepressor (type 3)	HR increases and BP increases	BP decreases throughout tilt period	BP collapse with only a slight decrease in HR
Dysautonomia	Gradual decrease in BP	Gradual and progressive decrease in BP, with only a small change in HR	BP collapse accompanied by drop in HR
POTS	Early and sustained modest increase in HR	Continued increase in HR, with progressive decrease in BP	Abrupt collapse in BP and HR

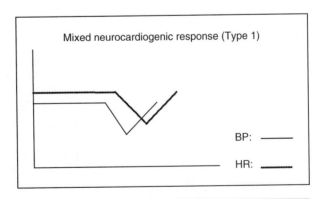

Figure 6-5 **Mixed response (type 1) tilt-table test results.**

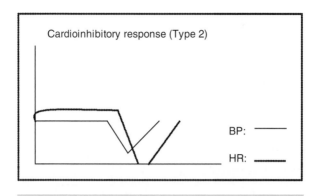

Figures 6-6 **Cardioinhibitory response (type 2) tilt-table test results.**

3. *Vasodepressor response (type 3)*: Hypotension heralds the onset of syncope, with a concomitant reduction in the heart rate to >40 beats per minute for >10 seconds. Figure 6-7 portrays this syndrome.
4. *Orthostatic response*: On assumption of the upright position, the patient develops hypotension with an appropriate increase in heart rate.

On the other hand, patients with a dysautonomia demonstrate a gradual and progressive decrease in blood pressure, usually with a small or insignificant change in heart rate which represents a failure of the cardiovascular system to adapt to the hemodynamic stress of upright posture. In contrast, patients with POTS demonstrate an early and sustained increase in heart rate, often associated with a progressive decrease in blood pressure.

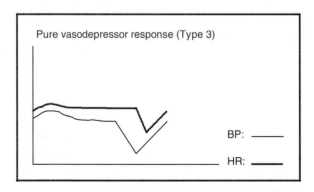

Figure 6-7 **Vasodepressor response (type 3) tilt-table test results.**

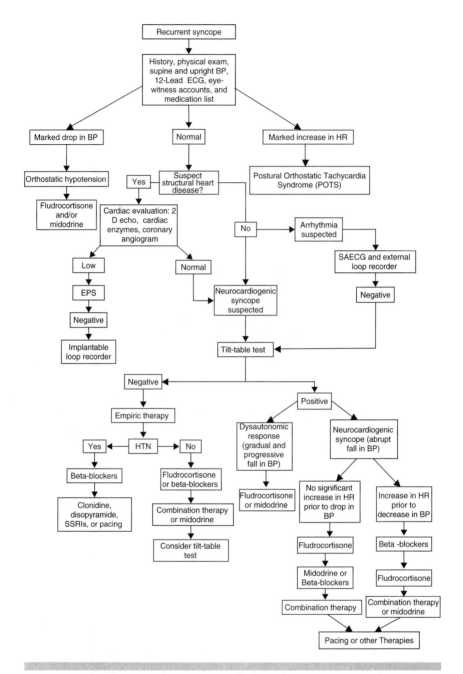

Figure 6-8 **Syncope testing and therapy algorithm.**

Although uncommon, the episode of tachycardia can be associated with a dramatic decrease in blood pressure and frank syncope.

Adenosine Triphosphate Test

Adenosine triphosphate (ATP) has been suggested to aid in the diagnosis of patients with unexplained syncope caused by transient atrioventricular (AV) block. The patient is kept supine with continuous electrocardiographic monitoring, and 20 mg of ATP is administered intravenously. Asystole lasting longer than 6 seconds or AV block lasting longer than 10 seconds is indicative of a positive test for transient AV block. ATP testing to determine transient block is still considered an investigational tool.

Carotid Sinus Massage

Carotid sinus massage (CSM) is recommended in patients over 40 years of age presenting with syncope of unknown cause. CSM is performed while monitoring both the electrocardiogram and blood pressure. CSM should be performed while the patient is in the supine and standing positions, and for a minimum of 5 minutes but no longer than 10 minutes. CSM should be avoided in patients at risk of stroke and those with carotid bruits. Figure 6-8 presents an algorithm for the work-up and treatment (discussed later) of recurrent synoscope.

CURRENTLY AVAILABLE PHARMACOLOGIC THERAPY AND PATIENT FOLLOW-UP

Pharmacologic Therapy

When considering the use of pharmacologic agents in the treatment of neurocardiogenic syncope, it is important to remember that the various components comprising this entity are reflex-mediated.

The body's sodium content determines the volume of extracellular fluid, including plasma. Therefore, the initial treatment of this spectrum of disorders involves increasing one's intravascular volume in an attempt to mute the hemodynamic impact of venous pooling. This may be accomplished by increasing one's dietary salt and fluid intake. Patients must be counseled to avoid recognizable triggers (i.e., extreme heat, dehydration, or postexertional standing).

In most instances, however, pharmacotherapy in combination with conservative management is required for effective treatment. The following agents are used in the treatment of neurocardiogenic syncope.

BETA-ADRENERGIC BLOCKING AGENTS

This class of pharmacologic agents have been the most widely used agents in the treatment of neurocardiogenic syncope. These agents mute the effects of the high level of circulating catecholamines and work to block the stimulation of the cardiac mechanoreceptors. Although widely used, there have been no prospective trials testing the efficacy of these agents in the treatment of this spectrum of disorders.

Side effects associated with the use of these agents include fatigue, symptomatic bradycardia, sexual dysfunction, bronchospasm, and rarely AV block.

FLUDROCORTISONE

Fludrocortisone is a mineralocorticoid commonly used to treat patients with neurocardiogenic syncope secondary to a significant vasodepressor component. Fludrocortisone acts by increasing the renal absorption of sodium resulting in an increase in intravascular volume. As in all volume expanders, care must be taken in treating patients with hypertension. Fludrocortisone may increase the sensitivity of the peripheral vascular circulation to circulating catecholamines, thereby augmenting the vasoconstrictive effects of norepinephrine.

Side effects associated with fludrocortisone include hypertension, peripheral edema, acne, depression, and (in rare instances) hypokalemia. Data supporting the value of fludrocortisone for the treatment of vasodepressor syncope are limited. Despite this, because fludrocortisone is not associated with serious organ toxicity, it is often considered early in the management of neurocardiogenic syncope.

ALPHA$_1$-AGONISTS

Midodrine is a selective alpha$_1$-adrenergic agonist, whose action increases the peripheral vascular resistance and decreases venous capacitance. Side effects associated with midodrine include scalp itching, paresthesias, chills, urinary retention, and supine hypertension.

Although midodrine and etilefrine are both peripherally acting alpha-adrenergic agonists, etilefrine was not shown to be effective in preventing syncope. It is unclear why midodrine is effective in preventing this disorder.

Methylphenidate is a central nervous system stimulant that has peripheral vasoconstrictor properties, making it attractive for patients with vasodepressor (type 3) syncope.

Dextroamphetamine, a potent central and peripheral adrenergic agonist, has been evaluated for the treatment of vasodepressor syncope. Despite being a potent vasoconstrictor, its potential for abuse may make it an unattractive option.

Prospective clinical trial data have confirmed the efficacy of midodrine in the treatment of vasodepressor syncope.[1]

SELECTIVE SEROTONIN REUPTAKE INHIBITORS

Serotonin is believed to play a role in the development of hypotension and bradycardia during vasovagal syncope. Selective serotonin reuptake inhibitors (SSRIs) prevent reuptake of serotonin at the synaptic cleft. This produces a downregulation in postsynaptic serotonin receptor density in response to increased intrasynaptic serotonin concentrations, therefore, attenuating the response to serotonin. This class of agents includes sertraline, fluoxetine, and paroxetine. The efficacy of paroxetine has been shown in a prospective clinical trial in the treatment of neurocardiogenic syncope.[5]

Side effects associated with SSRIs include anxiety, insomnia, somnolence, headache, anorexia, drowsiness, and fatigue.

Alternative Pharmacologic Therapy

DISOPYRAMIDE

Disopyramide, a class IA antiarrhythmic agent, is considered beneficial in the treatment of neurocardiogenic syncope. The negative inotropic, anticholinergic, and direct peripheral vasoconstrictive effects of disopyramide are useful in the treatment of this disorder. Disopyramide has been found to be useful in patients who have failed beta-blockers therapy, especially if treatment with beta-blockers is associated with bradycardia or asystole.

Side effects associated with disopyramide stem from its anticholinergic action, which includes dry mouth, blurred vision, constipation, and urinary retention. Rarely, patients on disopyramide can develop torsades de pointes. As a direct result of its side effect profile and proarrhythmic potential, disopyramide is not considered first-line therapy, and is reserved for the subset of patients refractory to other treatments.

CLONIDINE

Clonidine, a selective alpha$_2$-adrenergic receptor agonist, has been proposed in the treatment of neurocardiogenic syncope. The ability of clonidine to reduce venous capacitance is thought to be the potential mechanism of action. However, there are no prospective data proving this drug's efficacy in the treatment of this syndrome. Potential side effects include hypotension and profound hypertension on drug withdrawal.

ROLE OF ALTERNATIVE NONPHARMACOLOGIC THERAPY

Vasovagal syncope is rarely life threatening, however, one potential risk factor for SCD is documented asystole during a spontaneous episode. In contrast, asystole during TTT is not associated with a higher mortality. Although mortality is not increased, patients with frequent vasovagal syncope have a poor quality of life. In terms of physical and psychosocial function, patients with recurrent syncope have a level of impairment comparable to patients afflicted with severe rheumatoid arthritis, chronic low-back pain, and institutionalized psychiatric patients.[3]

Several clinical studies have demonstrated that patients are much less likely to faint after receiving a permanent pacemaker.[9,10] In principle, the role of cardiac pacing is to overcome the transient bradycardia, which occurs during syncope, providing enough heart rate support to compensate for the transient hypotension that often accompanies cardioinhibitory syncope.

It is imperative, following the insertion of a permanent pacemaker, that one programs an effective pacing strategy once bradycardia is detected. It should be noted that patients who do not exhibit significant bradycardia during neurally mediated syncope are not likely to benefit from the insertion of a permanent pacemaker.

The simplest overall pacing strategy is to pace empirically with single-chamber devices programmed at a fixed lower rate. With advancements in pacemaker programmability more options are currently available. The three programming options include rate smoothing, rate hysteresis, and rate-drop response. Independent of the programming feature used, 50% of patients have no further fainting spells and the remainder have shown significant clinical improvement.[10]

Alternate sensing strategies, such as monitoring the QT interval, right ventricular pressure, core temperature, and various indices of contractility, are under investigation. The latter can be estimated with online impedance cardiography or online ventricular lead accelerometry. The theory behind contractility sensors is that neurocardiogenic syncope might be preceded by small but significant increases in contractility due to a sympathetic surge. These pacemakers increase pacing rates in response to rises in apparent contractility, and then slowly decrease their rates after contractility returns to baseline.

Pacemakers should be considered for patients with frequent and medically refractory neurally mediated syncope, especially if they exhibit a significant cardioinhibitory component. In equivocal cases, TTT with invasive hemodynamic monitoring (e.g., arterial line) and temporary atrial and ventricular pacing may document the benefit of pacing in drug refractory patients.

Indications for Hospitalization

The decision to hospitalize a patient with syncope is a complex process. In patients with structural heart disease and syncope it is prudent that the work-up be undertaken in the in-patient setting. Risk stratification in a monitored setting is imperative. Patients with strong family history of SCD who exhibit exertional syncope, and have suffered significant injuries should also be hospitalized.

Patients with no significant cardiac dysfunction, a normal baseline 12-lead ECG, and a high probability of neurocardiogenic syncope are at low risk of SCD. An outpatient work-up is more appropriate for this patient population.

CONCLUSION

Long-standing diabetes predisposes to an increased risk of development of renal dysfunction, cardiovascular disease, peripheral vascular disease, primary cardiomyopathy, retinal damage, and syncope. The above treatise focused on the work-up of the patient who presents following an episode of syncope. In the patient with the structural heart disease the work-up includes appropriate risk stratification for SCD. Paradoxically, the work-up and determination of the cause of syncope in a patient with no apparent heart disease is often elusive. Especially in the elderly diabetic patient, postural adaptation is often less brisk than in the younger or nondiabetic patient. The above discussion attempted to focus the practitioner in the available therapies for patients suffering from the various positional and neurally mediated syndromes.

REFERENCES

1. Grubb BP, Sutton R, Bloomfield DM, et al. A symposium: treatment for patients with vasovagal syncope. *Am J Cardiol* 1999;84:1Q–39Q.

2. Grubb BP. Neurocardiogenic syncope and related disorders of orthostatic intolerance. *Circulation* 2005;111:2297–3006.

3. Grubb BP. Neurocardiogenic syncope. *N Engl J Med* 2005;352:1004–1010.

4. Kapoor WN. Syncope: review article. *N Engl J Med* 2000;343:1856–1862.

5. Grubb BP, Jorge SdC. A review of the classification, diagnosis, and management of autonomic dysfunction syndromes associated with orthostatic intolerance. *Arq Bras Cardiol* 2000;74(6):545–552.

6. Krahn AD, Klein GJ, Yee R, et al. Cost implications of testing strategy in patients with syncope (RAST). *J Am Coll Cardiol* 2003;42:495–501.

7. Krahn AD, Klein GJ, Yee R, et al. Final results from a pilot study with an implantable loop recorder to determine the etiology of syncope in patients with negative noninvasive and invasive testing. *Am J Cardiol* 1998;82(1):117–119.

8. Krahn AD, Klein GJ, Yee R, et al. Use of extended monitoring strategy in patients with problematic syncope. *Circulation* 1999;99:406–410.

9. Connoly SJ, Sheldon R, Roberts R, et al. The North American Vasovagal Pacemaker Study: a randomized trial of permanent cardiac pacing for the prevention of vasovagal syncope. *J Am Coll Cardiol* 1999;333:16–20.

10. Benditt DG, Petersen M, Lurie KG, et al. Cardiac pacing for prevention of recurrent vasovagal syncope. *Ann Intern Med* 1995;122:204–209.

DIABETIC
CARDIOMYOPATHY

Judith E. Mitchell

ESSENTIALS OF DIAGNOSIS

- Diabetic cardiomyopathy is generally regarded as a unique pathologic and clinical entity marked by diffuse myocardial fibrosis and hypertrophy that may result in the emergence of progressive left ventricular dysfunction and congestive heart failure (HF).
- It is diagnosed by evidence of left ventricular dysfunction in the absence of structural heart disease (e.g., coronary, hypertensive, valvular, and congenital) or other cause of secondary cardiomyopathy (e.g., toxic, infectious, and familial).
- Patients may present with typical signs and symptoms of congestive HF: dyspnea, edema, and effort intolerance.
- However, patients may be also be asymptomatic:
- Echocardiographic parameters of diastolic dysfunction precede change in ejection fraction but may go unnoticed due to the absence of symptoms.
- Electrocardiogram, chest x-ray, and brain natriuretic peptide levels may be normal before the onset of HF or left ventricular hypertrophy.
- Diabetic patients are also at high risk of developing concomitant cardiovascular disease (CVD), especially hypertension and coronary heart disease (CHD), which creates a combined clinical presentation including left ventricular hypertrophy and HF.
- Diabetic cardiomyopathy is common in patients with both type 1 (insulin-dependent) and type 2 (non-insulin-dependent) diabetes mellitus and, because of its high prevalence, should even be suspected in patients with impaired glucose tolerance (prediabetes).
- The presence of microalbuminuria increases the likelihood of diabetic cardiomyopathy.

GENERAL CONSIDERATIONS

HF affects an estimated 5 million people and 550,000 new cases are diagnosed each year. The direct and indirect costs due to HF total $27.9 billion.[1] Its incidence has been rising and is expected to double and affect an estimated 10 million people in the next 25 years (Fig. 7-1).[2]

Hospital discharges for HF rose by 157% for a total of 970,000 discharges in 2002, and almost 58,000 people died of HF in 2001. Compared to the overall death rate increase (7.7%), HF-related mortality has increased 35.5% in the last decade alone and the prognosis is grim after congestive HF is diagnosed. One in five patients die within 1 year and the majority of patients die within 8 years.[1]

Although its prevalence is similar in men and women (2.6% and 2.1% of the general population, respectively), its prevalence increases with age. At age 40, women have a higher lifetime risk of HF than men, which may be attributed to their longer life expectancy. Interestingly, women and the

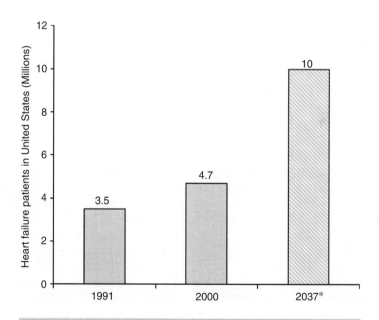

Figure 7-1 *Epidemiology of heart failure in the United States.* (Source: Adapted from American Heart Association. Heart Disease and Stroke Statistics—2005 Update. Dallas, TX: American Heart Association, 2005; Rich MW. Epidemiology, pathophysiology, and etiology of congestive heart failure in older adults. J Am Geriatr Soc 1997;45:968–974.)

elderly are two populations whose survival has not improved. In fact, women account for 60% of all HF-related deaths and fewer than 15% of women survive longer than 8–12 years of a HF diagnosis.[1]

HF also disproportionately affects minorities. It affects 3.1% and 3.5% of black men and women, respectively, who are also at increased risk of mortality. In comparison to the overall death rate for congestive HF (18.7), death rates were 21.7 for black males, 19.6 for white males, 18.8 for black females, and 18.1 for white females.[1] African Americans, Hispanics, and American Indians also have a higher prevalence of HF hospitalization than that of whites.[3]

Diabetes is a growing epidemic in the United States that is expected to worsen (Fig. 7-2).[4] Diabetes contributes to HF development and its prognosis, like HF, is expected to worsen. It currently affects over 18 million people, about one-third of whom are unaware that they even have the disease, and its prevalence is expected to nearly double over the next 25 years.[5,6] This dramatic growth is due in part to the aging of the population and the increasing prevalence of obesity and physical inactivity.[6]

Diabetes and hypertension are two of the most important risk factors in the development of HF; 75% of cases have antecedent hypertension and, among women, the presence of diabetes was the most powerful risk factor in predicting CHD.[1] Importantly, both diabetic and prediabetic individuals are at substantially increased risk of developing CVD and there may be underlying processes responsible for the high prevalence of hypertension, dyslipidemia, and CVD in diabetic patients.[5,7] CVD is the leading cause of diabetes-related death, responsible for up to three-fourths of all diabetic mortality.[1]

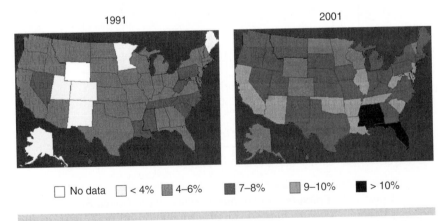

Figure 7-2 **Prevalence of diabetes among adults in the United States.** (*Source: Adapted from Mokdad AH, Ford ES, Bowman BA, et al. Prevalence of obesity, diabetes, and obesity-related health risk factors, 2001. JAMA 2003; 289:76–79.*)

Rubler et al. first described a distinctive cardiomyopathy in diabetic patients without hypertension or coronary or valvular disease in 1972 (Fig. 7-3).[8] The Framingham Heart Study later found that HF was twice as common in diabetic men and five times as common in diabetic women as in age-matched controls.[9] The overall prevalence of diabetes in major clinical HF trials is more than three times higher than that in the general American population, 22% compared with 6.3%.[5,10] Moreover, HF may actually have been underrepresented in these clinical trials, since exclusion criteria, such as impaired renal function, are often used that bias selection against diabetes. Registry data in hospitalized HF patients suggest that the prevalence of diabetes in HF patients may be as high as 44%.[11] Registry data have shown that the prevalence and impact of diabetes in the African

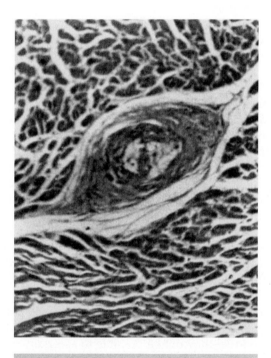

Figure 7-3 **Section of myocardium showing a small intramural coronary arteriole with thickening of the wall due to fibrosis and accumulation of acid-staining mucopolysaccharide material.** *(Source: Adapted from Rubler S, Dlugash J, Yuceoglu YZ, et al. New type of cardiomyopathy associated with diabetic glomerulosclerosis. Am J Cardiol 1972;30: 595–602.)*

American population may be even greater. In a registry of 286 patients, 92% black, consecutively admitted with HF, approximately 50% of the patients hospitalized with HF had diabetes.[12] The contribution of diabetes to the development and progression of HF in African Americans with the associated worsened prognosis should be of particular concern to the physician.

The earliest discernable evidence of diabetic cardiomyopathy is increased diastolic myocardial stiffness in the presence of normal left ventricular systolic function and mass. The incidence of left ventricular diastolic dysfunction has been reported to be as high as 50–60% even in patients with well-controlled type 2 diabetes and without hypertension, structural heart disease, or HF.[13,14] Similarly, in a large unselected community population, 48% of all diabetic individuals were found to have measurable left ventricular diastolic dysfunction.[15]

The evidence continues to mount in other trials. A large, nationwide, case-control study found that patients diagnosed with idiopathic cardiomyopathy characterized by decreased systolic function and ventricular dilatation were 75% more likely to have diabetes than control subjects.[16] The Strong Heart Study observed that diabetic subjects had significantly reduced echocardiographic parameters of left ventricular systolic function when compared to nondiabetic subjects.[17] A longitudinal study in Uppsala County, Sweden, found that the presence of factors associated with insulin resistance, such as proinsulin levels, in 50-year-old men without heart disease predicted the development of left ventricular systolic dysfunction (ejection fraction <40%) 20 years later at age 70.[18] Evidence of subclinical systolic dysfunction has also been reported as an early manifestation of diabetic cardiomyopathy in diabetic patients with no overt CVD and preserved systolic function (ejection fraction >50%). Systolic function was inversely related to glycated hemoglobin A1c (HbA1c) levels.[19–21] Because of the large amount of data, the presence of diabetic cardiomyopathy is generally accepted.

Isolated diabetic cardiomyopathy can also result in left ventricular hypertrophy. However, since more than 70% of diabetic patients have concomitant hypertension,[5] the specific etiology of left ventricular hypertrophy in a diabetic individual may not be possible to ascertain. Furthermore, isolated diabetic cardiomyopathy is rarely symptomatic in the absence of hypertension or myocardial ischemia.[22] The Framingham Heart Study found that hyperglycemia and insulin resistance, the primary markers of type 2 diabetes, were related to left ventricular mass, especially in women.[23] Thirty-two percent of patients with type 2 diabetes were found to have evidence of left ventricular hypertrophy independent of blood pressure.[24] Interestingly, even in nondiabetic individuals with borderline or mild hypertension, insulin sensitivity was found to be related to left ventricular mass independent of blood pressure.[25]

PATHOGENESIS

Both type 1 and 2 diabetes lead to chronic hyperglycemia and type 2 diabetes leads to compensatory hyperinsulinemia. Left ventricular diastolic dysfunction associated with diabetic cardiomyopathy is primarily due to qualitative and quantitative changes in interstitial collagen.[22] In the presence of chronic hyperglycemia, collagen becomes irreversibly bound to advanced glycosylation end products (AGEs) that, in turn, form covalent cross-links throughout the collagen molecule, increase myocardial stiffness, and decrease ventricular compliance.[26] AGEs may also promote increased fibrosis through specific AGE cell surface receptors that upregulate the expression of prosclerotic cytokines.[27]

In addition to these structural changes, functional changes in diastolic relaxation may also occur. Cyclical diastolic removal of intracellular calcium can be slowed through the inhibition of sarcoplasmic reticulum calcium ATPase (SERCA2) activity by AGE binding and SERCA2 downregulation.[28] Hyperinsulinemia also contributes to left ventricular diastolic dysfunction by stimulating myocardial hypertrophy, possibly through growth factor receptor activation or increased sympathetic nervous system activity.[25]

A metabolic hypothesis has been proposed to explain the progression of diabetic cardiomyopathy from early diastolic abnormalities to the eventual development of contractile dysfunction. Intracellular fatty acids are increased in the early insulin-resistant state, and cardiac myocytes respond to this increase by upregulating the expression of the enzymes necessary for their disposal. These enzymes are controlled by the nuclear transcription factor peroxisome proliferator-activated receptor alpha (PPARα) that increases in response to diabetic hyperlipidemia.

During the progression of diabetes, however, the expression of PPARα undergoes a dramatic decrease and cardiac myocytes are unable to metabolize their increased fatty acid load. The subsequent accumulation of intracellular lipids can result in the increased production of the toxic lipid product ceramide, which is associated with increased oxidative stress, apoptosis, and decreased contractile function.[29] In an experimental animal model of diabetes marked by intracellular triglyceride accumulation, high ceramide levels, and apoptosis, the PPARα agonist troglitazone reduced myocardial triglycerides, ceramide, and evidence of apoptosis and preserved normal contractile function.[30] Other mechanisms have been proposed to account for decreased systolic function in diabetic cardiomyopathy. These include ischemia due to microvascular disease or dysregulation, altered myocardial energy metabolism, and hyperglycemia-induced increases in protein kinase C (PKC)-β_2 activity and oxidative stress. Increased PKC activity ultimately results in myocardial necrosis and fibrosis and oxidative stress leads to a wide variety of potentially harmful responses including myocardial inflammation, defective calcium transport, mitochondrial dysfunction, and apoptosis.[22,29,31]

PREVENTION

Well-controlled diabetes is the goal in every diabetic patient and due to the high incidence of asymptomatic diabetic cardiomyopathy in diabetic patients, every effort should be made to retard the development of systolic dysfunction and clinical HF by intensive glycemic control and aggressive blood pressure management. In addition to pharmacologic therapy, non-pharmacologic measures such as smoking cessation, diet, and exercise may help maintain glycemic control. The American Diabetes Association recommends that HbA1c levels be maintained below 7%.[32] Controlling for other CVD risk factors such as hypertension, dyslipidemia, and obesity is also important. The seventh report of the Joint National Committee on Prevention, Detection, Evaluation, and Treatment of High Blood Pressure (JNC 7) recommends blood pressure <130/80 mmHg in diabetic patients[33] and the National Cholesterol Education Project Adult Treatment Panel (NCEP ATP III) recommends total cholesterol <200 mg/dL and high-density lipoprotein cholesterol (HDL) ≥60 mg/dL. Optimal low-density lipoprotein cholesterol (LDL) levels are determined by a patient's CHD risk level and diabetic patients with CVD, who are in the highest risk category, are advised to keep LDL levels <70 mg/dL (Table 7-1).[34,35] The use of agents that ameliorate the morphologic changes seen in diabetic cardiomyopathy, which are discussed in the treatment section, may help prevent or at the very least delay its onset.

Table 7-1 **Current Treatment Recommendations for Patients with Type 2 Diabetes**

Parameter	Goal
Total cholesterol	200 mg/dL
Triglycerides	<150 mg/dL
LDL cholesterol	<100 mg/dL (optional goal: <70 mg/dL)
HDL cholesterol	>45 mg/dL, men
	>55 mg/dL, women
HbA1c	<7%
Preprandial plasma glucose	<90–130 mg/dL
Blood pressure	<130/80 mmHg

Source: Data compiled from Refs. 32–35.

CLINICAL FINDINGS

Symptoms and Signs

Diabetic cardiomyopathy may have a long asymptomatic period, especially in patients with type 2 diabetes, and its earliest presentation may often be due to concomitant hypertension or CHD. Left ventricular diastolic dysfunction is indicated by a decreased rate of early diastolic filling and a compensatory increase in late diastolic filling with a greater dependence on atrial systole for left ventricular filling as well as a prolongation of isovolumetric relaxation.[36] The subsequent presentation of systolic dysfunction is indistinguishable from other dilated cardiomyopathies with variable symptoms of congestive HF including exertional dyspnea, orthopnea, effort intolerance, fatigue, and peripheral edema. However, diabetic patients with clinical HF as well as those with asymptomatic left ventricular systolic dysfunction have been found to have significantly worse outcomes including myocardial infarction (MI), angina, pulmonary edema, HF hospitalization, and death than their nondiabetic counterparts.[37] An asymptomatic diabetic patient may show subtle signs of diabetic cardiomyopathy related to decreased left ventricular compliance and/or left ventricular hypertrophy. Physical examination may demonstrate prominence of an "a" wave in the jugular venous pulse, and the cardiac apical impulse may be overactive or sustained throughout systole rather than normally tapping. Auscultation may reveal a fourth heart sound. After the development of systolic dysfunction, left ventricular dilatation, and symptomatic HF, the jugular venous pressure may become elevated, the apical impulse displaced downward and to the left, and a third heart sound may be heard as well as a systolic mitral valve murmur.

Laboratory Findings

Several laboratory studies may also be useful. The likelihood of developing clinical HF has been strongly correlated to the degree of chronic hyperglycemia as indicated by HbA1c levels in large observational studies. The Kaiser-Permanente study of nearly 50,000 adults with predominantly type 2 diabetes who were followed for an average of 2.2 years observed an independent, graded association between hyperglycemia and the incidence of HF. Each 1% increase in HbA1c was associated with an 8% increased risk of developing HF.[38] Similarly, the United Kingdom Prospective Diabetes Study (UKPDS) reported that the incidence of HF increased from 2.3 cases per 1000 person-years for HbA1c levels <6% to 11.9 cases per 1000 person-years for HbA1c levels ≥10%. In addition to HF, HbA1c levels predict CHD events in patients with type 2 diabetes.[39] In the European Prospective Investigation into Cancer in Norfolk (EPIC-Norfolk), a prospective population study of 4662 men

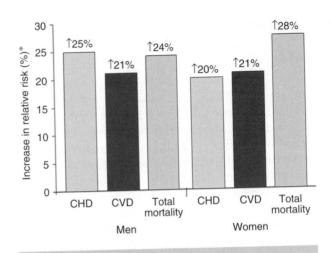

Figure 7-4 **EPIC-Norfolk Study: every 1% increase in HbA1c increased cardiovascular risk. *Multivariate regression adjusted for age and risk factor.** (Source: Adapted from Khaw KT, Wareham N, Bingham S, et al. Association of hemoglobin A1c with cardiovascular disease and mortality in adults: the European Prospective Investigation into Cancer in Norfolk. Ann Intern Med 2004;141:413–420.)

and 5570 women followed for 6 years, every 1% increase in HbA1c increased the risk of cardiovascular events dramatically (Fig. 7-4).[40]

Each 1% decrease in HbA1c was associated with decrease a number of adverse outcomes, including death.[41] Albuminuria has also been found to be associated with left ventricular dysfunction in type 2 diabetes. In the Strong Heart Study, Doppler echocardiographic parameters of both diastolic and systolic functions were significantly related to the presence of micro- and macroalbuminuria in over 1500 type 2 diabetic subjects.[42] UKPDS also found microalbuminuria to be associated with abnormal electrocardiograms in type 2 diabetics.[43]

Imaging Studies

Several studies have documented a variety of electrocardiographic changes that may be associated with diabetic cardiomyopathy in as many as 60% of patients without structural heart disease, although usually not in the early asymptomatic phase. The P-wave may be prolonged and notched with greater terminal negativity or have increased amplitude, and the PR interval may be prolonged. The QRS axis may be shifted to the left, and the QT_C interval may lengthen. There may also be a reduction in R- and T-wave voltage.[44,45] Although the findings are nonspecific in the general population, an abnormal ECG in the diabetic patient should prompt a cardiac evaluation.

TREATMENT

The presence of diabetes is so strongly associated with the development of HF in persons without overt CVD as well as its progression in those with established left ventricular dysfunction that the American College of Cardiology and American Heart Association (ACC/AHA) Joint Guidelines for the Evaluation and Management of Chronic Heart Failure has classified patients with diabetes as stage A HF patients (Fig. 7-5).[46] Patients with diabetes and established left ventricular systolic dysfunction but without clinical HF are classified as stage B HF patients, and those with symptomatic HF are considered stage C HF patients.

Accordingly, the pharmacologic treatment of diabetic patients, especially those with other cardiovascular risk factors, should be aimed at retarding the development and progression of left ventricular dysfunction in order to reduce the risk of cardiovascular morbidity and mortality. The high prevalence of diabetic cardiomyopathy in diabetic individuals and the increased

	Stage	Patient description
A	High risk for developing HF	• Hypertension • CAD • Diabetes mellitus • Family history of cardiomyopathy
B	Asymptomatic HF	• Previous MI • Left ventricular systolic dysfunction • Asymptomatic valvular disease
C	Symptomatic HF	• Known structural heart disease • Shortness of breath and fatigue • Reduced exercise tolerance
D	Refractory end-stage HF	• Marked symptoms at rest despite maximal medical therapy (e.g., those who are recurrently hospitalized or cannot be safely discharged from the hospital without specialized interventions)

Figure 7-5 **New approach to the classification of heart failure from the American College of Cardiology/American Heart Association. CAD, coronary artery disease.** *(Source: Adapted from Hunt SA, Abraham WT, Chin MG, et al. ACC/AHA 2005 Guideline Update for the Diagnosis and Management of Chronic Heart Failure in the Adult: a report of the American College of Cardiology/American Heart Association Task Force on Practice Guidelines, 2005.)*

cardiovascular risk from coexisting hypertension and CHD require that long-term management utilize a combined approach that maximizes treatment of diabetes, hypertension, and CHD.

Glycemic Control

The evidence from large observational studies cited in the preceding section demonstrates that the level of chronic hyperglycemia is strongly related to the risk of developing HF in patients with type 2 diabetes and provides a compelling reason for aggressive and early glycemic control. Results from UKPDS also show that pharmacologic control of hyperglycemia may lower the incidence of HF as well as the risk of diabetes-related death. These studies compared intensive glycemic control with oral hypoglycemic agents (sulfonylureas or metformin) or insulin to conventional dietary therapy over a 10-year follow-up period. Mean HbA1c levels were reduced to 7.0–7.4 with intensive drug therapy compared to 7.9–8.0 with conventional treatment. Patients treated with hypoglycemic therapy had a lower incidence of HF than those treated with conventional therapy. Patients receiving insulin or metformin had a 20% lower incidence of HF than conventionally treated patients. However, patients receiving sulfonylureas were not shown to demonstrate a consistent reduction in HF.[47,48]

Thiazolidinediones (TZDs), including pioglitazone and rosiglitazone, are effective oral antihyperglycemic drugs widely used to treat patients with type 2 diabetes. A third TZD, troglitazone, was withdrawn from clinical use due to severe hepatoxicity. TZDs are PPARα agonists that have been shown to prevent intracellular myocardial lipid accumulation, apoptosis, and systolic dysfunction in experimental animals. TZD use in patients with evidence of established HF is controversial because of their tendency to cause fluid retention, experienced mostly as peripheral edema. However, diabetic patients with established HF also appear to largely tolerate TZDs well without significant fluid retention, and the development of TZD-related fluid retention is not necessarily a sign of increased cardiac decompensation.[49] A large retrospective study using health insurance claims found that TZD use was associated with about a 60% relative increase in the risk of new-onset HF over a 40-month follow-up period for a 1.1% absolute annual risk increase.[50] However, a recent study of more than 1600 matched pairs of patients receiving pioglitazone or insulin for 2 years reported that TZD use was associated with significantly lower rates of new-onset HF than insulin (2% vs. 4%; hazard ratio 0.5; $P < 0.001$).[51] TZDs may be particularly useful in the early management of diabetic hyperglycemia in patients with dilated cardiomyopathy (DCM) but should be used cautiously in patients with severe symptomatic HF.

The nonpharmacologic management of diabetes through diet, weight loss, and exercise may be sufficient in some patients to adequately control HbA1c levels. Exercise, even without weight loss, has been shown to improve insulin sensitivity and decrease HbA1c as well as attenuate athero-genic dyslipidemia.[52,53]

Lipid-Lowering Agents

Intensive lipid management should be employed to lower CHD risk because diabetes is a powerful risk factor and MI is a major factor that advances asymptomatic diabetic cardiomyopathy to clinical HF. Diabetic patients often have an atherogenic dyslipidemia and symptomatic HF may emerge in diabetic patients with diabetic cardiomyopathy due to the clinical expression of CHD, especially MI. The primary goal, as in high-risk nondiabetics, is to achieve LDL levels <100 mg/dL at the very least and optimally to <70 mg/dL. A prospective study from UKPDS found that, of a number of factors, increased LDL and decreased HDL levels were the most important predictors of CHD, suggesting that diabetic patients may benefit from lipid-lowering therapy to a greater extent than the general population.[54]

Pharmacologic strategies aimed at preventing primary and secondary CHD events have been moderately successful, particularly through the widespread use of statins, which are the preferred drug to lower LDL. On average, statins are associated with a 30% reduction in LDL cholesterol levels and a 29% decrease in CHD mortality. Clinical trial data reveal that cholesterol-lowering therapies including statins were associated with a 17–42% decrease in CHD risk in diabetic patients. This decrease is comparable to the 21–32% risk reduction shown for nondiabetic subjects.[34]

A subgroup analysis of the Scandinavian Simvastatin Survival Study (4S) in 4242 patients with previous MI or angina examined 6-month survival in diabetic versus nondiabetic patients. Despite a similar lipid-lowering effect, nondiabetic patients had a 4% absolute survival difference (92% with treatment vs. 88% with placebo) whereas diabetic patients had a 15% survival difference (84% with simvastatin vs. 69% with placebo). The absolute benefit of statin therapy may actually be greater in diabetic than nondiabetic persons because diabetes significantly increases the risk of CHD-related death and cholesterol is a powerful predictor of CHD-related death in diabetic patients.[55]

These findings are further reinforced by data from the Heart Protection Study (HPS)[56] and the Collaborative Atorvastatin Diabetes Study (CARDS). In the 5-year, placebo-controlled HPS, lipid lowering with simvastatin 40 mg qd reduced cardiovascular morbidity and mortality to a similar or greater degree in diabetic compared with nondiabetic patients. Diabetic patients ($n = 5963$) who received simvastatin experienced a 22% reduction in major coronary events ($P < 0.0001$) and the results were consistent even when adjusted for differences in baseline patient characteristics; diabetic patients without occlusive coronary disease experienced a 33% reduction ($P = 0.0003$). CARDS exclusively studied 2838 diabetic patients without a history of CVD and found that atorvastatin 10 mg qd reduced major cardiovascular events by 36% ($P = 0.001$) and all-cause mortality by 27% compared with placebo after 4 years of follow-up.[57]

Bile acid sequestrants or ezetimibe may be added if statin therapy is insufficient. If baseline LDL levels are already <100 mg/dL but triglyceride levels are >200 mg/dL, a fibrate or low-dose niacin can be employed. Niacin also has been shown to significantly raise HDL levels. Although niacin may reduce insulin sensitivity, it has a modest effect on glycemic control and does not affect HbA1. Both fibrates and niacin can be combined with a statin, if necessary, to normalize blood lipid levels.[34]

Antihypertensives

The degree of blood pressure lowering achieved in hypertensive diabetic patients importantly impacts the reduction in cardiovascular complications including HF, MI, and death. UKPDS randomized 1148 hypertensive patients with type 2 diabetes to "tighter" (<150/85 mmHg) or "less tight" (<180/105 mmHg) blood pressure control for a mean treatment period of 8 years. Patients assigned to tighter blood pressure control experienced significantly lower rates of HF and diabetes-related death than those assigned to less stringent blood pressure control.[58] Similarly, 18,790 patients in the Hypertension Optimal Treatment (HOT) trial were randomized to three different diastolic blood pressure goals: ≤90, ≤85, or ≤80 mmHg. The trial included 1501 patients with diabetes who showed a decline in major cardiovascular events in relation to the assigned blood pressure target. Patients randomized to diastolic blood pressure ≤80 mmHg experienced half the incidence of MI, stroke, or death of those randomized to diastolic blood pressure ≤90 mmHg.[59]

However, the relative efficacy of specific antihypertensive agents is under debate and JNC 7 recommends the use of certain drugs in patients with diabetes (Table 7-2).[33] Hypertensive patients with type 2 diabetes in UKPDS ($n = 1148$) were randomized to receive treatment with either the angiotensin-converting enzyme (ACE) inhibitor captopril or the beta-blocker atenolol. After 9 years, both treatment regimens were associated with comparable reductions in cardiovascular events including HF, fatal and nonfatal MI, and death.[60] The Antihypertensive and Lipid Lowering Treatment to Prevent Heart Attack Trial (ALLHAT) is the largest randomized clinical hypertension trial. Performed to date in 10,000 patients, it found that after 8 years of treatment, the thiazide diuretic chlorthalidone resulted in larger reductions of cardiovascular endpoints in diabetic patients including HF and CHD events than the ACE inhibitor lisinopril or the calcium channel blocker (CCB) amlodipine.[61] However, in aggregate, most clinical trials suggest that the level of blood pressure lowering achieved is more important than the individual agent administered.

The blood pressure-lowering effects of ACE inhibitors and angiotensin receptor blockers (ARBs) have been found to be comparable to other antihypertensive agents in improving mortality risk,[62,63] and ACE inhibitors and

Table 7-2 **JNC 7 Treatment Recommendations**

Compelling Indication	Recommended Drug					
	Diuretic	Beta-Blocker	ACE Inhibitor	ARB	CCB	Aldosterone Antagonist
HF	X	X	X	X		X
Post-MI		X	X			X
High coronary disease risk	X	X	X		X	
Diabetes	X	X	X	X	X	
Chronic kidney disease			X	X		
Recurrent stroke prevention	X		X			

Source: Data compiled from Ref. 33.

ARBs have demonstrated important mortality and morbidity advantages beyond their hypotensive effects in high-risk patients, including those with diabetes. The Heart Outcomes Prevention Evaluation (HOPE) randomized over 9000 patients considered to be at high cardiovascular risk, including 3577 persons with diabetes, to ramipril or placebo for 5 years. Despite modest blood pressure lowering (2/3 mmHg), ramipril-treated patients with diabetes experienced a 37% reduction in cardiovascular death, a 22% reduction in MI, and a 20% reduction in HF compared with placebo-treated patients. Also, significantly fewer ramipril-treated patients developed overt nephropathy. Mean HbA1c levels increased 2.2% over 2 years with placebo treatment but fell 0.1% with ramipril treatment.[64]

The EURopean trial On reduction of cardiac events with Perindopril in stable coronary Artery disease (EUROPA) also evaluated treatment with perindopril in a randomized placebo-controlled study of 12,218 patients with established CHD, of whom 12% were diabetic. Cardiovascular endpoints were significantly reduced by the ACE inhibitor and were comparable in diabetic and nondiabetic subjects at the end of 4 years. Blood pressure reductions were not great, although somewhat more than in HOPE (5/2 mmHg).[65]

Diabetic patients with hypertension and left ventricular hypertrophy ($n = 1195$) treated with the ARB losartan in Losartan Intervention For Endpoint reduction in hypertension study (LIFE) experienced reductions in all-cause (39%) and cardiovascular mortality (37%) compared with patients treated with the beta-blocker atenolol, despite dramatic blood pressure lowering in both groups (29/17 mmHg). In addition, losartan-treated patients were less likely to develop new-onset diabetes after 4.7 years of follow-up.[66,67]

ACE inhibitors and ARBs also confer a renoprotective benefit in the management of diabetes. Diabetes is the leading cause of chronic renal failure, dialysis, and kidney transplantation in the United States and both classes of drugs have been shown to slow the development and progression of renal disease. ACE inhibitors and ARBs slow the elevation of serum creatinine, reverse or reduce proteinuria and albuminuria, and retard progression to end-stage renal disease and diabetic nephropathy.[68-70] ARBs have been also shown to slow progression to microalbuminuria.[69,71] ACE inhibitors or ARBs may be preferred because of their demonstrated renoprotective effects and can be added to thiazide diuretics to help lower blood pressure. ACE inhibitors also reduce cardiovascular events in high-risk patients. CCBs or beta-blockers may also be needed to lower blood pressure to target levels.[33] Most patients require at least three antihypertensives to successfully control blood pressure to target levels of <130/80 mmHg.[72]

Heart Failure Management

There is currently no generally established effective treatment for left ventricular diastolic dysfunction associated with diabetic cardiomyopathy. However, an investigational agent (ALT-711) that breaks collagen cross-links formed in the diabetic myocardium under the influence of AGEs may eventually prove to be efficacious and safe in diabetic cardiomyopathy.[27] Early studies with this agent found it improved left ventricular function and optimized ventriculovascular coupling in older nondiabetic primates and improved arterial compliance in older human subjects.[73]

Antiplatelet therapy with aspirin is now generally used for primary as well as secondary CHD prevention. The large Antiplatelet Trialists' Collaboration overview of 142 clinical studies of aspirin in high-risk patients found no significant difference between outcomes in diabetic compared to nondiabetic patients,[74] despite the increase in prothrombotic factors reported to be associated with diabetes. National HF guidelines recommend that all patients be treated with an ACE inhibitor or an ARB in the absence of intolerance or contraindications and diuretics as required, once left ventricular systolic dysfunction or clinical HF has developed. All patients should also receive beta-blocker therapy.[46] Although most beta-blockers increase insulin resistance and HbA1c levels and may exacerbate atherogenic lipid abnormalities, the nonspecific vasodilating beta-blocker carvedilol with alpha properties improves insulin sensitivity and may reduce triglyceride and raise HDL levels. ACE inhibitor ARBs and nonspecific beta-blockers are agents that may also reduce or reverse microalbuminuria and retard the progression of renal dysfunction.

Although diabetic patients in the landmark Studies of Left Ventricular Dysfunction (SOLVD) had a higher risk for the combined endpoint of death or HF hospitalization than nondiabetic patients, those receiving enalapril had significantly better outcomes than those receiving placebo (54% vs. 67% odds ratio, respectively). In addition, treated diabetic patients with symptomatic HF had a similar absolute improvement in the combined endpoint to nondiabetic subjects, 12% and 8%, respectively. However, when compared with placebo-treated patients, enalapril-treated diabetic patients with asymptomatic left ventricular systolic dysfunction actually improved significantly more than their nondiabetic counterparts (10% vs. 3% reduction).[37] These data suggest that ACE inhibitors may benefit patients with preclinical diabetic cardiomyopathy. Expectedly, the addition of beta-blockers further reduced mortality in diabetic patients in the SOLVD Prevention Trial.[75]

Bisoprolol, carvedilol, and metoprolol tartrate are the only three beta-blockers indicated for the treatment of HF. Bisoprolol reduced mortality by 34% in the Cardiac Insufficiency Bisoprolol Study II (CIBIS-II)[76]; carvedilol reduced mortality by 17–65% in the Carvedilol Or Metoprolol European Trial (COMET),[77] Australia/New Zealand Heart Failure Trial (ANZ),[78] Carvedilol Prospective Randomized Cumulative Survival Study (COPERNICUS),[79] and the U.S. Carvedilol Heart Failure Study[80]; and metoprolol succinate reduced mortality by 34% in the Metoprolol Controlled-Release Randomized Intervention Trial in Congestive Heart Failure (MERIT-HF).[81]

Although beta-blockers are recommended for most patients with HF caused by left ventricular systolic dysfunction, diabetic patients are less likely to receive this class of drugs, in part due to their adverse effects on glycemic control and blood lipids; the same reservations hold true for their use in treating hypertension.[82] Both nonselective beta-blockers such as propranolol and beta$_1$-selective blockers such as atenolol and metoprolol have been consistently shown to increase insulin resistance and raise serum insulin levels. In addition, these older beta-blockers exacerbate the proatherogenic profile of blood lipids, raise triglycerides, and lower HDL levels. Nevertheless, beta-blocker therapy significantly improves clinical outcomes in diabetic patients with established CHD.[83]

However, use of the vasodilating beta-blocker carvedilol has not been associated with these adverse metabolic effects.[84] Compared to metoprolol, which decreased insulin sensitivity by 14%, carvedilol increased insulin sensitivity by 9%.[85] A randomized 24-week trial compared carvedilol and atenolol in 45 patients with type 2 diabetes being treated for hypertension. Whereas atenolol-treated patients experienced a decrease in insulin sensitivity and HDL and an increase in serum insulin and triglycerides, carvedilol-treated patients demonstrated an increase in insulin sensitivity and HDL and a decrease in serum insulin and triglycerides. Atenolol was also associated with a 4% rise in HbA1c levels compared to a 1.4% decrease with carvedilol.[86]

In the COMET study of 3029 HF patients, those treated with carvedilol had a 22% lower incidence of diabetes-related adverse events, including decreased glucose tolerance or hyperglycemia, and an 11% lower rate of mortality or worsening HF than patients treated with metoprolol tartrate after a 5-year follow-up period.[87] Furthermore, Glycemic Effects in Diabetes Mellitus: Carvedilol-Metoprolol Comparison in Hypertensives (GEMINI) compared carvedilol and metoprolol tartrate in 1235 diabetic patients with hypertension and found that carvedilol not only stabilized insulin resistance and HbA1c levels but also reduced or reversed microalbuminuria compared to metoprolol tartrate despite comparable blood pressure reduction.[88]

Aldosterone antagonists such as spironolactone and eplerenone have improved clinical outcomes in patients with HF due to left ventricular systolic dysfunction.[89,90] Their benefit in left ventricular diastolic dysfunction is believed to result from the profibrotic effect of aldactone.[91] The placebo-controlled Eplerenone PostAcute Myocardial Infarction Heart Failure Efficacy and Survival Study (EPHESUS) evaluated eplerenone in addition to an ACE inhibitor or ARB and beta-blocker in 6600 patients with left systolic ventricular dysfunction and clinical HF due to MI; diabetes was present in one-third of randomized subjects. In the clinical endpoints of the study, all-cause mortality and cardiovascular death or hospitalization were both significantly improved by the addition of eplerenone after 16 months of follow-up. All-cause mortality was reduced by 15% in all patients treated with eplerenone.[90] The patients in EPHESUS with diabetes ($n = 2122$) also benefited from aldosterone blockade and there was no significant heterogeneity with respect to mortality benefit between diabetic and nondiabetic patients.[90]

PROGNOSIS

The long asymptomatic stage of diabetic cardiomyopathy makes early intervention problematic. However, its high prevalence in diabetic patients should encourage clinical awareness and promote attentive evaluation for its presence. In the absence of a correct diagnosis and effective intervention, the development of systolic dysfunction may lead to clinical HF with the dismal prognosis associated with DCM. One-half of patients with severe HF die within 1 year and the majority of patients die within 8 years.[1] While there are no available therapies to correct the underlying physiologic abnormalities in early diabetic cardiomyopathy, all diabetic patients require aggressive management to reduce the high risk of CVD engendered by the high prevalence of coexisting hypertension and CHD, especially HF, MI, and stroke. Physicians should be especially vigilant about helping minimize modifiable risk factors since the majority of diabetic patients do not achieve optimal treatment goals and are underutilizing life-saving therapies.[92] Long-term intensive interventions aimed at modifying all of the known risk factors may reduce the likelihood of cardiovascular complication by as much as 50%.[93]

REFERENCES

1. American Heart Association. Heart Disease and Stroke Statistics—2005 Update. Dallas, TX: American Heart Association, 2005.

2. Rich MW. Epidemiology, pathophysiology, and etiology of congestive heart failure in older adults. *J Am Geriatr Soc* 1997;45:968–974.

3. Mensah GA, Mokdad AH, Ford ES, et al. State of disparities in cardiovascular health in the United States. *Circulation* 2005;111:1233–1241.

4. Mokdad AH, Ford ES, Bowman BA, et al. Prevalence of obesity, diabetes, and obesity-related health risk factors, 2001. *JAMA* 2003;289:76–79.

5. U.S. Department of Health and Human Services, Centers for Disease Control and Prevention. National diabetes fact sheet: general information and national estimates on diabetes in the United States, 2002. Atlanta, GA: American Diabetes Association, 2003.

6. Wild S, Roglic G, Green A, et al. Global prevalence of diabetes: estimates for the year 2000 and projections for 2030. *Diabetes Care* 2004;27:1047–1053.

7. Haffner SM, Lehto S, Ronnemaa T, et al. Mortality from coronary heart disease in subjects with type 2 diabetes and in nondiabetic subjects with and without prior myocardial infarction. *N Engl J Med* 1998;339:229–234.

8. Rubler S, Dlugash J, Yuceoglu YZ, et al. New type of cardiomyopathy associated with diabetic glomerulosclerosis. *Am J Cardiol* 1972;30:595–602.

9. Kannel WB, Hjortland M, Castelli WP. Role of diabetes in congestive heart failure: the Framingham study. *Am J Cardiol* 1974;34:29–34.

10. Bobbio M, Ferrua S, Opasich C, et al. Survival and hospitalization in heart failure patients with or without diabetes treated with beta-blockers. *J Card Fail* 2003;9:192–202.

11. Adams KF, Fonarow GC, Emerman CL, et al. Characteristics and outcomes of patients hospitalized for heart failure in the United States: rationale, design, and preliminary observations from the first 100,000 cases in the Acute Decompensated Heart Failure National Registry (ADHERE). *Am Heart J* 2005; 149:209–216.

12. Mitchell JE, Caboral MF, Feng J, et al. Prevalence and impact of diabetes mellitus in black patients hospitalized with heart failure with impaired or preserved systolic function. *J Card Fail* 2004;10:S130.

13. Poirier P, Bogaty P, Garneau C, et al. Diastolic dysfunction in normotensive men with well-controlled type 2 diabetes: importance of maneuvers in echocardiographic screening for preclinical diabetic cardiomyopathy. *Diabetes Care* 2001; 24:5–10.

14. Valle R, Bagolin E, Canali C, et al. The BNP assay does not identify mild left ventricular diastolic dysfunction in asymptomatic diabetic patients. *Eur J Echocardiogr* 2006;7:40–44.

15. Redfield MM, Jacobsen SJ, Burnett JC Jr, et al. Burden of systolic and diastolic ventricular dysfunction in the community: appreciating the scope of the heart failure epidemic. *JAMA* 2003;289:194–202.

16. Bertoni AG, Tsai A, Kasper EK, et al. Diabetes and idiopathic cardiomyopathy: a nationwide case-control study. *Diabetes Care* 2003;26:2791–2795.

17. Devereux RB, Roman MJ, Paranicas M, et al. Impact of diabetes on cardiac structure and function: the strong heart study. *Circulation* 2000;101:2271–2276.

18. Arnlov J, Lind L, Zethelius B, et al. Several factors associated with the insulin resistance syndrome are predictors of left ventricular systolic dysfunction in a male population after 20 years of follow-up. *Am Heart J* 2001;142:720–724.

19. Fang ZY, Yuda S, Anderson V, et al. Echocardiographic detection of early diabetic myocardial disease. *J Am Coll Cardiol* 2003;41:611–617.

20. Vinereanu D, Nicolaides E, Tweddel AC, et al. Subclinical left ventricular dysfunction in asymptomatic patients with type II diabetes mellitus, related to serum lipids and glycated haemoglobin. *Clin Sci (Lond)* 2003;105:591–599.

21. Fang ZY, Najos-Valencia O, Leano R, et al. Patients with early diabetic heart disease demonstrate a normal myocardial response to dobutamine. *J Am Coll Cardiol* 2003;42:446–453.

22. Bell DS. Diabetic cardiomyopathy. *Diabetes Care* 2003;26:2949–2951.

23. Rutter MK, Parise H, Benjamin EJ, et al. Impact of glucose intolerance and insulin resistance on cardiac structure and function: sex-related differences in the Framingham Heart Study. *Circulation* 2003;107:448–454.

24. Struthers AD, Morris AD. Screening for and treating left-ventricular abnormalities in diabetes mellitus: a new way of reducing cardiac deaths. *Lancet* 2002; 359:1430–1432.

25. Phillips RA, Krakoff LR, Dunaif A, et al. Relation among left ventricular mass, insulin resistance, and blood pressure in nonobese subjects. *J Clin Endocrinol Metab* 1998;83:4284–4288.

26. Brownlee M, Cerami A, Vlassara H. Advanced glycosylation end products in tissue and the biochemical basis of diabetic complications. *N Engl J Med* 1988; 318:1315–1321.

27. Candido R, Forbes JM, Thomas MC, et al. A breaker of advanced glycation end products attenuates diabetes-induced myocardial structural changes. *Circ Res* 2003;92:785–792.

28. Bidasee KR, Zhang Y, Shao CH, et al. Diabetes increases formation of advanced glycation end products on Sarco(endo)plasmic reticulum $Ca2^+$-ATPase. *Diabetes* 2004;53:463–473.

29. Young ME, McNulty P, Taegtmeyer H. Adaptation and maladaptation of the heart in diabetes: part II: potential mechanisms. *Circulation* 2002;105:1861–1870.

30. Zhou YT, Grayburn P, Karim A, et al. Lipotoxic heart disease in obese rats: implications for human obesity. *Proc Natl Acad Sci USA* 2000;97:1784–1789.

31. Diamant M, Lamb HJ, Groeneveld Y, et al. Diastolic dysfunction is associated with altered myocardial metabolism in asymptomatic normotensive patients with well-controlled type 2 diabetes mellitus. *J Am Coll Cardiol* 2003;42:328–335.

32. American Diabetes Association. Standards of medical care for patients with diabetes mellitus. *Diabetes Care* 2003;26(Suppl 1):S33–S50.

33. Chobanian AV, Bakris GL, Black HR, et al. The Seventh Report of the Joint National Committee on Prevention, Detection, Evaluation, and Treatment of High Blood Pressure: the JNC 7 report. *JAMA* 2003;289:2560–2572.

34. Third Report of the National Cholesterol Education Program (NCEP) Expert Panel on Detection, Evaluation, and Treatment of High Blood Cholesterol in Adults (Adult Treatment Panel III) final report. *Circulation* 2002;106:3143–3421.

35. Grundy SM, Cleeman JI, Merz CN, et al. Implications of Recent Clinical Trials for the National Cholesterol Education Program Adult Treatment Panel III Guidelines. *Circulation* 2004;110:227–239.

36. Schannwell CM, Schneppenheim M, Perings S, et al. Left ventricular diastolic dysfunction as an early manifestation of diabetic cardiomyopathy. *Cardiology* 2002;98:33–39.

37. Shindler DM, Kostis JB, Yusuf S, et al. Diabetes mellitus, a predictor of morbidity and mortality in the Studies of Left Ventricular Dysfunction (SOLVD) Trials and Registry. *Am J Cardiol* 1996;77:1017–1020.

38. Iribarren C, Karter AJ, Go AS, et al. Glycemic control and heart failure among adult patients with diabetes. *Circulation* 2001;103:2668–2673.

39. Kuusisto J, Mykkanen L, Pyorala K, et al. NIDDM and its metabolic control predict coronary heart disease in elderly subjects. *Diabetes* 1994;43:960–967.

40. Khaw KT, Wareham N, Bingham S, et al. Association of hemoglobin A1c with cardiovascular disease and mortality in adults: the European Prospective Investigation into Cancer in Norfolk. *Ann Intern Med* 2004;141:413–420.

41. Stratton IM, Adler AI, Neil HA, et al. Association of glycaemia with macrovascular and microvascular complications of type 2 diabetes (UKPDS 35): prospective observational study. *BMJ* 2000;321:405–412.

42. Liu JE, Robbins DC, Palmieri V, et al. Association of albuminuria with systolic and diastolic left ventricular dysfunction in type 2 diabetes. The Strong Heart Study. *J Am Coll Cardiol* 2003;41:2022–2028.

43. UKPD Study Group. UK Prospective Diabetes Study 6. Complications in newly diagnosed type 2 diabetic patients and their association with different clinical and biochemical risk factors. *Diabetes Res* 1990;13:1–11.

44. Uusitupa M, Mustonen J, Siitonen O, et al. Quantitative electrocardiographic and vectorcardiographic study on newly-diagnosed non-insulin-dependent diabetic and non-diabetic control subjects. *Cardiology* 1988;75:1–9.

45. Casis O, Echevarria E. Diabetic cardiomyopathy: electromechanical cellular alterations. *Curr Vasc Pharmacol* 2004;2:237–248.

46. Hunt SA, Abraham WT, Chin MH, et al. ACC/AHA 2005 Guideline Update for the Diagnosis and Management of Chronic Heart Failure in the Adult: a report of the American College of Cardiology/American Heart Association Task Force on Practice Guidelines (Writing Committee to Update the 2001 Guidelines for the Evaluation and Management of Heart Failure), 2005.

47. UK Prospective Diabetes Study (UKPDS) Group. Intensive blood-glucose control with sulphonylureas or insulin compared with conventional treatment and risk

of complications in patients with type 2 diabetes (UKPDS 33). *Lancet* 1998;352: 837–853.

48. UKPD Study Group. Effect of intensive blood-glucose control with metformin on complications in overweight patients with type 2 diabetes (UKPDS 34). UK Prospective Diabetes Study (UKPDS) Group. *Lancet* 1998;352:854–865.

49. Tang WH, Francis GS, Hoogwerf BJ, et al. Fluid retention after initiation of thiazolidinedione therapy in diabetic patients with established chronic heart failure. *J Am Coll Cardiol* 2003;41:1394–1398.

50. Delea TE, Edelsberg JS, Hagiwara M, et al. Use of thiazolidinediones and risk of heart failure in people with type 2 diabetes: a retrospective cohort study. *Diabetes Care* 2003;26:2983–2989.

51. Rajagopalan R, Rosenson RS, Fernandes AW, et al. Association between congestive heart failure and hospitalization in patients with type 2 diabetes mellitus receiving treatment with insulin or pioglitazone: a retrospective data analysis. *Clin Ther* 2004;26:1400–1410.

52. Boule NG, Haddad E, Kenny GP, et al. Effects of exercise on glycemic control and body mass in type 2 diabetes mellitus: a meta-analysis of controlled clinical trials. *JAMA* 2001;286:1218–1227.

53. Duncan GE, Perri MG, Theriaque DW, et al. Exercise training, without weight loss, increases insulin sensitivity and postheparin plasma lipase activity in previously sedentary adults. *Diabetes Care* 2003;26:557–562.

54. Turner RC, Millns H, Neil HA, et al. Risk factors for coronary artery disease in non-insulin dependent diabetes mellitus: United Kingdom Prospective Diabetes Study (UKPDS: 23). *BMJ* 1998;316:823–828.

55. Pyorala K, Pedersen TR, Kjekshus J, et al. Cholesterol lowering with simvastatin improves prognosis of diabetic patients with coronary heart disease. A subgroup analysis of the Scandinavian Simvastatin Survival Study (4S). *Diabetes Care* 1997;20:614–620.

56. Collins R, Armitage J, Parish S, et al. MRC/BHF Heart Protection Study of cholesterol-lowering with simvastatin in 5963 people with diabetes: a randomised placebo-controlled trial. *Lancet* 2003;361:2005–2016.

57. Colhoun HM, Betteridge DJ, Durrington PN, et al. Primary prevention of cardiovascular disease with atorvastatin in type 2 diabetes in the Collaborative Atorvastatin Diabetes Study (CARDS): multicentre randomised placebo-controlled trial. *Lancet* 2004;364:685–696.

58. UKPD Study Group. Tight blood pressure control and risk of macrovascular and microvascular complications in type 2 diabetes: UKPDS 38. UK Prospective Diabetes Study Group. *BMJ* 1998;317:703–713.

59. Hansson L, Zanchetti A, Carruthers SG, et al. Effects of intensive blood-pressure lowering and low-dose aspirin in patients with hypertension: principal results of the Hypertension Optimal Treatment (HOT) randomised trial. HOT Study Group. *Lancet* 1998;351:1755–1762.

60. UKPD Study Group. Efficacy of atenolol and captopril in reducing risk of macrovascular and microvascular complications in type 2 diabetes: UKPDS 39. UK Prospective Diabetes Study Group. *BMJ* 1998;317:713–720.

61. ALLHAT Collaborative Research Group. Major outcomes in moderately hyperc-holesterolemic, hypertensive patients randomized to pravastatin vs usual care: The Antihypertensive and Lipid-Lowering Treatment to Prevent Heart Attack Trial (ALLHAT-LLT). *JAMA* 2002;288:2998–3007.

62. Sawicki PT. Do ACE inhibitors offer specific benefits in the antihypertensive treatment of diabetic patients? 17 years of unfulfilled promises. *Diabetologia* 1998;41:598–602.

63. Siebenhofer A, Plank J, Horvath K, et al. Angiotensin receptor blockers as anti-hypertensive treatment for patients with diabetes mellitus: meta-analysis of con-trolled double-blind randomized trials. *Diabet Med* 2004;21:18–25.

64. Effects of ramipril on cardiovascular and microvascular outcomes in people with diabetes mellitus: results of the HOPE study and MICRO-HOPE substudy. Heart Outcomes Prevention Evaluation Study Investigators. *Lancet* 2000;355: 253–259.

65. Fox KM. Efficacy of perindopril in reduction of cardiovascular events among patients with stable coronary artery disease: randomised, double-blind, placebo-controlled, multicentre trial (the EUROPA study). *Lancet* 2003;362:782–788.

66. Lindholm LH, Ibsen H, Dahlof B, et al. Cardiovascular morbidity and mortality in patients with diabetes in the Losartan Intervention For Endpoint reduction in hypertension study (LIFE): a randomised trial against atenolol. *Lancet* 2002;359: 1004–1010.

67. Lindholm LH, Ibsen H, Borch-Johnsen K, et al. Risk of new-onset diabetes in the Losartan Intervention For Endpoint reduction in hypertension study. *J Hypertens* 2002;20:1879–1886.

68. Parving HH, Lehnert H, Brochner-Mortensen J, et al. The effect of irbesartan on the development of diabetic nephropathy in patients with type 2 diabetes. *N Engl J Med* 2001;345:870–878.

69. Brenner BM, Cooper ME, de Zeeuw D, et al. Effects of losartan on renal and car-diovascular outcomes in patients with type 2 diabetes and nephropathy. *N Engl J Med* 2001;345:861–869.

70. Should all patients with type 1 diabetes mellitus and microalbuminuria receive angiotensin-converting enzyme inhibitors? A meta-analysis of individual patient data. *Ann Intern Med* 2001;134:370–379.

71. Lewis EJ, Hunsicker LG, Clarke WR, et al. Renoprotective effect of the angiotensin-receptor antagonist irbesartan in patients with nephropathy due to type 2 diabetes. *N Engl J Med* 2001;345:851–860.

72. Bakris GL. The importance of blood pressure control in the patient with diabetes. *Am J Med* 2004;116(Suppl 5A):30S–38S.

73. Kass DA, Shapiro EP, Kawaguchi M, et al. Improved arterial compliance by a novel advanced glycation end-product crosslink breaker. *Circulation* 2001;104: 1464–1470.

74. Antiplatelet Trialists' Collaboration. Collaborative overview of randomised trials of antiplatelet therapy—I: prevention of death, myocardial infarction, and stroke by prolonged antiplatelet therapy in various categories of patients. *BMJ* 1994;308:81–106.

75. Exner DV, Dries DL, Waclawiw MA, et al. Beta-adrenergic blocking agent use and mortality in patients with asymptomatic and symptomatic left ventricular systolic dysfunction: a post hoc analysis of the Studies of Left Ventricular Dysfunction. *J Am Coll Cardiol* 1999;33:916–923.

76. CIBIS-II Investigators. The Cardiac Insufficiency Bisoprolol Study II (CIBIS-II): a randomised trial. *Lancet* 1999;353:9–13.

77. Poole-Wilson PA, Swedberg K, Cleland JG, et al. Comparison of carvedilol and metoprolol on clinical outcomes in patients with chronic heart failure in the Carvedilol or Metoprolol European Trial (COMET): randomised controlled trial. *Lancet* 2003;362:7–13.

78. Australia/New Zealand Heart Failure Research Collaborative Group. Randomised, placebo-controlled trial of carvedilol in patients with congestive heart failure due to ischaemic heart disease. Australia/New Zealand Heart Failure Research Collaborative Group. *Lancet* 1997;349:375–380.

79. Packer M, Coats AJ, Fowler MB, et al. Effect of carvedilol on survival in severe chronic heart failure. *N Engl J Med.* 2001;344:1651–1658.

80. Packer M, Bristow MR, Cohn JN, et al. The effect of carvedilol on morbidity and mortality in patients with chronic heart failure. U.S. Carvedilol Heart Failure Study Group. *N Engl J Med* 1996;334:1349–1355.

81. MERIT-HF Investigators. Effect of metoprolol CR/XL in chronic heart failure: Metoprolol CR/XL Randomised Intervention Trial in Congestive Heart Failure (MERIT-HF). *Lancet* 1999;353:2001–2007.

82. Lithell HO. Effect of antihypertensive drugs on insulin, glucose, and lipid metabolism. *Diabetes Care.* 1991;14:203–209.

83. Jonas M, Reicher-Reiss H, Boyko V, et al. Usefulness of beta-blocker therapy in patients with non-insulin-dependent diabetes mellitus and coronary artery disease. Bezafibrate Infarction Prevention (BIP) Study Group. *Am J Cardiol* 1996;77: 1273–1277.

84. Hauf-Zachariou U, Widmann L, Zulsdorf B, et al. A double-blind comparison of the effects of carvedilol and captopril on serum lipid concentrations in patients with mild to moderate essential hypertension and dyslipidaemia. *Eur J Clin Pharmacol* 1993;45:95–100.

85. Jacob S, Rett K, Wicklmayr M, et al. Differential effect of chronic treatment with two beta-blocking agents on insulin sensitivity: the carvedilol-metoprolol study. *J Hypertens* 1996;14:489–494.

86. Giugliano D, Acampora R, Marfella R, et al. Metabolic and cardiovascular effects of carvedilol and atenolol in non-insulin-dependent diabetes mellitus and hypertension. A randomized, controlled trial. *Ann Intern Med* 1997;126:955–959.

87. Torp-Pedersen C, Cleland JG, Metra M, et al. Effect of long-term treatment with carvedilol compared to metoprolol on heart failure morbidity and diabetes in COMET. Presented at the American College of Cardiology (ACC) 53rd Annual Scientific Sessions; March 7–10, 2004; New Orleans, LA: Tracking number 04-A-294565-ACC. *J Am Coll Cardiol* 2004;43.

88. Bakris GL, Fonseca V, Katholi RE, et al. Metabolic effects of carvedilol vs metoprolol in patients with type 2 diabetes mellitus and hypertension: a randomized controlled trial. *JAMA* 2004;292:2227–2236.

89. Pitt B, Zannad F, Remme WJ, et al. The effect of spironolactone on morbidity and mortality in patients with severe heart failure. Randomized Aldactone Evaluation Study Investigators. *N Engl J Med* 1999;341:709–717.

90. Pitt B, Remme W, Zannad F, et al. Eplerenone, a selective aldosterone blocker, in patients with left ventricular dysfunction after myocardial infarction. *N Engl J Med* 2003;348:1309–1321.

91. Chatterjee K. Primary diastolic heart failure. *Am J Geriatr Cardiol* 2002;11:178–187.

92. Saydah SH, Fradkin J, Cowie CC. Poor control of risk factors for vascular disease among adults with previously diagnosed diabetes. *JAMA* 2004;291:335–342.

93. Giles TD, Sander GE. Diabetes mellitus and heart failure: basic mechanisms, clinical features, and therapeutic considerations. *Cardiol Clin* 2004;22:553–568.

TREATMENT

OF DYSLIPIDEMIA

OF TYPE 2 DIABETES

Clinton D. Brown
John C. LaRosa

INTRODUCTION

People with type 2 diabetes are at a far greater risk for developing micro- and macrovascular disease.[1-3] Type 2 diabetes is the leading cause of end-stage renal disease,[4] blindness,[5] limp amputation,[6] and atherosclerotic cardiovascular disease.[7] Dyslipidemia is a major risk factor for cardiovascular disease in type 2 diabetes; one that is amenable to aggressive intervention.[8,9]

The prevalence of diabetes mellitus is increasing worldwide mainly due to the pandemic of obesity.[10] It is estimated that by the year 2025, the number of individuals to contract diabetes will approximate 300 million.[11] According to the U.S. Centers for Disease Control and Prevention, 12 million people in the United States have diabetes and remarkably another 5.2 million Americans are undiagnosed.[12] The number of Americans diagnosed with type 2 diabetes is projected to more than double to approximately 29 million by 2050.[13]

The U.S. financial burden for the treatment of diabetes including its complications is enormous. For example, indirect cost of premature death, loss of wages, and disability are $40 billion, whereas no less than $92 billion spent annually to cover direct medical costs.[14]

Once considered a disease associated with industrialized countries, type 2 diabetes is fast becoming a major health problem in developing countries. As countries become modernized and urbanized, studies have shown that there is increased consumption of calorie-dense foods, decreased physical activity, and a rising incidence and prevalence in overweight and obesity.[15]

Consequently, lifestyles (i.e., Western) perceived to be desirable include changing the types of foods consumed and activity levels in rural areas and developing countries.[16]

Longitudinal studies worldwide have confirmed the strong linkage between type 2 diabetes and overweight/obesity.[17,18] The correlation between the amount of fatness and the frequency of type 2 diabetes is shown in Fig. 8-1.

About 8 out of 10 type 2 diabetic individuals are overweight/obese and the risk of developing type 2 diabetes increases progressively as the body mass index (BMI) or more specifically, as visceral adiposity, increases. In fact, the atherogenic dyslipidemic profile of insulin resistance (IR) and type 2 diabetes is closely associated with intra-abdominal (visceral) fat distribution.[19,20]

Underpinning the global rise in overweight/obesity is the expression of multiple, so-called, "thrifty" genes that produced the "thrifty" phenotype. It has been hypothesized that this genetic expression enabled our ancestors to survive prolonged periods when food was scarce.[10,21] This survival advantage is primarily determined by single nucleotide polymorphisms and is characterized by storage of fat in subcutaneous and visceral compartments in the abdomen and, economic use of this energy source. One can consider the gene that encodes for the hormone leptin to fall in this category of a thrifty gene in that its action is to maintain adiposity and to influence body metabolism. It is the loss of adipose tissue during starvation and attendant

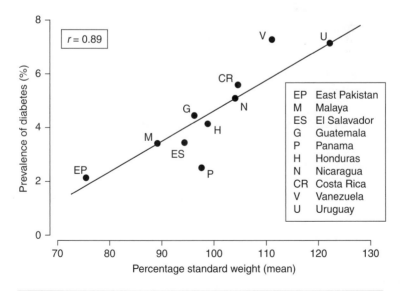

Figure 8-1 **Diabetes prevalence strongly correlates with the degree of fatness.**

fall in leptin levels that triggers increased appetite and reduced metabolic rate.[10,22] Adipose tissue, besides playing a passive role as a storage depot for fats, also functions as an endocrine organ that signals peripheral tissue and the brain by producing hormones and cytokines (Table 8-1).[23]

The nuclear hormone receptor, peroxisome proliferator-activated receptor gamma (PPARγ) mediates differentiation and maturation of adipocytes (adipogenesis)[21,24] which enables mature adipocytes to produce a number of hormones and cytokines. Some adipocyte factors such as adiponectin and leptin promote insulin sensitivity, whereas other factors such as tumor necrosis factor alpha (TNF-α) and nonesterified free fatty acids (FFA) are potent inhibitors of insulin sensitivity. Blood levels of these mediators are increased in obese individuals. In contrast, with weight reduction, the plasma concentration of the insulin sensitizer, adiponectin, is increased significantly in patients with type 2 diabetes.[25]

Elevated ambient glucose concentration results in increased levels of advanced glycation end products (AGEs) and generation of reactive oxygen species (ROS).[26,27] AGE and ROS modify low-density lipoprotein (LDL) and make it more atherogenic. Clearance of glycated LDL by native LDL receptors is impaired. Glycated LDL is preferentially taken up by the scavenger receptor of the macrophage, internalized, stored, and eventually the macrophage is transformed into a foam cell (Table 8-2).[28] Oxidized LDL may be atherogenic in many ways in addition to its uptake by the macrophage; it is chemotactic for circulating monocytes thereby fostering their accumulation in the vessel wall where they can become foam cells (Table 8-2). Furthermore, both AGE and ROS have been shown to cause endothelial dysfunction by suppressing nitric oxide (NO) production.[29]

Table 8-1 **Effects of Adipose Tissue-Derived Hormones and Cytokines on Insulin Resistance**

Adipose-Derived Protein	Effects on IR	Other Source
Leptin	Improvement	None
Adiponectin	Improvement	None
Adipsin/ASP	Decline	None
Resistin	Decline	Macrophage
TNF-α	Decline	Macrophage
IL-6	Decline	Macrophage
PAI-1	Decline	Liver
MCP-1	Decline	Macrophage
Angiotensinogen	Decline	Liver

Abbreviations: MCP-1, macrophage monocyte chemoattractant protein-1; PAI-1, plasminogen activator inhibitor-1; IL-6, interleukin-1.

Source: Adapted from Ref. 10.

Table 8-2 **Proatherogenic Characteristics of Oxidized* and Glycosylated† LDL**

- Increased uptake by macrophage leading to foam cell formation[*,†]
- Impaired recognition by the LDL receptor [*,†]
- Stimulation of platelet aggregation[*,†]
- Chemotaxis for blood monocytes[*]
- Impaired vascular response to NO[*]
- Stimulates synthesis of MCP-1[*]

Source: Adapted from Refs. 28 and 82. *Oxidized LDL, †Glycosylate LDL

With excellent control of blood sugar one might expect prevention of long-term diabetes-induced complication. In deed, there is evidence that tight glycemic control is beneficial in treating microvascular disease (retinopathy and nephropathy), however, macrovascular disease (coronary heart disease [CHD] and stroke) appear to be far less responsive to therapeutic glucose control.[30]

Modification of risk factors for cardiovascular disease such as hypertension[31] and blood lipids in patients with type 2 diabetes have resulted in significant improvement in cardiovascular morbidity and mortality.[32-34] This review will focus on strategies for treating the dyslipidemia associated with type 2 diabetes.

LIPOPROTEINS AND LIPIDS

In type 2 diabetes there are both lipid and lipoprotein abnormalities. A variety of dyslipidemias can be seen in diabetic patients (Table 8-3). The most common patterns are elevated triglycerides (TGs), low high-density lipoprotein (HDL), and small dense LDL.[35] Elevated cholesterol with or without increased very low-density lipoprotein (VLDL) and TGs is common in diabetic patients with proteinuria, especially in cases of massive proteinuria seen in diabetes-associated nephrotic syndrome.[36] Also seen in diabetic individuals with proteinuria is an elevated level of the atherogenic lipoprotein, lipoprotein (a) (Lp (a)).[37] Central obesity, through its endocrine function and release of cytokines, initiates IR by increasing circulating nonesterified FFA which directly interferes with glucose transport (i.e., $\downarrow$ GLUT-4) in skeletal muscle (Fig. 8-2).[38] In the adipocyte, insulin normally suppresses hormone sensitive lipase and postprandial lipolysis; however, in IR, there is an inappropriate release of FFAs after meals.[39] Elevated FFA content in the hepatocyte results in TG-rich VLDL and high plasma TG concentration. Associated

Table 8-3   **Lipoprotein/Lipid Abnormalities Characteristic of Type 2 Diabetes**

Elevated VLDL
Hypertriglyceridemia
Low HDL (low apo AI)
Low HDL-C
Small dense LDL
LDL-C usually not elevated
Elevated LDL*
Increased Lp (a)
Glycosylated LDL
Oxidized LDL

*Elevated apoB-100.

Source: Adapted from Refs. 35–37 and 82.

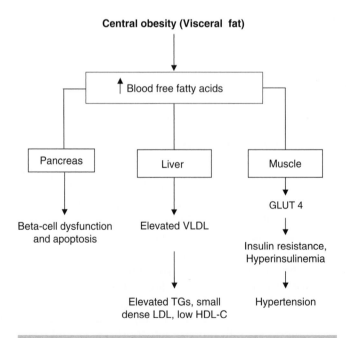

Figure 8-2   **Metabolic effects of elevated free fatty acids (derived from visceral fat).**

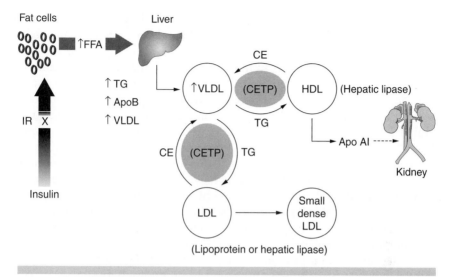

Figure 8-3 **Mechanisms relating to insulin resistance and dyslipidemia.**

with the rise in TGs in diabetic patients is a decrease in HDL-C levels and the production of small dense LDL. TG-induced lowering of HDL-C is caused by the exchange of TG (from VLDL and VLDL remnants) for cholesterol ester (CE) in HDL (and LDL). This process is mediated by the enzyme cholesterol ester transfer protein (CETP). As HDL becomes more TG enriched, it is acted on by the enzyme hepatic lipase (HL) that removes TG and produces an HDL particle that is small, dense, and cholesterol depleted. In addition, there is evidence that small dense HDL and apoprotein (apo) AI are rapidly cleared by the kidney, thereby causing further reduction in HDL plasma concentration (Fig. 8-3).[40] Also, small dense LDL particles undergo glycation and/or oxidation which make LDL, in patients with type 2 diabetes, particularly atherogenic.[41]

Another consequence of elevated TGs and FFA levels is pancreatic beta-cell dysfunction and apoptosis that results in insulinopenia, and necessitates treatment with exogenous insulin.[42]

TREATMENT

Dietary Intervention

There are opposing points of view in regards to the most appropriate diet for patients with diabetes and dyslipidemia or with metabolic syndrome. Although LDL-cholesterol (LDL-C) can be markedly increased in diabetes-associated nephrotic syndrome, usually LDL-C is normal or slightly elevated in diabetic patients without proteinuria. The typical lipid and lipoprotein profile abnormalities are elevated TGs (including elevated VLDL and VLDL remnants), low HDL-C, and small dense LDL. In this scenario, LDL may undergo changes in composition as mentioned above, and therefore can be more atherogenic compared to LDL of nondiabetic patients.[43] Therefore, one dietary approach to treating a patient with type 2 diabetes and dyslipidemia according to the Adult Treatment Panel III (ATP III),[44] and the American Diabetes Association (ADA),[45] would be to initiate a diet in which saturated fat has been reduced to less than 7% of total daily calories, and total calories restricted to promote weight loss. In fact, prospective studies have shown that weight reduction of approximately 10% of initial body weight dramatically improves glycemic control and blood lipids.[46] Even modest reduction in body weight of about 3% sustained over a prolonged period is associated with significant risk reduction in developing diabetes in overweight individuals.[47]

On the other hand, proponents of the low carbohydrate diet point out that reducing dietary carbohydrates will improve lipids by lowering TGs. Foster et al. report a 28% reduction of TGs after a 12-month trial of a low carbohydrate diet in obese adults.[48] A third approach would involve using a high protein (30% of total calories) and moderate amount of carbohydrate (40% of calories) and 30% of calories from fat (10:10:10, P:S:M, respectively) in type 2 diabetic patients have been shown to improve glycemic control over the short term without having an affect on lipids or renal function.[49]

By incorporating elements of each diet mentioned (i.e., reduction in saturated fats and restriction of simple sugars, starch, and alcohol) into one that promotes weight loss (when weight loss is indicated) can be quite effective in lowering TGs, cholesteraol, and improving glycemic control.[50]

Omega-3 Oil

Purified Omega-3 oil (Omacor, Reliant) has been shown to significantly reduce TGs while having a neutral effect on LDL-C and HDL-C in diabetic patients, and to significantly reduce mortality in postmyocardial infarction survivors.[8,51] Omega-3 oil regulates activity of nuclear receptors which results in directing fatty acid metabolism toward beta-oxidation and away from TG storage. This action is mediated by omega-3 oil-associated reduced expression of sterol regulatory element binding protein 1c (SREBP 1c), a dominant lipogenic gene regulator controlling lipogenesis.[52,53] Omega-3 oil also stimulates lipoprotein lipase activity resulting in delipidation of VLDL. Because of the efficient removal of TG from VLDL and conversion of VLDL to LDL, there is a modest rise of LDL-C especially in diabetic patients with marked hypertriglyceridemia. However, the LDL particle generated by this mechanism is large, buoyant, and thought to be less atherogenic.

In addition, Omega-3 oil has antithrombotic and vasodilatory effect by interfering with platelet aggregation, and providing substrate for increasing the production of thromboxane A_3 (a poor vasoconstrictor) in favor of the potent vasoconstrictor, thromboxane A_2.[54] And there is speculation, stemming from results of one clinical trial, that omega-3 oil may have life-saving antiarrhythmic properties.[8]

For the reasons mentioned above, isocalorically substituted omega-3 oil (1–4 g/day) or increasing fish consumption to two dishes per week may be a desirable addition to the therapeutic regimen designed to treat the dyslipidemia of type 2 diabetes.

Physical Activity

Exercise is an important adjunct to therapy for type 2 diabetes and obesity. Unfortunately, the word "exercise" like "diet" often is associated with negative connotations as the U.S. population become more sedentary, overweight/obese, and diabetic. We know that adolescents' participation in physical activity is very poor and that this lifestyle carries over into adulthood. There is a direct correlation between the hours spent watching TV and childhood and adolescent obesity.[55] Overall, 26% of the U.S. children aged 8–16 years watch 4 hours or more of TV every day and 67% watch at least 2 hours daily. African American boys and girls compared to other ethnic groups surveyed, had the highest rate of watching 4 or more hours of TV per day at 42%.[56]

A concerted effort must be made by the clinician and the health care team to initiate and sustain a safe exercise program for patients with type 2 diabetes. Studies have shown that participation in physical activity on a regular basis in patients with type 2 diabetes can result in reduced total and abdominal fat,[57] improved insulin sensitivity and glycemic control,[58–60] improved left ventricular diastolic function, arterial compliance,[61] and improved control of blood pressure and lipids. For example, aerobic exercise training has been shown to significantly lower plasma TGs and increase HDL-C.[62] Weight loss through exercise training and controlled diet may have metabolic advantages over diet only-induced weight loss. In fact, studies have shown that type 2 diabetes can be prevented by approximately 60% with regular aerobic exercise in obese subjects with glucose intolerance.[63,64] The exercise prescription for patients with type 2 diabetes depends on their individual level of fitness. The therapeutic goal is to achieve a daily aerobic exercise regimen that is commensurate with level of fitness for the individual patient[65,66] (Table 8-4).

While regular exercise has many benefits for patients with type 2 diabetes, there are some attendant hazards that can occur. Patients with type 2 diabetes are considered to have underlying coronary artery disease (CAD) and therefore, aerobic exercise may place the patient at risk for cardiac arrhythmia or myocardial infarction. Diabetic patients may have peripheral neuropathy, which predisposes them to foot and joint injury as a result of high impact during exercise. Also, loss of vision in patients with diabetic retinopathy due to heavy impact or increased intracranial pressure has been

Table 8-4 **Prescribing Exercise for the Individual Patient**

Prescription Parameters	Sedentary	Not regular Exercise	Regular Exercise
Exercise level	Moderate	Moderate to vigorous	Vigorous
Frequency	5–7 days/week	≥3 days/week	3–5 days/week
Intensity	40–60% MHR	50–65% MHR	65–85% MHR
Duration	30 min	20–60 min	30–60 min
Progression	Inc. duration 5%/week	Inc. freq. by 1 day/week	Maint. or inc.*

Abbreviation: MHR, maximum heart rate.

Source: Modified from Ref. 66.

reported.[67,68] Metabolic complications caused by exercise in diabetic patients include hyperglycemia and ketosis due to increased liver production of glucose, or hypoglycemia resulting from exercise-induced improved insulin sensitivity and enhanced glucose uptake.[69]

To begin an exercise program that is effective and safe the diabetic patient should first undergo cardiac evaluation, which includes an assessment of exercise tolerance and risk stratification. An individualized exercise prescription for each patient can be achieved with the service of an exercise physiologist.[70] The podiatrist plays a key role in assessing foot care and prescribing suitable foot ware for exercising.

Complications of glycemic control caused by aerobic exercise can be avoided by paying close attention to the diabetic regimen (adjusting the dose of insulin or oral hypoglycemic agents and self-monitoring of blood glucose).

PHARMACOLOGIC TREATMENT

Statins

Controlled clinical trials show greater cardiovascular benefits from statin therapy in patient subgroups with type 2 diabetes, impaired fasting glucose, and metabolic syndrome.[32,33] According to the ATP III and ADA guidelines, statins are the first-line drugs for the treatment of dyslipidemia of diabetes.[44,45] This class of drug is the most effective in reducing LDL-C; it lowers TGs (20–30%) and raises HDL-C moderately (5–10%).[71,72] Statin-induced rise in HDL is thought to be caused by inhibiting the geranylgeranyl pyrophosphate (GGPP) pathway and prenylation of Rho proteins which indirectly lead to PPARα activation.[73] Statin-induced reduction in plasma concentration of LDL and VLDL is due to enhanced clearance by the LDL receptor.[74]

There are currently six statins available for clinical use in the United States. In terms of drug potency, statins can be grouped into two categories: less potent, LDL-C reduction 20–40% (fluvastatin, pravastatin, and lovastatin); more potent, LDL-C reduction 30–60% (simvastatin, atorvastatin, and rosuvastatin). In general, selection of a statin depends on the patient's CHD risk and the patient's target LDL-C. All statins are remarkably safe. Currently, there is no evidence that one statin is more or less safe than the other.

In the Heart Protection Study, 5963 patients with type 2 diabetes and total cholesterol >135 mg/dL were enrolled. In that study, patients assigned to simvastatin 40 mg/day demonstrated a 22% reduction in the event rate of cardiac events.[75] This risk reduction was similar among all LDL subcategories. In the Collaborative Atorvastatin Diabetes Study (CARDS) trial, 2838 patients with type 2 diabetes with retinopathy, albuminuria, or hypertension were randomized to atorvastatin 10 mg or placebo. The primary endpoint was first coronary event, coronary revascularization, or stroke. In the treated group, LDL-C was reduced by 40% and the median LDL-C was 78 mg/dL. This study was stopped prematurely at 3.9 years because of a 37% reduction in primary endpoints in the treated group (Fig. 8-4).[32] Other clinical trials

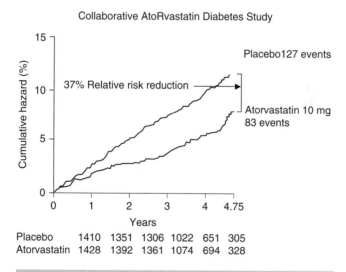

Figure 8-4 **CARDS: atorvastatin reduces primary outcome in patients with diabetes.** (Source: Adapted from Colhoun HM, Betteridge DJ, Durrington PN, et al. Primary prevention of cardiovascular disease with atorvastatin in type 2 diabetes in the Collaborative Atorvastatin Diabetes Study (CARDS): multicentre randomized placebo-controlled trial. Lancet 2004;364:685–696.)

using statins have included small numbers of diabetic patients that show similar outcomes as seen in the Heart Protection Study and in CARDS.

The therapeutic goal for LDL-C in diabetic patients without clinical CHD is <100 mg/dL, and for those patients with CHD the goal should be <70 mg/dL.[43] After achieving the desired level of LDL-C, the next target should be lowering non-HDL-C to 30 mg/dL, above the of LDL-C goal (Table 8-5).[71]

Statin-Induced Proteinuria

Proteinuria associated with statin therapy has been shown to occur with all statins, most frequently with rosuvastatin taken at the 80 mg/day dose. Statin-induced proteinuria was in general transient and not associated with worsening renal function.[76] In fact, there is mounting evidence that statins may be renoprotective.[77]

Receptor-mediated endocytosis is the mechanism responsible for the renal proximal tubule uptake of albumin and other, smaller molecular weight proteins. Statins variably inhibit the synthesis of mevalonate, which is necessary for the generation of isoprenoid pyrophosphates (i.e., GGPP). GGPP is required for prenylation of the guanosine triphosphate (GTP)-binding protein needed to stabilize proximal tubule protein receptors, cubulin, and megalin.[74] Therefore, statin inhibition of hydroxymethylglutaryl- coenzyme A (HMG-CoA) reductase can impair receptor-mediated endocytosis and this may result in tubular proteinuria in some patients.[79,80] This type of proteinuria should not be confused with glomerular proteinuria, which is an indicator of significant renal dysfunction. Moreover, statin treatment has been shown to be safe and to significantly lower the incidence of major cardiac events in subjects with microalbuminuria and metabolic syndrome (mean follow-up 46 months).[81]

Table 8-5 **ATP III: Management of Diabetic Dyslipidemia**

Primary target of therapy: LDL-C
Diabetes: CHD risk equivalent
Goal for persons with diabetes and no CHD: <100 mg/dL
Goal for persons with CHD and diabetes: <70 mg/dL
Therapeutic options:
LDL-C 100–129 mg/dL: increase intensity of TLC; intensify statin therapy, add drug to modify atherogenic dyslipidemia (ezetimibe, fibrate, or nicotinic acid)
LDL-C (130 mg/dL simultaneously initiate TLC and LDL-C-lowering drugs
After LDL-C goal is met: non-HDL-C (<100 mg/dL for persons with CHD and <130 mg/dL for persons without CHD) becomes secondary target

Source: Adapted from Refs. 43 and 71 TLC-Therapeutic lifestyle change.

Bile Acid Sequestrants

Bile acid sequestrants (BAS; e.g., cholestyramine, colestipol, and coleseve-lam) bind bile acids in the intestines and increase fecal excretion of acidic sterols that lead to reduction in the hepatic bile acid pool. Reduction of the hepatic bile acid pool lifts the feedback inhibition of cholesterol 7-alpha hydroxylase and hepatic cholesterol is converted to bile acid. In addition, in response to the BAS interruption of the enterohepatic circulation, two other homeostatic mechanisms are triggered. There is upregulation in LDL recep-tor, and increased cholesterol and VLDL synthesis.

BAS can lower LDL-C in diabetic and nondiabetic patients alike by approximately 20%. However, diabetic patients typically have hypertriglyc-eridemia and, BAS increase plasma TGs. For this reason, hypertriglyc-eridemia will limit the use of BAS in type 2 diabetic patients.[82]

Fibrates

Gemfibrozil and fenofibrate are the two drugs in this class that are avail-able in the United States. These drugs are ligands for PPARα. PPARα acti-vation results in increase beta-oxidation of fatty acids, reduction in plasma TG levels by enhancing lipoprotein lipase activity, and increased HDL-C (by activating genes encoding for apo AI and apo AII). Fibrates lower TGs about 40–50% and raise HDL-C about 10%.[83] Similar to omega-3 ethyl esters, the effect of fibrates on LDL-C plasma concentration is vari-able and this variability depends on the efficiency of conversion of VLDL to LDL by the action of lipoprotein lipase, and on how well LDL is removed from circulation by the LDL receptor.[84] Therefore, it is not uncommon to see a modest rise in LDL-C after treatment with a fibrate in patients with type 2 diabetes and moderate to severe hypertriglyc-eridemia. The LDL generated by this mechanism is a large, less dense, and a less atherogenic particle.

When baseline TGs are not elevated fibrates will lower LDL-C by about 10%.[79] Favorable outcomes (i.e., significant reduction in nonfatal coronary events of 24% in patients with prior history of CAD) from clinical trials were noted in small subsets of diabetic patients in which fibrates were used.[83,85] However, in a more recent report in which fenofibrate monotherapy com-pared to placebo plus usual care in the treatment of dyslipidemia in nearly 10,000 patients with type 2 diabetes, revealed significant prevention in non-fatal heart attacks but a trend toward increased total mortality in the treat-ment group.[86] During the trial 17% of patients randomized to the placebo plus usual care group were on statins, compared to 8% in the treated group. The discrepancy in the use of statins among the study groups during trial may have confounded the primary and secondary outcomes. Nevertheless, the investigators of the FIELD Trial[86] conclude that long-term use of fibrates should be in combination with a statin in type 2 diabetic patients with per-sistent hypertriglyceridemia.

Fibrates increase serum creatinine and are contraindicated in patients with significant renal impairment.[87] Fibrates are highly bound to albumin and displace warfarin. Patients on warfarin require close monitoring when fibrates are used or discontinued. By increasing bile lithogenicity, fibrates therapy raises the risk for gallstone formation. Also, fibrates have been shown to raise homocysteine by 35%; however, the clinical significance of this side effect is unknown.[88]

Nicotinic Acid (NIACIN)

Niacin is unique in that it favorably affects all lipid and lipoprotein abnormalities. Niacin is available in three formulations: immediate release (IR), extended release (ER), and long acting (LA). IR niacin is quickly absorbed and excreted. It reaches peaked blood levels in 30–60 minutes. Like IR, LA niacin is sold over-the-counter and it has delayed absorption that exceeds 12 hours. ER niacin is absorbed over 8–12 hours. There are Food and Drug Administration (FDA)-approved IR and ER niacin formulations but no FDA-approved LA formulation.

Niacin inhibits mobilization of FFAs from adipose tissue and thereby lowers TG synthesis in the liver. In addition, it lowers hepatic apoB content which leads to reduced VLDL synthesis and secretion.[89] Niacin significantly lowers LDL-C by 5–15% and TGs by 20–50%. Niacin is one of a few agents that significantly lowers plasma levels of the atherogenic lipoprotein, Lp (a).[86,90] Other agents that lower the Lp (a) are estrogen and ezetimibe.[91]

Niacin has a profound effect in raising HDC-C by inhibiting hepatic receptor uptake of this lipoprotein, thereby allowing it to remain in circulation longer to further participate in reverse cholesterol transport.[92] HDL-C is increased by niacin from 15 to 30%. Because of niacin's effect on HDL-C metabolism, it is the best drug available to treat patients with isolated low HDL-C.

The drawback in using niacin is its side effect profile. Most common side effects are itching and flushing (prostaglandin mediated) (Table 8-6). It is recommended that patients started on IR or ER niacin should be started on a low dose and gradually titrated upward to a daily dose of 2–3 g. Alternatively,

Table 8-6 **Side Effects of Nicotinic Acid**

Skin	Gastrointestinal	Metabolic	Other
Flushing	Gastritis	Glucose intolerance	Cardiac arrhythmias
Itching	Peptic ulcer disease	Hyperuricemia, gout	Toxic amblyopia
Acanthosis nigricans	Hepatitis	Hyperhomocysteinemia	

Source: Adapted from Refs. 86–91.

taking an aspirin (325 mg) 30 minutes before taking niacin will prevent or minimize flushing.

Other side effects include elevated uric acid, aggravation of peptic ulcer disease, and glucose intolerance. Because it causes glucose intolerance, niacin's use for treating dyslipidemia in type 2 diabetes has been limited. However, niacin may be added with caution to statin therapy in mixed dyslipidemia and persistent elevation in TGs. Niacin is indicated for the treatment of severe hypertriglyceridemia associated with eruptive xanthoma or abdominal pain caused by pancreatitis. Under these circumstances, hypoglycemic therapy may need to be reinforced to maintain glycemic control in patients with type 2 diabetes.

Ezetimibe

Ezetimibe is a selective inhibitor of intestinal absorption of cholesterol (dietary and biliary) through a mechanism dependent on the Nieman Pick C_1 like 1 protein (NPC 1L1). Its major effect, as monotherapy, is to lower LDL-C about 18%.[91] However, when used in combination it dramatically enhances the potency of statins.[93] Ezetimibe also lowers Lp (a) about 7.5%.[87] There are no clinical trial data on the use of ezetimibe in combination therapy in type 2 diabetes. Ezetimibe is very well tolerated as monotherapy and when used in combination with statins transaminase elevations occurred in 1.3% of patients compared to 0.4% of patients on statin monotherapy.

FURTHER PHARMACOLOGIC CONSIDERATIONS

If LDL-C goal is not achieved after initiating statin therapy in the diabetic patient, treatment options include increasing the dose of statin or adding ezetimibe to existing statin therapy. If there is persistent elevation of TGs despite statin use (with or without ezetimibe), one should consider adding a fibrate or nicotinic acid (Fig. 8-5). There is however, no clinical trial evaluation of the latter drug combinations. And one must keep in mind the risk for developing myopathy increases when statins and fibrates (especially gemfibrozil) are combined. Gemfibrozil is to be avoided for combination therapy because of its interference with the glucuronidation, a pathway for the elimination of active hydroxy acid metabolites of statins. Blockade of this pathway results in raised plasma concentrations of the active acid form of statins. Fenofibrate has significantly less glucuronide inhibitory action, and this might explain why there is less drug interaction between it and statins. Fenofibrate is the preferred fibrate for combination therapy with a statin. The statin dose should remain low in combination therapy.[82]

If TGs are very elevated (400 mg/dL or greater), a fibrate or nicotinic acid should be prescribed to minimize the risk of acute pancreatitis (Fig. 8-6). The use of nicotinic acid requires close monitoring of blood sugar since this drug

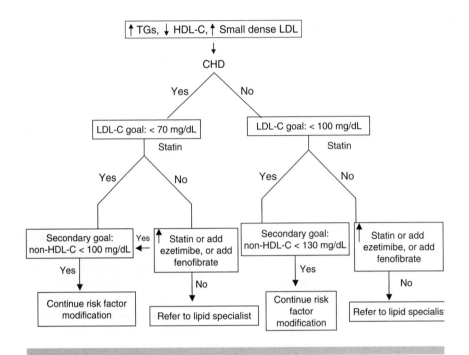

Figure 8-5 **Treatment of diabetic dyslipidemia.**

will cause glucose intolerance as well as other complications (Table 8-6). However, low doses of nicotinic acid (2 g/day or less) may not have much of a deleterious effect on glycemic control while being effective in lowering TGs and raising HDL-C.[45]

Adding omega-3 oil to statin therapy is another variation of combined therapy, which may be useful in treating the dyslipidemia of type 2 diabetes. This combination poses no drug-drug interaction, as omega-3 has no effect on the liver CYP P450 enzyme pathway. This combination has been shown to significantly lower C-reactive protein better than either agent when given as monotherapy in a group of patients with combined dyslipidemia.[94] In another study, the combination of omega-3 oil and atorvastatin resulted in significant reduction in small dense LDL particles compared to atorvastatin monotherapy.[95] In 59 patients with established CHD, taking simvastatin (10–40 mg/day), and randomized to placebo or omega-3 oil (4 g/day) for 1 year, resulted in a 40% reduction in plasma TGs. In this trial, patients with type 2 diabetes did as well as nondiabetic patients. It is also important to note that there was no significant change in fasting glucose concentration or HbA1c in either diabetic or nondiabetic patients receiving omega-3 oil.[96] Finally, in a small group of obese type 2 diabetic men, treatment with atorvastatin 40 mg/day and 4 g/day of omega-3 oil (Omacor, Reliant) significantly improved serum TGs, non-HDL-C, VLDL, and apoB-100.[97]

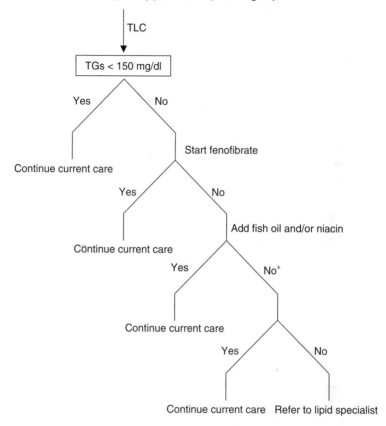

Isolated severe hypertriglyceridemia (≥ 400 mg/dL)

TLC

TGs < 150 mg/dl

Yes — Continue current care

No — Start fenofibrate

Yes — Continue current care

No — Add fish oil and/or niacin

Yes — Continue current care

No*

Yes — Continue current care

No — Refer to lipid specialist

Figure 8-6

CONCLUSION

Abdominal/visceral obesity is a key factor contributing to the atherogenic lipid profile of type 2 diabetes as well as other sequelae, such as hypertension, hyperinsulinemia, and beta-cell apoptosis. A global strategy is required to replace inactivity with healthy active lifestyles and to adapt a diet that provides sufficient calories to achieve and maintain an acceptable lean body weight. In the United States, community-based programs focused on obesity/overweight and type 2 diabetes prevention and treatment will benefit a lot of people by spreading culturally relevant messages while implementing healthy lifestyle programs. A combined effort from health care providers, community leaders, local organizations, legislators, industry, nutrition policy makers, and community residents is necessary in order to tackle the complex

Table 8-7 **Treatment of the Lipid/Lipoprotein Components of Diabetic Dyslipidemia in Adults**

LDL-C lowering

First choice: HMG-CoA reductase inhibitor (statin)
Second choice: fibrates or ezetimibe (used with statin)

HDL-C raising

Behavior interventions such as weight loss, increased physical activity, and
  smoking cessation
Glycemic control
Nicotinic acid* (most effective agent), fibrates

TG lowering

Glycemic control first priority
Fibrates, fish oil, nicotine acid*
Statins are moderately effective at high dose in hypertriglyceridemic subjects
  who also have high LDL-C

*Glycemic regimen may need reinforcement since nicotinic acid causes glucose intolerance.

Source: Adapted from Ref. 95.

and multifaceted problem of obesity, and obesity-related IR, type 2 diabetes, and dyslipidemia.

Pharmacologic treatment of the dyslipidemia of type 2 diabetes should be directed primarily at lowering LDL-C with statin therapy (Table 8-7).[98] If TGs are >400 mg/dL, achieving good glycemic control with diet and hypoglycemic agents (sulfonaureas, thiazolidinediones [TZDs], and insulin) is key. Starting pharmacologic therapy with a fibrate or nicotinic acid because of severe hypertrigyceridemia and the risk of acute pancreatitis, or in cases of eruptive xanthoma, is strongly advised. Combination therapy using a statin and nicotinic acid or a fibrate may be used in patients with elevations in TGs and LDL-C that cannot be corrected to therapeutic goals by a statin alone, however, these regimens have not be evaluated in long-term clinical trials for safety and clinical outcomes.

REFERENCES

1. Haffner SM. Epidemiological studies on the effects of hyperglycemia and improvement of glycemic control on macrovascular events in type 2 diabetes. *Diabetes Care* 1999;22:C54–C56.

2. Laakso M. Hyperglycemia and cardiovascular disease in type 2 diabetes. *Diabetes* 1999;48:937–942.

3. Wild SH, Dunn CJ, McKeigue PM, et al. Glycemic control and cardiovascular disease in type 2 diabetes: a review. *Diabetes Metab Rev* 1999;15:197–204.

4. U.S. Renal Data System, USRDS 2004 Annual data Report Atlas of End-Stage Disease in the United States, National Institutes of Health, National Institute of Diabetes and Digestive and Kidney Diseases, Bethesda, MD, 2004. United Kingdom Prospective Diabetes Study Group. Intensive blood-glucose control with sulfonylureas or insulin compared with conventional treatment and risk of complications in patients with type 2 diabetes. *Lancet* 1998;352:837–853.

5. Klein R, Klein BE, Moss E. The Wisconsin epidemiological study of diabetic retinopathy: a review. *Diabetes Metab Rev* 1989;5:559–570.

6. Chait A, Bierman E. In: Khan CR, Weir GC, eds., *Joslin's Diabetes Mellitus.* Philadelphia, PA: Lea & Febiger, 1994: 648–664.

7. Haffner SM, Leehto S, Ronnema T, et al. Mortality from coronary artery disease from subjects with type 2 diabetes and in nondiabetic subjects with and without prior myocardial infarction. *N Engl J Med* 1998;339:229–234.

8. GISSI-Prevenzione Investigators. Dietary supplementation with n-3 polyunsaturated fatty acids and vitamin in 11,324 patients with myocardial infarction: results of the GISSI-Prevenzione trial. *Lancet* 1999;354:447–455.

9. Yokoyama M. Effects of eicosapentaenoic acid (EPA) on major cardiovascular events in hypercholesterolemic patients: the Japan EPA Lipid Intervention Study (JELIS). American Heart Association Scientific Sessions. Dallas, TX: Late Breaking Clinical Trials II, 2005.

10. Lazar MA. How obesity causes diabetes: not a tall tale. *Science* 2005;307:373–375.

11. King H, Aubert RE, Herman WH. Global burden of diabetes, 1995-2005: prevalence, numerical estimates, and projections. *Diabetes Care* 1998;21:1414–1431.

12. Centers for Disease Control and Prevention. Diabetes, National Diabetes Fact Sheet: General Information and National on Diabetes in the United States, 2003. U.S. Department of Health and Human Services, National Center for Disease Control and Prevention, Atlanta, GA, 2004.

13. Boyle JP, Honeycutt A, Narayan VKM, et al. Projection of diabetes burden through 2050. *Diabetes care* 2001;24:1936–1940.

14. National Center for Health Statistics. Health, United States, 1998. Hyattsville, MD: Public Health Service, 1999.

15. Popkin BM, Horton S, Kim S, et al. Trends in diet, nutritional status, and diet-related noncommunicable disease in China and India: the economic costs of the nutrition transition. *Nutr Rev* 2001;59:379–390.

16. Yusuf S, Reddy S, Ounpuu S, et al. Global burden of cardiovascular disease. *Circulation* 2001;104:2746–2758.

17. Folsom AR. Associations of general and abdominal obesity with multiple health outcomes in older women: the Iowa Women's Health Study. *Arch Intern Med* 2000;160:2117–2128.

18. Ohlson LO. The influence of body fat distribution on the incidence of diabetes mellitus: 13.5 years of follow-up of the participants in the study of men born in 1913. *Diabetes* 1985;34:1055–1058.

19. Nieves DJ, Cnop M, Retzlaff B, et al. The atherogenic lipoprotein profile associated with obesity and insulin resistance is largely attributable to intra-abdominal fat. *Diabetes* 2003;52:172–179.

20. Pouliot MC, Depres JP, Moorjani S, et al. Visceral obesity in men: association with glucose tolerance, plasma insulin, and lipoprotein levels. *Diabetes* 1992;41:826–843.

21. Auwerx J. PPARγ, the ultimate thrifty gene. *Diabetologia* 1999;42:1033–1049.

22. Schwartz MW, Porte D Jr. Diabetes, obesity, and the brain. *Science* 2005;307: 375–379.

23. Kershaw EE, Flier JS. Adipose tissue as an endocrine organ. *J Clin Endocrinol Metab* 2004;89:2548–2556.

24. Maeda N, Masahiko T, Funahashi T, et al. PPARγ ligands increase expression and plasma concentrations of adiponectin, an adipose-derived protein. *Diabetes* 2001; 50:2094–2099.

25. Hotta K, Funahashi T, Takahashi M, et al. Plasma concentrations of a novel, adipose-specific protein, adiponectin, in type 2 diabetic patients. *Arterioscler Thromb Vasc Biol* 2000;20:1595–1599.

26. Schimdt A, Sheetz MJ, King GL. Molecular understanding of hyperglycemia's adverse effects for diabetic complications. *JAMA* 2002;288:2579–2588.

27. Brownlee M. Biochemistry and molecular cell biology of diabetic complications. *Nature* 2001;414:813–820.

28. Witzum JL, Sternberg D. Role of oxidized low density lipoprotein in atherogenesis. *J Clin Invest* 1991;88:1785–1792.

29. Devaraj S, Vega-Lopez S, Jialal I. Antioxidants, oxidative stress, and inflammation in diabetes. In: Marso SP, Stern DM, eds., *Diabetes and Cardiovascular Disease.* Philadelphia, PA: Lippincott Williams & Wilkins 2004, 19–37.

30. United Kingdom Prospective Diabetes Study Group. Intensive blood-glucose control with sulfonylureas or insulin compared with conventional treatment and risk of complications in patients with type 2 diabetes. *Lancet* 1998;352:837–853.

31. The ALLHAT Officers and Coordinators for the ALLHAT Collaborative Research Group. Major outcomes in high-risk hypertensive patients randomized to angiotensin-converting enzyme inhibitor or calcium channel blocker vs diuretic: the Antihypertensive and Lipid-Lowering Treatment to Prevent Heart Attack Trial (ALLHAT). *JAMA* 2002;288:2981–2997.

32. Colhoun HM, Betteridge DJ, Durrington PN, et al. Primary prevention of cardiovascular disease with atorvastatin in type 2 diabetes in the Collaborative Atorvastatin Diabetes Study (CARDS): multicentre randomized placebo-controlled trial. *Lancet* 2004;364:685–696.

33. Collins R, Armitage J, Parish S, et al. MRC/BHF Heart Protection Study of cholesterol-lowering with simvastatin in 5963 people diabetes: a randomized placebo-controlled trial. *Lancet* 2003;361(9374):2005–2016.

34. The Scandinavian Simvastatin Survival Study Group. Randomized trial of cholesterol lowering in 4444 patients with coronary heart disease: the Scandinavian Simvastatin Survival study (4S). *Lancet* 194;344:1383–1389.

35. Ginsberg HN. Treatment for patients with the metabolic syndrome. *Am J Cardiol* 2003;91:29E–39E.

36. Newmark SR, Anderson CF, Donadio FV, et al. Lipoprotein profiles in adult nephrotics. *Mayo Clin Proc* 1975;50:359–365.

37. Karadi I, Romics L, Heimburger O, et al. Lipoprotein (a) concentration in serum of patients with heavy proteinuria of different origin. *Clin Chem* 1994;35(10): 2121–2123.

38. Boden G, Chen X, Ruiz J, et al. Mechanisms of fatty acid-induced inhibition of glucose uptake. *J Clin Invest* 1994;93:2438–2446.

39. Coppack SW, Jensen MD, Miles JM. In vivo regulation of lipolysis in humans. *J Lipid Res* 1994;35:177–193.

40. Horowitz BS, Goldberg IJ, Mecrab J, et al. Increased plasma and renal clearance of an exchangeable pool of apolipoprotein A-I in subjects with low levels of high-density lipoprotein cholesterol. *J Clin Invest* 1993;91:1743–1760.

41. Eckel RH, Grundy SM, Zimmet PZ. The metabolic syndrome. *Lancet* 2005;356: 1415–1428.

42. Fonseca V. The metabolic syndrome, hyperlipidemia, and insulin resistance. *Clin Cornerstone* 2005;7(2/3):61–72.

43. Grundy SM, Cleeman JI, Metz CN, et al. Implications of recent clinical trial for the National Cholesterol Education Program Adult Treatment Panel III guidelines. *Circulation* 2004;110:227–239.

44. Expert Panel on Detection, Evaluation, and Treatment of High Blood Cholesterol in Adults (Adult Treatment Panel III). Executive, and Treatment of the Third Report of the National Cholesterol Education Program (NECP). *JAMA* 2001; 285:2486–2497.

45. American Diabetes Association. Dyslipidemia management in adults with diabetes. *Diabetes Care* 2004;27:S68–S71.

46. Marcul M, Blair EH, Watanabe R, et al. Caloric restriction per se is a significant factor in improvements in glycemic control and insulin sensitivity during weight loss in obese NIDDM patients. *Diabetes Care* 1994;17:30–36.

47. Resnick HE, Halter JB, Lin X. Relation of weight gain and weight loss on subsequent diabetes risk in overweight adults. *J Epidemiol Community Health* 2000; 54:596–602.

48. Foster GD, Wyatt HR, Hill JO, et al. A randomized trial of a low-carbohydrate diet for obesity. *N Engl J Med* 2003;348;2082–2090.

49. Nuttall FQ, Gannon M. Metabolic response of people with type 2 diabetes to a high protein diet. *Nutr Metab* 2004;1:6–15.

50. American Diabetes Association. Nutrition principles and recommendations in diabetes (Position Statement). *Diabetes Care* 2004;27(Suppl 10):S36–S46.

51. Holub BJ. Clinical nutrition: 4. Omega-3 fatty acids in cardiovascular care. *CMAJ* 2002;166(5):608–615.

52. Thomas J, Bramlett KS, Montrose C, et al. A chemical switch regulates fibrate specificity for peroxisome proliferators-activated receptor alpha (PPAR alpha) versus liver X receptor. *J Biol Chem* 2003;278:2403–2410.

53. Jump DB. The biochemistry of n-3 polyunsaturated fatty acids. *J Biol Chem* 2002;277:8755–8758.

54. Connor WE. Importance of n-3 fatty acids in health and disease. *Am J Clin Nutr* 2000;71(Suppl):171S–175S.

55. Crespo CJ, Smith E, Troiano RP, et al. Television watching, energy intake, and obesity in US children: results in from the third National Health and Nutrition Examination Survey, 1988-1994. *Arch Pediatr Adolesc Med* 2001;155:360–365.

56. Andersen RE, Crespb CJ, Barlett SJ, et al. Relationship of physical activity and television watching with body weight and level of fatness among children. Results from the Third National Health and Nutrition Examination Survey. *JAMA* 1998;279:938–942.

57. Wing RR, Hill JO. Successful weight loss maintenance. *Annu Rev Nutr* 2001; 21:323–341.

58. Mikines KJ, Sonne B, Tronier B, et al. Effects of acute exercise and detraining on insulin action trained men. *J Appl Physiol* 1989;166:604–711.

59. Rosenthal M, Haskell WL, Solomon R, et al. Demonstration of a relationship between level of physical training and insulin-stimulated glucose utilization in normal humans. *Diabetes* 1983;32:408–411.

60. Watts NB, Spanheimer RG, DiGirolamo M, et al. Prediction of glucose response to weight loss in patients with non-insulin-dependent diabetes mellitus. *Arch Intern Med* 1990;150:803–806.

61. McGavock J, Mandic S, Lewanczuk R, et al. Cardiovascular adaptations to exercise training in postmenopausal women with type 2 diabetes mellitus. *Cardiovsc Diabetol* 2004;3:3–15.

62. Durstine JL, Grandjean PW, Cox CA, et al. Lipids, lipoproteins, and exercise. *J Cardiopulm Rehabil* 2002;22:385–398.

63. Tuomilehto J, Lindsrom J, Eriksson JG, et al., for the Finnish Diabetes Prevention Study Group. Prevention of type 2 diabetes mellitus by changes in lifestyle among subjects with impaired glucose tolerance. *N Engl J Med* 2001;344: 1343–1350.

64. Knowler WC, Barrett-Connor E, Fowler SE, et al. Diabetes Prevention Program Research Group. Reduction in the incidence of type 2 diabetes with lifestyle intervention or meformin. *N Engl J Med* 2002;346:393–403.

65. Di Loreto, Fanelli C, Lucidi P, et al. Make your diabetic patients walk. *Diabetes Cares* 2005;28:1295–1302.

66. Anderson RE, Blair SN, Cheskin LJ, et al. Encouraging patients to become more physically active: the physician's role. *Ann Intern Med* 1997;129:395–400.

67. Bell DS. Exercise for patients with diabetes. Benefits, risks, precautions. *Postgrad Med* 1992;92(1):187–190.

68. Chipkin SR, Klugh SA, Chasan-Taber L. Exercise and diabetes. *Cardiol Clin* 2001;19(3):498–505.

69. Horton ES. Exercise and diabetes mellitus. *Med Clin North Am* 1988;72:1301–1321.

70. King CN, Senn MD. Exercise testing and prescription. Practical recommendations for the sedentary. *Sports Med* 1996;21:326–336.

71. Grundy SM, Cleeman JI, Daniels SR, et al. Diagnosis and treatment of the metabolic syndrome. *Circulation* 2005;112:2735–2752.

72. McKenney JM, Jones PH, Adamczyk MA, et al. Comparison of the efficacy of rosuvastatin versus atorvastatin, simvastatin and pravastatin in achieving lipid goals: results from the STELLAR trail. *Curr Med Res Opin* 2003;19(8): 557–566.

73. Martin G, Duez H, Blanquart C, et al. Statin-induced inhibition of the Rho-signaling pathway activates PPRARα and induces HDK apo A-I. *J Clin Invest* 2001;107:1423–1432.

74. Bilz S, Wagner S, Schmitz M, et al. Effects of atorvastatin versus fenofibrate on apoB-100 and apoA-I kinetics in mixed hyperlipidemia. *J Lipid Res* 2001;45: 174–185.

75. Heart Protection Study Collaborative Group: MRC/BHF Heart Protection Study of cholesterol-lowering with simvastatin in 5963 people with diabetes: a randomized placebo controlled trial. *Lancet* 2003;361:2005–2016.

76. Brewer HB. Benefit-risk assessment of rosuvastatin 10 to 40 milligrams. *Am J Cardiol* 2003;92:23K–29K.

77. Fried LF, Orchard TJ, Kasiske BL. Effect if lipid reduction on the progression of renal disease: a meta-analysis. *Kidney Int* 2001;59:260–269.

78. Christensen EL. Pathophysiopogy of protein and vitamin handling in the proximal tubule. *Nephrol Dial Transplant* 2002;17(Suppl 9):57–58.

79. Sidaway JE, Davisdon RG, McTaggart F. Inhibitors of 3-hydroxyl-3-methylglutaryl CoA reductase reduce receptor-mediated endocytosis in opossum kidney cells. *J Am Soc Nephrol* 2004;15:2258–2265.

80. Verhulst A, D'PC, DE Broe ME. Inhibitors of HMG-CoA reductase reduce receptor-mediated endocytosis in human kidney proximal tubular cells. *J Am Soc Nephrol* 2004;15:2249–2257.

81. Geluk CA, Asselbergs FW, Hillege HL, et al. Impact of statins in microalbuminuric subjects with the metabolic syndrome: a substudy of the PREVENT Intervention Trial. *Eur Heart J* 2005;26(13):1314–1320.

82. Stone NJ, Blum CB. *Management of Lipids in Clinical Practice*, 5th ed. West Islip, NY: Professional Communication Publisher, 2005: 311.

83. Frick MH, Elo O, Haapa K, et al. Helsinki Heart Study: primary prevention trial with Gemfibrozil in middle-aged men with dyslipidemia. Safety of treatment, changes in risk factors, and incidence of coronary heart disease. *N Engl J Med* 1987;317:1237–1245.

84. Insua A, Massari F, Rodriguez M, et al. Fenofibrate or gemfibrozil for treatment of types IIa and IIb primary hyperlipoproteinemia: a randomized, double-blind, crossover study. *Endocr Pract* 2002;8:96–101.

85. Rubins HB, Robins SJ, Collins D, et al. Gemfibrozil for the secondary prevention of coronary heart disease in men with low levels of high-density lipoprotein cholesterol. Veterans Affairs High-Density Lipoprotein Cholesterol Intervention Trial Study Group. *N Engl J Med* 1999;341:410–418.

86. Keech A, Simes RJ, Best J, et al. Effects of long-term fenofibrate therapy on cardiovascular events I 9795 people with type 2 diabetes mellitus (the FIELD study). *Lancet* 2005;366(9500):1849–1861.

87. Yadav D, Pitchumoni CS. Issues in hyperlipidemic pancreatitis. *J Clin Gastroenterol* 2003;36:54–62.

88. Giral P, Bruckert E, Jacob N, et al. Homocysteine and lipid lowering agents. A comparison between atorvastatin and fenofibrate in patients with mixed hyperlipidemia. *Atherosclerosis* 2001;154:421–427.

89. Garg R, Malinow M, Pettinger M, et al. Niacin treatment increases plasma homocyst(e)ine levels. *Am Heart J* 1999;138:1082–1087.

90. Grundy SM, Mok HY, Zech L, et al. Influence of nicotinic and acid on metabolism of cholesterol and triglycerides in man. *J Lipid Res* 1981;22:24–36.

91. McKenney J. Niacin. Niacin for dyslipidemia: considerations in product selection. *Am J Health Sys Pharm* 2003;60(10):995–1005.

92. Knopp RH, Gitter H, Truitt T, et al. Effects of ezetimibe, a new cholesterol absorption inhibitor, on plasma lipids in patients with primary hypercholesterolemia. *Eur Heart J* 2003;24:729–741.

93. McKenney J. New perspectives on the use of niacin in the treatment of lipid disorders. *Arch Intern Med* 2004;164:697–705.

94. Ballantyne CM, Houri J, Norarbartolo A, et al. Ezetimibe Study Group. Effect of ezetimibe coadministered with atorvastatin in 628 patients with primary hypercholesterolemia: a prospective, randomized, double-blind trial. *Circulation* 2003;107: 2409–2415.

95. American Diabetes Association. *Diabetes Care* 2000;23(Suppl 1):S57–S60.

96. Harris WS. N-3 fatty acids and serum lipoproteins: human studies. *Am J Clin* 1997;65:1645–1654.

97. Nordoy A, Hansen JB, Brox J, et al. Effects of atorvastatin and omega-3 fatty acids on LDL sub-fractions and postprandial hyperlipidemia in patients with combined hyperlipidemia. *Nutr Metab Cardiovasc Dis* 2001;11:7–16.

98. Durrington PN, Bhatnagar D, Mackness MI, et al. An omega-3 polyunsaturated fatty acid concentrate administered for one year decreased triglycerides in simvastatin treated patients with coronary heart disease and persisting hypertriglyceridaemia. *Heart* 2001;85:544–548.

99. Chan DC, Watts GF, Barrett HR, et al. Regulatory effects of HMG CoA reductase inhibitor and fish oils on apolipoprotein B-100 kinetics in insulin-resistant obese male subjects with dyslipidemia. *Diabetes* 2005;51:2377–2386.

MANAGEMENT OF HYPERTENSION IN PATIENTS WITH DIABETES MELLITUS

Michael A. Weber

BACKGROUND: THE CONNECTION BETWEEN HYPERTENSION AND DIABETES

Hypertension and diabetes mellitus frequently coexist. Both of these conditions can be manifestations of the cardiovascular (CV) metabolic syndrome which is rapidly growing in prevalence in the United States and many other countries. In turn, this syndrome is closely linked to obesity, another condition that is becoming far more common.[1,2]

There are clear mechanistic reasons for how obesity can lead to the features of the metabolic syndrome, including hypertension and diabetes. As reviewed in detail previously,[3] subcutaneous and particularly visceral fat cells associated with obesity—often now referred to as adipocytes—produce growth factors and cytokines that predispose both to increases in blood pressure and to insulin resistance. Among the stimuli that can increase blood pressure are enhanced sympathetic drive as well as the sodium and water retention that often characterize obesity.[4] And, at the same time, there is compelling evidence linking obesity to insulin resistance by a variety of mechanisms that can eventually produce clinical type 2 diabetes mellitus.[3] So, it is not surprising that many hypertensive patients have insulin resistance with an increased risk for diabetes; and it is also not surprising that many diabetic patients have elevated blood pressures. In patients whose diabetes progresses to the development of nephropathy, hypertension almost invariably will become apparent.

Published recommendations for the management of diabetes have had the effect of yet further adding to the likelihood of these conditions existing concomitantly, for it is believed that CV events, stroke, and renal outcomes in diabetic people can best be prevented by aggressive management of high blood pressure. Whereas hypertension usually is diagnosed when blood pressure is 140/90 mmHg or above, the guidelines now recommend that in diabetic patients this diagnostic criterion be set at 130/80 mmHg, thus leading to further increases in the prevalence of hypertension in diabetes.[5,6]

Other risk factors such as lipid disorders likewise are commonly associated with diabetes and hypertension; they are dealt with elsewhere in this book. This chapter will focus on the interactions between diabetes and hypertension, and in particularly will explore the evidence supporting aggressive reduction of blood pressure in diabetes. It will also examine evidence indicating that interrupting the actions of the renin-angiotensin system (RAS) could be a critical part of therapeutic strategies. As well, there is growing evidence that drugs which block the effects of angiotensin II may be beneficial in decreasing the incidence of new-onset diabetes in patients at risk of this condition, and this information will also be examined. Some of the most interesting clinical trials in patients with diabetes have been performed in those with diabetic nephropathy; these clinical trials likewise shed light on the management of hypertension in diabetic patients.

THE COMBINED EFFECTS OF DIABETES MELLITUS AND HYPERTENSION ON CARDIOVASCULAR RISK

Epidemiologic studies demonstrate that the effects of CV risk factors are at least additive when combined. The data in Fig. 9-1 demonstrate the impact of increasing levels of systolic blood pressure (SBP) on the probability of CV mortality.[7] In nondiabetic people, compared with SBPs below 120 mmHg, for instance, values in the range 160–180 mmHg triple the probability of major adverse outcomes. But, in diabetic patients, CV mortality rates at each level of blood pressure are increased two- to threefold compared with nondiabetic individuals.[7] Looking at the same relationship in a different way, the findings in Fig. 9-2 show the effect of hypertension compared with normal blood pressure, separately for men and women, on the likelihood of diabetic patients having myocardial infarctions (MI), strokes, or left ventricular hypertrophy (LVH).[8] It is clear that the presence of hypertension in diabetic patients dramatically increases the probability of these adverse outcomes.

A more precise demonstration of the joint effects of blood pressure and diabetes on CV endpoints is shown in Fig. 9-3. These data show the hazard ratios for diabetic endpoints for death attributed primarily to diabetes and for all-cause mortality in diabetic patients as a function of differing blood pressure levels.[9] It is evident that increases in blood pressure in the range

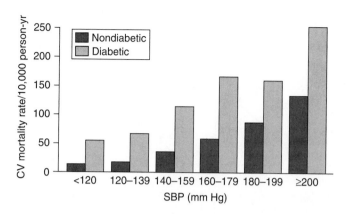

Figure 9-1 **The relationship between SBP and CV mortality across a range of normal and hypertensive blood pressure values in diabetic and nondiabetic patients.** *(Source: Adapted from Stamler J, Vaccaro O, Neaton JD, et al. Diabetes, other risk factors, and 12-yr cardiovascular mortality for men screened in the Multiple Risk Factor Intervention Trial.* Diabetes Care *1993;16(2):434–444.)*

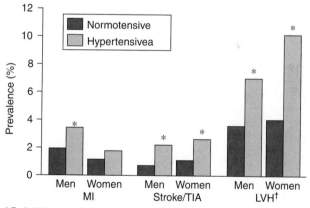

*P<0.05 hypertensive vs normotensive.
†ECG criteria for LVH.

Figure 9-2 **The effects of hypertension (as compared with normal blood pressure, <140/90 mmHg) on MI, strokes, and LVH (as defined by electrocardiographic criteria) in men and women.** *(Source: Data from Hypertension in Diabetes Study (HDS): 1. Prevalence of hypertension in newly presenting type 2 diabetic patients and the association with risk factors for cardiovascular and diabetic complications.* J Hypertens *1993;11:309–317.)*

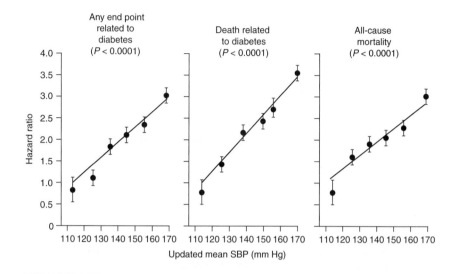

Figure 9-3 **Hazard ratios for all diabetic events, diabetes-related death, and all-cause mortality as a function of increasing deciles of SBP in diabetic patients.** *(Source: Adapted from Adler A, Stratton IM, Neil HA, et al. Association of systolic blood pressure with macrovascular and microvascular complications of type 2 diabetes (UKPDS 36): prospective observational study.* BMJ *2000; 321(7258):412–419.)*

110–170 mmHg increase the risk of these adverse events in a linear fashion; compared with the lowest level of blood pressure in these diabetic patients, the highest value is associated with approximately a fourfold increase in risk. Although epidemiologic data such as these do not necessarily justify treatment recommendation, they nevertheless are strongly consistent with evidence (see later) that achieving the lowest possible blood pressures in patients with diabetes is of clinical value.

CARDIOVASCULAR EFFECTS OF TREATING HYPERTENSION IN PATIENTS WITH DIABETES

It is now almost 40 years since the seminal work of Freis et al. demonstrated that treating hypertension significantly reduced mortality and major CV events.[10] As far as the treatment of hypertension in diabetes is concerned, some compelling early work came from studies of diabetic kidney disease demonstrating that improved control of hypertension resulted in a reduction in the rate of deterioration of renal function.[11] Since then, a number of large-scale clinical trials have more clearly defined the effects of blood pressure treatment on CV outcomes in patients with diabetes mellitus. Some of these studies have been hypertension trials in which diabetic patients formed specified subgroups.

One of the most interesting studies of this type was the Systolic Hypertension in the Elderly Program (SHEP) that was designed to examine the effects on outcome events of treatment of isolated systolic hypertension (SBPs >160 mmHg with diastolic blood pressures <90 mmHg) in elderly patients.[12] Since there had been no previous data addressing this question, the study was placebo-controlled; patients were randomized to treatment with either placebo or the thiazide-like diuretic, chlorthalidone (with an option to add the beta-blocker, atenolol, if needed to reduce SBP below 140 mmHg). The topline results of the trial are found in Fig. 9-4. This figure shows the effects of active treatment on cumulative CV event rates, although the main benefits within this composite endpoint were for reductions in stroke and heart failure. It is interesting that both the nondiabetic and diabetic patients exhibited closely similar treatment benefits, approximately 34% relative reductions in event rates. It is also evident, however, that the

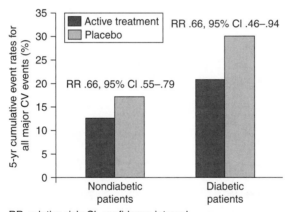

RR, relative risk; CI, confidence interval.

Figure 9-4 **Effects in the SHEP of active treatment (chlorthalidone-based) as compared with placebo in elderly hypertensive patients with isolated systolic hypertension on 5-year event rates for major CV outcomes. Data are shown separately for diabetic and nondiabetic patients. RR, relative risk.** *(Source: Adapted from Curb JD, Pressel SL, Cutler JA, et al. Effect of diuretic-based antihypertensive treatment on cardiovascular disease risk in older diabetic patients with isolated systolic hypertension. Systolic Hypertension in the Elderly Program Cooperative Research Group. JAMA 1996; 276(23):1886–1892.)*

incidence of events in the diabetic patients, regardless of whether they received placebo or active drug, were clearly higher than in the nondiabetic cohort. So, while the two patient groups had similar relative benefits from active treatment, the diabetic patients had a greater absolute benefit.[12]

Another illustrative study, also in an elderly population with predominantly systolic hypertension, was the Systolic Hypertension in Europe (Syst-Eur) trial.[13] This European-based study compared the calcium channel blocker, nitrendipine (combined, when necessary for blood pressure control, with an angiotensin-converting enzyme [ACE] inhibitor) with placebo. Like SHEP,[12] the results for the overall study cohort strongly favored active treatment over placebo, particularly for stroke prevention; the full potential benefits of treatment could not be completely explored because the study was ended prematurely on ethical grounds owing to the early and obvious superiority of the drug therapy.[13] Major endpoints for the study are shown in Fig. 9-5, including data shown separately for the subgroup of diabetic patients included in the trial. Although nondiabetic patients had benefits for stroke reduction and composite CV events, the diabetic patients experienced significantly more powerful results. In fact, as shown in Fig. 9-5, cardiac events and

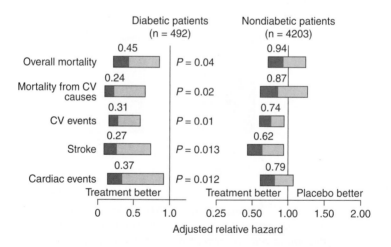

Figure 9-5 **Effects in the Syst-Eur trial of active treatment (nitrendipine-based) as compared with placebo in elderly hypertensive patients with predominant systolic hypertension on mortality from CV causes and nonfatal CV, stroke, and cardiac events. Data are shown separately for diabetic and nondiabetic patients.** (Source: Adapted from Tuomilehto J, Rastenyte D, Birkenhager WH, et al. Effects of calcium-channel blockade in older patients with diabetes and systolic hypertension. Systolic Hypertension in Europe Trial Investigators. N Engl J Med 1999;340(9):677–684.)

mortality were significantly reduced by treatment in the diabetic patients as well as the stroke and composite benefits seen for the full study group. Despite the relatively small number of patients in the diabetic subgroup, this study raised the possibility that diabetic patients might benefit to an even greater extent than nondiabetic patients from effective reduction of blood pressure.

Diabetic patients have been included in several hypertension trials beyond SHEP and Syst-Eur, and many of these are included in a recent meta-analysis of hypertension studies that strongly confirms the benefits of blood pressure reduction in diabetic patients with hypertension.[14] In addition, though, it is important to point out results in the Heart Outcomes Prevention Evaluation (HOPE) study, largely because this is such a well-known and widely cited trial.[15] Although HOPE was not primarily a hypertension study, and patients were not required to have high blood pressures to be enrolled in the trial, the presence of diabetes mellitus was an important inclusion criterion.[15] Other patients were included on the basis of histories of coronary disease, prior strokes, and other evidence for major vascular disease. Patients continued taking medications appropriate to their various conditions. The study examined the effects on major clinical endpoints of an ACE inhibitor, ramipril, compared with placebo, when added to the ongoing treatments.

Figure 9-6 shows the main results in the diabetic and nondiabetic patients in HOPE.[15] As would be expected, the absolute incidence of the primary

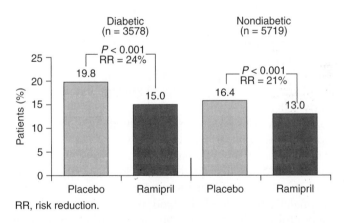

RR, risk reduction.

Figure 9-6 **Effects in the HOPE study of ramipril as compared with placebo in high-risk CV patients on the composite of MI, stroke, or CV death. Data are shown separately for diabetic and nondiabetic patients.** *(Source: Adapted from Yusuf S, Sleight P, Pogue J, et al. Effects of an angiotensin-converting-enzyme inhibitor, ramipril, on cardiovascular events in high-risk patients. The Heart Outcomes Prevention Evaluation Study Investigators. N Engl J Med 2000;342:145–153.)*

endpoint (MI, strokes, or CV death) was higher in diabetic than nondiabetic patients; and the relative treatment-induced reduction in clinical outcomes was at least as high in the diabetic patients as in the nondiabetics. So, as in SHEP,[12] the absolute reduction in events in the diabetic patients was, if anything, greater than for the overall cohort. Following publication of HOPE, there has been active discussion as to whether the benefits associated with treatment reflected ACE inhibition as such, or whether the blood pressure reductions produced by the ACE inhibitor could explain some or most of its observed benefits. It is likely that both of these mechanisms played a part, so HOPE can still be regarded as further evidence that diabetic patients benefit from effective blood pressure reduction.

WHAT IS THE APPROPRIATE BLOOD PRESSURE TARGET IN DIABETES MELLITUS?

The major guidelines for the management of hypertension both in the United States and in Europe recommend a treatment target of <140/90 mmHg for hypertensive patients in general, but a target of <130/80 mmHg for people with diabetes.[5,6] Like most guidelines recommendations, these criteria are based on the judgment of experts using available evidence from well-conducted clinical trials. Only a few studies have examined whether there might be an incremental advantage in terms of reducing major clinical endpoints if outcomes in patients randomized to more aggressive blood pressure control regimens are compared with those in patients getting less aggressive regimens. The two most credible examples of such studies are the Hypertension Outcomes Trial (HOT)[16] and the United Kingdom Prospective Diabetes Study (UKPDS).[17]

The HOT study was designed to examine whether there were outcomes differences among patients randomized to target diastolic blood pressure levels of 90, 85, or 80 mmHg. Treatment was based on a calcium channel blocker and an ACE inhibitor, and additional drugs could be added as required to help achieve the appropriate target level in patients randomized to each of the three target arms. Unfortunately, the intended blood pressure differentials among the groups were not fully realized, for the 90 mmHg group finished with a value slightly less than that level, whereas the 80 mmHg group finished slightly higher than its target. For the patients as a whole, there were no significant differences among the three treatment arms in clinical events. However, as shown in Fig. 9-7, there was a significant trend for event rates in the diabetic subgroup in this study. Indeed, the relatively small difference in diastolic blood pressure across the three groups was associated with approximately a 40% relative difference in event rates between the highest and lowest blood pressure groups.[16]

The UKPDS study was entirely a type 2 diabetes study and was carried out mainly by primary care physicians in Great Britain.[17] This study asked

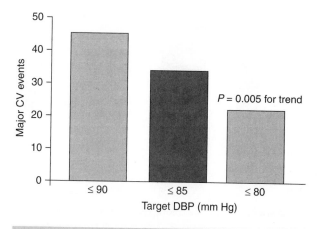

Figure 9-7 **Effects of differing degrees of intensity of blood pressure control in diabetic hypertensive patients on major CV endpoints in the HOT study.** *(Source: Adapted from Hansson L, Zanchetti A, Carruthers S, et al. for the HOT study group. Effects of intensive blood-pressure lowering and low-dose aspirin in patients with hypertension: principal results of the Hypertension Optimal Treatment (HOT) randomized trial. Lancet 1998;351:1755–1762.)*

two basic questions: first, is there a meaningful difference in clinical events when using more aggressive as compared with less aggressive blood pressure treatment? And, second, is there any clinical benefit associated with more aggressive as compared with less aggressive control of blood glucose levels? As far as blood pressure control was concerned, physicians could use either an ACE inhibitor-based regimen or a beta-blocker-based regimen, and patients were randomized—regardless of the regimen used—into a "usual control" as compared with a "tight control" treatment arm. Blood pressures were reduced in all patients, but by the end of the study the "tight control" group had blood pressures that averaged 10/6 mmHg less than the other patients. The results of this study are shown in Fig. 9-8. It is quite clear that tight blood pressure control produced dramatic reductions in stroke, diabetes-related deaths, and other clinical diabetic endpoints. It was also interesting that tight blood pressure control seemed to be even more effective than tight glucose control in preventing these important outcomes.

All the studies discussed so far in the context of hypertension management have demonstrated clear clinical benefits when hypertension is effectively treated in diabetic patients. As well, the evidence points to additional advantages when blood pressure is treated aggressively, though we still do

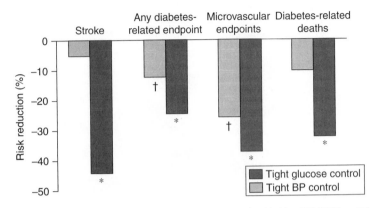

*$P < 0.02$, tight BP control (achieved BP 144/82 mm Hg) vs less tight control (achieved BP 154/87 mm Hg).
†$P < 0.03$, intensive glucose control (achieved HbA$_{1c}$ 7.0%) vs less intensive control (achieved HbA$_{1c}$ 7.9%).

Figure 9-8 **Effects of tight blood pressure and tight glucose control (as compared with usual levels of control) in patients with type 2 diabetes mellitus and hypertension in the UKPDS.** *(Source: Adapted from UK Prospective Diabetes Study Group. Tight blood pressure control and risk of macrovascular and microvascular complications in type 2 diabetes: UKPDS 38.* BMJ *1998;317:703–713.)*

not have definitive information on precisely the most advantageous target for patients with diabetes. Even so, the recommendations of guidelines committees that blood pressures in these patients be reduced to below 130/80 mmHg appear reasonable for preventing CV and other clinical diabetic endpoints.

TREATING HYPERTENSION IN THE DIABETIC PATIENT WITH RENAL INVOLVEMENT

Both hypertension and diabetes predispose to kidney damage, so it is not surprising that diabetic patients with hypertension—a combination that is highly prevalent—are particularly at risk of proteinuria and renal dysfunction. Studies in patients with diabetic nephropathy have been particularly useful in illuminating the value of antihypertensive therapy.

One of the most important early studies in this area was a single-site long-term observation.[11] This study was carried out in a small number of patients with proteinuria and chronic kidney disease. Although this was a nonblinded study, and did not have a control group, the results as shown in Fig. 9-9 are particularly interesting. Following a period during which renal function and proteinuria clearly were deteriorating rapidly, intensive blood pressure-lowering therapy was begun. Of note, together with the resulting

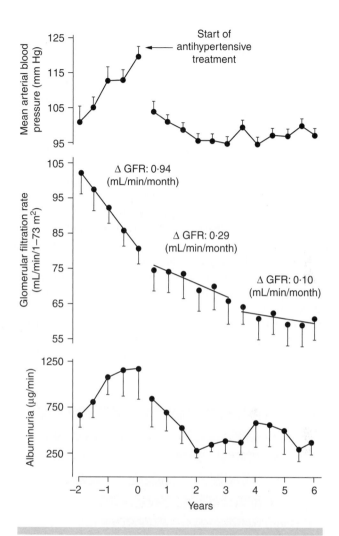

Figure 9-9 **Effects of starting antihypertensive treatment in patients with chronic kidney disease on mean blood pressure, glomerular filtration rate, and albuminuria during a 6-year observation.** *(Source: Adapted from Parving HH, Andersen AR, Smidt UM, et al. Effect of antihypertensive treatment on kidney function in diabetic nephropathy.* Br Med J (Clin Res Ed) *1987;294(6585):1443–1447.)*

reduction in blood pressure, proteinuria was strongly decreased and there was a reduction in the rate of deterioration of renal function.[11] This small but classic study was one of the first to point to the importance of blood reduction in preserving renal function in patients with nephropathy.

Microalbuminuria

Before considering the issues of renal protection, it is interesting to consider the important prognostic signals associated with the appearance of microalbuminuria (urinary albumin excretion between 30 and 300 mg/day). For instance, the investigators of the HOPE study,[15] the trial in high-risk CV patients discussed earlier, noted that microalbuminuria was the single most powerful predictor of adverse CV outcomes in their patient cohort. These data are demonstrated in Fig. 9-10, and emphasize the importance of this physical sign.

It is also known that microalbuminuria often progresses to macroalbuminuria (urinary albumin excretion >300 mg/day), which in turn is termed nephropathy and is an indicator of progression to renal dysfunction and, ultimately, end-stage renal disease (ESRD). Accordingly, therapeutic interruptions of these unwanted progressions have been regarded as critical in the management of diabetic patients, particularly those with high blood pressure. The data shown in Fig. 9-11 show the results of one such study in which an angiotensin receptor blocker was tested in patients with diabetes and microalbuminuria.[18] Compared with control therapy (effective blood pressure medications that did not include angiotensin receptor blockers or ACE inhibitors), the angiotensin receptor blocker effectively—and in dose-dependent fashion—prevented progression of microalbuminuria to

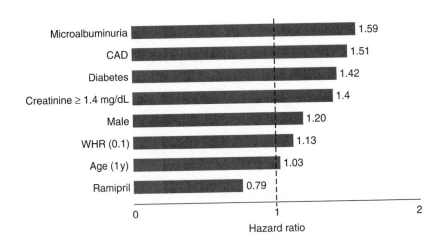

Figure 9-10 **Effects of differing risk factors on the probability of fatal and nonfatal CV outcomes in high-risk patients enrolled in the HOPE study.** (Source: Adapted from Yusuf S, Sleight P, Pogue J, et al. Effects of an angiotensin-converting-enzyme inhibitor, ramipril, on cardiovascular events in high-risk patients. The Heart Outcomes Prevention Evaluation Study Investigators. N Engl J Med 2000;342:145–153.)

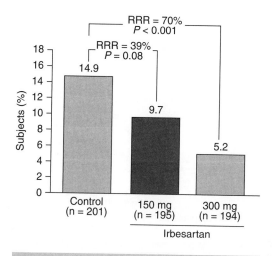

Figure 9-11 **Effects on progression of microalbuminuria to overt nephropathy in patients with type 2 diabetes of control (antihypertensive therapy not including blockers of the RAS) or irbesartan in doses of 150 or 300 mg daily.** (Source: Adapted from Parving HH, Lenhert H, Brochner-Mortensen J, et al. The effect of irbesartan on the development of diabetic nephropathy in patients with type 2 diabetes. N Engl J Med 2001;345(12):870–878.)

nephropathy. This study was important in demonstrating that blockade of the RAS, as well as blood pressure reduction, was important in optimizing renal protection in such patients.

Diabetic Nephropathy

Even though most observations discussed in this chapter pertain to patients with type 2 diabetes, the first important trial to examine the potential benefits of selective antihypertensive therapy in patients with diabetic nephropathy was carried out in those with type 1 diabetes.[19] This pivotal trial compared the ACE inhibitor, captopril, with non-ACE inhibitor antihypertensive agents in such patients. As demonstrated clearly in Fig. 9-12, treatment with this type of agent reduced the composite endpoint of mortality and ESRD by close to 50%. Based on this trial, it is now considered mandatory that patients with type 1 diabetes and nephropathy be treated with an ACE inhibitor.

A more recent trial in patients with type 2 diabetes and nephropathy has extended these observations in two critical ways, showing that beyond RAS

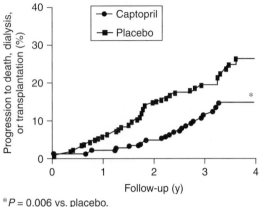

*P = 0.006 vs. placebo.

Figure 9-12 **Effects in patients with type 1 diabetes mellitus and chronic kidney disease of
captopril or placebo on progression to death,
dialysis, or transplantation during a 4-year
treatment period.** (*Source: Adapted from Lewis
EJ, Hunsicker LG, Bain RP, et al. The effect of
angiotensin-converting-enzyme inhibition on diabetic nephropathy. The Collaborative Study
Group.* N Engl J Med *1993;329(20):1456–1462.*)

blockade reductions in blood pressure and proteinuria each contribute to
renal protection. The Irbesartan Diabetic Nephropathy Trial (IDNT) compared the effects of an angiotensin receptor blocker, a calcium channel
blocker, and antihypertensive therapy (not including the principal drug
types used in the other two arms) in patients with type 2 diabetes and
nephropathy.[20] By the end of this study, which had a duration of approximately 4.5 years, patients randomized to irbesartan had significantly less
progression to ESRD, doubling of serum creatinine, or death than in the
other two groups (see Fig. 9-13). However, beyond showing the value of an
angiotensin receptor blocker in such patients, two further pieces of information of therapeutic value were revealed.

The first of these extra findings was related to reduction of proteinuria.
In this trial, the angiotensin receptor blocker was significantly more effective
than the other two treatment strategies in reducing proteinuria throughout
this study.[20] This may have been a critical observation, for in this study, as
well as in a similar trial conducted with the angiotensin receptor blocker,
losartan, those patients whose protein excretions were lowest during therapy had the best outcomes as far as progression to ESRD was concerned.[21]

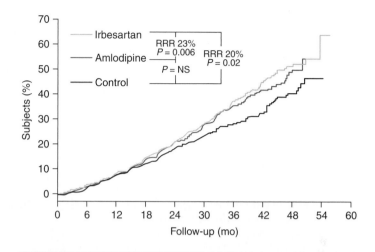

Figure 9-13 **Effects in patients with type 2 diabetes and nephropathy of treatment with antihypertensive agents (control, excluding calcium channel blockers or blockers of the RAS), amlodipine-based therapy, or irbesartan-based therapy on the prevalence of doubling of serum creatinine, ESRD, or death.** *(Source: Adapted from Lewis EJ, Hunsicker LG, Clarke WR, et al. for the Collaborative Study Group. Renoprotective effect of the angiotensin-receptor antagonist irbesartan in patients with nephropathy due to type 2 diabetes. N Engl J Med 2001;345:851–860.)*

The relationships between on-treatment levels of proteinuria and renal or CV endpoints, during losartan treatment, are shown in Fig. 9-14.[22]

A second important discovery in the IDNT study, beyond the apparent benefits of RAS blockade, was the importance of blood pressure reduction. Analysis of renal outcomes in patients in the IDNT study according to quartiles of blood pressure reduction demonstrated, regardless of the type of antihypertensive treatment being used, that patients with the lowest achieved blood pressures during therapy had the best renal prognosis.[23] Figure 9-15 shows clearly, beyond drug type, blood pressure effects of treatment play a significant part in optimizing outcomes.

In summary, these and other studies of patients with diabetic nephropathy appear to have established three important factors in maximizing renal protection in patients with diabetic nephropathy. First, as discussed throughout this chapter, effective control of blood pressure is a major determinant of renal protection. Second, reduction of proteinuria, apparently independent of other treatment effects, is also a major determinant of renal

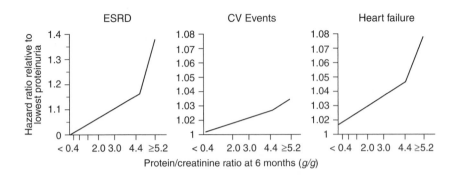

Figure 9-14 **Effects in patients with type 2 diabetes and nephropathy of differing levels of achieved protein:creatinine ratios on the hazard ratios of
ESRD, CV events, or heart failure.** *(Source: Adapted from De Zeeuw D,
Remuzzi G, Parving HH, et al. Proteinuria, a target for renoprotection in patients
with type 2 diabetic nephropathy: lessons from RENAAL. Kidney Int 2004;65:
2309–2320.)*

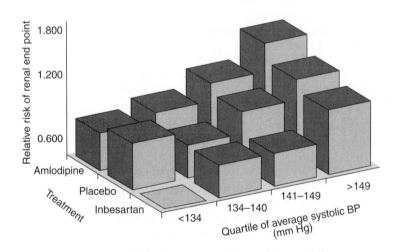

Figure 9-15 **Effects in patients with type 2 diabetes and
nephropathy on renal endpoints of treatments based on placebo
(antihypertensive drugs not including calcium channel blockers
or blockers of the RAS), amlodipine, or irbesartan according to
quartiles of achieved SBPs in the IDNT.** *(Source: Data from Pohl MA,
Blumenthal S, Cordonnier DJ, et al. Independent and additive impact
of blood pressure control and angiotensin II receptor blockade on
renal outcomes in the Irbesartan Diabetic Nephropathy Trial: clinical
implications and limitations. J Am Soc Nephrol 2005;16(10):
3027–3037.)*

outcomes, indicating that reduction of proteinuria should, of itself, be a key goal of treatment. And, third, there appears to be strong evidence both in type 1 and type 2 diabetes that drugs that interrupt the RAS, for the same degree of blood pressure control, may be more effective than other classes of antihypertensive drugs in providing renal protection. Despite this, there is still some debate about the importance of RAS blockade in managing hypertension in patients with diabetes, and this should now be briefly considered.

IS IT NECESSARY TO BLOCK THE RENIN-ANGIOTENSIN SYSTEM?

Despite the apparently convincing evidence that blockers of the RAS have an advantage when compared with other antihypertensive drug classes in providing renal protection in patients with diabetic nephropathy, it is still not clear whether the use of RAS blockers provides similar advantages in reducing endpoints with other organ systems. Indeed, a large-scale meta-analysis that included 27 randomized trials in hypertension with 33,395 diabetic patients and 125,314 nondiabetic patients appeared to find little, if any, evidence for overall benefits of RAS blockers in diabetic patients.[14]

In this analysis, head-to-head comparisons of angiotensin receptor blockers with other drug classes, for instance, demonstrated a modest advantage for the angiotensin receptor blockers in preventing heart failure in diabetic patients, but not for any other important endpoints. Likewise, for ACE inhibitors there did not appear to be any particular benefits in diabetic patients for these agents when compared with other drug classes for preventing CV events or strokes.[14] However, caution must be employed in interpreting the results of large meta-analysis. For instance, this particular study included data from the Antihypertensive and Lipid-Lowering treatment to prevent Heart Attack Trial (ALLHAT)[24] that was biased against ACE inhibitor treatment owing to study design features that caused a significant blood pressure disadvantage to patients being treated in this way. Since even modest blood pressure differences can amplify into important effects on clinical outcomes, this issue could have affected the findings of the meta-analysis.[23] In fact, one interesting finding from this work lends support to the importance of blood pressure differences, for in diabetic patients—as compared with nondiabetic patients—more intense as opposed to less intense treatment of hypertension produced significant endpoint benefits.

It is of interest to consider another widely cited study. The Losartan Intervention for Endpoints Reduction (LIFE)[25] trial is an example of an angiotensin receptor blocker-based trial with nonrenal endpoints that appeared to provide specific benefits for this type of agent in diabetic patients. For the total study cohort of high-risk hypertensive patients, nondiabetics plus diabetics, the angiotensin receptor blocker, losartan, for the same blood pressure

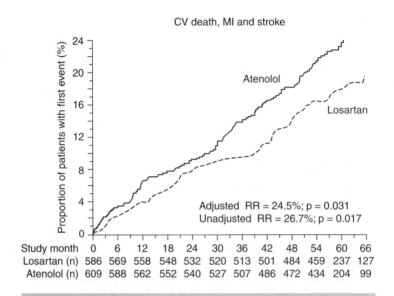

CV death, MI and stroke

Adjusted RR = 24.5%; p = 0.031
Unadjusted RR = 26.7%; p = 0.017

Study month	0	6	12	18	24	30	36	42	48	54	60	66
Losartan (n)	586	569	558	548	532	520	513	501	484	459	237	127
Atenolol (n)	609	588	562	552	540	527	507	486	472	434	204	99

Figure 9-16 **Effects in patients with diabetes mellitus and hypertension (with ECG evidence for LVH) on CV death, MI, and stroke of treatment with losartan or atenolol during a 5-year period in the LIFE study.** *(Source: Adapted from Lindholm LH, Ibsen H, Dahlof B, et al. for the LIFE Study Group. Cardiovascular morbidity and mortality in patients with diabetes in the Losartan Intervention For Endpoint reduction in hypertension study (LIFE): a randomized trial against atenolol. Lancet 2002;359:1004–1010.)*

effect had a 12% advantage over the beta-blocker, atenolol, in reducing the composite endpoint of fatal and nonfatal coronary events and strokes. This finding was driven primarily by a 25% greater reduction in stroke produced by the angiotensin receptor blocker. When considered alone, however, the diabetic patients had a greater benefit than the overall cohort. As shown in Fig. 9-16, the composite endpoint in the diabetic patients was reduced by 25% by the angiotensin receptor blocker as compared with the beta-blocker.[25] Moreover, unlike the findings for the full cohort, the benefits for the angiotensin receptor blocker were seen separately for stroke, coronary events, and mortality.

TREATING HYPERTENSION: REDUCING THE INCIDENCE OF NEW-ONSET DIABETES

A large proportion of people with hypertension also have evidence for the metabolic syndrome, including findings of insulin resistance and lipid abnormalities in addition to excess body weight. Since many of the patients with this syndrome can progress to the full manifestation of type 2 diabetes, treatment strategies for hypertensive patients that could prevent or at least delay the appearance of this condition are naturally of interest. The choice of drugs used in treating hypertension appears to be important in this respect.

In general, it is believed that blockers of the RAS like ACE inhibitors or angiotensin receptors blockers can reduce the incidence of new-onset diabetes, whereas drugs like thiazide diuretics and beta-blockers might accelerate its appearance. In the HOPE study, for instance, the patients treated with an ACE inhibitor, as compared with placebo, were 30% less likely to have a diagnosis of new-onset diabetes by the end of the trial.[15] Again, in the LIFE study, patients treated with the angiotensin receptor blocker, as compared with a beta-blocker, were approximately 25% less likely to be diagnosed with diabetes by the end of the 4–5 years of treatment.[25] More recently, the Anglo-Scandinavian Cardiac Outcomes Trial (ASCOT), a study carried out in relatively high-risk hypertensive patients, compared so-called newer antihypertensive agents (a calcium channel blocker combined with an ACE inhibitor) with older agents (a beta-blocker combined with a thiazide); the incidence of new-onset diabetes by the end of this 5-year study was about 30% lower in the patients receiving the newer agents.[26]

One of the more interesting studies in this context was the ALLHAT study. The effects of the three separate treatments: diuretic-based, calcium channel blocker-based, and ACE inhibitor-based regimens, on fasting glucose and incident type 2 diabetes are shown in Fig. 9-17.[27] For those patients

Normal FG at baseline (<110 mg/dl)

	Chlorthalidone	Amlodipine	Lisinopril
FG at 4 years:	102.0*	99.8	98.8
Incident diabetes	11.5*	8.3%	7.6%

Impaired FG at baseline (110–125 mg/dl)

	Chlorthalidone	Amlodipine	Lisinopril
FG at 4 years:	138.8**	135.0	122.9
Incident diabetes	52.5%	45.5%	36.8%

* $P < 0.006$ vs. both other drugs; **$P < 0.001$ vs. lisinopril

Figure 9-17 **Effects in high-risk hypertensive patients with normal or impaired fasting glucose (FG) at baseline on FG or new-onset diabetes after 4 years of treatment with chlorthalidone, amlodipine, or lisinopril in the ALLHAT study.** (Source: Data from Barzilay JI, Pressel S, Davis BR, et al. Risk and impact of incident glucose disorders in hypertensive older adults treated with an ACE inhibitor, a diuretic, or a calcium channel blocker: a report from the ALLHAT trial. Am J Hypertens 2004;17:1A.)

with normal baseline fasting glucose values (defined as <110 mg/dL), the incidence of new-onset diabetes was 18% lower in the calcium channel blocker arm than in the diuretic arm, and 43% relatively lower in the ACE inhibitor arm.[24] Of particular note, however, in patients who entered ALL-HAT with impaired fasting glucose (values between 110 and 125 mg/dL), there was a particularly high incidence of new diabetes during the trial. Although this outcome was lower in patients receiving the calcium channel blocker or the ACE inhibitor than in those taking the diuretic, conversion of these patients to type 2 diabetes was still remarkably high in all three groups.[27] One factor that might have contributed to this finding was that most patients in the study, regardless of their primary drug assignment, received a beta-blocker if a second agent was required for blood pressure control.

The original ALLHAT report claimed that the development of new-onset diabetes did not appear to be associated with an increase in CV events.[24] It is likely, though, that this surprising finding could be explained by the fact that patients were not followed for a sufficiently long period following the onset of their diabetes; it has been clearly demonstrated by other investigators that the adverse CV outcomes associated with new-onset diabetes take at least 5 years to become apparent.[28]

Perhaps the best example of the potential protective effects against incident diabetes by a RAS blocker was demonstrated in the Valsartan Antihypertensive Long-term Use Evaluation (VALUE) study.[29] In that clinical trial, the angiotensin receptor blocker, valsartan, was compared with the calcium channel blocker, amlodipine. This calcium channel blocker is known not to adversely affect glucose metabolism, so the apparent benefit of the angiotensin receptor blocker shown in Fig. 9-18 appears to demonstrate that a blocker of the RAS truly has protective effects against the appearance of clinical diabetes. The mechanisms for this effect include increasing insulin sensitivity in the periphery as well as beneficial effects on pancreatic beta-cell function. A more detailed discussion of this issue can be found elsewhere in this Book.

TREATMENT STRATEGIES FOR CONTROLLING HYPERTENSION AND DIABETES

Before considering practical approaches for hypertension treatment it is important to remember that diabetic patients usually have other risk factors as well. Beyond the obvious need to control glucose levels as tightly as possible, it should be noted that a majority of diabetic patients also have lipid abnormalities. Indeed, in the ASCOT-Lipid Lowering Arm (ASCOT-LLA), it was reported that the use of a low-dose statin agent in hypertensive patients, even those who were not diabetic nor had meaningful lipid abnormalities,

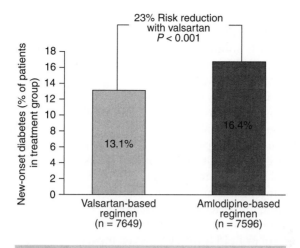

Figure 9-18 **Incidence of new-onset diabetes in previously nondiabetic high-risk hypertensive patients treated with valsartan or amlodipine-based therapies in the VALUE trial.** *(Source: Adapted from Julius S, Kjeldsen SE, Weber M, et al. for the VALUE trial group. Outcomes in hypertensive patients at high cardiovascular risk treated with regimens based on valsartan or amlodipine: the VALUE randomized trial.* Lancet *2004;363:2022–2031.)*

produced significant reductions in major CV events.[30] So, it should be assumed that the treatment of hypertension and diabetes will almost invariably call for concomitant lipid management as well, usually looking to achieve low-density lipoprotein (LDL) cholesterol levels below 100 mg/dL. It is also vital to utilize appropriate lifestyle changes. Weight loss, in particular, will aid diabetes management as well as blood pressure and lipid treatment. Cigarette smoking adds enormously to the risk burden in these patients, and smokers must be encouraged as a matter of urgency to quit this habit.

The following are some practical comments on managing hypertension:

- *Goal of treatment.* Based on the previous discussion in this chapter, the blood pressure target should be <130/180 mmHg; if proteinuria is present (>1 g daily), some experts would recommend getting the SBP down to 125 mmHg.[5]
- *Combination therapy.* To achieve appropriate blood pressure targets in diabetes, most patients will require combination therapy. Guidelines recommend starting with combination treatment if a reduction of 20 mmHg

or more in SBP is needed. This means that for diabetic patients a pre-treatment value of 150 mmHg or more should trigger the use of combination therapy. It should be remembered that treating hypertension in diabetic patients with renal disease can be particularly difficult, and it is not uncommon to require three to six drugs to achieve control.

- *RAS blockers.* In general, the published guidelines[5,6] recommend the use of angiotensin receptors blockers or ACE inhibitors for initiating antihypertensive therapy in diabetic patients. For those patients in whom combination treatment is appropriate, most usually a diuretic would be used with the RAS blocker, although combinations of RAS blockers with calcium channel blockers are becoming popular.

- *Diuretics.* Many physicians are reluctant to routinely use thiazide diuretics for treating hypertension in diabetes. They fear that these agents could cause unwanted effects on key metabolic measurements such as glucose control or lipid levels. However, most of the clinical trials cited in this chapter have shown that diuretics, particularly when added to other agents, have been associated with positive clinical outcomes. It appears that the blood pressure-lowering benefits of the thiazides clearly outweigh any negative impacts of their metabolic side effects.

- *Calcium channel blockers.* These agents also have shown that they contribute valuable protection against CV endpoints in diabetic patients, even when not combined with RAS blockers.[13,29] Together with RAS blockers and low-dose thiazides, calcium channel blockers typically would help comprise the three-drug regimen required for blood pressure control in a large proportion of diabetic patients.

- *Beta-blockers.* Some physicians are concerned that beta-blockers, perhaps because of unwanted effects on glucose and lipid measurements, may only have limited value in treating high-risk patients. Admittedly, in some of the trials cited earlier these agents did not perform as well in preventing CV endpoints as RAS blockers.[25,26] On the other hand, when tight control of blood pressure with beta-blockers was achieved in the UKPDS,[17] the endpoint benefits were at least equal to those achieved with an ACE inhibitor. Beta-blockers can certainly be an effective part of a multidrug regimen in treating hypertension in diabetic patients.

- *Other drug types.* When treatment with the previously mentioned drug classes has still not successfully achieved blood pressure targets, some older agents can be considered. Among these are clonidine which, when administered as a transdermal patch, is both efficacious and well tolerated. Hydralazine can also provide additional antihypertensive effects, though it is important when using this drug to check regularly for sign of lupus. Another direct-acting vasodilator is minoxidil. It is most effective when combined with a powerful diuretic and a sympatholytic agent; one of its main side effects is that it causes unwanted hair growth, which can be particularly of concern in women patients. Reserpine is another agent to be considered; in low doses its known depressive effects are less problematic.

- *Loop diuretics.* Although not as convenient as thiazides, agents like furosemide are usually necessary to produce effective diuresis and blood pressure effects in patients with impaired renal function. Many patients with diabetic nephropathy will require this type of therapy.

- *Unusual combinations.* In difficult-to-control patients it is sometimes necessary to consider unconventional drug combinations. For instance, if a patient is already receiving a dihydropyridine calcium channel blocker, adding a nondihydropyridine can provide further antihypertensive efficacy. Similarly, in a patient already receiving a maximum dose of an angiotensin receptor blocker, adding an ACE inhibitor can enhance antihypertensive efficacy. This combination of two RAS blockers is particularly popular with nephrologists for producing maximum reductions in proteinuria. At the same time, it is important when using this type of therapy to be vigilant in monitoring potassium levels.

REFERENCES

1. United States Department of Health and Human Services, Public Health Service. The Surgeon General's Call to Action to Prevent and Decrease Overweight and Obesity. Rockville, MD: U.S. Department of Health and Human Services, Public Health Service. Office of the Surgeon General, 2001.

2. Ehtisham S, Barrett TG, Shaw NJ. Type 2 diabetes mellitus in UK children: an emerging problem. *Diabetes Med* 2000;17:867–871.

3. Weber MA. The metabolic syndrome. In: Antman E, ed., *Cardiovascular Therapeutics*. Philadelphia, PA: Elsevier, 2006, in press.

4. Weber MA, Neutel JM, Smith DHG. Contrasting clinical properties and exercise responses in obese and lean hypertensive patients. *J Am Coll Cardiol* 2001;37:169–174.

5. The Seventh Report of the Joint National Committee on Prevention, Detection, Evaluation, and Treatment of High Blood Pressure: the JNC 7 report. *JAMA* 2003;289:2560–2572.

6. European Society of Hypertension, European Society of Cardiology guidelines for the management of arterial hypertension. *J Hypertens* 2003;21:1011–1054.

7. Stamler J, Vaccaro O, Neaton JD, et al. Diabetes, other risk factors, and 12-yr cardiovascular mortality for men screened in the Multiple Risk Factor Intervention Trial. *Diabetes Care* 1993;16(2):434–444.

8. Hypertension in Diabetes Study (HDS): 1. Prevalence of hypertension in newly presenting type 2 diabetic patients and the association with risk factors for cardiovascular and diabetic complications. *J Hypertens* 1993;11:309–317.

9. Adler A, Stratton IM, Neil HA, et al. Association of systolic blood pressure with macrovascular and microvascular complications of type 2 diabetes (UKPDS 36): prospective observational study. *BMJ* 2000;321(7258):412–419.

10. Freis ED. A history of hypertension treatment. In: Oparil S, Weber MA, eds., *Hypertension: A Companion to Brenner and Rector's The Kidney*, 2nd ed. Philadelphia, PA: Elsevier, 2005.

11. Parving HH, Andersen AR, Smidt UM, et al. Effect of antihypertensive treatment on kidney function in diabetic nephropathy. *Br Med J (Clin Res Ed)* 1987;294 (6585):1443–1447.

12. Curb JD, Pressel SL, Cutler JA, et al. Effect of diuretic-based antihypertensive treatment on cardiovascular disease risk in older diabetic patients with isolated systolic hypertension. Systolic Hypertension in the Elderly Program Cooperative Research Group. *JAMA* 1996;276(23):1886–1892.

13. Tuomilehto J, Rastenyte D, Birkenhager WH, et al. Effects of calcium-channel blockade in older patients with diabetes and systolic hypertension. Systolic Hypertension in Europe Trial Investigators. *N Engl J Med* 1999;340(9):677–684.

14. Effects of different blood pressure-lowering regimens on major cardiovascular events in individuals with and without diabetes mellitus. Results of prospectively designed overviews of randomized trials. *Arch Intern Med* 2005;165:1410–1419.

15. Yusuf S, Sleight P, Pogue J, et al. Effects of an angiotensin-converting-enzyme inhibitor, ramipril, on cardiovascular events in high-risk patients. The Heart Outcomes Prevention Evaluation Study Investigators. *N Engl J Med* 2000;342: 145–153.

16. Hansson L, Zanchetti A, Carruthers S, et al. for the HOT study group. Effects of intensive blood-pressure lowering and low-dose aspirin in patients with hypertension: principal results of the Hypertension Optimal Treatment (HOT) randomized trial. *Lancet* 1998;351:1755–1762.

17. UK Prospective Diabetes Study Group. Tight blood pressure control and risk of macrovascular and microvascular complications in type 2 diabetes: UKPDS 38. *BMJ* 1998;317:703–713.

18. Parving HH, Lenhert H, Brochner-Mortensen J, et al. The effect of irbesartan on the development of diabetic nephropathy in patients with type 2 diabetes. *N Engl J Med* 2001;345(12):870–878.

19. Lewis EJ, Hunsicker LG, Bain RP, et al. The effect of angiotensin-converting-enzyme inhibition on diabetic nephropathy. The Collaborative Study Group. *N Engl J Med* 1993;329(20):1456–1462.

20. Lewis EJ, Hunsicker LG, Clarke WR, et al. for the Collaborative Study Group. Renoprotective effect of the angiotensin-receptor antagonist irbesartan in patients with nephropathy due to type 2 diabetes. *N Engl J Med* 2001;345:851–860.

21. Brenner BM, Cooper ME, De Zeeuw D, et al. for the RENAAL Study Investigators. Effects of losartan on renal and cardiovascular outcomes in patients with type 2 diabetes and nephropathy. *N Engl J Med* 2001;345:861–869.

22. De Zeeuw D, Remuzzi G, Parving HH, et al. Proteinuria, a target for renoprotection in patients with type 2 diabetic nephropathy: lessons from RENAAL. *Kidney Int* 2004;65:2309–2320.

23. Pohl MA, Blumenthal S, Cordonnier DJ, et al. Independent and additive impact of blood pressure control and angiotensin II receptor blockade on renal outcomes

in the Irbesartan Diabetic Nephropathy Trial: clinical implications and limitations. *J Am Soc Nephrol* 2005;16(10):3027–3037.

24. The ALLHAT Officers and Coordinators for the ALLHAT Collaborative Research Group. Major outcomes in high-risk hypertensive patients randomized to angiotensin-converting enzyme inhibitor or calcium channel blocker vs diuretic. The Antihypertensive and Lipid-Lowering treatment to prevent Heart Attack Trial (ALLHAT). *JAMA* 2002;288:2981–2997.

25. Lindholm LH, Ibsen H, Dahlof B, et al. for the LIFE Study Group. Cardiovascular morbidity and mortality in patients with diabetes in the Losartan Intervention For Endpoint reduction in hypertension study (LIFE): a randomized trial against atenolol. *Lancet* 2002;359:1004–1010.

26. Dahlof B, Sever PS, Poulter NR, et al. for the ASCOT Investigators. Prevention of cardiovascular events with an antihypertensive regimen of amlodipine adding perindopril as required versus atenolol adding bendroflumethiazide as required, in the Anglo-Scandinavian Cardiac Outcomes Trial-Blood Pressure Lowering Arm (ASCOT-BPLA): a multicentre randomized controlled trial. *Lancet* 2005;366:895–906.

27. Barzilay JI, Pressel S, Davis BR, et al. Risk and impact of incident glucose disorders in hypertensive older adults treated with an ACE inhibitor, a diuretic, or a calcium channel blocker: a report from the ALLHAT trial. *Am J Hypertens* 2004;17:1A.

28. Verdecchia P, Reboldi G, Angeli F, et al. Adverse prognostic significance of new diabetes in treated hypertensive subjects. *Hypertension* 2004;43:1–7.

29. Julius S, Kjeldsen SE, Weber M, et al. for the VALUE trial group. Outcomes in hypertensive patients at high cardiovascular risk treated with regimens based on valsartan or amlodipine: the VALUE randomized trial. *Lancet* 2004;363:2022–2031.

30. Sever PS, Dahlof B, Poulter NR, et al. for the ASCOT Investigators. Prevention of coronary and stroke events with atorvastatin in hypertensive patients who have average or lower-than-average cholesterol concentrations, in the Anglo-Scandinavian Cardiac Outcomes Trial–Lipid Lowering Arm (ASCOT-LLA): a milticentre randomized controlled trial. *Lancet* 2003;361:1149–1158.

FITNESS AND EXERCISE REHABILITATION FOR THE HEART DISEASE PATIENT WITH DIABETES MELLITUS

CLINICAL ISSUES PRIOR TO, DURING, AND FOLLOWING EXERCISE TRAINING

Roseann Chesler

Diabetes is the seventh leading cause of death in the United States.[1] Approximately 6% of the population in the United States currently has diabetes and 1,500,000 new cases are diagnosed every year. Women have a higher prevalence of diabetes compared with males. African Americans and Hispanic Americans have nearly twice the incidence of type 2 diabetes compared with whites.[2]

The rate of diabetes is expected to reach epidemic proportions within the next several decades, increasing 165% within the next 50 years.

Over the years, the age-adjusted prevalence of diabetes has risen dramatically from 2.6% of adults over age 45 in 1960, to 7% in 1990, and it is still rising.[3,4]

According to the latest report on teen health from the American Heart Association, approximately 1 million U.S. teens are at high risk for future coronary heart disease (CHD) mediated by the increased diagnosis of hypertension and diabetes secondary to obesity. This has tripled since 1960 (4.2% of 12–19 years old in the United States currently have metabolic syndrome). It has been proposed that this trend is expected to continue to rise as our population becomes more overweight, obese, and physically inactive.[5]

As compelling as these statistics appear, it underestimates the impact of diabetes and its association with an increased mortality. The complications associated with an inability to utilize glucose places an individual at a greater risk of developing microvascular disease, neuropathy, and macrovascular disease.

CHD resulting from an accelerated form of atherosclerosis is common among individuals with both major forms of diabetes mellitus (DM). In the Multiple Risk Factor Intervention Trial, the age-adjusted incidence of CHD was four times greater among those with diabetes[6] and CHD is responsible for approximately 65% of deaths and the onset of CHD generally occurs at a younger age.[7]

Several cardiovascular complications have been identified in the diabetic coronary patient and these include an increased incidence in patient fatality rates following an acute myocardial infarction (MI),[8,9] increased mortality in the months following discharge from an acute MI,[10] cerebrovascular disease,[11] peripheral vascular disease,[12] and chronic congestive heart failure.[13]

In addition, patients diagnosed with diabetes and concomitant cardiovascular disease (CVD) have a more frequent occurrence of silent myocardial ischemia which places them at a greater risk for an adverse exercise-induced cardiovascular event (e.g., MI and sudden cardiac death) and the prevalence of angina is higher.[14]

Although an overwhelming number of epidemiologic investigations have provided convincing evidence to demonstrate a direct relationship between overt diabetes and CVD and many theories have been proposed.[8,9,13,15] To date, the causality between diabetes and atherosclerosis remain undetermined.

It has been postulated that rather than being a complication of DM, CHD and DM share common genetic and environmental antecedents.[16,17] They share many CHD risk factors, and a possible link between them appears to be insulin resistance syndrome, otherwise known as the metabolic syndrome or syndrome X (Fig. 10-1).[18]

As illustrated, an interaction of multiple factors appear to be involved such as hypertension, dyslipidemia, hyperinsulinemia, and the majority of patients who manifest this syndrome have abdominal obesity. In the San Antonio Heart Study, it was noted that obesity, specifically waist circumference, was an independent risk factor for DM and evidence suggests that

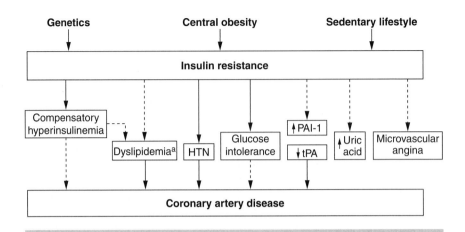

Figure 10-1 **Components of insulin resistance syndrome. Solid arrow (→)
indicates probable or established causal relationship. Dotted arrow (⋯→) indicates association present but causal relationship not determined.
ᵃDyslipidemia includes increased triglyceride levels, decreased HDL-C levels, small dense LDL particles, and large postprandial triglyceride-rich
lipoprotein particles. HTN, hypertension, PAI-1, plasminogen activator
inhibitor, type 1; tPA, tissue plasminogen activator.** *(Source: Adapted from
Erhman JK. Clinical Exercise Physiology. Champaign, IL: Human Kinetics, 2003:
129–152. Original source: Davidson MB. Diabetes Mellitus Diagnosis and
Treatment, 4th ed. Philadelphia, PA: W.B. Saunders, 1998:267–298.)*

abdominal obesity, rather than generalized obesity, is a stronger cardiovascular risk factor.[19]

Elevations in blood pressure (BP) and disturbances in the lipid-lipoprotein
profile, commonly associated with diabetic nephropathy and renal failure secondary to diabetes, will further accelerate the atherosclerotic process.[20,21]

The Framingham data show that hyperlipidemia (higher very low-density
lipoprotein [VLDL] and triglycerides with lower high-density lipoproteins
[HDLs]) is commonly associated with diabetes and it is considered a major
determinant in the development of coronary artery disease.[22] The Scandinavian
Simvastatin Survival Study notes that lowering the low-density lipoprotein
(LDL) in diabetic patients with heart disease significantly decreases cardiac
mortality and events.[23]

Corrective strategies for improving lipoprotein profiles among those
patients with diabetes continues to be investigated. The Diabetes
Atherosclerosis Intervention Study will shed light on whether this corrective
strategy will reduce the CHD mortality and morbidity among those with
type 2 DM.[24]

Although controversial, degree and duration of hyperglycemia have
been implicated as a cause of macrovascular disease. In the patient with

non-insulin-dependent diabetes mellitus (NIDDM), it has been noted that the likelihood of other cardiovascular risk factors precedes the development of hyperglycemia.

The recent findings presented by the Diabetes Complications Trial (DCT) have concluded that vascular complications can be dramatically reduced by intensive glucose control in patients with insulin-dependent diabetes mellitus (IDDM). It is uncertain whether this exists for the patient with NIDDM. There is little doubt that it does not apply to the non-insulin-dependent diabetic, although it appears that in the patient with NIDDM, abnormalities in several other CVD risk factors may be more influential. The data presented by the DCT did not establish whether vascular complications associated with diabetes can be reduced by glycemic control in the older, insulin-dependent diabetic patient.[25]

Several studies have supported evidence to demonstrate that among adult males and females, a low fitness level seems to coincide with an increasing clustering of the metabolic abnormalities associated with the insulin resistance syndrome.[26,27] Based on this, those individuals with type 2 diabetes should derive the greatest benefit from a regimen of regular exercise.

The scope of this chapter is to provide an overview of the role of exercise and fitness in the clinical management of the diabetic patient with heart disease. Several important areas will be addressed:

- Disease-related factors for impaired exercise performance
- Pre-exercise assessment for the diabetic patient
- Review of the acute exercise response in healthy compared with diabetic individuals
- Safe and effective recommendations for endurance and resistance exercise training
- Special disease-related considerations for aerobic and resistance exercise programming
- Potential exercise-related training benefits associated with aerobic and resistance training with a focus on the special needs in the heart disease patient with diabetes
- Special issues regarding exercise compliance and patient education
- Pedometer training as an alternative means of improving physical activity

DISEASE-RELATED EFFECTS ON EXERCISE PERFORMANCE: A MULTIFACTORIAL PROBLEM

Cardiovascular disease and diabetes are multifactorial diseases which ultimately exert a negative impact on exercise performance and functional capacity. In fact, the magnitude of the functional impairment will be largely dictated by the complications associated with both diseases.

Some of the limitations include extent of glycemic control and involvement of peripheral vasculature for the diabetic patient combined with the amount and location of myocardial damage and the nature of the blood supply to the remaining viable myocardium for the patient with underlying heart disease.

It has been reported that patients with uncomplicated type 2 diabetes have an impaired peak exercise performance compared with age- and activity matched controls.[28,29] In previous studies which examined submaximal and maximal oxygen consumption responses during graded exercise, it was demonstrated that in the patient with type 2 diabetes the relationship between oxygen consumption and workload is blunted and there is a slower increase in oxygen consumption at submaximal exercise. This response is similar to that which is observed for patients with congestive heart failure and peripheral vascular disease. In addition, the lactate threshold is lower at submaximal and maximal exercise and there is a greater propensity for early anaerobic metabolism and the onset of dyspnea and/or leg fatigue.[30]

Regensteiner et al. examined the degree of impairment during submaximal and maximal exercise among 10 sedentary patients with uncomplicated, NIDDM compared with healthy controls. While the hemodynamic measurements were not significantly different at maximal exercise, diabetic patients had a 24% lower maximal walking time and a 20% lower oxygen consumption, even after correcting for body mass index (BMI). During graded exercise at submaximal workloads the oxygen consumption per workload was 16% lower compared with nondiabetic controls (Fig. 10-2).[31]

In addition, absolute VO_2 at lactate threshold was lower in the diabetic patient at any given minute of exercise. Therefore, the diabetic patient was working above the lactate threshold and this can limit functional capacity due to early onset of dyspnea or skeletal muscle fatigue (Fig. 10-3).[31]

Based on their findings several possible mechanisms were proposed to explain the reduced submaximal and maximal oxygen consumption among the diabetic patients and they include the following:

1. The reduced rate of circulatory adjustment to an increased workload can be reflective of impaired oxygen delivery that is characteristic of several disease states (e.g., peripheral vascular disease and chronic congestive heart failure). The finding that submaximal VO_2 of diabetic patients was lower than that of controls at submaximal work suggests the possibility that impaired oxygen delivery may limit exercise performance in those with uncomplicated diabetes.[30,31]

2. It has been noted that diabetics also have an impaired cardiac output response to increasing workloads compared with nondiabetics. This occurs even among those with an intact autonomic function.[32]

3. Reduced skeletal muscle strength and weakness is more common among patients with long-term DM compared with age-matched controls[32,33]

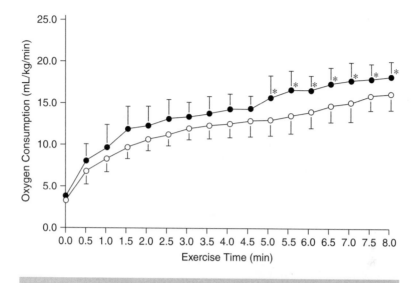

Figure 10-2 **Oxygen consumption during submaximal exercise in diabetic (open circles) and control (closed circles) subjects. The diabetic subjects had a lower oxygen consumption than the nondiabetic subjects. *P < 0.05 between time points.** *(Source: Adapted from Regensteiner JG, Sippel J, McFarling ET, et al. Effects of non-insulin-dependent diabetes on oxygen consumption during treadmill exercise. Med Sci Sports Exerc 1995;27(6):875–881.)*

and this is also a common manifestation shared by those patients with clinical heart disease.

Additional disease-related characteristics resulting from other investigations may be present that help to explain an impaired oxygen transport and reduced exercise tolerance:

1. Cameron et al. and Stephenson et al. demonstrated that muscle atrophy, disruption in contractile proteins, motor neuropathy, and impaired blood flow to skeletal muscles are important factors contributory to skeletal muscle weakness and poor exercise capacity among diabetic patients.[13,14,18,34,35]
2. Blockage of the blood vessels to the heart and periphery, which commonly occurs in the diabetic cardiac patient results in intermittent claudication and impaired exercise tolerance. During large muscle exercise, for example, walking or cycling, the capacity for oxygen transport is essential for the ability to perform prolonged exercise.[36]

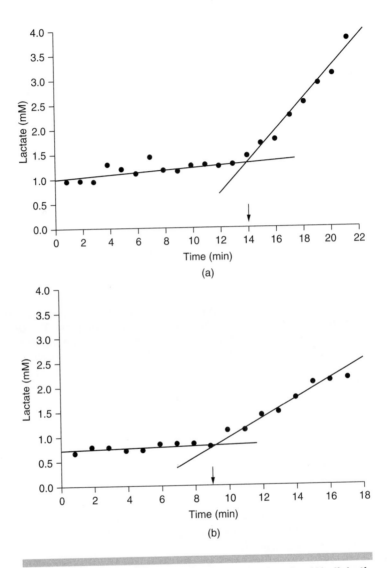

Figure 10-3 **Representative lactate thresholds for (A) diabetic and (B) control subjects. Lines through data points represent regression of the data below and above the lactate threshold. The inflection point for each subject is considered to be the threshold (as indicated by the arrow). The VO_2 at that minute of exercise was identified as the VO_2 of the threshold.** *(Source: Adapted from Regensteiner JG, Sippel J, McFarling ET, et al. Effects of non-insulin-dependent diabetes on oxygen consumption during treadmill exercise. Med Sci Sports Exerc 1995;27(6):875–881.)*

3. Peripheral neuropathy will typically affect the legs. Over time, patients will experience loss of tendon reflexes. As the disease progresses, patients become high risk for foot injuries. Muscle weakness and atrophy can also result.[37]

4. Diabetic autonomic neuropathy has the potential to occur in any system of the body, including cardiovascular, respiratory, or neuroendocrine, all of which are integral to the ability to perform exercise.[38]

5. Cardiovascular autonomic neuropathy is manifested by resting tachycardia, attenuated heart rate (HR) response during exercise, abnormal BP response during and following exercise, and an impaired redistribution of blood flow response. This too can contribute to an impaired functional capacity.[18,38]

MANAGEMENT OF DM: INTRODUCTION TO EXERCISE PROGRAMMING

The medical management for the heart disease patient with DM is a lifetime affair which involves several lifestyle changes. Some of the treatment goals which are important to the heart disease patient with diabetes include improving functional capacity and quality of life, eliminating symptoms related to their disease state, and preventing or reducing the severity of chronic complications associated with both comorbidities.

The four essential therapeutic modalities include medication management, dietary counseling, regular exercise, and improved habitual physical activity. Although several leading health organizations have supported the use of exercise for the patient with DM, many have focused on the beneficial effects of exercise on glycemic control and few mention the improvements in cardiovascular health.

Since diabetes and heart disease are commonly associated with metabolic syndrome, optimal therapeutic management will also target additional atherogenic risk factors such as obesity (BMI and abdominal circumference), hypertension, and hyperlipidemia in order to retard the continued progression of CVD.

In addition, exercise training plays an important role in preserving cardiovascular health because it has been associated with improvements in several characteristics of cardiovascular function and structure including left ventricular (LV) diastolic function,[39–41] endothelial function,[42–45] arterial stiffness,[46–49] and inflammation (C-reactive protein, interleukin [IL]-6).[50–52] All of which are common manifestations of diabetes and coronary disease and they are all factors related to impaired exercise performance.

Pre-exercise Assessment

It is essential to perform a thorough evaluation involving several systems prior to allowing the patient to begin an exercise program. Table 10-1 lists the key essential components for the preexercise evaluation.

Pre-progamming Assesment

Silent myocardial ischemia is very common in the diabetic patient and this can have serious implications, particularly in those with preexisting heart disease. In addition to the screening for vascular and neurologic complications, it is important to also screen for silent ischemia along with assessing the severity of underlying clinical heart disease.

A graded exercise test is strongly recommended in the patients with heart disease and diabetes. Since these patients quite often have abnormal resting ECGs and many are prone to a positive response to exercise (e.g., 1–1.5 mm ST depression) at a moderate stress level (7–10 metabolic equivalents [METS]), it is recommended that the patients undergo a graded exercise test which includes some form of imaging (echocardiography or single photon emission computed tomography [SPECT] nuclear imaging) (Table 10-2).

If the graded exercise test results are to be applied to an individualized systematic exercise program, it is desirable to have the test performed under

Table 10-1 **Components of the Preexercise Assessment**

Cardiovascular status
BP
Evidence of micro- or macrovascular disease (peripheral)
Clinical status (stable CHD)
Optimal management

Neurologic
Neuropathy

Musculoskeletal
Joints
Feet

Ophthalmologic
Retinopathy

Renal
Nephropathy

Table 10-2 **Guidelines for Graded Exercise Testing in the Diabetic Patient**

1. Previously sedentary individual with diabetes aged >35 years; or sedentary at any age and having diabetes >10 years
2. Having type 1 diabetes >15 years or type 2 diabetes >10 years
3. Having additional major risk factors for coronary artery disease, such as the presence of smoking, hyperlipidemia, obesity, and being sedentary
4. Displaying clinically advanced peripheral vascular or renal disease, microvascular disease, cardiomegaly, or congestive heart failure
5. Presence of advanced autonomic, renal, or cerebrovascular disease
6. Patients with known advanced coronary artery or carotid occlusive disease

Source: Adapted from Ref. 53.

conditions similar to those that the patient will exercise under (e.g., time of day and on medications). Specifically, there should be a coordination between testing time and meals, insulin administration, or oral antihyperglycemic agents. In addition, if patients are on cardiac medications, they should also be tested on medications (particularly beta-blockers) to better obtain an accurate target HR and to evaluate BP response during exercise.

Patients should only be considered for exercise if they demonstrate glycemic control. Testing should be avoided if the patient's glucose levels are above 250 mg/dL and ketosis is present or if glucose levels are above 300 mg/dL. If glucose levels are below 100 mg/dL, then the patient should be given glucose prior to testing to prevent exercise-induced hypoglycemia.[53]

If the primary objective of the exercise test is diagnostic, then medications such as antianginal and beta-blockers (which have the potential to mask ischemia due to their blunting effects on myocardial oxygen consumption) should be avoided 2 days prior to the test.[53]

However, these results cannot be applied to the exercise prescription since HR response is different for beta-blockers. Therefore, it may be necessary to test the patient a second time, on medications, to obtain an accurate target HR for exercise training.

The diabetic patient can undergo graded exercise testing using a number of modalities. Certain common modalities such as the treadmill is a more familiar modality and patients tend to achieve a higher exercise capacity compared to a leg cycle ergometer. On the other hand, for those who may have peripheral arterial disease or neuropathy it is recommended to avoid weight-bearing activities. A leg cycle may be a more appropriate modality.

Before initiating the graded exercise test, neurologic problems, eye problems, foot problems, and peripheral vascular problems should all be assessed because they can have a negative impact on the testing protocol as well as dictate the modality of testing.

Table 10-3 **Abnormal Exercise-Induced Cardiovascular Parameters in Patients with Diabetes Having Autonomic Neuropathy**

Parameter	Abnormality or Possible Etiology
Nervous system	Impaired sympathetic
	Impaired parasympathetic
Electrocardiogram	Resting tachycardia (>100 bpm)
	Decreased resting beat-to-beat variation
	Prolonged QT intervals
	Attenuated chronotropic response
	Ischemia: ST-T depression
Arrhythmias	Ischemia potentially secondary to exercise-induced hypoglycemia and its stimulation of the sympathetic nervous system
Diastolic function	Abnormal
LV ejection fraction	Impaired, both at rest and with exercise
Rate-pressure product	Higher resting; lower at exercise maximum
BP	Hypertension with exercise
	Hypotension with exercise
Orthostasis (↓ SBP >20 mmHg on standing)	Decreased release of catecholamines with increased vasoconstrictive effect
Silent ischemia	Advanced coronary artery disease

Source: Adapted from Ref. 53.

Autonomic neuropathy is common among diabetics and it can also present major complications for the patient with coronary disease. Table 10-3 lists some of those abnormal cardiovascular parameters that may manifest during the graded exercise test.

DIABETIC EXERCISE PHYSIOLOGY

The use of exercise as a therapeutic intervention for DM was first noted in the early 1950s. Since that time, an abundant amount of research has isolated the effects of exercise on blood glucose regulation in patients with both types of diabetes.[54]

The physiologic response to exercise depends on several factors including type of diabetes, degree of glycemic control, bioavailability of insulin, diet, and baseline cardiorespiratory fitness level. Patients who have lost the normal compensatory decrease in insulin secretion (IDDM) that accompanies exercise are faced with unique challenges before, during, and after exercise to avoid metabolic decompensation (see "Endurance Exercise," below).[55]

Endurance Exercise

During exercise, whole-body oxygen consumption can increase as much as 20-fold to meet the energy needs of skeletal muscle utilization and this energy demand for oxygen-rich blood is met through a cascade of events which involve the cardiovascular, respiratory, and metabolic systems.

Systemic Adaptations

At the onset of endurance exercise the integrated response directed at meeting the need for oxygen to skeletal muscle involves a shunting of blood from nonactive areas (e.g., hepatosplanchnic and gastrointestinal vascular beds) to working muscle and this is done in a dose-responsive manner. This process is mediated by an enhancement of sympathetic tone which causes generalized vasoconstriction of nonworking vasculature and local vasodilation to skeletal muscle. As a result, approximately 900 mL of blood is supplied to working muscle. In addition, there is an increased oxygen extraction from blood perfusing working muscle.[56] This represents an important component in the adaptive exercise response and it is one of the key limitations for the patient with CVD and microvascular complications associated with the diabetic state.

Central Adaptations

Another essential component for the adaptive response during acute exercise is an increased cardiac output (i.e., HR and stroke volume), which rises linearly with an increase in work output. In the untrained individual, the increase in cardiac output is initially met by a predominant increase in stroke volume (up to approximately 50–60% of oxygen consumption) followed by an increase in HR occurring at higher workloads.

With continued exercise, the body's total oxygen consumption is a reflection of the cardiac output and the skeletal muscles ability to extract oxygen. Since these responses are highly dependent on an intact local muscle metabolic response as well as a peripheral vascular response to sympathetic stimuli, these mechanisms can be significantly impaired in the cardiac patient with concomitant DM.

Metabolic Adaptations

Exercise is a physiologic state which requires a rapid mobilization and redistribution of metabolic fuels to ensure adequate energy supply for skeletal muscle contraction.[57]

During the onset of exercise, muscle glycogen serves as an immediate source of energy which is directly available to contractile tissue. With continued exercise, glycogen stores become depleted and glucose (carried in bloodstream) assumes an important role. Skeletal muscle can consume a significant amount of glucose transported in the blood (70–90%) and this can last up to 48 hours during recovery from a single bout of exercise.

Moderate- or high-intensity exercise will rapidly reduce plasma glucose levels due to the fact that glucose uptake and oxygen consumption is increasing 20 times over resting levels and accounting for 25–40% of the total fuel for oxidative requirements.

In the healthy nondiabetic individual, there is a precise coordination between metabolic and hormonal events during exercise which result in glucose homeostasis. Blood glucose levels remain unchanged or slightly decrease during the initial 40 minutes of exercise.

The predominant fuels for muscular contraction are glucose and free fatty acids. Their relative contributions are dependent on the duration and intensity of exercise, nutritional, and hormonal status of the individual and degree of cardiorespiratory fitness. Trained athletes utilize glucose more efficiently compared with untrained, healthy individuals.

Exercising skeletal muscle will increase glucose uptake as a result of glycogenolysis (utilizing livers' glucose stores), gluconeogenesis (conversion of protein or fat to glucose), lipolysis (glycogen and triglycerides as well as free fatty acids derived from the breakdown of adipose tissue triglycerides and glucose released from the liver), and the stimulation of hepatic glucose output.

At rest, the skeletal muscle is dependent on the oxidation of free fatty acids. With continued exercise, oxidative fuels are utilized in the following sequence:

1. Initially, muscle glycogen is a primary energy source.
2. With continued exercise, local glycogen stores become depleted and blood-borne glucose takes on an important role.
3. With an increase in glucose uptake and utilization, there is an increased production of glucose in the liver, initially due to glycogenolysis and with continued exercise glyconeogenesis.
4. With prolonged exercise, plasma-free fatty acids become a major source of energy yielding substrate. The contribution of free fatty acid to oxidative metabolism may be two times that of glucose at this point in exercise. Diabetic patients are more efficient at utilizing free fatty acids for fuel.

The oxidation of fat-derived fuels is not sufficient to fully replace the utilization of glucose even during prolonged exercise. Therefore, the limiting factor during prolonged exercise (e.g., marathon running) is the availability of circulating glucose. Exercise performance will become diminished once hepatic glucose production becomes inadequate to prevent hypoglycemia.

Hypoglycemia rarely occurs in the nondiabetic individual. The replenishment of glycogen stores usually takes 24–48 hours and the postexercise recovery, especially following exhaustive exercise, is characterized by enhanced insulin sensitivity. However, if exercise continues for a long enough period of time, blood glucose will eventually fall, despite these mechanisms.

It has been noted that exercise endurance increases when muscle glycogen stores are high and there is a positive correlation between the amount of glycogen in skeletal muscle and exercise capacity.[58]

Hormonal Adaptations

The metabolic adjustments that preserve normoglycemia are hormonally mediated. The hormonal responses to exercise include a decreased insulin secretion and a concomitant increase in circulating counter-regulatory hormones (e.g., catecholamines, glucagon, growth hormone, and cortisol).

Insulin plays the most important role in mediating the exercise-induced metabolic adaptations, because it facilitates hepatic glucose production and the mobilization of free fatty acids from the adipose tissue.

Glucose is transported across the skeletal muscle membrane through a series of glucose transporters, one of these transporters is GLUT-4. Insulin and exercise can independently increase the translocation of GLUT-4 to the cell membrane.[59]

The mechanism by which insulin increases glucose transport is by activating the insulin receptor. This results in the phosphorylation of several intracellular proteins (insulin receptor substrate-1). This will initiate the biochemical signals for the translocation of GLUT-4 and subsequently glucose uptake and this occurs as a result of the activation of adenosine monophosphate (AMP)-activated protein kinase by biochemical pathways independent of insulin. This not only occurs during exercise in the healthy individual, but also occurs in those with type 2 diabetes.[60]

In order to maintain these beneficial effects, it is essential to exercise at least every other day. It has been shown that endurance training can improve glucose transport and storage by increasing the activity of hexokinase II and glycogen synthase.[61–63]

Glucagon and epinephrine also play a significant role in maintaining glucose homeostasis during exercise. Glucagon exerts its influence by stimulating and maintaining increased hepatic glucose production during exercise. This will prevent hypoglycemia from occurring as a consequence of increased skeletal muscle glucose uptake. It has been shown that glucagon is responsible for approximately 75% of the increase in exercise-induced hepatic glucose production.[64]

Epinephrine plays a role by preserving circulating glucose levels. This occurs via three mechanisms: (1) exerts a similar effect on liver glucose production, (2) inhibits glucose uptake by skeletal muscle, and (3) stimulates lipolysis in adipose tissue resulting in an increase in free fatty acid production, making it an available alternative substrate for exercising muscle.

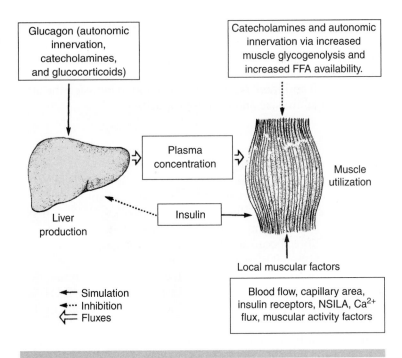

Figure 10-4 **Glucose homeostasis during exercise.** *(Source: Adapted from Zinman B, Vranic M. Diabetes and exercise. Med Clin North Am 1985;69(1):145–157.)*

Figure 10-4 provides a summary of the metabolic and hormonal adaptations during exercise.[57]

The obvious complexity associated with the metabolic and hormonal adaptations during exercise in the healthy individual presents many physiologic challenges for the diabetic patient. This is most evident for the insulin-dependent diabetic patient.

A most distinguishing feature which differentiates the insulin-dependent and the non-insulin-dependent diabetic is that those with insulin-dependent diabetes have lost the hormonal adaptations during exercise. Therefore, they rely predominantly on exogenous insulin injections. As a result, in the insulin-dependent diabetic patient the exercise response will be highly dependent on:

- Type of insulin used
- Time between insulin injections and onset of exercise
- Time between exercise and last meal
- Site of insulin injection (skeletal muscle or abdominal muscle)

Those patients with non-insulin-dependent diabetes characteristically have abnormalities in insulin sensitivity and secretion and although they are also prone to abnormalities in metabolic regulation during exercise, if in glycemic control, adverse affects are not as common.

In the type 1 diabetic, the metabolic response to exercise is influenced by the metabolic state prior to exercise. As a consequence, when patients have too little circulating insulin due to inadequate therapy or if ketosis is present, exercise will result in an increase in plasma glucose and accelerated ketone formation. This occurs because the exercise-induced increase in muscle glucose uptake with exercise is insulin-dependent and in the presence of an insulin deficiency the usual muscle glucose uptake with exercise is inhibited. Insulin deficiency also results in an increased free fatty acid mobilization and this will accelerate ketone body formation by the liver. Therefore, exercise performed by a patient who is insulin deficient should be avoided since it will result in undesirable metabolic consequences as a result of excessive release of counter-insulin hormones during exercise and this may increase already high levels of glucose and ketone bodies, precipitating ketoacidosis.

On the other hand, the presence of high levels of insulin, due to exogenous insulin administration, can attenuate or even prevent the increased mobilization of glucose and other substrates because the elevated insulin levels cause an inhibition of hepatic glucose production. Although the muscle glucose uptake increases with exercise, the liver is unable to increase its production of glucose to replenish the loss of glucose from circulation. As a result, there is a precipitous fall in plasma glucose and hypoglycemia ensues.

This metabolic consequence can also occur if precipitated by a rapid absorption of depot insulin during exercise. Absorption from the injection site increases if exercise involves those muscle groups at the injection site. The elevated insulin levels will inhibit glycogenolysis and gluconeogenesis resulting in a rapid fall in blood glucose levels.

Patients with type 1 diabetes typically have an abnormal glucose excursion with meals resulting from the inadequate matching of depot insulin absorption from the subcutaneous injection site with that of carbohydrate absorption from the gastrointestinal tract. Exercise results in increased glucose utilization by skeletal muscle.

Caron et al. set out to determine whether exercise following a meal could significantly improve postprandial hyperglycemia among type 1 diabetes. The patients were tested under two conditions (at rest and during 45 minutes of leg cycle at 50% of VO_2 max 30 minutes following breakfast). Based on their findings, it appeared that there was a marked improvement in glucose excursion with breakfast in the majority of patients studied. It was also determined that the responses were variable.[65]

Patients should be encouraged to exercise following meals and this may reduce the need for extra caloric supplementation following exercise. Although it is prudent to caution patients about the possibility of a delayed hypoglycemic response which can occur several hours following exercise.

The response to exercise is more unpredictable in patients with type 1 diabetes, since they are more prone to excessive shifts in plasma glucose levels during exercise and the degree of glycemic control during exercise will vary from one patient to another. During exercise, the type 2 diabetic is also susceptible to hypoglycemia, however, it tends to be less of a problem in these patients due to the fact that the major problem associated with this form of diabetes is insulin resistance. Table 10-4 lists some recommendations for the exercise programming in the diabetic patient.

Acute Exercise in the Type 2 Diabetic Patient

For the patient with type 2 diabetes, obesity, excessive caloric intake, and physical inactivity significantly contribute to the onset of type 2 diabetes. Therefore, exercise as a therapeutic modality in this population of patients is targeted at facilitating glycemic control and promoting weight loss.

Exercise causes significant decreases in plasma glucose levels in response to 45 minutes of moderate-intensity exercise. This is related to an increased glucose uptake by skeletal muscle that is retained in nondiabetic and type 2 diabetic patients for approximately 48 hours during recovery from a single bout of exercise. This response is mediated by a combined effect of increased insulin sensitivity and an endogenous increase in GLUT-4 transporters on the sarcolemmas of the exercised muscle fibers.

The exercise-induced increase in insulin sensitivity is greatest during exercise involving a larger skeletal muscle mass.[66] However, for those unaccustomed to exercise, particularly if the type of exercise is eccentric (e.g.,

Table 10-4 **Exercise Program Guidelines for the Diabetic Patient**

- Before your patient starts an exercise program, perform a complete history and physical examination. Evaluate diabetes control and screening for proliferative retinopathy and CVD.
- Prescribe moderate workloads that increase slowly.
- Self blood glucose monitoring can be used to document individual glycemic responses to different circumstances, since changes in insulin or food intake before exercise may be required.
- When possible, the patient should be encouraged to schedule exercise so as to improve postprandial hyperglycemia.
- Discourage the patient from exercising during peak insulin action.
- Exercising extremities should not be used as insulin injection sites.
- Patients should be alerted about the possibility of delayed exercise-induced hypoglycemia, which may occur several hours after the completion of exercise.

Source: Adapted from Ref. 57.

running downhill and weight lifting) the muscle damage associated with this form of exercise causes a transient decrease in insulin sensitivity.[67]

Exercise for the type 2 diabetic should be concentric, rhythmic, and involve large muscle mass. In addition, those sedentary patients beginning an exercise program should start with a low level of exercise, even if it does not provoke target heart rate reserve (HRR). This will allow for a gradual adaptive response and reduce the onset of skeletal muscle soreness.

Studies have noted that the improvements in blood glucose associated with acute exercise will dissipate within 72 hours of the previous exercise bout. This emphasizes the need for consistent exercise participation.[29]

RECOMMENDATIONS FOR EXERCISE PRESCRIPTION

When formulating the exercise prescription it is essential to consider the topic of fitness versus the health benefits acquired with exercise training. An important goal of any exercise program is to improve maximal oxygen uptake. However, this is not the only goal since changes in health status are not always parallel with increases in maximal oxygen consumption. This is an essential point to remember for training the cardiac patient with diabetes because risk factor management is the primary target and this can be achieved with light moderate-intensity exercise which will not have an optimal effect on maximal oxygen consumption.[18]

When prescribing exercise for the diabetic patient it is important to remember that the selection of the mode of exercise should be based on the following: activities that are enjoyable by the patient, activities which are appropriate for the health and fitness status of the individual, and the activities should be ones that can be performed regularly.

Table 10-5 lists the American College of Sports Medicine (ACSM) recommendations for those with DM.[53]

All exercise sessions should be preceded by a warm-up period and followed by a cool-down period. The warm-up period should consist of 5–10 minutes of low-intensity aerobic exercise (e.g., slow walking and unloaded cycling). The rationale behind the warm-up is to prepare the skeletal muscles, heart, and lungs for a progressive increase in exercise intensity and raise skeletal muscle temperature. The muscles involved in the warm-up should be the same muscles that will be used during the exercise training session. Following the exercise session a cool-down should be performed and it can be structured the same way as the warm-up. The cool-down period should last 5–10 minutes and gradually bring the HR down to preexercise levels. After the cooldown session, muscles should be gently stretched for 5–10 minutes.[53]

As mentioned earlier, patients with coronary disease and diabetes have lower oxygen consumption compared with healthy age-matched individuals and many will be obese and unfit. Some patients will be unable to initially

Table 10-5 **Aerobic Training**

Mode	Intensity	Duration	Frequency	Time to Training Goal
Large muscle groups (e.g., walking and swimming)	60–75% HRR or intermittent*	30–60 min continuous Expend at least 1000 kcal/week	4–5 days/week	4–6 months

*HRR = (peak HR − resting HR) + resting HR, intermittent = 10-min sessions, two to three times per day until patient can exercise continuously.

Source: Adapted from Ref. 53.

complete 30 minutes of continuous exercise and will be unable to reach the 1000 kcal weekly energy expenditure. It may be essential to divide the exercise duration into three 10-minute sessions performed two to three times per day until the patient can reach a fitness level, which allows for continuous exercise.

In addition, to better adjust food intake and insulin or oral hyperglycemics the energy requirements of the activities should be quantified.

Resistance training is an effective exercise modality to increase muscle strength and local muscle endurance. Therefore, a resistance training program is paramount for the patient with heart disease and diabetes since muscle atrophy and weakness are manifestations of both diseases and it should be combined with an aerobic exercise program (Table 10-6).[68,69]

For diabetic patients without retinopathy, it is important to instruct them on the proper weight lifting technique (avoid a Valsalva) to prevent an exaggerated BP response (>200 mmHg).[53]

One of the most difficult tasks associated with resistance training is establishing a proper intensity (percentage of the 1-repetition maximum [1 RM]). The 1 RM indicates a weight that a patient can lift one time. The 1 RM should be assessed several times starting at a weight that is 50% of the 1 RM and increasing the weight until an actual 1 RM is lifted. The alternative method for establishing a 1 RM would be to use a 10 RM, which involves lifting a weight for 10 repetitions while monitoring the HR and BP. This weight can be adjusted over several days or weeks until an appropriate workload is established. This is a preferred method for those diabetic patients with coronary disease and those with diabetic complications.

For the diabetic patient with underlying coronary disease it is recommended to control the intensity and duration of the isometric component of the skeletal muscle contraction and the simultaneous pressor response. This

Table 10-6 **Recommendations for Resistance Training in the Diabetic Patient**

Type: resistance

Mode: free weights, machines, elastic bands
Frequency: at least two times per week but never on consecutive days
Duration: 10–15 repetitions per set, one to two sets per type of specific
resistance exercise
Intensity; approximately 60% of 1 RM
Time to training goal: 4–6 months

Type: range of motion

Mode: static stretching
Frequency: postaerobic exercise
Duration: 10–30 s per exercise of each major muscle group

Source: Adapted from Ref. 69.

can be done by selecting lighter resistance loads and performing exercises
which will utilize a smaller amount of muscle mass.[70]

To date, there have been no known adverse effects when exercising
patients with diabetic retinopathy (DR). It has been recommended that severe
endurance exercise and strenuous resistance training be contraindicated
because it may result in retinal hemorrhage and retinal separation. Table 10-7
lists precautions for the diabetic patient with retinopathy.[60,71]

Table 10-7 **Precautions for the Diabetic Patient with Retinopathy**

1. Bending over so that the head is positioned lower than the waist
2. Valsalva-type maneuvers
3. Near-maximal isometric contractions
4. Weight lifting with high resistance and low repetition
5. Rapid eye-head movements (contact sports)
6. Strenuous upper-extremity exercises (rowing, arm cycle ergometry)
7. Vigorous bouncing
8. Parachuting and scuba diving
9. Yoga, as many of the postures used increases intraocular pressure

Source: Data from Graham C, Lasko-McCartney P: Exercise options for persons with diabetic complications.
Diabetes Educ 1990; 16:215.

RISKS AND PRECAUTIONS FOR EXERCISE

Three most common risks associated with exercise training in the patient with diabetes, particularly the insulin-dependent diabetic are: hypoglycemia and hyperglycemia with ketoacidosis and chronic degenerative complications.

Exercise is metabolic (muscle glycogen, bloodborne glucose, and free fatty acids are a primary fuel source), therefore, it is essential that the patient demonstrates a history of satisfactory glycemic control prior to embarking on an exercise program (optimal preexercise glucose level 120–180 mg/dL).

Exercise-induced hypoglycemia is common for those on endogenous insulin and it has also been observed in those on oral sulfonylureas.

It is unclear what the clinical utility is of exercise for glycemic control in the type 1 diabetic patient. Exercise can have a harmful effect by triggering a potentially adverse dual response in glycemic balance. The training-induced enhancement of glucose uptake by skeletal muscle and the enhanced exogenous insulin distribution by an increased circulation provoked with exercise could worsen the glucose supply and usage balance.

To prevent this, it is essential to educate patients on the importance of self-glucose monitoring before and after exercise and as the patient becomes trained, an adjustment in their medications (sometimes 50–90% of the daily dose) may be necessary. At times, extra carbohydrates may be required before, during, and after exercise.

Hyperglycemia is also a common finding particularly in insulin-dependent patients as well as poorly managed diabetic patients. It is usually an adverse response in the under-insulinized state.

If the preexercise glucose levels are above 250 mg/dL, the acute effect of exercise is to augment the release of counter-regulatory hormones (e.g., catecholamines and glucagon) and as a result excess hepatic glucose production will exceed blood glucose uptake in the skeletal muscle due to the lack of insulin. This explains the reason behind postponing exercise if glucose is 250 mg/dL or greater and to begin once the glucose levels are better controlled. Excess glucose levels may also contribute to excessive urinary ketones which can be dangerous and fatal.[53]

Timing of the Exercise Session

To reduce the likelihood that the patient will become hypoglycemic following exercise it is suggested that the patient exercise at the same time of day during each session. It is crucial for the patient to avoid performing exercise during peak insulin action because the exercise will behave like insulin and it will promote peripheral glucose uptake. Therefore, the combination of exercise and insulin will increase the chance that the patient will become hypoglycemic. Because of this, it is more likely that the hypoglycemia will occur following exercise rather than prior to exercise or during exercise. The exercise session should not be scheduled late in the evening when insulin and oral hyperglycemic agents may peak. This will increase the risk of hypoglycemia while the patient is sleeping. Table 10-8 lists the guidelines for preventing hypoglycemia.

The exercise recommendations for the patient with DR will be contingent on the stage of complication and should focus on limiting the increase in systolic blood pressure (SBP) and excluding any type of jarring activities. Table 10-9 lists the general guidelines which incorporate the appropriate activites based on the severity of the retinopathy. It is recommended that exercise be conducted in a supervised environment if retinopathy is significant.

Table 10-8 **Guidelines for Preventing Hypoglycemia**

1. Monitor blood glucose immediately before and 15 min after prolonged exercise.
2. If blood glucose is <100 mg/dL before starting an exercise session, consume 15–20 g of carbohydrates and wait 15–30 min; recheck blood glucose levels and delay exercise until blood glucose is >100 mg/dL.
3. If symptoms appear during exercise, stop immediately and assess BP.
4. If blood glucose monitoring is not possible during exercise, patients should exercise at no more than moderate intensity and supplement with 10–30 g of carbohydrates during exercise of 40–50 min duration.
5. Consume 15–30 g of carbohydrates as soon as possible if blood glucose following exercise is <60 mg/dL.
6. Do not initiate exercise if blood glucose is >250 mg/dL and urinary ketones are present or if blood glucose is >300 mg/dL, even if ketones are not present.
7. Avoid exercising at the time of peak insulin action.
8. Avoid injecting insulin in an extremity that will be exercised. Use the abdominal wall.
9. Reduce insulin dosage prior to exercise:
   a. For moderate-intensity exercises of 45–60 min, reduce insulin dose 15–40%, if exercise is performed during peak time of insulin action.
   b. For CSII, decrease basal insulin infusion rate during an activity and/or preworkout meal bolus.
10. Avoid exercising late at night to avoid hypoglycemic episodes during sleep.

Abbreviation: CSII, continuous subcutaneous insulin infusion.

Source: Adapted from Ref. 60.

Table 10-9 *Considerations for Activity Limitations in the Patient with DR*

Level of DR	Acceptable Activities	Discouraged Activities	Ocular and Activity Reevaluation
No DR	Dictated by medical status	Dictated by medical status	12-months
Mild NPDR	Dictated by medical status	Dictated by medical status	6–12 months
Moderate NPDR	Dictated by medical status	Activities that dramatically increase blood such as power lifting, heavy Valsalva maneuver	
Severe NPDR		Limit systolic blood, Valsalva maneuvers, active jarring, boxing, heavy competitive sports	2–4months (may require laser surgery)
PDR	Low-impact cardiovascular conditioning: swimming (not diving); walking; low-impact aerobics; stationary cycling; endurance exercises	Low-impact cardiovascular jarring; Weight lifting, jogging, high-impact aerobics, racquet sports, strenuous trumpet playing	1–2 months (may require laser surgery)

BP = blood pressure; DR = diabetic retinopathy; NPDR = nonproliferative diabetic retinopathy; PDR = proliferative diabetic retinopathy.

Source: Adapted from Ref. 53.

SPECIAL CONSIDERATIONS

Peripheral Neuropathy

The exercise prescription must be individualized and carefully formulated with consideration given to risks and benefits. The consequences of the patients' disuse that may have resulted from heart disease combined with the complications can lead to more disability than complications alone. A major consideration in patients with peripheral neuropathy is the loss of sensation in the feet and legs. If not considered, these can lead to musculoskeletal injury and infection. It is recommended that the patient be instructed on daily self-foot examinations before and after exercise. Proper footwear must be worn to prevent blisters. An inspection of the feet should be done during routine physician visits and the patient should be instructed not to exercise with blisters or other acute foot problems. Non-weight-bearing exercise is recommended (Table 10-10).

Cardiovascular Neuropathy

Cardiovascular autonomic neuropathy is a common finding in the diabetic patient and it becomes even more important for the patient with underlying coronary disease because it requires several modifications in the exercise plan.

It is manifested by abnormal HR, BP, and redistribution of blood flow resulting in patients having a higher resting HR and lower maximal HR during exercise. For the cardiac patient with coronary artery disease this condition may precipitate exercise-induced ischemia.

Cardiovascular autonomic neuropathy can be detected during the graded exercise test. If present, it would require modification of the exercise prescription. The estimation of peak HR using age-predicted formulas in this population may result in overestimation of the training HR range. In addition, warning signs of myocardial ischemia may be absent among these patients. In addition, the risk of exercise-induced hypotension and sudden death increases. This can have serious consequences especially in the patient with coronary disease.[18]

Hypotension

To avoid a postexercise hypotensive response, it is essential to have the patient perform an active cool-down (activities similar to that incorporated in the exercise session, but with less intensity). Exercise among patients that demonstrate postexercise hypotension should target lower-intensity activities where mild changes in HR and BP can be accommodated.

In addition, due to the problems with thermoregulation, diabetic patients should be instructed to stay hydrated and avoid exercise in extreme heat or cold.

Lipid-Lowering Medications: Muscle Weakness

It is very likely that the coronary diabetic patient will also be on a regimen of lipid-lowering medications (e.g., hydroxymethylglutaryl-coenzyme A [HMG-CoA] reductase inhibitors) which have the potential to cause muscle damage. It is quite common for a patient to attribute muscle pain and weakness to the exercise rather than a side effect of medication. Patients should be instructed to report any muscle pain or weakness to their physician.

EXERCISE-INDUCED TRAINING BENEFITS

Endurance Exercise

Exercise training has long been recognized as an important component for medically managing the patient with diabetes. The role of systematic physical activity and exercise training on glycemic control in patients with type 1 diabetes has not been clearly defined and it is still controversial.

Exercise does play a major role in glycemic control for the type 2 diabetic and studies have shown an improved glucose control.[28,72–74] These studies have documented training adaptations occurring within 6 weeks to 12 months, with the improvement in glucose tolerance occurring in as little as 7 consecutive days of training.[75]

Although differences have been noted between the type 1 and the type 2 diabetic patient (see Table 10-11), exercise training is still an essential component of the comprehensive management for both types of DM.

The majority of the benefits shared by all patients focus on improving cardiovascular risk profile, psychological well-being, and overall quality of life. These are hallmark goals for the cardiac patient with DM (Table 10-11).

METABOLIC CONTROL

In the type 2 diabetic, exercise training improves insulin-mediated glucose disposal. Improvements in insulin sensitivity of skeletal muscle and adipose tissue can occur with or without a substantial change in body composition.[76–78] This improvement in insulin sensitivity is one of the most important training-induced changes for the patient with type 2 diabetes.

Several training-induced mechanisms involving skeletal muscle, adipose tissue, liver, and pancreatic output have been implicated in the favorable change in insulin sensitivity and glycemic control. Alterations in muscle mass, capillary density, body composition, and glucose transporter (GLUT-4) have been associated with an improvement in insulin sensitivity.[79]

Figure 10-5 summarizes training-induced mechanisms responsible for an improved insulin action and blood glucose homeostasis.[80,81]

Weight loss is an important therapeutic goal in the diabetic patient. This is especially true in the type 2 diabetic patients, since approximately 80% of

Table 10-10 **Exercises for Patients with Diabetes and Loss of Protective Sensation**

Contraindicated Exercise	Recommended Exercise
Treadmill	Swimming
Prolonged walking	Bicycling
Jogging	Rowing
Step exercises	Chair exercises
	Arm exercises
	Other non-weight-bearing exercise

Source: Adapted from Ref. 72.

Table 10-11 **Effects of Exercise in DM**

Parameter	Type 1[*]	Type 2[*]
Cardiovascular		
Aerobic capacity or fitness level	⇑	⇑/⇔
Resting pulse rate and rate-pressure product	⇓	⇓
Resting BP in mild-moderate hypertensives	⇓	⇓
HR at submaximal loads	⇓	⇓
Lipid and lipoprotein alterations		
HDL	⇑	⇑
LDL	⇓/⇔	⇓/⇔
VLDL	⇓	⇓
Total cholesterol	⇔	⇔
Risk ratio (total cholesterol/HDL)	⇓	⇓
Anthropometric measures		
Body mass	⇓	⇓
Fat mass, especially in obese persons	⇓	⇓
Fat-free mass	⇑	⇑/⇔
Metabolic parameters		
Insulin sensitivity and glucose metabolic machinery	⇑	⇑
HbA1c	⇔	⇓
Postprandial thermogenesis or thermic effect of food	⇑	⇑
Presumed psychological aspects		
Self-concept and self-esteem	⇑	⇑
Depression and anxiety	⇓	⇓
Stress response to psychological stimuli	⇓	⇓

[*]⇑ indicates increase; ⇓ indicates decrease; and ⇔ indicates no change.

Source: Adapted from Ref. 53.

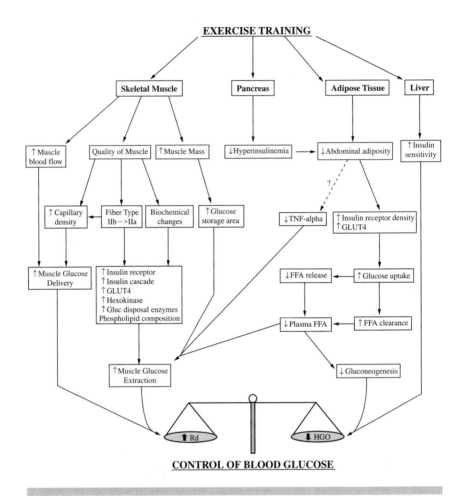

Figure 10-5 **Exercise training.** *(Source: Adapted from Ivy JL, Zderic TW, Fogt DL. Prevention and treatment of non-insulin dependent diabetes mellitus.* Exercise Sport Science Review *1999;27:1–35.)*

patients with type 2 diabetes are obese. A program which produces a moderate weight loss has been shown to improve glycemic control and decrease insulin resistance.[82,83] The benefits of training-related weight loss are more effective if combined with diet counseling. Visceral or abdominal fat (a significant risk factor associated with metabolic syndrome and CVD risk) is negatively associated with insulin sensitivity, therefore, a decrease in abdominal fat will increase peripheral insulin sensitivity.[84,85] Exercise training will result in preferential mobilization of visceral body fat and this is likely to contribute to metabolic improvements.[86]

The data regarding the effect of exercise training on lipids among those with diabetes demonstrate primarily positive results. An increase in aerobic capacity, induced by exercise training is related to a reduced atherogenic lipid profile. Improvements have been reported in triglycerides, total cholesterol, and the ratio between HDL cholesterol (HDL-C) and total cholesterol among type 2 diabetics.[87,88] Many of these studies also incorporated dietary modifications and it is difficult to determine whether diet or exercise had the most influence on atherogenic profile. To date, the information regarding the training-induced benefits and improvements in LDL cholesterol in the diabetic patient requires further investigation.

RESISTANCE TRAINING

The majority of evidence supporting the effects of regular exercise in enhancing insulin action have focused mainly on aerobic exercise. Although substantial evidence has been presented for the beneficial effects of resistance training on improving and developing muscular strength, endurance, power and muscle mass (hypertrophy), its beneficial affects on health-related factors and chronic disease has only recently been reported.

Previously, resistance training was not included in the recommended guidelines for exercise training and rehabilitation in the patient with diabetes and heart disease. Since 1990, investigations have provided evidence to support the profound effects of resistance training on general health and performance. It is now recommended, complementary with aerobic exercise, by several National health organizations including the American Heart Association, ACSM, and the American Diabetes Association (Table 10-12).

Aerobic and resistance exercise training encompasses several psychologic components associated with physical fitness such as cardiorespiratory endurance, body composition, skeletal muscle endurance, strength and power, flexibility, and balance and coordination. Although both training modalities elicit improvements in all of these, the emphasis for the specific physiologic benefits are different for each modality of training.

Pollock et al. in the publication of the *Research Digest* on "Resistance Training for Health" highlighted the health-related differences for the training-induced benefits comparing aerobic with resistance exercise (Table 10-13).[89]

For the coronary patient with DM, a combined program of aerobic and resistance exercise will facilitate all aspects of cardiovascular health.

The training-induced beneficial effects associated with aerobic exercise emphasizes the cardiorespiratory components specifically, improvements in maximal oxygen consumption and associated hemodynamic variables and the modulation of risk factors associated with metabolic syndrome and CVD. Conversely, some of the benefits associated with resistance training are additive to those obtained with aerobic training, however, some benefits

Table 10-12 **Health- and Performance-Related Improvements Due to Resistance Training**

Increases	Decreases
Muscle strength	BP
Muscle power	Cardiovascular demands to exercise
Local muscle endurance	LDL and total cholesterol
Muscle size	Sarcopenia
Motor performance (e.g., jumping ability, sprinting speed, and sports performance)	Risk of osteoporosis and colon cancer
	Body fat
Flexibility	Low back pain
Balance and coordination	
Functional capacity (e.g., stair climbing and walking)	
Aerobic capacity (circuit training programs)	
Basal metabolic rate and energy expenditure	
HDL-C	
Glucose tolerance and insulin sensitivity	
LV and septal wall thickness	
Bone mass and connective tissue strength	

Source: Adapted from Ref. 60.

obtained are unique to resistive exercise and cannot be achieved through aerobic activity alone.

Resistance training targets development of muscle strength, endurance, and muscle mass. This is particularly important to the patients with diabetes because of the increased propensity for skeletal muscle loss (sarcopenia) and abnormalities in skeletal muscle metabolism consequent to the burden of their disease. In addition, the effects of an upper and lower body strength training program will elicit improvements in daily function among those fail, elderly patients.

The following paragraphs will provide a brief review of the scientific literature related to the effectiveness of resistance exercise as a therapeutic modality for the diabetic patient with coronary disease, with an emphasis on:

Table 10-13 **Comparison of Effects of Aerobic Endurance Training with Strength Training on Health and Fitness Variables**

Variable	Aerobic Exercise*	Resistance Exercise*
Bone mineral density	↑↑	↑↑
Body composition		
% Fat	↓↓	↓
LBM	↔	↑↑
Strength	↔	↑↑↑
Glucose metabolism		
Insulin response to glucose challenge	↓↓	↓↓
Basal insulin levels	↓	↓
Insulin sensitivity	↑↑	↑↑
Serum lipids		
HDL-C	↑↔	↑↔
LDL-C	↓↔	↓↔
Resting heart rate	↓↓	↔
Stroke volume, resting and maximal	↑↑	↔
Blood pressure at rest		
Systolic	↓↔	↔
Diastolic	↓↔	↓↔
VO₂max	↑↑↑	↑↔
Submaximal and maximal endurance time	↑↑↑	↑↑
Basal metabolism	↑	↑↑

*↑, values increase; ↓, values decrease; ↔, values remain unchanged; ↑ or ↓, small effect; ↑↑ or ↓↓, medium effect; ↑↑↑ or ↓↓↓, large effect.

Source: Adapted from Ref. 89.

- Improved insulin sensitivity and glycemic control
- Decrease BP
- Weight control and reduced abdominal circumference
- Improved lipoprotein profile
- Improved muscular mass and quality of life

As with aerobic exercise, the benefits of participation are not entirely the same in the type 1 and the type 2 diabetic patients. The benefits of resistance training for those with type 1 DM are not yet clearly established. To date, only three studies have investigated the effects of resistance exercise on the type 1 diabetic patients[90–92] and among those studies only one study included an exercise protocol involving resistance exercise only.[90]

Currently, the Diabetes Aerobic and Resistance Exercise (T1-DARE) is ongoing with an expected completion date of September 2008. Its focus is on evaluating the effects of aerobic and resistance training on glycemic control (A1c) and to determine the effects of resistance and aerobic training on frequency of hypoglycemia, body composition, lipids, C-reactive protein, and quality of life.[93]

Just as was done previously for the cardiac patient, this form of training should be extensively studied from a risk/benefit perspective for the type 1 diabetic patient. One would speculate that the inclusion of resistance training for the type 1 diabetic patient merits more benefits than risks especially if the patient is adequately screened for overt disease-related complications. This review will focus primarily on the type 2 diabetic patients.

Strength Training: Effects on Metabolic and Cardiovascular Risk Factors

INSULIN RESISTANCE AND GLYCEMIC CONTROL

It has been argued that skeletal muscle is a primary target tissue for insulin and improvements in insulin action consequent to resistance training may be explained by a corresponding increase in skeletal muscle mass.[94] Two recent studies by Eriksson et al.[95] and Ishii et al.[96] documented benefits of strength training in improving insulin sensitivity and blood glucose control and these responses apparently were related to training-induced muscle hypertrophy.

Eriksson et al. enrolled eight participants with type 2 diabetes in a 3-month progressive resistance program consisting of 2 days a week of circuit training. The findings noted improvements in blood glucose with a significant increase in muscle mass.[95]

Ishii et al. reported the rate of blood glucose entry into skeletal muscles increased following a 6-week strength-training program at 40–50% of their 1 RM. More importantly, the training improved insulin sensitivity by 40%.[96]

Skeletal muscle is composed of fast-twitch glycolytic (type 2 a and b) and slow-twitch oxidative (type I) muscle fiber types and these differ in contractile as well as in metabolic properties. The fiber type that is most favorable for performing endurance exercise is the slow-twitch oxidative fiber (type I).

In those patients with a low functional capacity, as is present in the coronary diabetic patient, they demonstrate elevated levels of fast-twitch glycolytic fibers and a decreased number of slow-twitch oxidative fibers as a result of their physical inactivity.[97]

There is a significant correlation between muscle fiber type and glucose clearance rates among type 2 diabetic patients. The glucose transporter protein (GLUT-4) is found in larger amounts in slow-twitch fibers compared with fast-twitch fibers. Therefore, aerobic or moderate-intensity resistance impacts on insulin sensitivity by increasing GLUT-4 protein expression and enzymes responsible for phosphorylation, storage, and oxidation of glucose.[98,99]

There is evidence to suggest that the morphologic changes in skeletal muscle that accompany resistance training (increased capillary density and fiber-type conversion) are associated with changes in fasting insulin levels and glucose tolerance.[97,99]

BLOOD PRESSURE

Blood pressure is an important risk factor shared by the diabetic and coronary patient. A meta-analysis of 14 trials have provided evidence that demonstrates the efficacy of exercise training in lowering BP in the nondiabetic patient. Studies have shown the beneficial effects of aerobic exercise on BP in nondiabetic patients but less is known about the effects of exercise on BP or cardiovascular function among those with type 2 diabetes and hypertension.

In addition, it was only recently that strength training was included in the comprehensive exercise plan. It was generally not recommended for the management of hypertension and it was considered more of a detriment. However, this was based on limited and early scientific research.

Although the data pertaining to hypertensive patients are limited, the existing evidence demonstrates that patients can exercise safely and benefit from strength training.

ABDOMINAL OBESITY

Obesity, specifically abdominal obesity is a predictor of type 2 diabetes and metabolic syndrome/insulin resistance. Much of the ensuing metabolic disruption (insulin resistance, dyslipidemia) stems from alterations in free fatty acid metabolism resulting from abdominal obesity. It appears that a reduction in abdominal fat accumulation, whether through caloric restriction, aerobic or resistance training, or a combination of these will improve the metabolic disruption.

Exercise training will result in preferential loss of fat from central regions. While aerobic exercise is more effective in inducing weight loss and reducing truncal obesity (due to its greater effects on basal metabolic rate and caloric expenditure), resistance training will complement aerobic training for effective weight loss.

While caloric restriction and aerobic exercise is effective in reducing truncal obesity, sometimes lean body mass (LBM; skeletal muscle tissue) is lost in the process.

When resistance training is included as part of a weight loss program, LBM can be simultaneously preserved or gained. This will prove advantageous in the long term for the type 2 diabetic patients with metabolic syndrome.

It has been shown that LBM is associated with improved insulin sensitivity possibly because it provides additional glycogen storage capacity.[100]

Miller et al. studied changes in insulin action among older men following 16 weeks of a resistance training program. Their data revealed that resistance exercise was associated with a 40% improvement in nonoxidative glucose disposal. They concluded that resistance training resulted in an enhanced insulin action and the principal mechanism responsible was an increase in the pathways responsible for glycogen storage capacity. The response was similar to that reported for aerobic exercise training.[94]

LIPID PROFILE

It has been well established that aerobic, endurance exercise training favorably alters the HDL-C. Investigations concerning the effects of strength training on lipoprotein profile are not as clear and recent studies have produced conflicting findings.

Studies that have demonstrated a positive result typically involve higher volumes of training. Hurley et al. reported a 13% increase in HDL-C following a 16-week program of heavy strength training.[101,102] Goldberg et al. reported that emphasizing a program consisting of high volume with short rest periods increased HDL and subsequently decreased LDL and serum triglycerides.[103]

On the other hand, findings by Kokkinos et al.,[104] Kohl et al.,[105] and Smutok et al.,[106] have noted that strength training did not significantly alter serum lipid profiles.

Based on the evidence, it appears that the resistance training that best modifies lipoprotein profile incorporates larger muscle mass, multisegment exercise with a high total volume (reps × sets × load) prescription.[107] And the intensity associated with a possible improvement in lipoprotein profile is above the level of exercise that is performed by cardiac patients with diabetes, although this assumption may be too premature without further conclusive evidence. Additional training studies that control the body composition changes, day-to-day variations in lipoproteins, and dietary factors provide a more credible conclusion regarding the effect of resistance training on blood lipids and lipoproteins.

Strength Training: Effects on Disease-Related Functional Impairment

MUSCLE MASS

A physically inactive adult can lose 3–4% of muscle mass and strength per decade after age 40.

A large majority of the strength training research has focused on its role in the prevention of age-related loss of skeletal muscle mass and subsequent strength and function (sarcopenia).

It has been reported that up to a 50% decrease in leg strength and loss of muscle mass (sarcopenia) is common in patients with diabetes and it is also a hallmark finding in patients with underlying coronary disease (e.g., chronic congestive heart failure). The decrease in muscle strength leads to decreased mobility and greater frailty and incidence of falls.

Strength training is the only type of exercise that has been shown to reverse sarcopenia due to its direct effects on improving muscle mass, strength, and power.

Preserving muscle function, independence, and quality of life is a universal goal for all patients.

Strength Training: Safety Considerations for the Diabetic Patient with Coronary Disease

For the diabetic patient with coronary disease, the number of disease-related concerns regarding the safety of a resistance program is higher compared with the diabetic patient without coronary disease. Below is a list of contraindications for the diabetic coronary patient and the majority of the safety considerations relate to the clinical complications associated with cardiac disease.

The American Heart Association has composed a list of the following absolute contraindications for strength training[89]:

- Unstable angina
- Uncontrolled BP (systolic ≥160 mmHg, diastolic ≥100 mmHg)
- Uncontrolled arrhythmia
- Recent history of congestive heart failure
- Hypertrophic cardiomyopathy
- Severe stenotic or regurgitant valvular disease
- Certain stages of retinopathy (moderate, severe, and proliferated)

The guidelines for resistance training in the diabetic patient with coronary disease will be the same recommendations as for patients with various forms of overt coronary disease.

The major safety concern for resistance training in the diabetic patient without coronary disease relates mainly to the presence and extent of microvascular disease.

Resistance Training in Diabetic Patients with Cardiac Disease

PRESERVE LEFT VENTRICULAR SYSTOLIC FUNCTION

It is recommended that patients with moderate to good LV systolic function (≥45%) and a cardiorespiratory fitness level of 5–7 METS without anginal symptoms, evidence of exercise-induced ischemic ST-T wave changes, hypotension, or hypertensive response be permitted to engage in resistance training.[108,109]

Butler et al. compared the frequency of LV wall motion abnormalities among a group of patients with cardiac disease who cross-trained with aerobic and resistance exercise. Their findings revealed that resistance training at 40–60% of the 1 RM cause fewer wall motion changes compared with aerobic exercise.[110]

Those resistance programs which utilized lighter loads (30–50% of the 1 RM) did not produce anginal symptoms or sustained arrhythmias.[111]

IMPAIRED LEFT VENTRICULAR SYSTOLIC FUNCTION

Those patients diagnosed with chronic congestive heart failure, myocardial ischemia, poor LV function, or autonomic neuropathies must be carefully evaluated prior to initiating a strength-training program.

The isometric work associated with strength training may cause LV compromise if LV function is <45%.[112]

There is a lack of scientific evidence supporting the benefits and safety of resistance training among these patients; therefore, this form of training should either be avoided or patients should be referred to a supervised, monitored cardiac rehabilitation program.

Compliance Issues

Although exercise is integral to the comprehensive medical management of coronary disease and DM, a low prevalence of physical activity and exercise training has been reported among these patient populations.

Traditionally, the most common approach to an exercise prescription taken by clinicians has emphasized the physiologic principles associated with acute exercise and long-term exercise training. Most of the research evaluating this traditional approach has not been favorable in terms of long-term compliance.

More recently, contemporary theories and models associated with behavioral science have contributed greatly to the understanding of barriers associated with physical activity. These theories are being incorporated into the exercise prescription in an attempt to improve patient adherence.

Hays and Clark assessed physical activity behavior and correlated (i.e., physical activity knowledge, barriers, and performance and outcome expectations) among 260 adult type 2 diabetics. The majority of patients reported zero minutes of weekly physical activity. This was particularly true of older female patients. The most significant correlates of weekly physical activity were age, education, motivation, perceived health, and performance expectations.[113]

Previous studies have noted that the presence of underlying chronic disease is associated with a lower physical activity level. In addition, personal and environmental barriers have been consistently associated with nonadherence and an increased dropout rate.[114,115]

To effectively promote physical activity and improve compliance the following are recommended:

1. Telling patients what to do is not successful, especially in the long term. It is best to facilitate long-term changes by advising patients on how to change their lifestyle.
2. According to Bandura's Social Learning Theory,[116] behavioral changes are mediated by performance expectations. These will predict whether an individual will choose to engage in a behavior, the amount of effort spent on the behavior, and how persistent the individual will be despite

barriers or obstacles. Among perceived barriers, motivational barriers emerge as a significant factor. Exercise should be enjoyable, patients should choose activities they like, and vary the type of exercise and the setting.

3. A number of environmental (time constraint) and social factors can also affect physical activity behavior. The patient should exercise at a convenient time and location. The site should be near to the individual's home or work place.

   The patients' behavior should be reinforced by family, friends, and medical personnel. Family and friends can provide support and encouragement. Some patients will better comply with participation in exercise groups because of the camaraderie.

4. Knowledge about the activity and self-efficacy are also associated with greater compliance. Quantitative indices of progress to provide feedback is essential. The information should be easy to follow and meaningful to the patient. Oxygen consumption graphs will not have as much impact as a simple chart showing training-induced increases in exercise duration or decreases in body weight and fat percentage.

5. If patients do not see improvements with training, they will become frustrated and discontinue the exercise prescription. It is advisable to set small, attainable exercise goals. Goals which are unrealistically high should not be assigned.

Patient Education

The diabetic patient needs to know about the essential components of an exercise program with regard to the potential benefits and disease-related complications. It is also essential to instruct the patient to integrate their glycemic control with the adaptations related to regular exercise. The following guidelines are suggested:

1. If possible, the exercise should be performed daily and should be approximately the same intensity each time. This will allow downward adjustments in insulin or the use of an extra carbohydrate prior to exercise.

2. Patients should be educated about the signs and symptoms associated with hypo- and hyperglycemia. Patients should be instructed to postpone or discontinue the exercise session if it occurs. Indicators of hypoglycemia would require consuming carbohydrates. Patients should be told to always carry some form of carbohydrate with them when they are exercising.

3. Symptoms of chest pain, dizziness, unusual fatigue, visual disturbances, or nausea should alert the patient to discontinue the exercise and consult with his or her physician.

4. Exercise performed in extreme heat or cold should be avoided and a reduction in the duration of the exercise should be made in moderate heat. Diabetic patients are more susceptible to dehydration and hyperthermic consequences.

5. Patients should be advised to select an injection site for insulin remote from the exercising muscle group. This will reduce the likelihood of an inappropriate increase in serum insulin levels secondary to enhanced absorption.
6. Patients should be encouraged to have an alternative exercise plan for indoor exercise in case of inclement weather or a scheduling conflict with their health club.
7. Encourage lifestyle-based physical activity. This focuses on home, work, or community based participation in different forms of exercise that revolve around the patient's daily routine (e.g., walking the stairs instead of using the elevator, yard maintenance, home repair, walking partially during lunch, and performing stretches and calisthenics while reading or watching television). All are effective forms of lifestyle physical activity.

PEDOMETER TRAINING: ANOTHER ALTERNATIVE FOR IMPROVING PHYSICAL ACTIVITY IN THE DIABETIC PATIENT

Most of us would agree that with the age of computers and modern technology less attention has been devoted to the prevalence of a sedentary lifestyle and its relationship with DM. Some technologic changes have been positive while others have been negative.

One constant of American living has been that "America's famous past time" still is television watching. The average male spends 29 hours per week watching television and the average female spends approximately 34 hours per week.[117] In fact, over the past several decades with advent of the computer game era and cable satellite TV with well over 200 channels, the proportion of the U.S. population engaged in television watching or some other sedentary activity has increased significantly.

Pedometers have been in existence since 1926, but it is only recently that they have become a popular modality for monitoring habitual physical activity. Whether you go to the local supermarket or fast food chain restaurant they are distributing free pedometers with your purchase.

While pedometers have no inherent power to change behavior or increase physical activity, they do supply two essential ingredients of a lifestyle-based approach. First, they yield objective, cumulative, and quantitative measurements of the most common physical activities. Second, they provide a means of accountability for meeting daily activity goals.

Increasing evidence exists to support the health benefits of moderate walking in the diabetic patient. Walking appears to be a favorable exercise modality because it is accessible, inexpensive, and can be easily incorporated into daily routines.

Within various groups at high risk for diabetes (e.g., African-Americans, Hispanic, overweight, and elderly), walking has been reported to be a prevalent activity between 28 and 45% of individuals who reported walking at least on occasion.[118] In addition, based on large population data on diabetic patients, it was reported that walking was a preferred activity compared with a more conventional exercise like leg cycling or swimming.[114]

If nonvigorous activity (e.g., walking) was to be confirmed as having health benefits in the prevention of chronic diseases such as diabetes and coronary artery disease, it should be incorporated into the overall therapeutic plan. Particularly, because it is already a common and acceptable behavior among several patient populations.

Mayer-Davis et al. in the Insulin Resistance Atherosclerosis study examined 1467 men and women aged 40–60 years of African-American, Hispanic, and non-Hispanic white ethnicity with glucose tolerance ranging from normal to mild NIDDM. They demonstrated that increased participation in nonvigorous and vigorous exercise were significantly associated with an increased insulin sensitivity in the diabetic patients. Their findings further supported the current public health recommendations for increased moderate-intensity physical activity on most days of the week.[78]

Lauzon et al. examined the effectiveness of the pedometer-based lifestyle activity approach with type 2 diabetes patients. The study was designed to determine if a pedometer-based walking program could be successfully implemented in a diabetes education center and lead to an increase in physical activity and health-related outcomes.

The study population consisted of 136 type 2 diabetes patients with a mean age of 54 years, mean BMI of 36.1, and mean duration of diagnosed diabetes of 52 months. The subjects wore digital pedometers and recorded their total steps daily throughout the 16-week program. Over 16 weeks, the subjects succeeded in increasing their average daily step counts from 4364 at baseline to 8634 at program end, an improvement in their ambulatory activity level of nearly 98%. Positive changes (though not statistically significant) were also observed in BMI, waist circumference, BP, and resting HR.[119]

Tanasescu et al. noted that walking and walking pace were associated with a reduction in total mortality among men with type 2 diabetes. They reported that walking was inversely related to total mortality and faster walking pace was inversely associated with CVD and total mortality and this finding was independent of time spent in walking.[120]

For the great majority of patients, however, the pedometer-based lifestyle activity represents a simple, very inexpensive, and effective exercise prescription for treatment of obesity, insulin resistance, and type 2 diabetes.

Walking programs such as those found in "Small Steps, Big Rewards," a National Diabetes Education program which incorporates increased physical activity to improve diabetes control and general health has proven successful in type 2 diabetes. The goal of the program is to help a patient adopt an increased physical activity level.

The Diabetes Prevention Trials (DPT) have demonstrated that those who walked or exercised five times a week for 30 minutes lost 5–7% of their body weight and reduced their risk of diabetes by 58%. For those over the age of 60, the reduction in diabetes risk was 71%, and this result was better than for any drug used in the study.[121]

Increased physical activity is only one factor for a comprehensive medical treatment regime that physicians commonly prescribe for obese diabetic patients. One of the most common problems practitioners confront in this regard is the inability of the overweight, sedentary diabetic patient to comply with a structured, high-intensity exercise regimen. While many patients make the initial effort to participate, relatively few incorporate structured exercise routines into their daily lives on a permanent basis. Patients can benefit substantially from modest increases in routine physical activity through pedometer training. Weight loss is an important goal in the overall clinical management of the obese, diabetic patient with heart disease and pedometer training can be a successful alternative to structured exercise.

To study the impact of improving habitual physical activity on controlling obesity, Bassett et al. followed a sample of 98 Old Order Amish adults, aged 18–75 years (with a mean age of 33 years), who avoid reliance on modern "labor-saving" technologies.

The study participants wore digital pedometers for a 7-day period to measure and record their total steps each day. During this week the subjects averaged about 50 hours of walking and performing other moderate-intensity activities, and several more hours of performing more vigorous activities. These measurements showed that on average, Amish men accumulated 18,000 steps per day and Amish women accumulated 12,435 steps per day. These averages represent roughly three times the average number of steps taken by persons in modernized nations.

Only 4% of the Amish subjects were classified as obese and only 26% as overweight. By comparison, 31% of all Americans today may be classified as obese and almost 65% as overweight. Since the Old Order Amish are not noted for low-fat, low-calorie diets or attendance at trendy health clubs, it seems clear that their comparatively low rates of obesity and excess weight are primarily due to their habitual physical activity.[122]

Recent research clearly indicates that increases in moderate-intensity lifestyle activity can yield health benefits comparable to those produced by structured exercise programs, including improved cardiovascular fitness, reduced body fat, decreased total cholesterol and BP, and—most importantly—extended patient compliance. Patients are also encouraged to adopt a lifetime activity approach by increasing their cumulative daily activity.[123]

In lieu of these findings, groups as diverse as the Surgeon General, Centers for Disease Control (CDC), National Institutes of Health (NIH), and the ACSM have all published recent position statements endorsing the lifestyle activity approach.

Walking is a form of activity that we all do on a daily basis. Start by walking 10 minutes per day, 3–5 days per week and work your way up to 30–60 minutes of walking every day.

Recommendations

It is very important to keep in mind that the patients' step goal will be based on their initial fitness level. The number of steps will also vary according to their lifestyle activity and occupation.

To determine a starting number, have the patients wear the pedometer for 1 full normal week and record the total number of steps taken each day. They should add an additional 200 steps per day or take the highest per day step count and make that their starting goal. When they have comfortably established this new goal, they can set a new goal.

Most individuals see an improvement in their energy level, strength, and lung capacity if they increase by 2000 steps per day. That is equivalent to a mile or approximately 15–20 minutes of walking.

Step Training for Weight Reduction

Some individuals will get 3000 steps per day just performing their daily activity and they still will gain weight. To burn off those extra calories for weight loss, your goal should be to walk 10,000 steps per day for most days of the week. You may take several weeks to reach this goal. The key is to get to the goal progressively.

There are several models of pedometers ranging from free or inexpensive to expensive depending on how many functions it perform and how the data are stored and displayed.

Some pedometers require an initial setup which includes setting the pedometer to the individual's cadence and some pedometers will keep track of steps only or will display steps per day, cumulative distance traveled, and calories per day. The recommended pedometer should be one which is preset based on the individual's stride length, have a display of steps per day and kilocalories, and should have the ability to store up to 7 days of step data.

The estimated steps to distance conversion (Table 10-14) will vary for each individual depending on stride length. To obtain an exact distance measurement:

- Go to a local high school track (usually 1/4 mile)
- Set the pedometer to 0, walk normally for one lap (1/4 mile)
- Multiply the steps recorded on the pedometer by 4
- This will give steps per mile

Table 10-14 **Conversion Chart (Estimated Total Steps-Total Distance)**

Number of Steps	Distance (Miles)
500	$1/4$
1000	$1/2$
1500	$3/4$
2000	1
2500	$1 1/4$
3000	$1 1/2$
3500	$1 3/4$
4000	2
4500	$2 1/4$
5000	$2 1/2$
5500	$2 3/4$
6000	3
6500	$3 1/4$
7000	$3 1/2$
7500	$3 3/4$
8000	4
8500	$4 1/4$
9000	$4 1/2$
9500	$3 3/4$
10,000	5

Note: This is a rough estimate of steps-distance.

CONCLUSION

Physical activity brings about many immediate and long-term benefits for the cardiac diabetic patient. The benefits of physical activity in improving metabolic abnormalities as well as reducing risk factors associated with insulin resistance syndrome are vital to the comprehensive medical management and must remain top priority in the primary care setting.

A program of vigorous, structured exercise is no longer required to achieve health benefits. Regular, moderate levels of exercise, including walking and daily leisure activities are easily attainable for all patient populations and they are also associated with improvements in the clinical status.

The type 2 diabetic with underlying coronary disease can perform mostly every type of physical activity, provided they are medically screened and educated as to the guidelines and recommendations for safe and effective exercise. For the type 1 diabetic, an emphasis must focus on careful preexercise screening as well as adjustments in therapeutic regimens for safe participation in all forms of exercise.

Finally, future investigations into the behavioral approaches to physical activity and exercise are indicated so as to identify potential barriers to lifestyle behavior modification. This will help to guide the patient into a lifetime of good physical well-being and optimal quality of life.

REFERENCES

1. Harris MI, Flegal KM, Cowie CC, et al. Prevalence of diabetes, impaired fasting glucose, and impaired glucose tolerance in U.S. adults. The Third National Health and Nutrition Examination Survey, 1988-1994. *Diabetes Care* 1998;21: 518–524.

2. National Institute of Diabetes and Digestive and Kidney Diseases. Diabetes in African Americans. NIH Publication No. 02-3266. Bethesda, MD: US Department of Health and Human Services, National Institutes of Health, 2002.

3. Boyle JP, Honeycutt AA, Narayan KMV, et al. Projections of disease burden through 2050. *Diabetes Care* 2001;24:1936–1940.

4. National Institute of Diabetes and Digestive and Kidney Diseases. National diabetes statistics fact sheet: general information and national estimates on diabetes in the United States. NIH Publication No. 04-3892: Bethesda, MD: US Department of Health and Human Services, National Institutes of Health, 2004.

5. American Heart Association. Heart Disease and Stroke Statistics 2006 Update. A report from the American Heart Association Statistics Committee and Stroke Subcommittee. *Circulation* 2006;113:898–918.

6. Stamler J, Vaccaro O, Neaton J, et al. For the Multiple Risk Factor Intervention Trial Research Group: Diabetes, other risk factors, and 12-year cardiovascular mortality for men screened in the Multiple Risk Factor Intervention Trial. *Diabetes Care* 1993;16:434–444.

7. American Diabetes Association. Diabetes and coronary heart disease. *Diabetes Spectrum* 1999;12(2):80–83.

8. Barrett-Connor E, Wingard DL. Diabetes and cardiovascular risk factors: The Framingham Study. *Circulation* 1979;59:8–13.

9. Donahue RP, Abbott RD, Reed DM, et al. Postchallenge glucose concentration and coronary heart disease in men of Japanese ancestry. Honolulu Heart Program. *Diabetes* 1987;36:689–692.

10. Smith JW, Marcus FL, Serokeman R. Prognosis of patients with diabetes mellitus after myocardial infarction. *Am J Cardiol* 1984;54:718–721.

11. Abbott RD, Donahue P, MacMahon SE, et al. Diabetes and the risk of stroke: the Honolulu Heart Program. *JAMA* 1987;257:949–952.

12. Melton LI 3rd, Macken KM, Palumbo PJ, et al. Incidence and prevalence of clinical peripheral vascular disease in a population-based cohort of diabetic patients. *Diabetes Care* 1980;3:650–654.

13. Kannel WB, Hjortland M, Castelli WP. Role of diabetes in congestive heart failure: The Framingham Study. *Am J Cardiol* 1974;34:29–34.

14. Wingard DL, Barrett-Connor E. Heart disease and diabetes. In: Harris MI, ed., *Diabetes in American*, 2nd ed. Bethesda, MD: National Institutes of Health (NIH Publication No. 95-1468), 1995: 429–448.

15. Savage PJ. Cardiovascular complications of diabetes mellitus: What we know and what we need to know about their prevention. *Ann Intern Med* 1996;124(1 pt 2): 123–126.

16. Stern M. Do non-insulin dependent diabetes mellitus and cardiovascular disease share common antecedents? *Ann Intern Med* 1996;124(1 pt 2):110–116.

17. Jarrett RJ, Shipley MJ. Type 2 (non-insulin dependent) diabetes mellitus and cardiovascular disease—putative association via common antecedents; further evidence from Whitehall Study. *Diabetologia* 1988;31(10):737–740.

18. Erhman JK. *Clinical Exercise Physiology*. Champaign, IL: Human Kinetics, 2003: 129–152.

19. Stern MP, Morales PA, Valdez RA, et al. Predicting diabetes. Moving beyond impaired glucose tolerance. *Diabetes* 1993;40:706–714.

20. Laakso M, Ronnemaa T, Pyorala K, et al. Atherosclerotic vascular disease and its risk factors in non-insulin diabetic and non-diabetic subjects in Finland. *Diabetes Care* 1988;11:449–463.

21. Simonson DC. Etiology and prevalence of hypertension in diabetic patients. *Diabetes Care* 1988;11:821–827.

22. Kannel WB, McGee DL. Diabetes and cardiovascular disease: The Framingham Study. *JAMA* 1979;241:2035–2038.

23. Pyorala K, Pedersen TR, Kjekshus J, et al. Cholesterol lowering with simvastatin improves prognosis of diabetic patients with coronary heart disease: a subgroup analysis of the Scandinavian Simvastatin Survival Study (4S). *Diabetes Care* 1997;20:614–620.

24. Steiner G. The DAIS Project Group: The Diabetes Atherosclerosis Intervention Study (DAIS): a study conducted in cooperation with the World Health Organization. *Diabetologia* 1996;39:1655–1661.

25. The Diabetes Control and Complications Trial Research Group. The effect of intensive treatment of diabetes on the development and progression of long-term complications in insulin-dependent diabetes mellitus. *N Engl J Med* 1993;329: 977–986.

26. Whaley MH, Kampert JB, et al. Physical fitness and clustering of risk factors associated with the metabolic syndrome. *Med Sci Sports Exerc* 1999;31(2):287–293.

27. Despres JP. Visceral obesity, insulin resistance and dyslipidemia: contribution of endurance exercise training to the treatment of the plurimetabolic syndrome. *Exerc Sport Sci Rev* 1997;25:271–300.

28. Holloszy JO, Schultz J, Kusnierkiewicz JM, et al. Effects of exercise on glucose tolerance and insulin resistance. Brief review and some preliminary results. *Acta Med Scand* 1986;711(Suppl):S55–S65.

29. Schneider SH, Amorosa LF, Khachadurian AK, et al. Studies on the mechanism of improved glucose control during regular exercise in type 2 (non-insulin dependent) diabetes. *Diabetologia* 1984;26:335–360.

30. Hansen J, Sue DY, Oren A, et al. Relation of oxygen uptake to work rate in normal men and men with circulatory disorders. *Am J Cardiol* 1987;59: 669–674.

31. Regensteiner JG, Sippel J, McFarling ET, et al. Effects of non-insulin-dependent diabetes on oxygen consumption during treadmill exercise. *Med Sci Sports Exerc* 1995;27(6):875–881.

32. Roy TM, Peterson HR, Snider HL, et al. Autonomic influence on cardiovascular performance in diabetic subjects. *Am J Med* 1989;87:382–388.

33. Andersen H. Motor function in diabetic neuropathy. *Acta Neurol Scand* 1999;100(4):211–220.

34. Cameron NE, Cotter MA, Robertson S. Changes in skeletal muscle contractile properties in streptozocin-infused diabetic rats and role of polyol pathway and hypoinsulinemia. *Diabetes* 1990;39:460–465.

35. Stephenson GM, O'Callaghan A, Stephenson DG. Single-fiber study of contractile and biochemical properties of skeletal muscles in streptozotocin-induced diabetic rats. *Diabetes* 1994;43(5):622–628.

36. American Diabetes Association. In: Ruderman N, Devlin J, eds., *The Health Professional's Guide to Diabetes and Exercise*. Alexandria, VA: American Diabetes Association, 1995:71–158.

37. Davidson MB. *Diabetes Mellitus Diagnosis and Treatment*, 4th ed. Philadelphia, PA: W.B. Saunders, 1998:267–298.

38. Albright AL. Exercise precautions and recommendations for patients with autonomic neuropathy. *Diabetes Spectrum* 1998;11:231–237.

39. Takemoto KA, Bernstein L, Lopez JF, et al. Abnormalities of diastolic filling of the left ventricle associated with aging are less pronounced in exercise-trained individuals. *Am Heart J* 1992;124:143–148.

40. Levy WC, Cerqueira MD, Abrass IB, et al. Endurance exercise training augments diastolic filling at rest and during exercise in healthy young and older men. *Circulation* 1993;88:116–126.

41. Brenner DA, Apstein CS, Saupe KW. Exercise training attenuates age-associated diastolic dysfunction in rats. *Circulation* 2001;104:221–226.

42. Maiorana A, O'Driscoll G, Cheetham C, et al. The effect of combined aerobic and resistance exercise training on vascular function in type 2 diabetes. *J Am Coll Cardiol* 2001;38:860–866.

43. Lavrencic A, Salobir BG, Keber I. Physical training improves flow-mediated dilation in patients with polymetabolic syndrome. *Arterioscler Thromb Vasc Biol* 2000; 20:551–555.

44. Higashi Y, Sasaki S, Sasaki N, et al. Daily aerobic exercise improves reactive hyperemia in patients with essential hypertension. *Hypertension* 1999;33(Suppl 1, pt 2):591–597.

45. Paterick TE, Fletcher GF. Endothelial function and cardiovascular prevention: role of blood lipids, exercise and other risk factors. *Cardiol Rev* 2001;9:282–286.

46. Kingwell BA, Arnold PJ, Jennings GL, et al. Spontaneous running increases aortic compliance in Wistar-Kyoto rats. *Cardiovasc Res* 1997;35:132–137.

47. Kingwell BA, Arnold PJ, Jennings GL, et al. The effects of voluntary running on cardiac mass and aortic compliance in Wistar-Kyoto and spontaneously hypertensive rats. *J Hypertens* 1998;16:181–185.

48. Vaitkeicius PV, Fleg JL, Engel JH, et al. Effects of age and aerobic capacity on arterial stiffness in healthy adults. *Circulation* 1993;88(Suppl 4, pt 1):1456–1462.

49. Jensen-Urstad K, Bouvier F, Jensen-Urstad M. Preserved vascular reactivity in elderly male athletes. *Scand J Med Sci Sports* 1999;9:88–91.

50. Geffken D, Cushman M, Burke G, et al. Association between physical activity and markers of inflammation in a healthy elderly population. *Am J Epidemiol* 2001;153:242–250.

51. Mattusch F, Dufauz B, Heine O, et al. Reduction in plasma concentration of C-reactive protein following nine months of endurance training. *Int J Sports Med* 2000;21:21–24.

52. Adamopoulos S, Parissis J, Kroupis C, et al. Physical training reduces peripheral markers of inflammation in patients with chronic heart failure. *Eur Heart J* 2001;22:791–797.

53. American College of Sports Medicine. *ACSM's Resource Guidelines for Exercise Testing and Prescription*, 5th ed. Philadelphia, PA: Lippincott Williams & Wilkins, 2006.

54. Wallberg-Henriksson H. Exercise and diabetes mellitus. *Exerc Sports Sci Rev* 1992;20:339–368.

55. Birrer RB, Sedaghat VD. Exercise and diabetes mellitus: optimizing performance in patients who have type I diabetes. *Phys Sportsmed* 2003;31(5):1–11.

56. Stein RA, Goldberg N, Kalman F, et al. Exercise and the patient with type I diabetes mellitus. *Pediatr Clin North Am* 1984;31(3):663–669.

57. Zinman B, Vranic M. Diabetes and exercise. *Med Clin North Am* 1985;69(1):145–157.

58. Bergstrom J, Hermansen L, Hultmann E, et al. Diet, muscle glycogen and physical performance. *Acta Physiol Scand* 1967;71:140–150.

59. Kanawaka K, Higuchi M, Ohmori H, et al. Muscle contractile activity modulates GLUT-4 protein content in the absence of insulin. *Horm Metab Res* 1995;28:75–80.

60. Skinner JS. *Exercise Testing and Exercise Prescription for Special Cases: Theoretical Basis and Clinical Applications*, 3rd ed. Philadelphia, PA: Lippincott Williams & Wilkins, 2005: 223–235.

61. Koval JA, DeFronzo RA, O'Doherty RM, et al. Regulation of hexokinase II activity and expression in human muscle by moderate exercise. *Am J Physiol* 1998; 274:E304–E308.

62. Nakatani A, Han DH, Hansen PA, et al. Effect of endurance exercise training on muscle glycogen supercompensation in rats. *J Appl Physiol* 1997;82:711–715.

63. Musi N, Fujii N, Hirshman MF, et al. AMP-activated protein kinase (AMPK) is activated in muscle of subjects with type 2 diabetes during exercise. *Diabetes* 2001;50:921–927.

64. Wasserman DH, Lickley HL, Vranic M. Interactions between glucagon and other counterregulatory hormones during normoglycemic and hypoglycemic exercise in dogs. *J Clin Invest* 1984;74(4):1404–1413.

65. Caron D, Poussier P, Marliss EB, et al. The effect of postprandial exercise on meal-related glucose tolerance in insulin-dependent diabetic patients. *Diabetes Care* 1982;5:364–369.

66. Richter EA, Kiens B, Saltin B, et al. Skeletal muscle glucose uptake during dynamic exercise in humans: role of muscle mass. *Am J Physiol* 1988;254(17): E555–E561.

67. Rogberg RA, Roberts SO. *Fundamental Principles of Exercise Physiology for Fitness, Performance and Health.* New York: McGraw-Hill, 2000:191.

68. Sanchez OA. Resistance training for health and rehabilitation. In: Graves JE, Franklin BA, eds., *Resistance Exercise for Patients with Diabetes Mellitus.* Champaign, IL: Human Kinetics, 2001:295–318.

69. American Diabetes Association. In: Ruderman N, Devlin J, Schneider S, eds., *Handbook of Exercise in Diabetes.* Alexandria, VA: American Diabetes Association, 2002:269–288.

70. Soukup J, Kovaleski J. A review of the effects of resistance training for individuals with diabetes mellitus. *Diabetes Educ* 1993;19(4):307–312.

71. Graham C, Lasko-McCartney P. Exercise options for persons with diabetic complications. *Diabetes Educ* 1990;16:212–220.

72. American Diabetes Association. Physical activity, exercise and diabetes. *Diabetes Care* 1999;26:S58–S62.

73. Lampman RM, Schteingart DE. Effects of exercise training on glucose control, lipid metabolism and insulin sensitivity in hypertriglyceridemia and non-insulin diabetes mellitus. *Med Sci Sports Exerc* 1991;23:703–712.

74. Reitman JS, Vasquez B, Klimes I, et al. Improvement of glucose homeostasis after exercise training in non-insulin dependent diabetes. *Diabetes Care* 1984;7:434–441.

75. Rogers MA, Yamamoto C, King DS, et al. Improvement in glucose tolerance after 1 wk of exercise in patients with mild NIDDM. *Diabetes Care* 1988;11:613–618.

76. Horton ES. Exercise and physical training: effects on insulin sensitivity and glucose metabolism. *Diabetes Metab Rev* 1986;2:1–17.

77. Koivisto VA, Yki-Jarvinen H, Defronzo RA. Physical training and insulin sensitivity. *Diabetes Metab Rev* 1986;1:445–481.

78. Mayer-Davis EJ, D'agostino R, Karta AJ, et al. Intensity and amount of physical activity in relation to insulin sensitivity. *JAMA* 1998;279:669–674.

79. Albright A, Franz M, Hornsby G, et al. Exercise and type 2 diabetes. *Med Sci Sports Exerc* 2000;32:1345–1362.

80. McCardle WD, Katch FI, Katch VL. *Exercise Physiology Energy, Nutrition and Human Performance,* 5th ed. Philadelphia, PA: Lippincott Williams & Wilkins, 2001:441.

81. Ivy JL, Zderic TW, Fogt DL. Prevention and treatment of non-insulin dependent diabetes mellitus. *Exerc Sport Sci Rev* 1999;27:1–35.

82. Watts NB, Spanheimer RG, Digirolamo A, et al. Prediction of glucose response to weight loss in patients with non-insulin dependent diabetes mellitus. *Arch Intern Med* 1990;150:803–880.

83. Wing RR, Koeske R, Epstein LH, et al. Long-term effects of modest weight loss in type 2 diabetic patients. *Arch Intern Med* 1987;147:1749–1753.

84. Bjorntorp P. Portal adipose tissue as a generator of risk factors for cardiovascular disease and diabetes. *Arteriosclerosis* 1990;10:493–496.

85. Paternostro-Bayles M, Wing RR, Robertson RJ. Effect of life-style activity of varying duration on glycemic control in type 2 diabetic women. *Diabetes Care* 1989; 12:34–37.

86. Mourier A, Gauier JF, Dekerviler E, et al. Mobilization of visceral adipose tissue related to the improvement in insulin sensitivity in response to training in NIDDM. *Diabetes Care* 1997;20:385–392.

87. Barnard RJ, Lattimore L, Holly RG, et al. Response of non-insulin-dependent diabetic patients to an intensive program of diet and exercise. *Diabetes Care* 1982;5: 370–374.

88. Ruderman NB, Ganda OP, Johansen K. The effect of physical training on glucose tolerance and plasma lipids in maturity-onset diabetes. *Diabetes* 1979;28(Suppl 1): 89–92.

89. Pollock ML, Franklin BA, Balady GJ, et al. Resistance exercise in individuals with and without cardiovascular disease: benefits, rationale, safety and prescription. *Circulation* 2000;101:828–833.

90. Durak EP, Jovanovic-Peterson L, Peterson CM. Randomized cross-over study of effect of resistance training on glycemic control, muscular strength and cholesterol in type 1 diabetic men. *Diabetes Care* 1990;13:1039–1043.

91. Mandroukas K, Krotkiewski M, Holm G, et al. Muscle adaptations and glucose control after physical training in insulin dependent diabetes mellitus. *Clin Physiol* 1986;6:39–52.

92. Mosher PE, Nash MS, Perry AC, et al. Aerobic circuit exercise training: effect on adolescents with well-controlled insulin dependent diabetes mellitus. *Arch Phys Med Rehabil* 1998;79:652–657.

93. Canadian Diabetes Association. Clinical Trials Type I Diabetes Aerobic and Resistance Exercise (T1-DARE). Clinical Trials Identifier NCT00148538, *ClinicalTrials.gov*.

94. Miller WJ, Sherman WM, Ivy JL. Effect of strength training on glucose tolerance and post-glucose insulin response. *Med Sci Sports Exerc* 1984;16:539–543.

95. Eriksson J, Taimela S, Eriksson K, et al. Resistance training in the treatment of non-insulin dependent diabetes mellitus. *Int J Sports Med* 1997;18:242–246.

96. Ishii T, Yamakita T, Sato T, et al. Resistance training improves insulin sensitivity in NIDDM subjects without altering maximal oxygen uptake. *Diabetes Care* 1998;21:1353–1355.

97. Scheuermann-Freestone M, Madsen PL, Manners D, et al. Abnormal cardiac and skeletal muscle energy metabolism in patients with type 2 diabetes. *Circulation* 2003;107:3040–3046.

98. Daugaad JR, Rithcer FA. Relationship between muscle fiber composition, glucose transporter protein 4 and exercise training: possible consequences in non-insulin dependent diabetes mellitus. *Acta Physiol Scand* 2001;171:267–276.

99. Ivy JL. Role of exercise training in the prevention and treatment of insulin resistance and non-insulin-dependent diabetes mellitus. *Sports Med* 1997;24(5): 321–336.

100. Zacker RJ. Lifestyle and behavior: strength training in diabetes management. *Diabetes Spectrum* 2005;18:71–75.

101. Hurley BF, Hagberg JM, Goldberg AP, et al. Resistive training can reduce coronary risk factors without altering VO2 max or percent body fat. *Med Sci Sports Exerc* 1988;20:150–154.

102. Johnson CC, Stone MH, Lopez SA, et al. Diet and exercise in middle-aged men. *J Am Diet Assoc* 1982;81:695–701.

103. Goldberg L, Elliot DL, Schutz RW, et al. Changes in lipid and lipoprotein levels after weight training. *JAMA* 1984;252:504–506.

104. Kokkinos PF, Hurley BF, Vaccaro P, et al. Effects of low and high-repetition resistive training on lipoprotein-lipid profiles. *Med Sci Sports Exerc* 1988;20:50–54.

105. Kohl HW, Gordon HF, Scott CB, et al. Musculoskeletal strength and serum lipid levels in men and women. *Med Sci Sports Exerc* 1992;24:1080–1087.

106. Smutok MA, Reece C, Kokkinos PF, et al. Aerobic versus strength training for risk factor intervention in middle-aged men at high risk for coronary heart disease. *Metabolism* 1993;42:177–184.

107. Stone MH, Fleck SJ, Triplett NT, et al. Health and performance-related potential of resistance training. *Sports Med* 1991;11:210–231.

108. Franklin B, Hellenstein H, Gordon S, et al. Exercise prescription for the myocardial infarction patient. *J Cardiopulm Rehabil* 1986;6:62–79.

109. Fardy P. Isometric exercise and the cardiovascular system. *Physician Sports Med* 1981;9:43–56.

110. Butler R, Beierwaltes W, Rogers F. The cardiovascular response to circuit weight training in patients with cardiac disease. *J Cardiopulm Rehabil* 1987;7:402–409.

111. Keleman MH. Resistive training safety and assessment guidelines for cardiac and coronary prone patients. *Med Sci Sports Exerc* 1989;21:675–677.

112. Franklin B, Bonzheim K, Gordon S, et al. Resistance training in cardiac rehabilitation. *J Cardiopulm Rehabil* 1991;11:99–107.

113. Hays LM, Clark DO. Correlates of physical activity in a sample of older adults with type 2 diabetes. *Diabetes Care* 1999;22(5):706–712.

114. Ford ES, Herman WH. Leisure-time physical activity patterns in the U.S. diabetic population. *Diabetes Care* 1995;18:27–33.

115. Clark DO. Racial and educational differences in physical activity among older adults. *Gerontologist* 1995;35:472–480.

116. Bandura A. *Social Learning Theory*. Englewood Cliffs, NJ: Prentice Hall, 1986.

117. Neilson Report on Television. Northbrook, IL: AC Neilsen Co, Media Research Division, 1998.

118. Seigel PZ, Brackbill RM, Heath GW. The epidemiology of walking for exercise: implications for promoting activity among sedentary groups. *Am J Public Health* 1995;85:706–710.

119. Lauzon NL, Tudor-Locke CT, et al. Increased physical activity and improved health measures with a pedometer-based physical activity intervention for type 2 diabetes. *Diabetes* 2003;52:A236.

120. Tanasescu M, Leitzmann MF, Rimm EB, et al. Physical activity in relation to cardiovascular disease and total mortality among men with type 2 diabetes. *Circulation* 2003;107:2435–2439.

121. The Diabetes Prevention Program Research Group: The Diabetes Prevention Program: design and methods for a clinical trial in the prevention of type 2 diabetes. *Diabetes Care* 1999;22:623–631.

122. Bassett DR, Schneider PL, Huntington GE. Physical activity in an Older Amish Community. *Med Sci Sports Exerc* 2004;1:79–84.

123. Dunn AL, Marcus BH, Garcia ME, et al. Comparison of lifestyle and structured interventions to increased physical activity and cardiorespiratory fitness: a randomized trail. *JAMA* 1999;281(4):327–334.

INTERNET RESOURCES

American College of Sports Medicine Position Stands: http://www.acsm.org/publications/positionstands.htm

American Diabetes Association: Diabetes and Cardiovascular Disease. http://s2mw.com/heartofdiabetes/cardio.html

American Diabetes Association. http://www.diabetes.org/for-health-professionals-and-scientists/professionals.jsp

American Society of Diabetes Educators. http://www.aadenet.org/ProfessionalEd/index.html

Centers for Disease Control and Prevention: National Center for Chronic Disease Prevention and Health Promotion: Diabetes Public Health Resource. http://www.cdc.gov/diabetes/index.htm

National Institutes of Health and National Heart, Lung, and Blood Institute: Clinical Guidelines on the Identification, Evaluation, and Treatment of Overweight and Obesity in Adults. http://www.nhlbi.nih.gov/guidelines/obesity/ob_home.htm

American Heart Association: Scientific Statements and Practice Guidelines List. http://www.americanheart.org/presenter.jhtml?identifier=2158

American Association for Cardiovascular and Pulmonary Rehabilitation. http://www.aacvpr.org

National Clinical Guideline Clearinghouse. http://www.guideline.gov

American Diabetes Association: Clinical Practice Recommendations. http://care.diabetesjournals.org/content/vol27/suppl_1/, http://care.diabetesjournals.org/content/vol26/suppl_1/

THE ASSESSMENT AND REDUCTION OF CARDIAC RISK IN DIABETICS UNDERGOING NONCARDIAC SURGERY

Jason M. Lazar
Louis Salciccioli

INTRODUCTION

Diabetics are increasingly being referred for noncardiac surgery. Diabetes confers an increased risk for postoperative cardiac complications due to a higher prevalence of coronary artery disease (CAD) and the need for higher risk surgeries required to treat the complications of diabetes. The symptoms of cardiac disease are often atypical in this patient population, making preoperative evaluation more difficult. The benefits of therapies aimed at reducing perioperative risk in diabetics have mostly been determined by subgroup analysis of larger studies of unselected patients. Preoperative evaluation is dependent on consideration of clinical predictors and functional capacity of the patient and, the specific risk of the type of surgical operation and whether the surgery is elective or emergent. Diabetes must be integrated into the evaluation. Cardiac risk stratification and management are summarized below.

EPIDEMIOLOGY

It is estimated that 25 million surgical procedures are currently performed annually in the United States.[1] While data addressing the exact number are lacking, a substantial proportion of the surgical patients have diabetes. Patients with diabetes have been estimated to have a 50% lifetime chance of requiring a surgical procedure. Moreover, the number of diabetics referred for surgical procedures in the United States will almost certainly rise due to the growing numbers of surgical procedures and the rapidly rising prevalence of diabetes. In addition, the microvascular and macrovascular complications of diabetes frequently require surgical treatment. Bariatric surgery has become an established treatment for morbid obesity, which is strongly associated with diabetes. Although a number of reviews address glycemic and metabolic control, few address cardiac risk of diabetic patients undergoing noncardiac surgery.[2,3] Cardiovascular complications are common in patients undergoing noncardiac surgery despite refinements in surgical techniques and improvements in anesthesia and perioperative management. Postoperative cardiac events occur in approximately 5% of patients and carry a 50% short-term mortality rate.[4] Perioperative cardiovascular events are also more strongly predictive of poorer long-term prognosis than are nonoperative cardiovascular events.[1]

The presence of CAD poses the highest risk for perioperative cardiac events.[4] Diabetes is presently considered a CAD equivalent because the incidence of myocardial infarction (MI) in diabetics without prior MI was found similar to that of nondiabetics with prior MI during 7-year follow-up.[5] The purpose of this chapter is to review the principles of preoperative cardiovascular risk stratification and risk reduction and make them applicable to the diabetic population.

Studies addressing surgical risk in diabetics have for the most part relied on subgroup analysis of larger studies of unselected patients. Their interpretation is further made difficult by the heterogeneity of diabetic patients and by the wide variety of surgical procedures across a spectrum of cardiac risk. In addition, the studies span several decades and differ by study methodologies, incorporation of disease management programs, and by inclusion in the medical, surgical, cardiovascular, anesthesia, and endocrinology publications. Moreover, variability in combined cardiac endpoints further complicate the matter. The following endpoints that have been evaluated alone or in combination: death, unstable angina, MI, pulmonary edema, stroke, and arrhythmias. Moreover, event rates such as MI will be impacted by whether the endpoint was established by clinical criteria retrospectively or by prospective surveillance using routine blood draws for cardiac enzyme determination and/or electrocardiography. The American College of Cardiology, American Heart Association, American College of Physicians, and other groups have published position papers addressing cardiovascular risk in noncardiac surgery.[6-8] There is frequent disagreement in guideline-guided management in patients referred for surgery.[9]

PATHOPHYSIOLOGY

Cardiovascular events related to noncardiac surgery are chiefly related to the development of myocardial ischemia provoked by the stress of surgery in patients with preexisting CAD. Whereas the vast majority of MIs unrelated to surgery are caused by atherosclerotic plaque rupture and intracoronary thrombosis, perioperative MI is felt to be related to increased oxygen demand that exceeds supply.[10] In a study of 26 fatal postoperative MIs, plaque rupture was present in only 46% of cases.[11] It is noteworthy that thrombus occurred at the site of high-grade stenoses (>50% cross-sectional area) in 33% of cases.

Both anesthesia and surgery evoke a number of metabolic, hemodynamic, and autonomic responses.[12,13] Surgery elicits a stress response that is proportional to the degree of tissue trauma. Anesthetic agents are cardioinhibitory, and result in vasodilation, and increased sympathetic tone. The postoperative period is characterized by neurohormonal activation, increased cortisol and catecholamine levels, and reduced production of tissue plasminogen activator. Postoperative pain, physiologic, and emotional stress may all contribute to cause tachycardia, hypertension, increase in cardiac output, and fluid shifts. These changes serve to increase myocardial oxygen demand, resulting in subendocardial ischemia and eventual MI. Inflammation and increased wall stress in association with platelet activation may lead to plaque disruption and coronary thrombosis.[10] Most perioperative MI are non-ST-segment elevation MIs, but carry a high mortality (Table 11-1).

Metabolic changes related to surgery lead to relative insulin hyposecretion, insulin resistance, and increased protein catabolism. Anesthesia further inhibits glucose metabolism but also directly suppresses insulin secretion. Relative functional insulin deficiency results in hyperglycemia and ketogenesis.[12,13]

A number of factors confer diabetic patients more susceptible to perioperative ischemia. Diabetes is associated with premature CAD, which is more extensive and more diffuse in nature than in nondiabetics.[14] Diabetics often exhibit painless myocardial ischemia, which makes clinical detection more difficult. Cardiovascular autonomic dysfunction renders the diabetic patient

---

Table 11-1 **Pathophysiology of Perioperative Cardiac Events**

Tissue trauma	$\rightarrow$	increased sympathetic tone				
Anesthesia	$\rightarrow$	increased cortisol	$\rightarrow$	increased	$\rightarrow$	myocardial
Postoperative pain	$\rightarrow$	platelet activation	$\rightarrow$	oxygen demand	$\rightarrow$	ischemia and MI

Table 11-2 **Paradigm of Perioperative Risk in Diabetics**

CAD + cardiovascular autonomic dysfunction + anesthesia + surgical stress + postoperative pain → perioperative risk

more susceptible to hemodynamic compromise precipitated by illness, surgery, and anesthesia (Table 11-2).[15]

It is controversial as to whether diabetes confers an increased risk of perioperative cardiac complications as a number of studies have provided conflicting results.[16-18] Although optimal glycemic control has been shown to reduce infectious complications of surgery and to hasten convalescence, it remains controversial as to whether tighter glycemic control reduces perioperative cardiovascular events.[19-21] In the setting of MI unrelated to surgery, admission blood glucose levels have been found elevated in a number of nondiabetic patients.[22] It is possible that hyperglycemia may be more predictive of adverse outcomes than the diagnosis of diabetes itself. One small study found no relationship between glucose control and short-term postoperative cardiovascular events,[18] whereas another study found hyperglycemia a univariate but not multivariate predictor of all-cause mortality at 14-month follow-up.[23] Amongst 1258 high-risk surgical patients, two-thirds of whom had prior cardiac disease, tight glycemic control resulted in a 48% reduction in mortality.[24] Conceivably, the recent practice of achieving tighter glycemic control could reduce the increased risk portended by diabetes.

Vascular Surgery

Patients requiring vascular surgery frequently have diabetes. In this setting, CAD may be asymptomatic because of reduced exercise capacity due to pre-existing noncardiac conditions including stroke or claudication. Diabetics with peripheral vascular disease have a high prevalence of significant coronary disease. Nesto et al studied 30 diabetic patients with peripheral vascular disease without suspected coronary disease and found 57% had scintigraphic evidence of myocardial ischemia or infarct.[25] While early studies of patients referred for vascular surgery showed worse short- and long-term outcomes for diabetics,[26] more recent large-scale studies have found similar outcomes in diabetics and nondiabetics.[27] Amongst 6500 patients undergoing major vascular surgery over a 10-year period, mortality rates were approximately 1% in the diabetic and nondiabetic groups.[27] Low cardiac event rates were attributed to a coordinated multidisciplinary approach, but were based on a clinical diagnosis of MI. Patients were not followed by routine serial electrocardiograms or by measurement of cardiac enzymes. Although perioperative outcomes were favorable, the same study showed the long-term prognosis is poor. During 5-year follow-up, diabetic patients had a 50% mortality rate, compared with about a 25% rate among the other patients in the series. Among the diabetic patients referred for vascular surgery, another study found older age and prior cardiac disease as specific risk factors for postoperative events.[28] A more recent study confirmed prior ischemic heart disease, urgent surgery, and American Society of Anesthesiologists (ASA) class as independent predictors of death up to 10 months after noncardiac surgery.[29] In summary, cardiovascular complications are the major cause of perioperative and late morbidity and mortality in patients undergoing major vascular surgery and are related to the frequent presence of underlying CAD rather than to diabetes itself.

Renal Transplantation

In multiple series, diabetics comprise the majority of patients referred for renal transplantation. Preexisting heart disease and age >50 years but not diabetes were found predictive of postoperative cardiac events.[30] These findings are similar to those found in vascular surgery. The perioperative cardiac event rate is 10% in diabetics undergoing renal transplantation.[31] Diabetes is also predictive of higher cardiac risk 2–3 years after renal transplantation.[32,33]

Bariatric Surgery

Bariatric surgery has become an increasingly performed treatment option for morbid obesity because of its efficacy in causing marked weight loss. A recent meta-analysis found up to 77% of patients had complete resolution of diabetes after bariatric surgery.[34] Although a number of techniques now exist for reducing stomach size, there is still a relatively high cardiac event rate, approaches 15%. As diabetes is tightly linked to obesity, cardiovascular evaluation and management is pertinent in diabetics. To date, studies addressing cardiovascular risk assessment and reduction strategies have not included patients referred for bariatric surgery. The presence of morbid obesity also confounds noninvasive cardiac testing because of artifact on nuclear stress testing and the recording of suboptimal images on stress echocardiography. Although the adjunct use of contrast agents with stress echo may improve endocardial delineation, this technique has not been evaluated with regard to risk stratification of bariatric surgical candidates.

Preoperative Cardiac Risk Stratification

Cardiac risk assessment is the goal of evaluation for patients undergoing noncardiac surgery. Over the past 25 years, a number of risk prediction schemes have been developed in order to use clinical criteria to estimate perioperative cardiac risk. Diabetes is considered a risk predictor in some but not all.[35–41]

The ASA classification is still used by anesthesiologists after its inception in 1963. It focuses on functional activity level rather than on specific aspects of organ function. These criteria were not designed to predict outcome but rather to quantify the degree of systemic disease before anesthesia. Accordingly, diabetes is not considered in this classification scheme.

In 1977, Goldman et al developed the first validated model to predict cardiac complications in a general surgical population.[35] Among 39 clinical variables, 9 were found predictive of the combined endpoint of cardiac death, MI pulmonary edema, and ventricular tachycardia. The individual criteria pertained to the presence of ischemic heart disease, congestive heart failure (CHF), cardiac arrhythmia, important aortic stenosis, general medical status, age, and type of surgery. A cardiac risk index was defined and patients were stratified into four risk classes. Diabetes was not found to be associated with higher perioperative risk.

Although this study was a landmark one, it had several limitations. Patients with angina were excluded and the study was criticized for a small number of endpoints, poor discriminative capability in patients rated as intermediate risk, its tendency to be institution-dependent, and its lower accuracy when applied to high-risk operations.[38]

In 1986, Detsky et al modified the original Goldman risk index to include the presence and severity of angina as well as the type of surgical procedure.[36] Since the Modified Cardiac Risk Index incorporated history, examination, and electrocardiographic features of the original Goldman criteria, diabetes was not considered as a predictive variable. Subsequently, Hollenberg et al identified five independent preoperative clinical predictors of postoperative myocardial ischemia: hypertension, electrocardiographic evidence of left ventricular hypertrophy (LVH), treated diabetes mellitus, documented CAD, and digoxin use.[37] The risk of postoperative myocardial ischemia increased along with the number of identified predictors: from 22% in patients without any predictors, 31% with one predictor, 46% with two predictors, 70% with three predictors, and 77% in patients with four predictors. Similarly, Larsen et al found diabetes in one of six clinical predictors (i.e., CHF, ischemic heart disease, diabetes mellitus, serum creatinine above 0.13 mmol/L, emergency operation, and the type of operation).[38] The American College of Physicians Guidelines Statement was originally published in 1997.[7] It is based on the Detsky modified risk index and the results of noninvasive testing such as dipyridamole thallium imaging or dobutamine stress echocardiography (DSE). In the ACC/AHA guideline, these factors are used to determine perioperative cardiac risk and whether or not additional preoperative testing is indicated.

In 1999, Lee et al studied 4315 patients 50 years of age or older who underwent elective major noncardiac surgery.[41] Factors associated with an increased risk of major cardiac complications (MI, pulmonary edema, ventricular fibrillation, complete heart block) included history of ischemic heart disease, history of CHF, history of cerebrovascular disease, an elevated creatinine level (≥ 2 mg/dL), and high-risk surgery. Diabetes was also a risk factor if insulin treatment was required. Rates of major complications with 0, 1,

Table 11-3 **Diabetes as an Independent Predictor in Perioperative Risk Stratification Indices**

Study	Index	Diabetes
American Society of Anaesthesiology (1963)	ASA classification	No
Goldman et al. (1977)	Original Cardiac Risk Index	No
Detsky et al. (1986)	Modified Cardiac Risk Index	No
Larsen et al. (1987)		Yes
Michel et al. (1990)		No
Hollenberg et al. (1992)		Yes, treated
L'Italien et al. (1996)	Combined clinical and nuclear	Yes
Lee et al. (1999)	Revised Cardiac Risk Index	Yes, insulin requiring
ACP guideline (1997)	Modified Cardiac Risk Index	No
ACC/AHA	Revised Cardiac Index	Yes, insulin requiring

2, ≥3 risk factors were: 0.5, 1.3, 4, and 9%, respectively. This index, known as the Revised Cardiac Risk Index was found superior to other risk prediction indexes (Table 11-3).

CLINICAL EVALUATION

In the ACC/AHA guidelines, a patient's risk for cardiac events during surgical procedures is estimated by consideration of three categories of information: clinical markers or predictors, level of functional capacity, and surgery-specific risks.[4] Clinical markers or predictors are divided into high, intermediate, and minor risk groups for perioperative cardiovascular complications. Diabetes is considered an intermediate clinical risk factor.[4] The patient at intermediate risk is often the most important but also the most challenging to further work-up prior to surgery. A patient's level of functional capacity is expressed by metabolic equivalents (METs) based on reported activities of daily living. Poor exercise capacity is the inability to achieve 4 METs (the equivalent of walking 4 mph on level ground, or climbing a flight of stairs). Poor exercise capacity is associated with a substantial increase in cardiac events after noncardiac surgical procedures. With regard to surgery-specific risks, high-risk operations (cardiac risk >5%) include major vascular procedures, major emergency procedures (particularly in the elderly), and prolonged procedures that involve large fluid shifts (Table 11-4).

The ACC/AHA guidelines advocate an algorithm based on asking the following five questions:

Table 11-4 **Clinical Markers of Increased Cardiovascular Risk**

CV Risk	Clinical Markers
High	Unstable angina, decompensated CHF, significant arrhythmias (high-grade AV block, ventricular arrhythmias, supraventricular tachyarrhythmias, severe valvular heart disease)
Intermediate	Stable angina, prior MI, compensated heart failure, diabetes
Low	Age >65 years, abnormal electrocardiogram (LVH, LBBB), low exercise capacity, prior CVA or TIA or uncontrolled hypertension

Abbreviations: LBBB, left bundle branch block; CVA, cerebrovascular accident; TIA, transient ischemic attack.

Source: Adapted from Ref 4 and 6.

1. Is there a need for emergency surgery? If the surgery is emergent, the procedure should be performed immediately and cardiovascular evaluation postponed until after the operation. If an emergency operation is not needed, step 2 should be proceeded with.
2. Has the patient undergone coronary revascularization during the last 5 years? If the patient has been revascularized, and is asymptomatic, then surgery may be proceeded with. If not, step 3 is next.
3. Has the patient had coronary angiography or a stress test within the last 2 years? If one or the other has been performed and the results were favorable, then surgery may be proceeded with. If not or if the results were unfavorable, step 4 is next.
4. Are major clinical predictors present? If they are present, then either an invasive or a noninvasive approach may be performed depending on the clinical situation and patient preferences. If no major clinical predictors are present, then step 5 is next.
5. Are intermediate clinical predictors present? If they are, then actions further are contingent on the patient's level of functional activity, surgery-specific risk. If deemed necessary, noninvasive and invasive testing.

Applying this algorithm to diabetics poses some caveats. Firstly, the symptoms of cardiac disease are often atypical in the diabetic population. A higher prevalence of silent ischemia in the diabetic population renders of a history of angina less reliable and would also impact questions 2 and 4. In addition, all diabetics would fall into the intermediate if not high-risk category and would therefore prompt either noninvasive or invasive testing.

A simplified version of the AHA/ACC algorithm suggests the use of non-invasive testing if the patient has at least two of the following risk factors:

- Intermediate clinical predictors: mild angina, prior MI, compensated or prior CHF, diabetes mellitus, renal insufficiency
- Poor functional capacity, defined as <4 METs
- High-risk surgery: emergency procedure, vascular surgery, prolonged procedure, or anticipated large fluid shifts or blood loss

Accordingly, most diabetics would fall into the intermediate risk category and be referred for noninvasive testing.

Cardiovascular Autonomic Neuropathy

Diabetics are well known to develop peripheral and autonomic neuropathy. Clinical manifestations of autonomic neuropathy are chiefly gastrointestinal (gastroparesis), urologic, and cardiovascular. Approximately, 20–40% of diabetics develop cardiac autonomic neuropathy (CAN) which is associated with an increased risk of cardiovascular events and a fivefold increase in overall mortality.[42,43] CAN is generally unrelated to age, duration of diabetes, or severity of microvascular complications. Symptoms of CAN include resting tachycardia due to involvement of parasympathetic nerve fibers, orthostatic hypotension and painless myocardial ischemia, and an impaired cardiovascular response to exercise and stress. CAN is also associated with an increased risk for ventricular arrhythmias and with impaired coronary flow reserve.

There exist a variety of methods to assess CAN in the diabetic patient ranging from simple bedside examination to Holter monitoring and cardiac imaging techniques.[44] Clinical assessment involves the determination of heart rate (HR) and blood pressure (BP) changes in response to a series of maneuvers including deep breathing, Valsalva, and upright posture. Indices of HR variability are reduced in CAN. Both short-term (15 minute) and long-term (24 hours) Holter monitoring have been used extensively to measure HR variability for investigational but not clinical purposes. Similarly, cardiac radionuclide imaging with metaiodobenzylguanidine (MIBG), an analog of norepinephrine has been used to evaluate cardiac sympathetic activity in clinical research studies.

The presence of CAN is associated with a two- to threefold increase in cardiovascular events in diabetics undergoing noncardiac surgery.[43,45] CAN increase the likelihood of hemodynamic instability due to impaired baroreceptor function.[15,43,45] Diabetics with CAN do not exhibit the normal responses of tachycardia and hypertension on induction of anesthesia and tracheal intubation. Cardiac output and hypotension may decrease precipitously in these patients. These changes render the diabetic less able to compensate for stress, blood loss, and cardiac depression.

Routine preoperative testing of autonomic function to detect CAN in diabetics has been advocated by some authors. Simple bedside assessment includes baseline assessment of clinical markers including resting tachycardia and a history of postural hypotension, silent MI, erectile dysfunction, abnormal sweating, and symptoms of gastroparesis or bladder disturbance. Autonomic neuropathy related to diabetes has been shown to be related to a prolonged QT interval and increased mortality rates in the setting of type 2 diabetes.[46] Peripheral neuropathy appears to be less important in the perioperative period than autonomic dysfunction. Although a number of variations have been proposed, a reasonable next step is the performance of a battery of simple bedside tests.[44]

HR RESPONSES

Valsalva maneuver

On Valsalva maneuver, HR increases and then subsequently decreases after cessation. The Valsalva ratio is derived from the maximal HR generated by Valsalva maneuver divided by the lowest HR following the maneuver. Normal values for the Valsalva ratio are ≥ 1.21, whereas abnormal is <1.21.

Deep breathing

On deep breathing, HR increases: normal ≥ 15 beats per minute, borderline: 11–14 beats per minute, and abnormal <10 beats per minute.

Standing up

While standing up, there is a tachycardia at 3–12 seconds followed by a bradycardia at 20 seconds. The initial cardioacceleration is an exercise reflex, while the subsequent tachycardia and bradycardia are baroreflex mediated. The 30:15 ratio, determined as the R-R interval at beat 30/R-R interval at beat 15, is an index of cardiovagal function. Values for the 30:15 ratio include: normal ≥ 1.04, borderline 1.01–1.03, and abnormal <1.00. More simply, a reduction of the normal tachycardic response to standing up can be used as a simple test. The HR should increase by more than 10% from the 15th to 30th beat on standing. Less than 10% may be considered abnormal.

BP RESPONSES

Sustained handgrip

On sustained handgrip, BP increases: normal is ≥ 16 mmHg, borderline is 11–15 mmHg, and abnormal is ≤ 10 mmHg.

Standing up

On standing up, BP falls. Normal is ≤ 10 mmHg, borderline is 11–29 mmHg, and an abnormal response of ≥ 30 mmHg (Table 11-5).

Table 11-5 **Indicators of Cardiovascular Autonomic Dysfunction**

Resting tachycardia
Orthostatic hypotension
Peripheral neuropathy
Silent myocardial ischemia or MI
QT prolongation
HR responses to Valsalva, deep breathing, standing up
BP responses to sustained handgrip, standing up

CARDIAC DIAGNOSTIC TESTING

Noninvasive and invasive testings are generally believed to improve the accuracy of risk stratification using clinical criteria. There exists a large and complex literature on the utility of cardiac diagnostic testing prior to noncardiac surgery including multiple meta-analyses on the subject. The ACC/AHA guidelines suggest that exercise stress testing is the preferred method for preoperative risk stratification.[4] Cardiac stress testing provides an objective measure of functional capacity, which is useful in preoperative evaluation. One meta-analysis showed that when stress testing is positive and leads to a coronary angiogram, there is a significant reduction of postoperative cardiac events.[47] However, the demonstration of ST depressions loses specificity in the presence of resting ST-segment and T-wave changes. These findings are rather common in diabetics. Accordingly, the guidelines advocate stress perfusion imaging and stress echocardiography as adjuncts to stress. Since a large proportion of patients are unable to exercise, dipyridamole perfusion imaging and dobutamine echocardiography are useful alternatives. A recent meta-analysis found DSE to result in half the number of false positive rates as compared with dipyridamole thallium imaging.[48] Another meta-analysis of studies pertaining to dipyridamole myocardial stress perfusion imaging prior to vascular surgery found that reversibility in <20% of myocardial segments did not change the likelihood of perioperative cardiac complications.[49] Accordingly, the greatest value in noninvasive testing lies in its high negative predictive value. The negative predictive value of stress thallium testing is 99% for MI and/or cardiovascular death, whereas the positive predictive value is 42%. Similarly, the negative predictive value of DSE is 93–100% and the positive predictive value is 17–43%. Exercise stress testing and stress imaging studies are most optimally used for risk stratification in intermediate risk patients.[4] Low- and high-risk patients would appear to benefit less and the ACC/AHA guidelines discourage the routine use of noninvasive testing in these groups of patients. Relatively few attempts have been made to collectively consider noninvasive and clinical data. Eagle et al. found dipyridamole thallium exercise imaging a useful method to risk stratify patients referred for vascular surgery.[50] There was a very low cardiac event rate in the absence of the following clinical parameters: Q waves on ECG, age >70 years, angina, premature ventricular contractions, or diabetes. Conversely, most diabetic patients referred for vascular surgery should be referred for noninvasive testing. The value of stress perfusion studies in the risk stratification of diabetics undergoing noncardiac surgery has been called into question. In diabetics referred for dipyridamole thallium scans preoperatively, scans were abnormal in 58% of without and in 93% of patients with clinical evidence of cardiac disease. Sixteen percent had perioperative cardiac complications in the latter group, whereas there were none in the former group.[31]

Several studies in the early 1990s have shown that cardiac morbidity in patients undergoing major, noncardiac surgery is best predicted by postoperative myocardial ischemia, rather than tradition preoperative clinical predictors. Early postoperative ischemia conferred a ninefold increased risk of early cardiac events and a twofold increased risk of long-term (2 years) events.[51] Ambulatory ECG monitoring for ischemia has also been examined as a tool for predicting adverse postoperative cardiac events. Ischemia on preoperative ambulatory ECG has been shown to correlate with cardiac complications with a positive predictive value of 38–67% and a negative predictive value of 86–99%. The technique is generally limited by the large number of patients with baseline electrocardiographic abnormalities. Furthermore, a recent meta-analysis of preoperative cardiac testing modalities concluded that ambulatory ECG monitoring for ischemia is less effective than other available modalities for predicting adverse cardiac outcomes after vascular surgery.[48]

RISK REDUCTION

Smoking cessation treatment with beta-blockers, centrally acting agents, statins, as well as revascularization have all been proposed useful and are utilized clinically to reduce the likelihood of perioperative events. Smoking cessation is well known to reduce pulmonary complications after surgery and to reduce cardiovascular events in patients not undergoing surgery. Recently, Moller et al. randomized 108 patients referred for elective orthopedic surgery to tobacco cessation.[52] Of the 60 patients in the treatment group, 36 stopped smoking entirely and 14 reduced smoking 6-8 weeks before surgery. Overall complication rates were lower in the intervention group (18% vs. 52%). This difference was driven mainly by a reduction in wound complication rates (5% vs. 31%). As diabetes is a risk factor for postoperative wound complications, it would appear imperative that diabetics undergo a smoking cessation program prior to surgery. The benefits of tobacco cessation with regard to cardiac risk reduction have not been specifically addressed in the diabetic population.

Beta-blockers are well known to reduce perioperative cardiac morbidity and mortality and are recommended in high-risk patients. Mangano et al. randomized 200 patients referred for elective, noncardiac surgery who had either a history of CAD or ≥ 2 Framingham risk factors including diabetes to receive atenolol versus placebo.[53] Atenolol was given intravenously (5 or 10 mg) or orally (50–100 mg) just before surgery and then daily until hospital discharge for a maximum of 7 days. During 2-year follow-up, there was a 55% relative risk (RR) reduction in total mortality and a 65% reduction in cardiovascular mortality in the atenolol group. Most of the advantage from atenolol occurred during the first 8 months (1 death in the atenolol group vs. 10 in the placebo group, 7 from cardiovascular causes). Thereafter, the survival curves became parallel. Interestingly, beta-blockers were not shown to reduce the in-hospital cardiac event rate. In this study, diabetes was an important consideration; 31% of patients were diabetic. Diabetes was an independent predictor of 2-year mortality, with a hazard ratio of 2.8 (95% CI 1.4–6.2). The risk related to diabetes was decreased by atenolol treatment as the hazard ratio for diabetes in atenolol-treated patients was only 1.2, whereas in the placebo group it was 4.0. There was significantly more beta-blocker used preoperatively, in the atenolol group, but also at hospital discharge and at 6 months, although these numbers were no longer statistically significant.

In another major study, Poldermans et al. screened 1351 patients and found 846 to have one or more cardiac risk factors.[54] Of the 846 patients, 173 had positive results on dobutamine echocardiography. Among 104 patients randomized to beta-blocker versus placebo, bisoprolol reduced perioperative mortality (3.4% vs. 34%, $P = 0.02$) and the frequency of nonfatal MI in high-risk patients who are undergoing major vascular surgery. Only 15% of patients in this study were diabetic.

A recent study evaluated the use of beta-blockers specifically in diabetic patients. The Diabetic Post-Operative Morbidity and Mortality (DIPOM) study randomized 921 diabetics undergoing major noncardiac surgery to receive metoprolol versus placebo[57] immediately prior to and up to 1 week after surgery. After 18-month follow-up, the primary composite endpoint of all-cause mortality, acute MI, unstable angina, or CHF was similar between the two groups: 21% versus 20%. All-cause mortality was identical between the groups: 16% versus 16%. A low (1%) hospital event rate as well as variable use of beta-blocker in the 2 postoperative days might have accounted for the lack of benefit. A larger study was proposed to further investigate this effect.

Despite the lack of benefit, there are ongoing studies evaluating the utility of beta-blockers. At present, perioperative beta-blockade in patients with major risk factors for CAD is a class IIa recommendation by the ACC/AHA. Diabetes mellitus requiring insulin therapy is a Cardiac Risk Index Criteria and is an indication for beta-blockade. Diabetes that does not require insulin is a minor criterion, and, in conjunction with other Framingham risk factors is an indication for beta-blockade (Table 11-6).

Table 11-6 **Studies Showing the Effect of Beta Blockers on Perioperative Outcomes**

Reference No.	N	Population	Diabetics (%)	Beta-blocker	Follow-up	Outcome	Result
Mangano et al. (1996)	200	Known CAD or two minor risk factors for CAD Major vascular, intra-abdominal, orthopedic, neurosurgical, and other	31	Atenolol	2 years	Mortality	10% vs. 21%
Poldermans et al. (1999)	112	More than 1 CV risk factor + inducible ischemia on dobutamine echo Abdominal aortic or infrainguinal arterial reconstruction	15	Bisoprolol	30 days	Death or nonfatal MI	3.4% vs. 34%, $P = 0.02$
Zaugg et al. (1999)	59	≥65 years of age Major abdominal, intrathoracic, or hip replacement	11	Atenolol	3 days	Myocardial ischemia; MI	
Urban et al. (2000)	107	CAD or >3 risk factors Knee replacement Elective total knee arthroplasty	10	Postoperative esmolol Followed by metoprolol	Myocardial ischemia; MI	6% vs. 15%, ns 2% vs. 6%, ns

Alpha agonists have been proposed as an alternative in patients with contraindications to beta-blockers. Alpha$_2$ receptor agonists reduce central sympathetic outflow and inhibit norepinephrine release from presynaptic nerve terminals. Clinically, this class of drug lowers resting HR and BP and enhances sedation and analgesia. Clonidine has been shown to reduce postoperative increases fibrinogen levels and antagonizes epinephrine-induced platelet aggregation. While a number of studies have suggested alpha agonists were effective in reducing perioperative events, a meta-analysis of including 9 coronary bypass and 12 noncardiac surgeries showed reduced mortality and MI rates (RR 0.47 and 0.66, respectively) in vascular surgery patients.[58] Although the 2002 ACC/AHA guidelines rate this class of drug a IIb recommendation, the use of alpha agonists have not to date become standard of care and have not been specifically examined in the diabetic population.

Preliminary studies suggest statins to reduce the risk of MI and death in the perioperative period.[59–64] Poldermans et al. retrospectively studied 2816 patients who underwent major vascular surgery and found statin use associated with a lower risk of perioperative mortality.[59] The odds ratios (OR) were 0.26 and 0.24 for diabetics and nondiabetics, respectively. While other studies have similarly demonstrated beneficial effects of statins in diabetics and nondiabetics, this issue has not been specifically addressed in diabetic patients (Table 11-7).

Revascularization

Although cardiac risk stratification may result in coronary revascularization, the clinical benefits portended by revascularization remain unproven. Accordingly, the updated ACC/AHA guidelines maintain that revascularization is rarely necessary to reduce the risk of noncardiac surgery alone.[4] The indications for revascularization prior to noncardiac surgery are generally the same as those in patients with CAD in the nonsurgical setting. Accordingly, revascularization strategies including percutaneous coronary intervention (PCI) and coronary bypass surgery should not be routinely considered to facilitate surgery. Relatively few observational studies have addressed the utility of prophylactic PCI prior to noncardiac surgery. The studies, which are small in size (40-207 patients) have shown cumulative mortality and MI rates of 6.9 and 5.4%, respectively. These studies have shown higher mortality and morbidity rates for surgery performed within 2–4 weeks of surgery, possibly related to the discontinuation of antiplatelet agents.[65–67] Therefore, it is recommended that elective surgery be delayed for 4–6 weeks after PCI (Table 11-8).

The Coronary Artery Revascularization Prophylaxis trial randomized 510 out of 5859 patients screened prior to undergoing vascular surgery who had CAD amenable to percutaneous or surgical revascularization versus no revascularization.[68] Patients with left main disease, severe left ventricular dysfunction, or aortic stenosis were excluded. Those who underwent revascularization had their vascular surgery delayed by 36 days. There were

Table 11-7 **Studies of Statins Prior to Noncardiac Surgery**

Study	N	Population	Diabetes Mellitus (%)	Outcome	Result
Amar et al. (2005)	131	Major lung or esophageal resection	1.5	Atrial fibrillation	
Kennedy et al. (2005)	3360	Retrospective cohort Carotid endarterectomy		Hospital mortality, in-hospital ischemic stroke or death	3.8% vs. 1.8% OR 0.53
Kertai et al. (2004)	570	Retrospective cohort Abdominal aortic aneurysms	6	30-day perioperative mortality and MI	3.7% vs. 11.7% OR 0.31
Durazzo (2004)	100	Prospective randomized Vascular surgery	17	6 months cumulative: cardiac death, nonfatal MI, unstable angina, stroke	8% vs. 26%
Poldermans et al. (2003)	2816	Case control Major vascular	36	Perioperative mortality	OR 0.22
O'Neill-Callahan et al. (2005)	1163	Carotid endarterectomy, aortic surgery, lower extremity revascularization	52	Death, MI, ischemia, CHF, ventricular tachyarrhythmias	

Table 11-8 **Studies of Coronary Stenting Prior to Noncardiac Surgery**

Study	No. of patients	Diabetes (%)	Deaths	Miscellaneous
Kaluza et al. (2000)	40	23	8	
Wilson et al. (2003)	207	28	6	Diabetes not a predictor of events
Sharma et al. (2004)	47		6	Diabetes not a predictor of major adverse cardiac events
Reddy and Vaitkus (2005)	56	57	4	

no significant differences in 30-day mortality (3.1% vs. 3.4%) or in mortality at 2.7 years follow-up (22% vs. 23%) between the groups.

Perioperative Monitoring

Perioperative monitoring encompasses a broad scope of monitoring and detection of myocardial ischemia. Monitoring ranges from the intraoperative use of the pulmonary artery (PA) catheter, transesophageal echocardiography, and continuous 12-lead electrocardiographic monitoring to detect myocardial ischemia. The use of PA catheterization is on the decline as observational studies have failed to confirm a benefit when used in critically ill patients. Recently, Sandham et al. conducted the first randomized trial addressing the utility of the PA catheter in 1994 patients undergoing noncardiac surgery.[69] Although more patients in the PA catheter group received inotropic agents, vasodilators, antihypertensive agents, packed red blood cell, and colloid transfusions, similar in-hospital mortality rates were observed in the PA catheter and control groups (7.8% vs. 7.7%, respectively). Similarly, there were no differences in in-hospital cardiac event rates or in mortality at 6- and 12-month follow-up. Therefore, use of the PA catheter does not improve perioperative outcomes. Although studies of patients undergoing vascular surgery have demonstrated efficacy of transesophageal echocardiography and continuous 12-lead electrocardiographic monitoring in detecting episodes of ischemia, a beneficial effect on clinical outcomes has not been well studied in diabetics alone or as a subgroup. There are no specific guidelines for intraoperative or perioperative monitoring or patients with CAD or valvular disease undergoing peripheral or aortic vascular procedures. Finally, although it has become common practice to draw cardiac enzymes or biomarkers to detect myocardial injury, the performance and timing of cardiac biomarkers including creatinine phosphokinase and troponins as well as the recording of 12-lead electrocardiograms are variable in clinical practice.

Current consensus guidelines recommend postoperative electrocardiographic surveillance in patients at relatively high risk of postoperative major cardiac complications. The value of postoperative electrocardiogram was confirmed in 3570 patients who underwent major noncardiac procedures and had electrocardiograms performed in the recovery room.[70] Rates of major cardiac complications (acute MI, pulmonary edema, ventricular fibrillation or primary cardiac arrest, and complete heart block) were higher in patients who had new postoperative electrocardiographic abnormalities consistent with ischemia (ST-T elevation or depression or T-wave abnormalities compatible with ischemia) compared with those without ischemia (6.7% vs. 1.9%, $P < 0.001$).[70] In this study, diabetics were more likely to have had electrocardiograms performed and were more likely to have major cardiac events. In another study, Charlson et al. found serial ECG recording on the first and second postoperative days was an excellent strategy for detecting perioperative myocardial ischemia and infarction.[71] In a study of patients undergoing major vascular surgery, diabetes was independent predictor of low but not high level troponin I elevation when drawn immediately after surgery and the first three mornings thereafter.[72] The yield of each determination was not reported for the diabetic group. In another study, troponin I elevation was associated with overall mortality 1 year after noncardiac surgery.[73] Interestingly, CAN measured by HR variability analysis was also an independent predictor, whereas diabetes itself was not.

SUMMARY

In summary, diabetics are increasingly being referred for noncardiac surgery. Diabetes confers an increased risk for postoperative cardiac complications due to a higher prevalence of CAD and the need for higher risk surgeries required to treat the complications of diabetes. The symptoms of cardiac disease are often atypical in this patient population, which serves to make preoperative evaluation more difficult. The benefits of therapies aimed at reducing perioperative risk in diabetics have for the most part been determined by subgroup analysis of larger studies of unselected patients. The risk of diabetes is chiefly related to the presence of CAD and cardiovascular autonomic dysfunction. Accordingly, diabetes is an intermediate clinical marker. Because stress myocardial perfusion imaging is indicated for perioperative cardiac risk stratification in intermediate risk patients, most diabetic patients will undergo testing. The indications for coronary revascularization are similar to those in the nonsurgical setting. Revascularization is seldom necessary to improve short-term perioperative outcome. Perioperative management with beta-blockers and statins may improve patients' perioperative and long-term outcome. A multidisciplinary approach including surgical, anesthesia, endocrine, as well as cardiology expertise is necessary in order to optimize perioperative outcomes.

REFERENCES

1. Mangano DT. Perioperative cardiac morbidity—epidemiology, costs, problems, and solutions. *West J Med* 1994;161(1):87–89.

2. McAnulty GR, Robertshaw HJ, Hall GM. Anaesthetic management of patients with diabetes mellitus. *Br J Anaesth* 2000;85:80–90.

3. Jacober SJ, Sowers JR. An update on perioperative management of diabetes. *Arch Intern Med* 1999;159:2405–2411.

4. Eagle KA, Berger PB, Calkins H, et al. ACC/AHA guideline update for perioperative cardiovascular evaluation for noncardiac surgery—executive summary: a report of the American College of Cardiology/American Heart Association Task Force on Practice Guidelines (Committee to Update the 1996 Guidelines on Perioperative Cardiovascular Evaluation for Noncardiac Surgery). *J Am Coll Cardiol* 2002;39:542–553, *Circulation* 2002,105:1257–1267.

5. Haffner SM, Lehto S, Ronnemaa T, et al. Mortality from coronary heart disease in subjects with type 2 diabetes and in nondiabetic subjects with and without prior myocardial infarction. *N Engl J Med* 1998;339(4):229–234.

6. ACC/AHA task force report. Special report: guidelines for perioperative cardiovascular evaluation for noncardiac surgery. Report of the American College of Cardiology/American Heart Association Task Force on practice guidelines (Committee on Perioperative Cardiovascular Evaluation for Noncardiac Surgery). *J Cardiothorac Vasc Anesth* 1996;10(4):540–552.

7. American College of Physicians. Guidelines for assessing and managing the perioperative risk from coronary artery disease associated with major noncardiac surgery. *Ann Intern Med* 1997;127:309–312.

8. Mangano DT. Perioperative medicine: NHLBI working group deliberations and recommendations. *J Cardiothorac Vasc Anesth* 2004;18(1):1–6.

9. Gordon AJ, Macpherson DS. Guideline chaos: conflicting recommendations for preoperative cardiac assessment. *Am J Cardiol* 2003;91(11):1299–1303.

10. Dawood MM, Gupta DK, Southern J, et al. Pathology of fatal perioperative myocardial infarction: implications regarding pathophysiology and prevention. *Int J Cardiol* 1996;57:37–44.

11. Cohen MC, Aretz TH. Histological analysis of coronary artery lesions in fatal postoperative myocardial infarction. *Cardiovasc Pathol* 1999;8(3):133–139.

12. Schade D. Surgery and diabetes. *Med Clin North Am* 1988;72:1531–1543.

13. Milaskiewicz RM, Hall GM. Diabetes and anaesthesia: the past decade. *Br J Anaesth* 1992;68:198–206.

14. Fallow GD, Singh J. The prevalence, type and severity of cardiovascular disease in diabetic and non-diabetic patients: a matched-paired retrospective analysis using coronary angiography as the diagnostic tool. *Mol Cell Biochem* 2004;261:263–269.

15. Latson TW, Ashmore TM, Reinhart DJ, et al. Autonomic reflex dysfunction in patients presenting for elective surgery is associated with hypotension after anaesthesia induction. *Anesthesiology* 1994;80:326–337.

16. Hjortuup A, Sorensen C, Dyremose E, et al. Influence of diabetes mellitus on operative risk. *Br J Surg* 1985;72:783–785.

17. Scherpereel P. Le diabète est-il un facteur de risque chez l'opéré? In: Conférences d'actualisation. Congrès National d'Anesthésie Réanimation, Masson Edit. Paris, 1991:31–40.

18. MacKenzie CR, Charlson MR. Assessment of perioperative risk in the patient with diabetes mellitus. *Surg Gynecol Obstet* 1988;167:293–299.

19. Alberti KG, Thomas DJB. The management of diabetes during surgery. *Br J Anaesth* 1979;51:693–710.

20. Thomas DJ, Platt HS, Alberti KG. Insulin-dependent diabetes during the perioperative period. An assessment of continuous glucose–insulin–potassium infusion, and traditional treatment. *Anaesthesia* 1984;39:629–637.

21. Hill Golden S, Peart-Vigilance C, Koa WH, et al. Perioperative glycemic control and the risk of infectious complications in a cohort of adults with diabetes. *Diabetes Care* 1999;22:1408–1414.

22. Malmberg K. Prospective randomised study of intensive insulin treatment on the long term survival after acute myocardial infarction in patients with diabetes mellitus. *BMJ* 1997;314:1512–1515.

23. Juul AB, Wetterslev J, Kofoed-Enevoldsen A, et al. The Diabetic Postoperative Mortality and Morbidity (DIPOM) trial: rationale and design of a multicenter, randomized, placebo-controlled, clinical trial of metoprolol for patients with diabetes mellitus who are undergoing major noncardiac surgery. *Am Heart J* 2004;147:677–683.

24. Van den Berghe G, Wouters P, Weekers F, et al. Intensive insulin therapy in critically ill patients. *N Engl J Med* 2001;345:1359–1367.

25. Nesto RW, Watson FS, Kowalchuk GJ, et al. Silent myocardial ischemia and infarction in diabetics with peripheral vascular disease: assessment by dipyridamole thallium-201 scintigraphy. *Am Heart J* 1990;120(5):1073–1077.

26. Treiman GS, Treiman RL, Foran RF, et al. The influence of diabetes mellitus on the risk of abdominal aortic surgery. *Am Surg* 1994;60:436–440.

27. Hamdan AD, Saltzberg SS, Sheahan M, et al. Lack of association of diabetes with increased postoperative mortality and cardiac morbidity: results of 6565 major vascular operations. *Arch Surg* 2002;137(4):417–421.

28. Zarich SW, Pierce ET, Nesto RW, et al. Age and history of cardiac disease as risk factors for cardiac complications after peripheral vascular surgery in diabetic patients. *Mayo Clin Proc* 2001;76(1):34–38.

29. Juul AB, Wetterslev J, Kofoed-Enevoldsen A. Long-term postoperative mortality in diabetic patients undergoing major non-cardiac surgery. *Eur J Anaesthesiol* 2004;21(7):523–529.

30. Humar A, Kerr SR, Ramcharan T, et al. Peri-operative cardiac morbidity in kidney transplant recipients: incidence and risk factors. *Clin Transplant* 2001;15(3):154–158.

31. Zarich SW, Cohen MC, Lane SE, et al. Routine perioperative dipyridamole 201Tl imaging in diabetic patients undergoing vascular surgery. *Diabetes Care* 1996;19(4):355–360.

32. Cortigiani L, Desideri A, Gigli G, et al. Clinical, resting echo and dipyridamole stress echocardiography findings for the screening of renal transplant candidates. *Int J Cardiol* 2005;103(2):168–174.

33. Chuang P, Gibney EM, Chan L, et al. Predictors of cardiovascular events and associated mortality within two years of kidney transplantation. *Transplant Proc* 2004;36(5):1387–1391.

34. Buchwald H, Avidor Y, Braunwald E, et al. Bariatric surgery. A systematic review and meta-analysis. *JAMA* 2004;292:1724–1737.

35. Goldman L, Caldera DL, Nussbaum SR, et al. Multifactorial index of cardiac risk in noncardiac surgical procedures. *N Engl J Med* 1977;297:845–850.

36. Detsky AS, Abrams HB, McLaughlin JR, et al. Predicting cardiac complications in patients undergoing non-cardiac surgery. *J Gen Intern Med* 1986;1:211–219.

37. Hollenberg M, Mangano DT, Browner WS, et al. Predictors of perioperative myocardial ischemia in patients undergoing noncardiac surgery: the study of perioperative ischemia research group. *JAMA* 1992;268:205–209.

38. Larsen SF, Olesen KH, Jacobsen E, et al. Prediction of cardiac risk in non-cardiac surgery. *Eur Heart J* 1987;8:179–185.

39. Michel LA, Jamart J, Bradpiece HA, et al. Prediction of risk in noncardiac operations after cardiac operations. *J Thorac Cardiovasc Surg* 1990;100:595–605.

40. L'Italien GJ, Paul SD, Hendel RC, et al. Development and validation of a Bayesian model for perioperative cardiac risk assessment in a cohort of 1,081 vascular surgical candidates. *J Am Coll Cardiol* 1996;27(4):779–786.

41. Lee TH, Marcantonio ER, Mangione CM, et al. Derivation and prospective validation of a simple index for prediction of cardiac risk of major noncardiac surgery. *Circulation* 1999;100:1043–1049.

42. Clarke BF, Ewing DJ, Campbell IW. Diabetic autonomic neuropathy. *Diabetologica* 1979;17:195–212.

43. Burgos LG, Ebert TJ, Asiddao C, et al. Increased intraoperative cardiovascular morbidity in diabetics with autonomic neuropathy. *Anesthesiology* 1989;70:591–597.

44. Piha SJ. Cardiac autonomic reflex tests normal responses and age related references values. *Clin Physiol* 1991;11:272–290.

45. Vohra A, Kumar S, Charlton AJ, et al. Effect of diabetes mellitus on the cardiovascular responses to induction of anaesthesia and tracheal intubation. *Br J Anaesth* 1993;71:258–261.

46. Pourmoghaddas A, Hekmatnia A. The relationship between QTc interval and cardiac autonomic neuropathy in diabetes mellitus. *Mol Cell Biochem* 2003;249: 125–128.

47. Beattie WS, Abdelnaem E, Wijeysundera DN, et al. A meta-analytic comparison of preoperative stress echocardiography and nuclear scintigraphy imaging. *Anesth Analg* 2006;102(1):8–16.

48. Mantha S, Roizen MF, Barnard J, et al. Relative effectiveness of four preoperative tests for predicting adverse cardiac outcomes after vascular surgery: a meta-analysis. *Anesth Analg* 1994;79:422–433.

49. Etchells E, Meade M, Tomlinson G, et al. Semiquantitative dipyridamole myocardial stress perfusion imaging for cardiac risk assessment before noncardiac vascular surgery: a meta-analysis. *J Vasc Surg* 2002;36(3):534–540.

50. Eagle KA, Coley CM, Newell JB, et al. Combining clinical and thallium data optimizes preoperative assessment of cardiac risk before major vascular surgery. *Ann Intern Med* 1989;110(11):859–866.

51. Mangano DT, Hollenberg M, Fegert G, et al. Perioperative myocardial ischemia in patients undergoing noncardiac surgery. I. Incidence and severity during the 4 day perioperative period. The Study of Perioperative Ischemia (SPI) Research Group. *J Am Coll Cardiol* 1991;17(4):843–850.

52. Moller A, Villebro N, Pedersen T, et al. Effect of preoperative smoking intervention on postoperative complications: a randomised clinical trial. *Lancet* 2002; 359(9301):114–117.

53. Mangano DT, Layug EL, Wallace A, et al. Effect of atenolol on mortality and cardiovascular morbidity after noncardiac surgery. Multicenter Study of Perioperative Ischemia Research Group. *N Engl J Med* 1996;335(23):1713–1720.

54. Poldermans E, Boersma E, Bax JJ, et al. The effect of bisoprolol on perioperative mortality and myocardial infarction in high-risk patients undergoing vascular surgery. Dutch echocardiographic cardiac risk evaluation applying stress echocardiography study group. *N Engl J Med* 1999;341:1789–1794.

55. Zaugg M, Tagliente T, Lucchinetti E. Beneficial effects from beta-adrenergic blockade in elderly patients undergoing noncardiac surgery. *Anesthesiology* 1999;91: 1674–1686.

56. Urban MK, Markowitz SM, Gordon MA, et al. Postoperative prophylactic administration of beta-adrenergic blockers in patients at risk for myocardial ischemia. *Anesth Analg* 2000;90:1257–1261.

57. Juul AB, Wetterslev J, Kofoed-Enevoldsen A, et al. The Diabetic Postoperative Mortality and Morbidity (DIPOM) trial: rationale and design of a multicenter, randomized, placebo-controlled, clinical trial of metoprolol for patients with diabetes mellitus who are undergoing major noncardiac surgery. *Am Heart J* 2004;147:677–683.

58. Wijeysundera DN, Naik JS, Beattie WS. Alpha-2 adrenergic agonists to prevent perioperative cardiovascular complications: a meta-analysis. *Am J Med* 2003;114(9): 742–752.

59. Poldermans D, Bax JJ, Kertai MD, et al. Statins are associated with a reduced incidence of perioperative mortality in patients undergoing major noncardiac vascular surgery. *Circulation* 2003;107(14):1848–1851.

60. Kertai MD, Boersma E, Westerhout CM, et al. A combination of statins and beta-blockers is independently associated with a reduction in the incidence of perioperative mortality and nonfatal myocardial infarction in patients undergoing abdominal aortic aneurysm surgery. *Eur J Vasc Endovasc Surg* 2004;28(4):343–352.

61. Kennedy J, Quan H, Buchan AM, et al. Statins are associated with better outcomes after carotid endarterectomy in symptomatic patients. *Stroke* 2005;36(10): 2072–2076.

62. O'Neil-Callahan K, Katsimaglis G, Tepper MR, et al. Statins decrease perioperative cardiac complications in patients undergoing noncardiac vascular surgery:

the Statins for Risk Reduction in Surgery (StaRRS) study. *J Am Coll Cardiol* 2005;45(3):336–342.

63. Amar D, Zhang H, Heerdt PM, et al. Statin use is associated with a reduction in atrial fibrillation after noncardiac thoracic surgery independent of C-reactive protein. *Chest* 2005;128(5):3421–3427.

64. Durazzo AE, Machado FS, Ikeoka DT, et al. Reduction in cardiovascular events after vascular surgery with atorvastatin: a randomized trial. *J Vasc Surg* 2004;39(5):967–975.

65. Kaluza GL, Joseph J, Lee JR, et al. Catastrophic outcomes of noncardiac surgery soon after coronary stenting. *J Am Coll Cardiol* 2000;35:1288–1294.

66. Wilson SH, Fasseas P, Orford JL, et al. Clinical outcome of patients undergoing non-cardiac surgery in the two months following coronary stenting. *J Am Coll Cardiol* 2003;42(2):234–240.

67. Sharma AK, Ajani AE, Hamwi SM, et al. Major noncardiac surgery following coronary stenting: when is it safe to operate? *Catheter Cardiovasc Interv* 2004;63(2): 141–145.

68. Reddy PR, Vaitkus PT. Risks of noncardiac surgery after coronary stenting. *Am J Cardiol* 2005;95(6):755–757.

69. McFalls EO, Ward HB, Moritz TE, et al. Coronary-artery revascularization before elective major vascular surgery. *N Engl J Med* 2004;351(27):2795–2804.

70. Sandham JD, Hull RD, Brant RF, et al. Canadian Critical Care Clinical Trials Group. A randomized, controlled trial of the use of pulmonary-artery catheters in high-risk surgical patients. *N Engl J Med* 2003;348(1):5–14.

71. Rinfret S, Goldman L, Polanczyk CA, et al. Value of immediate postoperative electrocardiogram to update risk stratification after major noncardiac surgery. *Am J Cardiol* 2004;94(8):1017–1022.

72. Charlson ME, MacKenzie CR, Ales K, et al. Surveillance for postoperative myocardial infarction after noncardiac operations. *Surg Gynecol Obstet* 1988;167(5):407–414.

73. Landesberg G, Mosseri M, Shatz V, et al. Cardiac troponin after major vascular surgery: the role of perioperative ischemia, preoperative thallium scanning, and coronary revascularization. *J Am Coll Cardiol* 2004;44(3):569–575.

74. Filipovic M, Jeger R, Probst C, et al. Heart rate variability and cardiac troponin I are incremental and independent predictors of one-year all-cause mortality after major noncardiac surgery in patients at risk of coronary artery disease. *J Am Coll Cardiol* 2003;42(10):1767–1776.

CARDIAC SURGERY
IN DIABETIC PATIENTS

Robert C. Lowery
Joshua Burack

INTRODUCTION

Over the past two decades, the incidence of diabetes mellitus has significantly increased worldwide, making it a major risk factor for coronary artery
disease.[1] The incidence of type 2 diabetes mellitus has paralleled the rise of
obesity in developed countries.[2] As of 2003, type 2 diabetes accounted for
90–95% of all diagnosed persons with diabetes.

According to the 2006 American Heart Association statistical update report,
the age-adjusted prevalence of diabetes for adults in the United States showed
an overall increase of 54% from 1994 through 2002.[3] The prevalence of diabetes
in African Americans aged 40–74 also increased at an alarming rate of 18.2%.

Much has been written about the adverse effects of this common disease
process on surgical intervention. It is often said that diabetic patients fare
worse when compared to their nondiabetic cohorts in most studies. This has
become part of the collective wisdom among those treating such patients.[4]

In this chapter, we explore the major types of cardiac surgery and explain
some of the techniques used in our discipline along with their rationale. The
role that diabetes may play in the genesis of the various disease states affecting the heart, the effect on surgical outcomes, and ways to reduce the risks
associated with hyperglycemia and diabetes are also addressed.

CORONARY ARTERY DISEASE

It is now well accepted that hypercholesterolemia is associated with the
inflammatory process that ultimately leads to the development of fatty
streaks, deposition of lipoproteins within the arterial wall, and subsequent
evolution into the atherosclerotic plaques. Modification of these lipids via

nonenzymatic glycosylation in patients with diabetes is of particular interest and persistent hyperglycemia may alter the function of the lipoproteins leading to accelerated atherosclerosis.[5] These lesions are responsible for one of the most frequently performed surgeries in the United States.

In 1967, while at the Cleveland Clinic, Rene Favolaro performed the first successful saphenous vein bypass thus ushering in the era of modern coronary artery bypass grafting (CABG).[6] Made possible by the use of the cardiopulmonary bypass machine, the technique enjoyed increasing success and during the 1980s became the most commonly performed procedure in the United States.[7]

From 1990 through 1992, Buffolo, Benetti, and then Pfister, searching for a cheaper alternative to using the pump, separately explored the possibility of performing bypass surgery without the use of the cardiopulmonary bypass circuit and oxygenator.[8–10] Though the initial impetus for this change was economic, it was soon suggested that "off-pump" might be a safer alternative as well.[11,12]

Although some studies have suggested that off-pump surgery conveys a mortality benefit when compared to on-pump,[13] others have shown only a decreased need for blood transfusion and a slightly decreased length of stay in the hospital.[14] Further, any survival benefit or quality-of-life advantage noted in the early postoperative period has disappeared by a few months and demonstrates no statistical advantage.[15] One large study using the New York State database evaluating nearly 70,000 patients, found that the observed mortality rate was lower in those patients done on-pump. However, again, any survival advantage disappeared in the last 2 years of that study as well.[16] Thus, despite several meta-analyses of the data, there has not been conclusive evidence to definitively support one technique over the other.[17,18] Some have suggested that it is possible that the improved mortality results noted in the off-pump series from a few large volume centers, may be the result of highly skilled surgeons performing the technically more demanding off-pump procedure more frequently.[19,20]

As of January 2005, 34% of surgeons surveyed around the world indicated that at least 50% of their procedures were done off-pump. Only about 15% reported performing "at least 90% of their revascularization procedures off-pump."[21] The actual number of patients receiving off-pump surgery is not known but in the United States has been estimated to be in the 20–30% range.

PERCUTANEOUS CORONARY INTERVENTION (PCI) VERSUS CORONARY ARTERY SURGERY

The Emory Angioplasty Versus Surgery Trial (EAST) and the Bypass Angioplasty Revascularization Investigation (BARI) were begun in 1987 and 1988, respectively, in an attempt to determine whether stenting was superior to bypass surgery. When the results of the BARI trial were reported in 1996, there was a significant 5-year survival advantage seen in the group of diabetic patients undergoing CABG rather than percutaneous therapy with stents.[22]

There is much anticipation of the results of ongoing trials to compare surgery with the results of current percutaneous revascularization techniques. In the Arterial Revascularization Therapies Study, diabetics had a 13% mortality rate when stented compared to an 8.3% rate when operated upon. Interestingly, there was no difference between diabetics and nondiabetics when both groups received an operation.[23]

CONDUITS

Vein Grafts

The first coronary grafts were performed using the saphenous vein. It is still the most commonly used conduit in the United States. Depending on the number of grafts required, it will be harvested from the thigh, the lower leg, or the entire leg. Since diabetic patients with coronary artery disease will often also be afflicted with peripheral vascular disease, the surgeon must take this into consideration. It has been our practice to restrict the vein harvest to the thigh unless the lower leg vein is the only conduit left. In patients with peripheral vascular disease, healing of the poorly perfused leg is usually marginal. The resultant poor healing can lead to amputations. Even when limited to the thigh, healing is often compromised leading to surgical site infections, longer lengths of stay, and higher rates of readmission (Fig. 12-1).

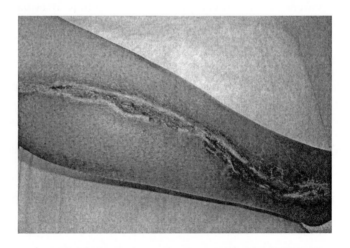

Figure 12-1 **Saphenous vein harvest site.** *(Courtesy of Robert C. Lowery, MD.)*

Endovascular vein harvesting is a recent development that has allowed for a decrease in the morbidity associated with standard harvesting techniques.[24] In addition to being "minimally invasive," it allows for much less a surgical insult when the vein is harvested (Figs. 12-2 and 12-3).

The long-term patency rate of many saphenous veins is about 80% at 1 year.[25] This is especially true in diabetics who have a greater risk of developing early graft closure. This leads to the potential need for either surgical- or catheter-based rerevascularization. Both are fraught with higher risk of mortality and cardiac injury related to distal embolization.[26]

There are a number of reasons given for the tendency for saphenous vein grafts to occlude at an accelerated rate. Among them are: thrombosis, neointima formation, and graft atherosclerosis.[27] Some have suggested that modulation of the vascular milieu of the saphenous using gene therapy could have an effect on improving the patency of these conduits.[28,29] However, such techniques remain experimental.[30]

By far, the best patency has been with arterial grafts. It has long been known that the internal mammary artery has enjoyed a much higher patency rate when compared to the saphenous vein.[31] Some of this advantage may be due to the higher expression of nitric oxide and other substances within the vessel wall and intima.[32,33]

Recent data have also shown an improved survival rate as well when at least the left internal mammary is used to bypass a diseased left anterior descending artery (LAD).

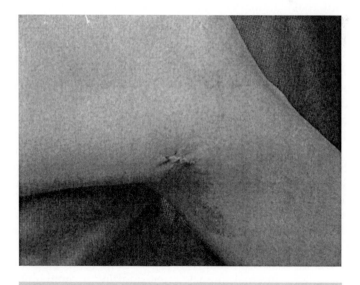

Figure 12-2 **Endovascular vein harvest site.** (Courtesy of Robert C. Lowery MD.)

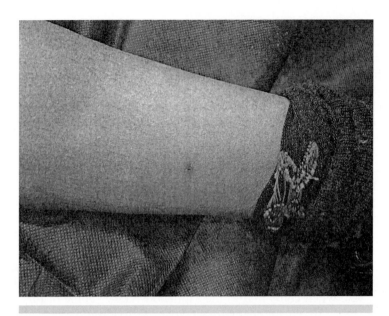

Figure 12-3 **Endovascular vein harvest sited at the ankle.**
(Courtesy of Robert C. Lowery, MD.)

Internal Mammary

When the internal mammary artery is placed to the LAD, the long-term mortality risk decreases in all patients when compared to saphenous vein grafting or bare metal stenting.[34] The use of bilateral mammaries has been shown to confer a survival advantage. In a retrospective study looking at over 10,000 patients having either an elective single or bilateral internal thoracic artery, those patients receiving two mammary grafts were found to have decreased risk of death, reoperation, and angioplasty.[35]

In diabetic patients, conventional surgical lore has found support in many studies suggesting an increase in morbidity when both mammaries are taken down in the diabetic patient. Therefore, the conduits are underutilized in this group of patients. The morbidity is usually related to an increase in sternal wound infections presumably because of the disruption of blood flow to the bone table.[36] Cosgrove et al. showed that there was a 5.7% prevalence of wound complication in those with diabetes versus 0.3% in those without.[37] Recent work by Endo et al. suggests that there may be no disadvantages to harvesting both vessels in the diabetic patient.[38] Further, Toumpoulis et al. have shown, in a retrospective propensity matched study comparing bilateral internal thoracic artery grafting to single internal thoracic artery grafting in diabetic patients, that long-term survival may also be increased in patients with diabetes aged 60–69 years.[39] Though the risk of sternal wound infections was slightly increased in diabetics versus nondiabetics (1.9% vs. 1.2%), survival was improved in diabetic patients after bilateral internal thoracic artery grafting.[40]

Skeletonization of the internal mammary artery has been considered a useful adjunct in decreasing the incidence of sternal wound complications associated with the use of this conduit. As mentioned, the skeletonization may be protective against feared sternal wound infections.[41] In performing this procedure, the internal mammary artery is dissected down from the chest wall without its investing fascia, muscle, accompanying veins, and fat. This has been shown to minimize disruption of the blood supply to the sternum, which should be of more benefit to diabetic patients at risk. Technically, somewhat more challenging, this technique takes longer to learn and there is greater time spent harvesting the conduits, especially when bilateral mammaries are used. Other advantages to the technique include a longer length of the mammary, less likelihood of disruption to flow related to axial orientation, and a greater possibility to use the graft for multiple arterial anastomoses. The technique has also been extended to routine use in diabetics by some authors.[42]

In an effort to increase the percentage of diseased vessels grafted with arterial conduits, there are a number of configurations used to attempt reaching the entire coronary arterial bed. A useful schema has been proposed by Muneretto et al. (Fig. 12-4).[43]

Newer methods of sternal protection are being evaluated. A novel animal study using basic fibroblast growth factor (bFGF) in diabetic rats showed some promise in increasing blood supply to the healing sternum and enhancing bone regeneration.[44] Prostaglandin E2 EP4 receptor agonist was applied to the posterior table of the sternum in Wistar rats resulting in accelerated healing in the study group.[45] With further research, some of these experimental possibilities may find their way into the clinical arena to further enhance our ability to prevent sternal wound infections in diabetics.

Therefore, despite the technical challenges involved in harvesting bilateral mammary arteries, the risk of early graft closure and the need for subsequent revascularization procedures have made saphenous vein a less desirable choice in recent years. Patency has always been a concern especially for venous conduits. Saphenous veins grafts unfortunately have a higher incidence of failure with patency rates as low as 57% at 10 years (Fig. 12-5).[46]

Although traditionally the conduit of choice, the risk of early closure and the potential need for subsequent revascularization procedures has made vein less desirable in recent years. Diabetics have an even greater predilection to close these grafts. Recent studies have shown that there is significantly more endothelial dysfunction leading to stenosis and graft closure in diabetic patients when compared to nondiabetics.[47] Arterial patency rates have been shown to be superior in a number of studies.[48,49] These factors have led to some use of other arterial conduits in an effort to improve long-term patency.

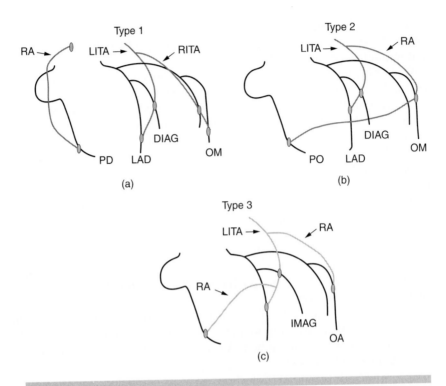

Figure 12-4 **Various configurations for total arterial grafting.** (Source: Reproduced with permission from Muneretto C, Negri A, Gianluigi B, et al. Is total arterial myocardial revascularization with composite grafts a safe and useful procedure in the elderly? Eur J Cardiothorac Surg 2003;23:657–664.)

Radial Artery

The radial artery has been used as both a primary graft and as part of a sequential arterial grafting strategy with varying degrees of success. Patency has ranged from 50 to 80%.[50,51] There have been randomized trials from Canada and Australia where 1-year patency was greater than 80% for the radial arteries.[52]

String Sign

Long-term angiographic data have occasionally been associated with narrowing of the radial conduit some time after its use.[50] Spasticity resulting in vasospasm has been frequently cited as the etiology.[53] Newer harvesting methods: ultrasonic dissection, minimal handling and use immediately after harvesting probably have allowed for some of the better recent results.

This conduit should not be used when there is potential for competitive flow. That is, when proximal target vessel stenoses that are estimated to be less than 70–80%.

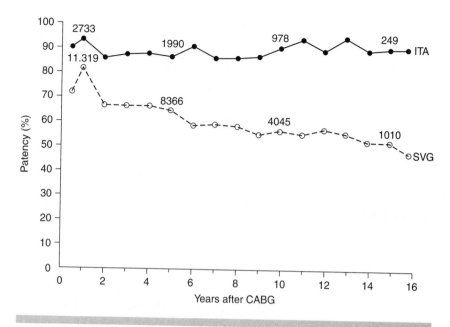

Figure 12-5 **Comparison of saphenous vein and internal thoracic artery graft patency by coronary system.**

It is important to realize that in 10–15% of patients, the radial artery is the dominant vessel to the hand and should not be used. Care should be taken in those patients who use their arms and hands as a means of livelihood (construction workers, plumbers, surgeons). Though the rate of complications is quite low, hand ischemia is quite debilitating. There may be a higher incidence of atherosclerosis of the radial artery in diabetic patients.[54]

MANAGEMENT OF GRAFT CLOSURE: VEINS

Once a patient becomes symptomatic and imaging studies show stenosis or occlusion of the venous conduit, an ideal strategy for dealing with these issues has not been completely elucidated. Many practitioners will approach this problem with the use of percutaneous techniques. Discussion of these is beyond the scope of this chapter.

Surgical approaches usually require resternotomy with its attendant risks. That risk is especially great when there are patent grafts in situ. A "no touch technique" should be adopted with respect to an occluded or stenotic vein graft. These old conduits will often be filled with a "cheesy" atherosclerotic material that has a propensity to embolize distally and cause infarctions. When possible, the coronary vessel subtended by these diseased conduits should be grafted using an arterial conduit.

In recent years, approaches other than sternotomy have also been employed. These include the MIDCAB (minimally invasive direct coronary artery bypass), a subxiphoid approach to LAD and right coronary artery distribution grafting and the so-called lateral MIDCAB.[55] The latter has been quite useful in cases where there is a need to regraft the posterior circulation of the heart when resternotomy is more dangerous than usual. Those instances would include the presence of a patent internal mammary artery or vein grafts to important coronaries which are then placed at jeopardy during sternal re-entry. This is especially true in patients having had multiple previous sternotomies.

OTHER ARTERIES

The gastroepiploic artery has also been used as an arterial conduit. Once harvested from around the stomach, it is brought through the diaphragm usually to supply the posterior descending branch of the right coronary artery. As a free graft, it can be used for other arterial beds as well. The patency has not been considered to be any better than that of saphenous vein grafts and because of its extremely variable size and flow rates, it may be prone to issues of competitive flow.[56]

OFF-PUMP SURGERY

Numerous studies have attempted to find an advantage of off-pump surgery when compared to on-pump surgery in diabetic patients as they are sicker and have a greater number of risk factors. Neurologic injury after conventional cardiac surgery has been shown to be around 6% of patients when rigorously searched for.[57] Although the etiology of this injury and that of other organ systems is varied, most often it has been attributed to particulate or gaseous embolization during cardiopulmonary bypass.[58] These emboli can enter the circulation via the pump or from aspirated blood from the surgical field.[59] The other likely candidate is atherosclerotic plaque from the aorta. Stratagems using arterial grafts are well suited to techniques that avoid touching the aorta all together.

Surgical Results

A recent analysis of the results of coronary bypass surgery in the Society of Thoracic Surgeons (STS) database has reaffirmed the observation that diabetic patients have significantly increased operative risk. In an analysis of over 500,000 surgical procedures nationwide, the overall operative mortality rate and major complication rate in nondiabetics compared to diabetics were 3.05 and 13.40%, respectively. In diabetics, particularly the insulin-dependent patients, there was a moderate increase in both the surgical mortality as well as each of the major types of postoperative morbidity (Table 12-1).[60]

Table 12-1 **Odds Ratios with 95% Confidence Intervals for CABG-Only Risk Models (1997–1999)***

Variable	Mortality OR (95% CI)	Stroke OR (95% CI)	Renal Failure (95% CI)	Prolonged Ventilation OR (95% CI)	Deep Sternal OR (95% CI)	Reoperation OR (95% CI)	Composite OR (95% CI)
Diabetes, oral treatment	1.15 (1.09, 1.21)	1.36 (1.28, 1.45)	1.35 (1.29, 1.42)	1.17 (1.13, 1.22)	1.53 (1.38, 1.70)	0.99 (0.96, 1.04)	1.14 (1.11, 1.17)
Insulin	1.50 (1.42, 1.58)	1.48 (1.37, 1.59)	2.26 (2.16, 2.37)	1.53 (1.47, 1.59)	2.74 (2.47, 3.03)	1.22 (1.17, 1.28)	1.59 (1.54, 1.64)

*Number of records = 403,325 CABG-only records (learning data set). For odds ratio (OR) only statistically significant risk factors are noted for each model with 95% confidence interval (CI). Composite; presence at any major morbidity or operative mortality.

Source: Adapted from Ref. 60.

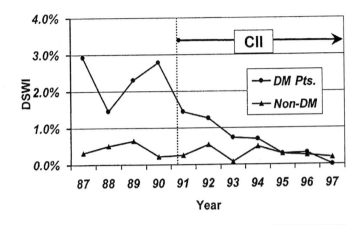

Figure 12-6 **Annual rates of deep sternal wound infections (DSWI) in diabetic and nondiabetic patients after cardiac surgical procedures at Providence St. Vincent Medical Center from 1987 through 1997. CII: continous insulin infusion.** *(Source: Reproduced with permission from Furnary AP, Zerr KJ, Grunkemeier GL, et al. Continuous intravenous insulin infusion reduces the incidence of deep sternal wound infection in diabetic patients after cardiac surgical procedures. Ann Thorac Surg 1999;67:352–360.)*

Glucose Control

The relationship between diabetes and the increased risk of infection is well described. In the patient recuperating from cardiac surgery, a sternal wound infection, as well as other septic events, is a feared and dangerous complication. As first described in 1997, the aggressive regulation of postoperative hyperglycemia, with intravenous insulin infusion to maintain blood glucose well below 200 mg/dL, has had a profound impact on the incidence of sternal wound infection (Fig. 12-6).[61]

In subsequent study, it has been shown that tight blood glucose control significantly reduces operative mortality, and that there is a direct correlation between hyperglycemia and mortality (Figs. 12-7 and 12-8).[61,62]

As better hyperglycemic control becomes widespread it is anticipated that many of the previous surgical risks ascribed to diabetes will be markedly reduced and the risk profile may approach that of the general population.

TRANSMYOCARDIAL LASER REVASCULARIZATION

The use of transmyocardial laser revascularization (TMR) has increased in the last few years. It is a surgical technique that allows creation of channels within the myocardium. There are now two technologies available: the CO_2

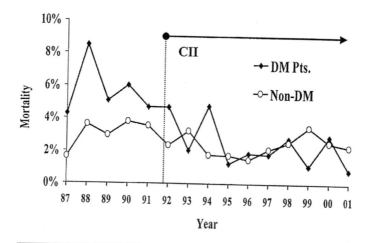

Figure 12-7 **Annualized Mortality in CABG Patients. CII: continous insulin infusion.** (Source: Reproduced with permission
from Furnary AP, Gao G, Grunkemeier GL, et al. Continuous
insulin infusion [CII] reduces mortality in patients with diabetes
undergoing coronary artery bypass grafting. J Thorac Cardiovasc
Surg 2003;125: 1007–1021.)

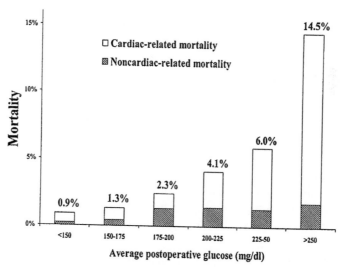

Figure 12-8 **Mortality among patients with diabetes mellitus
undergoing CABG by glucose quantile.** (Source: Reproduced
with permission from Furnary AP, Gao G, Grunkemeier GL, et al.
Continuous insulin infusion reduces mortality in patients with
diabetes undergoing coronary artery bypass grafting. J Thorac
Cardiovasc Surg 2003;125:1007–1021.)

and the holmium-yttrium-aluminum-garnet lasers. Initially utilized as a revascularization adjunct to bypass grafting procedures, favorable results in pain relief in patients who no longer have a graft option has led some to use the procedure as sole therapy via a small anterolateral thoracotomy or video-assisted thoracotomy.[63]

The precise mechanism of action is still debated. The leading candidates for the cause of the symptomatic improvement are laser-induced angiogenesis and laser-induced denervation of the myocardium. Horvath et al. showed that TMR-induced vascular endothelial growth factor (VEGF) expression is accompanied by an increase in tissue levels of VEGF mRNA.[64] Al-Sheik and others found that in the patients that they studied, there was an increase in sympathetic denervation indicated by positron emission tomography (PET) imaging using [11C] hydroxyephedrine. Whatever the mechanism, reduction in angina symptoms has been consistent across all laser wavelengths tested,[65] leading to a wider adoption for those patients without other surgical or percutaneous options.

Technique

Through a median sternotomy, a small anterior thoracotomy or a video-assisted thoracoscopic approach, multiple laser-created channels are made to traverse the myocardium. In diabetics with refractory angina without graftable vessels and who are no longer candidates for percutaneous techniques because of multiple restenoses or the diffuse nature of the coronary disease, this adjunct may provide some benefit. Indeed, Allen et al. showed that there was a greater than two class improvement in Canadian Cardiovascular Society angina scale in 88% of the TMR patients when compared to 44% in the medically managed group.[66]

GENE THERAPY

The promise of gene therapy is only now beginning to be realized. Several groups have begun clinical trials to look at the efficacy of this novel therapy.[67–69] Others have warned that current knowledge and techniques may not be adequate because of the pathophysiologic complexity of the processes involved.[70]

Valvular Heart Disease

Of the greater than 500,000 open heart surgeries performed in the United States yearly, 90,000 are valvular procedures.[3] The bulk of valve operations have been on the aortic valve. However, the number of mitral procedures has been increasing as repair techniques have become more standard in the operative armamentarium.[71] Operations on the tricuspid valve are third in prevalence followed by the pulmonic valve.

Patients with diabetes do not have a greater incidence of valvular heart disease in general. However, a significant proportion of diabetics are obese. Though no longer on the market, phentermine and fenfluramine (phen-fen) use in some patients led to the development of valvular lesions of the aortic, tricuspid, and mitral valves. These lesions mimicked those of carcinoid on the right side of the heart (Fig. 12-9) but are associated with a regurgitant valvulopathy of the aortic and mitral valves. Each lesion so caused can lead to the need for valve replacement.

It is hypothesized that involvement of 5-HT 2B receptors may be associated with these derangements.[72]

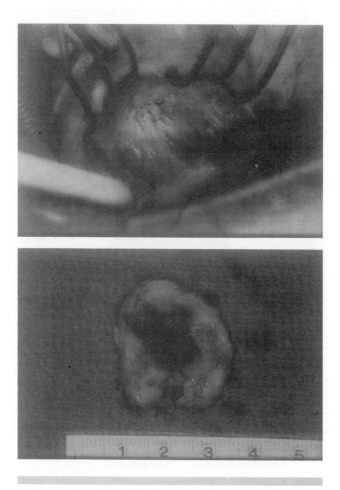

Figure 12-9 **Carcinoid of tricuspid valve.** (Courtesy of Robert C. Lowery, MD.)

TYPES OF REPLACEMENT VALVES

The first valves used to replace the human valve were human valves. They were preserved with a variety of chemicals, most notably glutaraldehyde. The first artificial valve to be used in humans was an elegant plastic construct implanted into the descending thoracic aorta to treat aortic insufficiency.

Today, replacement valves are either tissue or mechanical. Tissue valves are comprised of bovine pericardial, porcine valvular, and human valves—homografts.

The desire to avoid lifelong anticoagulation has led to the development of various techniques to mitigate the gradual degeneration of these tissue valves. Both bovine pericardial and porcine aortic valves are susceptible to calcification. Recent data have suggested a link between atherosclerosis and the accelerated degeneration of tissue valves implanted in younger patients. In one study, diabetes mellitus and elevated cholesterol were both independent risk factors for reoperation on implanted tissue valves.[73]

Mechanical Valves

Mechanical valves enjoy an overall increased freedom from structural deterioration over other types of valves. The first widely used mechanical valves were ball valves within a metal cage similar to valves used in industry. However, since the late 70s most successful valve designs have incorporated a bileaflet configuration (Fig. 12-10).

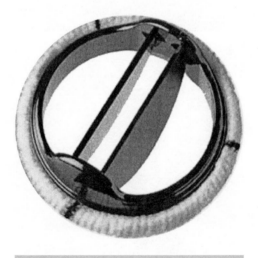

Figure 12-10 **Mechanical valve.** (Source: Reproduced with permission from The St. Jude. Corp, St. Paul, MN.)

These valves are constructed from a variety of materials but most frequently a carbon compound for the occluder discs, housing and Dacron, polypropylene, or Teflon for the sewing rings.

All mechanical valves have a central mechanism to control and allow flow to occur as naturally as possible. However, all designs have some degree of built in "regurgitation" which allows the valve mechanism to be "washed" thereby minimizing the bane of these valves, thromboembolic phenomena. Tissue valves have traditionally held an edge over mechanical valves in this regard. However, a recent long-term analysis of 2533 patients revealed similar rates of thromboembolism between one type of mechanical valve, St. Jude, and tissue valves.[74] Survival rates were similar in both mechanical and tissue valves over the 20-year study period. Tissue valves did exhibit an increased risk of reoperation over time. With newer techniques of tissue valve preservation, the useful life of some pericardial valves has been extended out to 17 years.[75]

The relatively new field of tissue engineering also holds promise for the development of "biologically correct" valves made from the patient's own cells. The premise is that a scaffold is prepared on to which are deposited mesenchymal or allogenic stem cells.[76] At least one commercial product has been developed as a decellularized homograft with the expectation that this matrix becomes "seeded" with compatible cells.[77] Prototypes have been developed for human valves.[78]

Valve Repair and Preservation

The aortic valve does not enjoy the fortuitous anatomic construction of the mitral which makes that valve so amenable to repair techniques. However, many methodologies have been developed in an attempt to avoid replacement in patients with aortic insufficiency. Existing techniques include commissural plication, partial cusp resection with plication, resuspension or cusp shortening, lengthening of the cusp with autologous pericardium, ultrasonic debridement of the calcified valve, and closure of cusp perforation with autologous or glutaraldehyde preserved bovine pericardium.

The results of these repairs have been variable. In some hands, however, the risk of reoperation for recurrent aortic insufficiency has been relatively low averaging about 8%.[79] In the case of aortic stenosis, debridement using standard surgical techniques as well as ultrasound technology has been used. Today, ultrasonic debridement has been abandoned altogether. An unacceptably high incidence of reoperation for restenosis as well as regurgitation has been the experience (Fig. 12-11).[80]

The gold standard for dealing with aortic insufficiency in the setting of aortic annular or root pathology has traditionally been the composite graft as described by Bentall and DeBono in 1968.[81] David and Yacoub independently developed techniques whereby an anatomically normal aortic valve

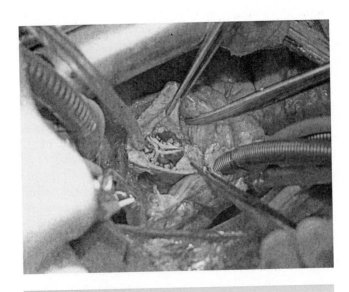

Figure 12-11 **Calcified aortic valve.** *(Courtesy of Robert C. Lowery, MD.)*

may be preserved in the event of type A dissections, aortic root, or sinus of Valsalva aneurysms (Fig. 12-12).[82,83]

These operations have gone through multiple refinements and there is a steep learning curve. There are as yet no guidelines for these procedures and because of the technical challenges encountered, have not enjoyed broad application.[84]

Though aortic operations are generally performed through a median sternotomy, smaller incisions are being utilized more frequently. Such incisions will, in experienced hands, allow procedures to be performed for most types of aortic pathology. These smaller incisions may be found to be associated with fewer sternal wound infections. This is an issue of particular concern in diabetics (Fig. 12-13).

Atrial Fibrillation

Although diabetes is not associated with atrial fibrillation per se, in combination, the two conditions are predisposing factors for congestive heart failure.[85] This has profound implications for patients with valvular disease who are already at risk because of their primary valve lesion. Moreover, recent studies have demonstrated that diabetes independently contributes to endothelial damage in patients with atrial fibrillation thus putting them at risk for thrombotic complications. This was especially true in patients with concomitant congestive heart failure.[86]

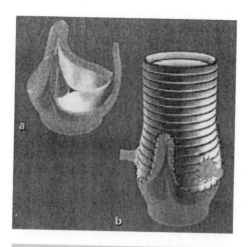

Figure 12-12 **Aortic root remodeling and valve preservation.** *(Source: Reproduced with permission from Albes JM, Stock UA, Hartrumpf M. Restitution of the aortic valve: what is new, what is proven, and what is obsolete?* Ann Thorac Surg *2005;80:1540–1549.)*

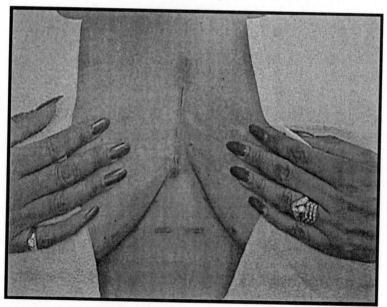

Figure 12-13 **Median sternotomy with small incision.** *(Courtesy of Robert C. Lowery, MD.)*

Surgical methods to treat atrial fibrillation have advanced significantly in recent years. The original procedure as developed by Cox et al. was designed to treat medically refractory atrial fibrillation.[87,88] Although the first "cut and sew" procedure, the Maze I proved to be efficacious in restoring sinus rhythm, there were problems with the need for permanent pacemakers, postoperative hemorrhage, and inadequate SA node response to exercise. That led to the development of the Maze III which also was less demanding technically.[89]

Now, in addition to the original procedure, multiple other methods of creating ablation lines have been developed. These include microwave, cryoablation, radiofrequency ablation as energy sources, and the recently developed ultrasonic ablation by the inventor of the original procedure. All are effective to varying degrees. Because atrial fibrillation can be so debilitating and is so common, refinements in surgical techniques designed to make this a safe, stand-alone procedure are developing rapidly.

HEART FAILURE AND CARDIAC TRANSPLANTATION

The incidence of heart failure has been rising in both males and females in the United States. For many patients, end-stage heart disease results in them being placed onto a cardiac transplant list. Traditionally, diabetes has been a relative contraindication to cardiac transplantation. In recent years, some

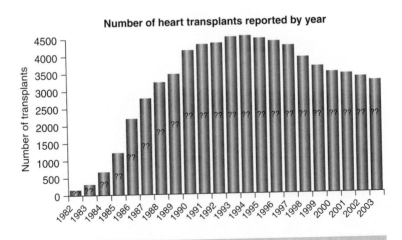

Figure 12-14 **Number of heart transplants reported by year.** (Source: Reproduced with permission from Taylor DO, Edwards LB, Boucek MM, et al. Registry of the International Society for Heart and Lung Transplantation: twenty-second official adult heart transplant report—2005. J Heart Lung Transplant 2005;24:945–955.)

programs have liberalized their criteria to allow certain diabetic patients to undergo the procedure. In one retrospective study done by a large transplant program, there were 76 diabetics who were transplanted. One and 3-year survival rates were similar to the nondiabetics and there were no differences between "low-risk and high-risk" diabetic patients.[90]

Postoperatively, the required administration of corticosteroids will often worsen the insulin requirements of transplanted diabetic patients. It is important then, to carefully consider the presence of end-organ damage before considering for transplantation.

The number of heart transplants performed worldwide has remained between 3000 and 4500 organs since 1990 (Fig. 12-14).[91]

The well-publicized shortage in donor hearts has made the use of left ventricular assist devices a real consideration that has attained traction since the publication of the REMATCH (Randomized Evaluation of Mechanical Assistance for the Treatment of Congestive Heart Failure) trial. A larger role is expected as these devices become smaller and more reliable.[92]

CONCLUSION

Diabetes remains a major public health issue. Though there have been some recent efforts to sway public opinion toward recognition of the danger, there is no evidence that our society is making any significant headway.[93,94]

There was a massive public health campaign and overarching public health initiatives that began in the mid-1960s to counteract the menace of tobacco such that cigarette smoking declined by half since 1965.[95] To date in the United States, there has been no such effort with respect to obesity and the risk factors leading to this condition. Such a commitment may be necessary, especially in lower income neighborhoods because there is a disproportionate percentage of low-cost, high-calorie, high-fat foods that are sold in such communities.[96–98] It has been estimated that in 1995 dollars, the direct costs associated with diabetes represented 5.7% of the national health expenditure in the United States.[99] One may easily theorize that a change in lifestyles could preclude the epidemic that now is obesity and type 2 diabetes mellitus. Such changes could impact the prevalence of coronary artery disease and the need for intervention. Until we are able to minimize the occurrence, aggressive management of hyperglycemia is necessary.

Pre-, intra-, and postoperative glucose control in diabetic patients not only has an effect on vein graft patency and infectious complications, it also appears to enhance survival. Therapies such as TMR and targeted gene therapy may allow for a better prognosis in this group of patients who are notorious for the degree of diffuse, difficult to treat atherosclerosis. The use of β-FGF or as yet to be discovered compounds may in the future mitigate sternal wound complications in diabetics and other patients.

There is evidence that CABG provides a survival advantage when compared to stenting during a previous era.[100] It remains to be determined whether drug-eluting stents will change this outlook, especially in the diabetic patient. Arterial conduits will play an increased role in those patients coming to operation. A randomized comparison between arterial grafting and drug-eluting stents is awaited.

It is likely that more diabetics will be transplanted in the future. However, due to the severe shortage of donor organs and the increased number of patients listed for transplant, it is inevitable that greater reliance will be placed on mechanical solutions, valve repair, and the promise of tissue engineering.

ACKNOWLEDGEMENT

We would like to thank Melissa Gunasekera, MSIII, SUNY Stonybrook, for her invaluable assistance in the preparation of this chapter.

REFERENCES

1. Beckman JA, Creager MA, Libby P. Diabetes and atherosclerosis: epidemiology, pathophysiology, and management. *JAMA* 2002;287:2570–2581.

2. National Center for Chronic Disease Prevention and Health Promotion. Diabetes Public Health Resource, Diabetes Surveillance System, 1999 Surveillance Report Chapter 1: The Public Health Burden of Diabetes Mellitus in the United States. Available at: http://www.cdc.gov/diabetes/statistics/survl99/chap1/prevalence.htm

3. Thom T, Haase N, Rosamond W, et al. American Heart Association Statistics Committee and Stroke Statistics Subcommittee. Heart disease and stroke statistics 2006 update: a report from the American Heart Association Statistics Committee and Stroke Statistics Subcommittee. Circulation 2006;113(6):e85–e151.

4. Nelligan P, Fleisher L. Obesity and diabetes: evidence of increased perioperative risk? *Anesthesiology* 2006;104:398–400.

5. Harrison's Internal Medicine Part 8. Disorders of the Cardiovascular System Section 4. Vascular Disease, Chapter 224. The Pathogenesis of Atherosclerosis 16th edition, Harrison's online.

6. Favaloro RG. Saphenous vein graft in the surgical treatment of coronary artery disease: operative technique. *J Thorac Cardiovasc Surg* 1969;58:178–185.

7. Eagle KA, Guyton RA, Davidoff R, et al. ACC/AHA 2004 Guideline Update for Coronary Artery Bypass Graft Surgery. A Report of the American College of Cardiology/American Heart Association Task Force on Practice Guidelines Committee to Update the 1999 Guidelines for Coronary Artery. Available at: http://www.acc.org/clinical/guidelines/cabg/index.pdf (last viewed 1-22-2006).

8. Buffolo E, Andrade JCS, Branco JNR, et al. Myocardial revascularization without extracorporeal circulation *1 seven-year experience in 593 cases. *Eur J Cardiothorac Surg* 1990;4:504–508.

9. Benetti FJ, Naselli G, Wood M, et al. Direct myocardial revascularization without extracorporeal circulation. Experience in 700 patients. *Chest* 1991;100:312–316.

10. Pfister AJ, Zaki MS, Garcia JM, et al. Coronary artery bypass without cardiopulmonary bypass. *Ann Thorac Surg* 1992;54:1085–1092.

11. Boyd WD, Desai ND, Del Rizzo DF, et al. Off-pump surgery decreases postoperative complications and resource utilization in the elderly. Ann Thorac Surg 1999;68:1490–1493.

12. Mack MJ. Pro: beating-heart surgery for coronary revascularization: is it the most important development since the introduction of the heart-lung machine? Ann Thorac Surg 2000;70:1774–1778.

13. Ascione R, Williams S, Lloyd CT, et al. Reduced postoperative blood loss and transfusion requirement after beating-heart coronary operations: a prospective randomized study. *J Thorac Cardiovasc Surg* 2001;121:689–696.

14. Puskas JD, Thourani VH, Marshall JJ, et al. Clinical outcomes, angiographic patency, and resource utilization in 200 consecutive off-pump coronary bypass patients. *Ann Thorac Surg* 2001;71:1477–1484.

15. van Dijk D, Nierich AP, Jansen EW, et al. Early outcome after off-pump versus on-pump coronary bypass surgery: results from a randomized study. *Circulation* 2001;104:1761–1766.

16. Racz MJ, Hannan EL, Isom OW, et al. A comparison of short- and long-term outcomes after off-pump and on-pump coronary artery bypass graft surgery with sternotomy. *J Am Coll Cardiol* 2004;43:557–564.

17. Reston JT, Tregear SJ, Turkelson CM. Meta-analysis of short-term and mid-term outcomes following off-pump coronary artery bypass grafting. *Ann Thorac Surg* 2003;76:1510–1515.

18. van der Heijden GJ, Nathoe HM, Jansen EW, et al. Meta-analysis on the effect of off-pump coronary bypass surgery. *Eur J Cardiothorac Surg* 2004;26:81–84.

19. Bonchek LI. Off-pump coronary bypass: is it for everyone? *J Thorac Cardiovasc Surg* 2002;124:431–434.

20. Magee MJ, Jablonski KA, Stamou SC, et al. Elimination of cardiopulmonary bypass improves early survival for multivessel coronary artery bypass patients. *Ann Thorac Surg* 2002;73:1196–1202.

21. Dullum MKC, Sergeant PT. CTSNet OPCAB Survey. Available at: http://www.ctsnet.org/sections/innovation/beatingheart/articles/article-22.html (last viewed 6-2-2006).

22. The Bypass Angioplasty Revascularization Investigation (BARI) Investigators. Comparison of coronary bypass surgery with angioplasty in patients with multivessel disease. *N Engl J Med* 1996;335:217–225.

23. Serruys PW, Ong ATL, van Herwerden LA, et al. Five-year outcomes after coronary stenting versus bypass surgery for the treatment of multivessel disease. The final analysis of the Arterial Revascularization Therapies Study (ARTS) randomized trial. *J Am Coll Cardiol* 2005;46:575–581.

24. Bonde P, Graham AN, MacGowan SW. Endoscopic vein harvest: advantages and limitations. *Ann Thorac Surg* 2004;77:2076–2082.

25. Fitzgibbon GM, Kafka HP, Leach AJ, et al. Coronary bypass graft fate and patient outcome: angiographic follow-up of 5,065 grafts related to survival and reoperation in 1,388 patients during 25 years. *J Am Coll Cardiol* 1997;29:706–707.

26. Borger MA, Rao V, Weisel RD, et al. Reoperative coronary bypass surgery: effect of patent grafts and retrograde cardioplegia. J Thorac Cardiovasc Surg 2001;121:83–90.

27. Loscalzo J. Vascular matrix and vein graft failure. Is the message in the medium? *Circulation* 2000;101:221–223.

28. Akowuah EF, Sheridan PJ, Cooper GJ, et al. Preventing saphenous vein graft failure: does gene therapy have a role? *Ann Thorac Surg* 2003;76:959–966.

29. George Sarah J, Lloyd CT, Angeline GD, et al. Inhibition of late vein graft neointima formation in human and porcine models by adenovirus-mediated overexpression of tissue inhibitor of metalloproteinase-3. *Circulation* 2000;101: 296–304.

30. Baker AH, Yim APC, Wan S. Opportunities for gene therapy in preventing vein graft failure after coronary artery bypass surgery. *Diabetes Obes Metab* 2006;8: 119–124.

31. Loop FD, Lytle BW, Cosgrove DM, et al. Influence of the internal-mammary-artery graft on 10-year survival and other cardiac events. *N Engl J Med* 1986;314:1–6.

32. Tarr FI, Sasvari M, Tarr M, et al. Evidence of nitric oxide produced by the internal mammary artery graft in venous drainage of the recipient coronary artery. *Ann Thorac Surg* 2005;80:1728–1731.

33. Archer SL, Gragasin FS, Wu X, et al. Endothelium-derived hyperpolarizing factor in human internal mammary artery IS 11,12-epoxyeicosatrienoic acid and causes relaxation by activating smooth muscle BKCa channels. Available at: http://cardiosrv1.uah.ualberta.ca/presentation/LIMA%20Circulation%20pap er.pdf (last viewed April 16, 2006).

34. Flaherty JD, Davidson CH. Diabetes and coronary revascularization. *JAMA* 2005;293:1501–1508.

35. Lytle BW, Blackstone EH, Loop FD, et al. Two internal thoracic artery grafts are better than one. *J Thorac Cardiovasc Surg* 1999;117:855–872.

36. Cohen AJ, Lockman J, Lorberboym M, et al. Assessment of sternal vascularity with single photon assessment of sternal vascularity with single photon emission computed tomography after harvesting of the internal thoracic artery. *J Thorac Cardiovasc Surg* 1999;118:496–502.

37. Cosgrove DM, Lytle BW, Loop FD, et al. Does bilateral internal mammary artery grafting increase surgical risk? *Circulation* 2003;108:1343–1349.

38. Endo M, Tomizawa Y, Nishida H. Bilateral versus unilateral internal mammary revascularization in patients with diabetes. *Circulation* 2003;108:1343–1349.

39. Toumpoulis IK, Anagnostopoulos CE, Balarum S, et al. Does bilateral internal thoracic artery grafting increase long-term survival of diabetic patients? *Ann Thorac Surg* 2006;81:599–607.

40. Stevens LM, Carrier M, Perrault LP, et al. Influence of diabetes and bilateral internal thoracic artery grafts on long-term outcome for multivessel coronary artery bypass grafting. *Eur J Cardiothorac Surg* 2005;7:281–288.

41. Lev-Ran O, Mohr R, Pevni D, et al. Bilateral internal thoracic artery grafting in diabetic patients: short and long-term results of a 515 patient series. *J Thorac Cardiovasc Surg* 2004;127:1:145–150.

42. Bical OM, Khoury W, Fromes Y, et al. Routine use of bilateral skeletonized internal thoracic artery grafts in middle-aged diabetic patients. *Ann Thorac Surg* 2004;78: 505–553.

43. Muneretto C, Negri A, Gianluigi B, et al. Is total arterial myocardial revascularization with composite grafts a safe and useful procedure in the elderly? *Eur J Cardiothorac Surg* 2003;23:657–664.

44. Iwakura A, Tabata Y, Tamura N, et al. Gelatin sheet incorporating basic fibroblast growth factor enhances healing of devascularized sternum in diabetic rats. *Circulation* 2001;104(12 Suppl 1):I325–I329.

45. Mauri A, Hirose K, Maruyama T, et al. Prostaglandin E2 EP4 receptor-selective agonist facilitates sternal healing after harvesting bilateral internal thoracic arteries in diabetic rats. *J Thorac Cardiovasc Surg* 2006;131:587–593.

46. Sabik III, Lytle BW, Blackstone EH, et al. Comparison of saphenous vein and internal thoracic artery graft patency by coronary system. *Ann Thorac Surg* 2005;79: 544–551.

47. Lorusso R, Pentiricci S, Raddino R, et al. Influence of type 2 diabetes on functional and structural properties of coronary artery bypass conduits. *Diabetes* 2003;52:2814–2820.

48. Tatoulis J, Buxton BF, Fuller JA. Patencies of 2,127 arterial to coronary conduits over 15 years. *Ann Thorac Surg* 2004;77:93–101.

49. Lytle BW, Loop FD, Cosgrove DM, et al. Long-term (5 to 12 years) serial studies of internal mammary artery and saphenous vein coronary bypass grafts. *J Thorac Cardiovasc Surg* 1985;89:248–258.

50. Khot UN, Friedman DT, Pettersson G, et al. Radial artery bypass grafts have an increased occurrence of angiographically severe stenosis and occlusion compared with left internal mammary arteries and saphenous vein grafts. *Circulation* 2004;109:2086–2091.

51. Possati G, Guadino M, Prati F, et al. Long-term results of the radial artery used for myocardial revascularization. *Circulation* 2003;108:1350–1354.

52. Buxton BF, Raman JS, Ruengsakulrach P, et al. Radial artery patency and clinical outcomes: five-year interim results of a randomized trial. *J Thorac Cardiovasc Surg* 2003;125:1363–1370.

53. Chardigny C, Jebara VA, Acar C, et al. Comparison with the internal mammary and gastroepiploic arteries with implications for coronary artery surgery. *Circulation* 1993;88(5 Pt 2):II115–II127.

54. Nicolosi AC, Pohl LL, Parsons P, et al. Increased incidence of radial artery calcification in patients with diabetes mellitus. *J Surg Res* 2002;102:1–5.

55. Stamou SC, Bafi AS, Boyce SW, et al. Coronary revascularization of the circumflex. *Ann Thorac Surg* 2000;70:1371–1377.

56. Sung LH, Tae KY, Nam YY, et al. Flow competition of right gastroepiploic artery graft. *Asian Cardiovasc Thorac Ann* 2001;9:264–268.

57. Roach GW, Kanchuger M, Mangano CM, et al. Adverse cerebral outcomes after coronary bypass surgery. Multicenter Study of Perioperative Ischemia Research Group and the Ischemia Research and Education Foundation Investigators. *N Engl J Med* 1996;335:1857–1863.

58. Stump DA, Rogers AT, Hammon JW, et al. Cerebral emboli and cognitive outcome after cardiac surgery. *J Cardiothorac Vasc Anesth* 1996;10:113–119.

59. Taylor RL, Borger MA, Weisel RD, et al. Cerebral microemboli during cardiopulmonary bypass: increased emboli during perfusionist interventions. *Ann Thorac Surg* 1999;68(1):89–93.

60. Shroyer ALW, Coombs LP, Peterson ED, et al. The Society of Thoracic Surgeons: 30 day operative mortality and morbidity risk models. *Ann Thorac Surg* 2003;75:1856–1865.

61. Furnary AP, Gao G, Grunkemeier GL, et al. Continuous insulin infusion reduces mortality in patients with diabetes undergoing coronary artery bypass grafting. *J Thorac Cardiovasc Surg* 2003;125:1007–1021.

62. Furnary AP, Zerr KJ, Grunkemeier GL, et al. Continuous intravenous insulin infusion reduces the incidence of deep sternal wound infection in diabetic patients after cardiac surgical procedures. *Ann Thorac Surg* 1999;67:352–360.

63. Allen GS. The Society of Thoracic Surgeons: mid-term results after thoracoscopic transmyocardial laser revascularization. *Ann Thorac Surg* 2005;80:553–558.

64. Horvath KA, Chiu E, Maun DC, et al. Up-regulation of VEGF mRNA and angiogenesis after transmyocardial laser revascularization. *Ann Thorac Surg* 1999;68:825–829.

65. Bridges CR (TMR Taskforce Chair), Horvath KA, Nugent WC, et al. The Society of Thoracic Surgeons Practice Guideline Series Transmyocardial Laser Revascularization. A Report from the Society of Thoracic Surgeons Workforce on Evidence-Based Medicine. The Society of Thoracic Surgeons 2003. *Ann Thorac Surg* 2004;77:1494–1502.

66. Allen KB, Dowling RD, Angell WW, et al. Transmyocardial revascularization: 5-year follow-up of a prospective, randomized multicenter trial. *Ann Thorac Surg* 2004;77:1228–1234.

67. Reilly JP, Grise MA, Fortuin FD, et al. Long-term (2-year) clinical events following transthoracic intramyocardial gene transfer of VEGF-2 in no-option patients. *J Intervent Cardiol* 2005;18(1):27–31.

68. Kastrup J, Jorgensen E, Ruck A, et al. Direct intramyocardial plasmit vascular endothelial growth factor-A 165 gene therapy in patients with stable severe angina pectoris. A randomized double-blind placebo-controlled study: the Euroinject One Trial. *J Am Coll Cardiol* 2005;45:982–988.

69. Rosengart TK, Lee LY, Patel SR, et al. Angiogenesis gene therapy phase I assessment of direct intramyocardial administration of an adenovirus vector expressing VEGF121 cDNA to individuals with clinically significant severe coronary artery disease. *Circulation* 1999;100:468–474.

70. Teng CJ, Lachapelle K, Chiu RCJ. Reappraisal of recent clinical trials of angiogenic therapy in myorcardial ischemia. *Asian Cardiovasc Thorac Ann* 2005;13: 90–97.

71. Savage EB, Ferguson TB, DiSesa VJ. Use of mitral valve repair: analysis of contemporary United States experience reported to the Society of Thoracic Surgeons National Cardiac Database. *Ann Thorac Surg* 2003;75:820–825.

72. Rothman RB, Baumann MH, Savage JE, et al. Evidence for possible involvement of 5-HT 2B receptors in the cardiac valvulopathy associated with fenfluramine and other serotonergic medications. *Circulation* 2000;102:2836–2841.

73. Nollert G, Miksch J, Kreuzer E, et al. Risk factors for atherosclerosis and the degeneration of pericardial valves after aortic valve replacement. *J Thorac Cardiovasc Surg* 2003;126:965–968.

74. Kahn SS, Trento A, DeRobertis M, et al. Twenty-year comparison of tissue and mechanical valve replacement. *J Thorac Cardiovasc Surg* 2001;122:257–269.

75. Banbury MK, Cosgrove DM III, Thomas JD, et al. Hemodynamic stability during 17 years of the Carpetier-Edwards aortic pericardial bioprosthesis. *Ann Thorac Surg* 2002;73:1460–1465.

76. Hoestrup SP, Kadner A, Melnitchouk S, et al. Tissue engineering of functional trileaflet heart valves from human marrow stromal cells. *Circulation* 2002;106: 1–143.

77. Bechtel JFM, Muller-Steinhardt M, Schmidtke C, et al. Evaluation of the decellularized pulmonary valve homograft SynerGraft. *J Heart Valve Dis* 2003;12: 734–739.

78. Elkins RC, Dawson PE, Goldstein S, et al. Decellularized human valve allografts. *Ann Thorac Surg* 2001;71(5 Suppl):S428–S432.

79. Minakata K, Schaff HV, Zehr KJ, et al. Is repair of aortic valve regurgitation a safe alternative to valve replacement? *J Thorac Cardiovasc Surg* 2004;127:645–653.

80. Weinschelbaum E, Stutzbach P, Oliva M,et al. Manual debridement of the aortic valve in elderly patients with degenerative aortic stenosis. *J Thorac Cardiovasc Surg* 1999;117:1157–1165.

81. Bentall H, DeBono A. A technique for complete replacement of the ascending aorta. *Thorax* 1968;23:338–339.

82. David TE, Armstrong S, Ivanov J, et al. Aortic valve sparing operations: an update. *Ann Thorac Surg* 1999;67:1840–1842.

83. Sarsam MA, Yacoub M. Remodeling of the aortic valve annulus. *J Thorac Cardiovasc Surg* 1993;105:435–438.

84. Albes JM, Stock UA, Hartrumpf M. Restitution of the aortic valve: what is new, what is proven, and what is obsolete? *Ann Thorac Surg* 2005;80:1540–1549.

85. Varughese GI, Tomson J, Lip GYH. Type 2 diabetes mellitus: a cardiovascular perspective. *Int J Clin Pract* 2005;59(7):798–816.

86. Varughese GI, Patel JV, Tomson J, et al. The prothrombotic risk of diabetes mellitus in atrial fibrillation and heart failure. *J Thromb Haemost* 2005;3(12):2811–2833.

87. Cox JL, Boineau JP, Schuessler RB, et al. Modification of the maze procedure for atrial flutter and atrial fibrillation: I. Rationale and surgical results. *J Thorac Cardiovasc Surg* 1995;110:473–484.

88. Cox JL, Boineau JP, Schuessler RB, et al. Successful surgical treatment of atrial fibrillation. Review and clinical update. *JAMA* 1991;266:1976–1980.

89. Cox JL. Atrial fibrillation II: rationale for surgical treatment. *J Thorac Cardiovasc Surg* 2003;126:1693–1699.

90. Lang CC, Beniaminovitz A, Edwards N, et al. Morbidity and mortality in diabetic patients following cardiac transplantation. *J Heart Lung Transplant* 2003;22: 244–249.

91. Taylor DO, Edwards LB, Boucek MM, et al. Registry of the International Society for Heart and Lung Transplantation: twenty-second official adult heart transplant report—2005. *J Heart Lung Transplant* 2005;24:945–955.

92. Rose EA, Gelijns AC, Moskowitz AJ, et al., the Randomized Evaluation of mechanical Assistance for the Treatment of Congestive Heart Failure (REMATCH) Study Group. Long-term use of a left ventricular assist device for end-state heart failure. *N Engl J Med* 2001;345:1435–1443.

93. Centers for Disease Control and Prevention. Overweight and obesity: obesity trends: U.S. obesity trends 1985–2004. Available at: http://www.cdc.gov/nccd-php/dnpa/obesity/trend/maps/ (last viewed 6–26–2006).

94. Henderson J, Low S. Center for the Study of Rural America. The Main Street Economist. Federal Reserve Bank of Kansas, 2006:1–4.

95. Giovino GA. Epidemiology of tobacco use in the United States. *Oncogene* 2002;21(48):7326–7340.

96. French SA, Harnack L, Jeffery RW. Fast food restaurant use among women in the pound of prevention study: dietary, behavioral and demographic correlates. *Int J Obes* 2000;24:1353–1359.

97. Weinsier RL, Hunter GR, Heini AF, et al. The etiology of obesity: relative contribution of metabolic factors, diet, and physical activity. *Am J Med* 1998;105(2): 145–150.

98. Drewnowski A, Specter SE. Poverty and obesity: the role of energy density and energy costs. *Am J Clin Nutr* 2004;79:6–16.

99. Wolf AM, Colditz GA. Current estimates of the economic cost of obesity in the United States. *Obes Res* 1998;6:97–106.

100. Hannan EL, Racz MJ, Walford G, et al. Long-term outcomes of coronary-artery bypass grafting versus stent implantation. *N Engl J Med* 2005;26;352: 2174–2183.

CHRONIC KIDNEY

DISEASE AND

CARDIORENAL

COMPLICATIONS

Nagarathna Manjappa
Amir Hayat
Moro O. Salifu

INTRODUCTION

Chronic kidney disease (CKD) is a major public health problem in the United States and worldwide. Emerging evidence suggests a strong relationship between CKD and cardiovascular disease (CVD) complications and that patients with CKD are more likely to die from CVD than progress to end-stage renal disease (ESRD).[1,2] Patients with CKD and CVD often share similar traditional risk factors such as diabetes and hypertension as their underlying comorbidity. However, CKD by itself and its associated complications are now being recognized as an independent risk factors for CVD. In fact, an intriguing paradoxical relationship exists between CKD and CVD. While CVD and cerebrovascular disease mortality has decreased over the last three decades, CKD-related mortality is on the rise,[3] largely due to excess CVD risk factors in this population. In this chapter, we will first explore CKD, pathophysiology of the cardiorenal link, and some CKD-specific risk factors for CVD.

DEFINITION AND CLASSIFICATION OF CKD

Chronic kidney disease terminology is used to define the presence of kidney damage for more than 3 months as confirmed by kidney biopsy or markers of kidney damage with or without decrease in glomerular filtration rate (GFR). An absolute GFR decline to ≤ 60 mL/min/1.73 m^2 of ≥ 3 months in duration is also diagnostic of CKD because it represents about 50% loss of renal mass. This definition is independent of the underlying cause of CKD such as diabetes (45%), hypertension (27%), glomerulonephritis (10%), cystic kidney disease (5%), and other causes. When renal mass is reduced by any mechanism (injury that chronically reduces GFR), the remaining nephrons undergo adaptive changes to restore GFR to its original values. First, the remaining nephrons hypertrophy and second, the filtration fraction of each individual nephron increases (hyperfiltration). If the injury permanently destroys nephrons, GFR will decline over time. Accordingly, the Work Group of the National Kidney Foundation[4] arbitrarily chose a cut-off time of greater than 3 months and classified CKD into five stages.

Stage 1 is characterized by kidney damage with a normal GFR (≥ 90 mL/min). The action plan is diagnosis and treatment; treatment of comorbid conditions, slowing of the progression of the kidney disease, and reduction of CVD risks. Stage 2 is characterized by kidney damage with a mild decrease in the GFR (60–90 mL/min). The action plan is estimation of the progression of kidney disease. Stage 3 is characterized by a moderately decreased GFR rate progression (30–59 mL/min). The action plan is evaluation and treatment of complications. Stage 4 is characterized by a severe decrease in the GFR (15–29 mL/min). The action plan is preparation for renal replacement therapy. Stage 5 is characterized by GFR <15 mL/min/1.73 m^2. The action plan is kidney replacement if the patient is uremic. Of note, once the GFR is <60 mL/min/1.73 m^2, progression to more advanced stages proceeds at a constant rate independent of the underlying disease. Each stage of kidney failure is associated with complications that are intricately associated with CVD as discussed below.

EPIDEMIOLOGY OF CKD

Assessment of worldwide prevalence of CKD is limited because most (>80%) patients undergoing renal replacement therapy live in North America, Europe, Australia, and Japan, whereas the rest of the world does not have adequate resources for early diagnosis, reporting, and management of this disease.[5] Furthermore, CKD is often asymptomatic until the disease is very advanced or death ensues, in developing nations, making worldwide estimates difficult. Population and disease registries in the United States and other developed countries have impacted our knowledge of CKD prevalence. In the United States for instance, data from National Health and Nutrition

Examination Survey (NHANES) and the Centers for Disease Control (CDC) show the prevalence of CKD to be 11% in the adult population of the United States. There are an estimated 10 million people with stage 1, 22 million with stage 2, 6 million with stage 3, 360,000 with stage 4, and about 450,000 people with stage 5 diseases receiving dialysis or kidney transplantation.[6] The number of patients receiving renal replacement therapy is growing at an alarming rate. It is estimated that by the year 2010, more than 650,000 patients will be receiving renal replacement therapy in the United States.[7]

Although the prevalence of CKD between stages 1 and 3 is astoundingly high, only about 2% of patients progress to stages 4 and 5. The elimination of a significant fraction of CKD patients before more advanced kidney failure is attributable to increased mortality secondary to CVD. Even among the group that ends up on renal replacement therapy due to advanced kidney failure, CVD remains a major cause of morbidity and mortality. It appears that CKD per se may be responsible for this excess CVD risk when compared to the general population. The incidence of various CVDs increases as the renal function deteriorates, even at stages with a GFR >60 mL/min/1.73 m².

Risk Factors for CKD and CVD

As shown in Table 13-1, traditional risk factors common to both CKD and CVD include diabetes, hypertension, obesity, dyslipidemia, smoking, and advanced age. These traditional risk factors may worsen during the course of CKD and

Table 13-1 **Traditional vs. CKD-Related Factors Potentially Related to an Increased Risk for CVD**

Traditional Risk Factors	CKD-related Risk Factors
Old age	Decreased GFR
Male gender	Proteinuria
White race	Renin angiotensin system
Family history of CVD	Extracellular fluid overload
Hypertension	Abnormal calcium and phosphorus metabolism
Elevated LDL-C	Dyslipidemia
Decreased HDL-C	Anemia
Diabetes mellitus	Malnutrition
Tobacco use	Inflammation
Physical inactivity	Infection
Menopause	Thrombogenic factors
Psychosocial stress	Oxidative stress
	Elevated homocysteine
	Uremic toxins

additional CKD-specific risk factors may develop imposing a greater risk for CVD in CKD patients than in the general population. Moreover, cardiovascular therapeutics and interventions (e.g., angiotensin-converting enzyme inhibitor [ACEI] and coronary angiography) are underutilized in patients with CKD because of fear or concerns of acute renal failure, hyperkalemia, and contrast-induced nephropathy raising their risk for CVD. Unique risk factors acquired through various stages of CKD, often termed as nontraditional risk factors include anemia, chronic inflammation, volume expansion, salt retention, hyperhomocysteinemia, hyperparathyroidism, hyperphosphatemia, endothelial dysfunction, and diastolic dysfunction.[9–12] Together, traditional and nontraditional risk factors compound each other leading to rapid development of CVD and death, a concept often termed accelerated atherosclerosis.[8] There has been increasing evidence that even minor decreases in renal function significantly increases the risk for CVD,[9] comparable in magnitude to diabetes[10] (in part due to addition of nontraditional risk factors).

PATHOPHYSIOLOGY OF CARDIORENAL COMPLICATIONS

In the normal physiologic state, the kidney and heart function in tandem to preserve extracellular volume and circulation, respectively. On the contrary, disease in one of these organs often leads to disease in the other, a phenomenon often termed as cardiorenal syndrome. It is simplistic to assume that a single phenomenon is responsible for the cardiorenal syndrome. An earlier description by Guyton[11] depicted in Fig. 13-1 provides a framework describing the physiologic relationship among cardiac output, extracellular volume, and blood pressure. In this model, volume expansion increases cardiac output, peripheral resistance, and blood pressure, a phenomenon that will culminate in cardiac hypertrophy,[12–14] blood vessel wall thickness[15–17], and clinically manifested as an increase in carotid or brachial pulse wave velocity,[18,19] and atherosclerosis.[20]

On the other hand, manifestations of low cardiac output in patients with cardiac failure stimulate renal salt and water reabsorption via activation of the renin angiotensin aldosterone system (RAAS), sympathetic nervous system (SNS), antidiuretic hormone (ADH), and enhanced proximal tubular reabsorption. These mechanisms result in expansion of the extracellular volume in an attempt to restore cardiac output but at a consequence of systemic vascular injury. In more advanced cardiac failure, renal hypoperfusion may result in deterioration of renal function, further activation of salt, and water retaining mechanism in a vicious cycle that often results in failure of both organs.[21,22] Other factors that have negative impacts on the hemodynamic response of the cardiorenal link include a possible role of oxidative stress, inflammation, and calcemic vasculopathy. In experimental models of apolipoprotein E knockout mice, renal dysfunction induces a state of accelerated atherogenesis due to reactive oxygen species (ROS).[23] Reactive oxidant species, the hallmark of oxidative stress, is generated in many cellular processes,

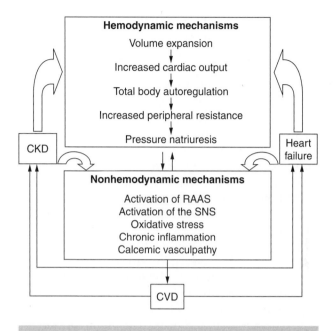

Figure 13-1 **Hemodynamic and nonhemodynamic factors related to an increased risk for CVD in patients with CKD. When one organ is diseased, a vicious cycle develops in which the RAAS, SNS, oxidative stress, chronic inflammation, and calcemic vasculopathy are activated directly or indirectly via hemodynamic mechanisms resulting in injury in the other and overall CVD morbidity.**

one of which is activation of nicotinamide adenine dinucleotide phosphate (NADPH)-oxidase activity by angiotensin II.[24] In patients with CKD, an imbalance exists where levels of ROS exceed nitric oxide (NO) in the circulation. This is due to excess activity of the RAAS, reactions of NO with oxygen radicals, as well as high concentrations of circulating levels of NO inhibitors such as asymmetric dimethyl arginine (ADMA). This imbalance induces oxidation of lipids, carbohydrates (advanced glycation end products) and proteins, leucocyte activation, triggering a state of chronic inflammation, cytokine release, endothelial injury, and atherosclerosis. This is supported by studies that implicate proinflammatory cytokines such as C-reactive protein (CRP), interleukin (IL)-1B, IL-6, and tumor necrosis factor alpha (TNF-α) as predictors of atherosclerosis in patients with CKD and CVD. Vascular calcification as discussed later, induced by hyperphosphatemia, hyperparathyroidism, and calcium contributes significantly to CVD in patients with CKD.

Thus, CKD is intricately connected with CVD via hemodynamic changes, and nonhemodynamic changes as shown in Fig. 13-1.[25]

ROLE OF CKD PER SE AS AN INDEPENDENT RISK FACTOR FOR CVD

Several studies have documented CKD as an independent risk factor for CVD. The Rotterdam study investigated whether the level of renal function, estimated by GFR, was associated with the risk of incident myocardial infarction among 4484 apparently healthy subjects (mean age, 69.6 years). The study showed that a 10 mL/min/1.73 m^2 decrease in GFR was associated with a 32% increased risk of myocardial infarction ($P < 0.001$) and that renal function is a graded and independent predictor of the development of myocardial infarction in an elderly population.[26] The Atherosclerosis Risk In Community (ARIC) study followed 15,350 subjects (45–65 years), stratified based on GFR (GFR by modified diet in renal disease formula). This study demonstrated that a decrease in GFR of 10 mL/min/1.73 m^2 was independently associated with a 5% increase in cardiovascular risk.[27] Other studies that support this finding are the Hypertension Optimal Trial,[28] Heart Outcomes Prevention Evaluation (HOPE) trial,[11] Hypertension Detection and Follow-up Study, and studies of renal function from the Framingham cohort.[29] The SYCOMORE study[30] evaluated the prognostic importance of renal insufficiency based on creatinine clearance, among patients with acute coronary syndromes (ACS). Patients with renal insufficiency who presented with ACS tended to have higher risk features, had greater disease burden, but received less aggressive treatment strategies and lesser use of medical therapy.[31] This paradox is mainly because of the concerns about contrast-induced nephropathy and risk of bleeding associated with procedures in patients with renal failure.

Role of CKD-Specific Risk Factors and CVD

MICROALBUMINURIA AND PROTEINURIA

Microalbuminuria and proteinuria are frequent modifiable complications of diabetic and nondiabetic CKD, respectively, and have been recognized as markers of cardiovascular and renal disease in patients with CKD. In fact, reduction in proteinuria has been associated with improved cardiovascular and renal outcomes in multiple studies. Microalbuminuria and proteinuria as markers of renal vascular damage may reflect the degree of systemic vascular damage in diabetes and hypertension. In nephrotic syndrome due to primary glomerular diseases, the association of proteinuria and hyperlipidemia with systemic vascular damage is less well understood, partly because some of these nephrotic syndromes are transient.[32] However, in more progressive forms of CKD due to nondiabetic or diabetic nephrotic syndrome, persistent proteinuria has been shown to worsen renal and cardiovascular outcomes. Data from the Framingham study,[33] and later from the European Prospective Investigation into Cancer (EPIC) trial,[34] prospective Hoorn study,[35] Prevention of Renal and Vascular

End Stage Disease (PREVEND) study,[36] and many more other studies all show that microalbuminuria is an independent indicator not only of cardiovascular risk and morbidity, but also of noncardiovascular morbidity. Endothelial dysfunction is proposed as the underlying mechanism for CVD in patients with microalbuminuria. The effect of renal insufficiency on CVD is immense in patients with microalbuminuria and early stages of kidney disease.[37]

ANEMIA AND CVD RISK IN PATIENTS WITH CKD

Anemia is a potentially modifiable risk factor for CVD in patients with CKD. In predialysis patients, the severity of anemia correlates with severity of GFR decline mainly because of deficiency or impaired action of erythropoietin (EPO).[38] However, other factors such as oxidative stress and chronic inflammation appear to play a role. Chronic inflammation is an underlying factor in severe anemia and hyporesponsiveness to EPO treatment. In these patients, inflammation and the acute phase response interact with the hematopoietic system at different levels, resulting in reduced erythropoiesis, accelerated destruction of red blood cells, and blunting of the erythrocyte response to EPO.[39] Anemia in CKD has been shown to increase the risk of left ventricular hypertrophy (LVH) and CVD. Reversal of LVH after correction of anemia has been documented.[40] Treatment of anemia in these patients has been shown to reduce LV mass and decrease CVD and all-cause mortality.[41] However, results from randomized-controlled trials (RCT) in dialysis patients are less conclusive.[42]

In other groups of patients such as those with heart failure, coronary artery disease, as well as in the general population, anemia appears to be an independent risk factor for poor CVD outcomes and treatment of anemia in heart failure and patients with CAD improve outcomes. In the ARIC study noted above, high serum creatinine (Scr) was associated with nearly a threefold increased risk of coronary heart disease (CHD) among middle-aged people with anemia, whereas no increased risk was found in people with high Scr in the absence of anemia. In the presence of anemia, CKD was associated with a substantially higher risk of stroke compared to no CKD ([RR] 5.43; 95% confidence interval [CI] 2.04–14.41). In contrast, when anemia was not present, CKD was associated with only a modest, nonsignificant elevation in stroke risk (RR 1.41; 95% CI 0.93–2.14). In this analysis of the ARIC population, the interaction between CKD and anemia on risk of stroke was statistically significant ($P <$ 0.01). These data further substantiate the notion that the combination of anemia and CKD substantially increase the risk of CVD. Early diagnosis is essential and therapy with EPO, iron, or a combination of both is essential in ameliorating the cardiovascular risk imposed by anemia in patients with CKD.

HYPERHOMOCYSTEINEMIA AND CVD RISK IN PATIENTS WITH CKD

Hyperhomocysteinemia occurs in the general population because of decreased conversion of homocysteine, a product of the amino acid methionine, to cystathione. The rate-limiting enzyme in this conversion, cystathione beta synthase requires folate, B_{12}, and B_6 for activation. Defects in this enzyme system, advanced age, decreased renal function (thereby impairing homocysteine metabolism or clearance), and deficiencies of folate, B_{12}, and B_6, alone or in combination, may account for the accumulation of homocysteine frequently observed in renal failure[43] although the exact mechanism is unclear. Hyperhomocysteinemia, as defined by total homocysteine (tHcy) >10 μM/L or >2 standard deviation above the mean after methionine load test[44] occurs in more than 90% of CKD patients and more than 70% of the tHcy is protein bound,[45] implying that nutritional status and serum albumin level, as well as the presence of inflammation and diabetes should be taken into consideration when evaluating tHcy as a risk factor for CVD in patients with CKD.[46] Epidemiologic studies link hyperhomocysteinemia with an increased risk of CVD in the general population[47] and in patients with CKD.[48,49] Prolonged exposure of endothelial cells to homocysteine impairs the production of NO and endothelium-dependent vasodilatation. Homocysteine also combines with low-density lipoprotein cholesterol (LDL-C) to produce aggregates that are taken up by vascular macrophages in the arterial intima (foam cells), produce aggregatory effects on the platelets, and decrease endothelial antithrombotic activity due to changes in thrombomodulin function.[50] Although CKD patients are at increased risk for hyperhomocysteinemia and CVD, therapy is difficult in this population. Patients with CKD are resistant to the routine doses of folic acid, vitamins B_6 and B_{12} used to correct hyperhomocysteinemia in the general population. tHcy levels decrease only partially in response to supraphysiologic dose therapy (folic acid doses of 5 mg or more).[50,51] In the absence of controlled clinical trials proving the benefit of lowering tHcy in CKD patients, no specific recommendations for the management of hyperhomocysteinemia are available at this time.

HYPERPHOSPHATEMIA, HYPERPARATHYROIDISM AND CVD RISK IN PATIENTS WITH CKD

Emerging evidence suggests that hyperphosphatemia[52–54] and hyperparathyroidism[55–58] are risk factors for CVD in patients with CKD. Soft-tissue and vascular calcification, often termed as calcemic vasculopathy is highly prevalent in ESRD. Vascular calcifications, manifesting as medial and intimal calcification of arteries are a hallmark of premature and accelerated atherosclerosis observed in uremia. The nature of vascular calcification is progressive, and is associated with arterial stiffness and increased cardiovascular mortality.

Age, duration of dialysis, and diabetes mellitus are clear determinants of the severity of vascular calcification. Disturbances of mineral metabolism such as hyperphosphatemia and hypercalcemia appear to contribute to progressive calcification, not only by passive precipitation but also by actively inducing changes in vascular smooth muscle cell behavior toward an osteoblast-like phenotype.[59] These physiologic changes that specifically arise from CKD account for the resulting high incidence and premature development of CVD.

Therapeutic strategies to lower serum phosphorus using phosphate binders and to lower parathyroid hormone (PTH) levels using vitamin D products or calcimimetics have been demonstrated to reduce CVD in patients with CKD.[60,61]

AGGRAVATION OF TRADITIONAL RISK FACTORS FOR CVD IN PATIENTS WITH CKD

Preexisting risk factors may be aggravated in CKD. Hypertension may worsen in CKD due to salt and water retenton and is usually difficult to manage without the use of diuretics. Hyperlipidemia is a frequent occurrence in patients with nephrotic syndrome, which may worsen in CKD. There is evidence to suggest that control of lipids slows progression of disease in patients with CKD and should be part of the treatment strategy.[62,63] Whether a preexisting risk factor is aggravated or not, control of all risk factors, with goals to: (1) lower blood pressure to normal with blockade of the RAAS as part of the antihypertensive regimen, (2) reduce lipid levels to normal with a statin, (3) reduce glycosylated hemoglobin A1c to less than 7%, (4) exercise and reduce weight, (5) discontinue smoking, and (6) restrict dietary protein to 0.8 g/kg (in patients with no evidence of malnutrition) are essential to reducing overall cardiovascular morbidity and mortality in this population.

SUMMARY

Cardiovascular disease and CKD are closely linked. Disease of one often results in disease of the other. Although both share similar traditional risk factors, there are CKD-specific risk factors, such as CKD per se, proteinuria, anemia, hyperhomocysteinemia, hyperphosphatemia, and hyperparathyroidism, making this population at higher and premature risk for CVD than the general population. The link between CVD and CKD is complex, involving all risk factors as well as well as hemodynamic and nonhemodynamic consequences of activation of the RAAS system. A growing body of evidence suggest that the RAAS system plays a major role in oxidative stress, inflammation, and cellular proliferation resulting in hypertrophy, endothelial dysfunction, and atherosclerosis. Strategies to reduce cardiorenal complications must be comprehensive, encompassing management of both traditional and nontraditional risk factors to their respective target goals of therapy.

REFERENCES

1. Sarnak MJ. Cardiovascular complications in chronic kidney disease. *Am J Kidney Dis* 2003;41(5 Suppl):11–17.

2. Levin A, Djurdjev O, Barrett B, et al. Cardiovascular disease in patients with chronic kidney disease: getting to the heart of the matter. *Am J Kidney Dis* 2001;38(6): 1398–1407.

3. National Heart, Lung, and Blood Institute. Morbidity and Mortality Chartbook on Cardiovascular Disease, Lung and Blood Diseases. Bethesda, MD: Public Health Service, 1998.

4. National Kidney Foundation: K/DOQI clinical practice guidelines for chronic kidney disease: evaluation, classification, and stratification. *Am J Kidney Dis* 2002;39(2 Suppl 1):S1–S266.

5. Moeller S, Gioberge S, Brown G. ESRD patients in 2001: global overview of patients, treatment modalities and development trends. *Nephrol Dial Transplant* 2002;17(12):2071–2076.

6. Schieppati A, Remuzzi G. Chronic renal diseases as a public health problem: epidemiology, social, and economic implications. *Kidney Int* 2005;68:S7–S10.

7. U.S. Renal Data System, USRDS 2005 Annual Data Report: Atlas of End-Stage Renal Disease in the United States, National Institutes of Health, National Institute of Diabetes and Digestive and Kidney Diseases, Bethesda, MD, 2005.

8. Mathur S, Devaraj S, Jialal I. Accelerated atherosclerosis, dyslipidemia, and oxidative stress in end-stage renal disease. *Curr Opin Nephrol Hypertens* 2002;11(2): 141–147.

9. Eberhard R, McClellan WM. Overview: Increased cardiovascular risk in patients with minor renal dysfunction: an emerging issue with far-reaching consequences. *J Am Soc Nephrol* 2005;15:513–516.

10. Mann JF, Gerstein HC, Pogue J, et al. Renal insufficiency as a predictor of cardiovascular outcomes and the impact of ramipril: the HOPE randomized trial. *Ann Intern Med* 2001;134(8):629–636.

11. Guyton AC. The surprising kidney-fluid mechanism for pressure control: its infinite gain! *Hypertension* 1990;16(6):725–730.

12. Rambausek M, Ritz E, Mall G, et al. Myocardial hypertrophy in rats with renal insufficiency. *Kidney Int* 1985;28(5):775–782.

13. Stefanski A, Schmidt KG, Waldherr R, et al. Early increase in blood pressure and diastolic left ventricular malfunction in patients with glomerulonephritis. *Kidney Int* 1996;50(4):1321–1326.

14. Amann K, Breitbach M, Ritz E, et al. Myocyte/capillary mismatch in the heart of uremic patients. *J Am Soc Nephrol* 1998;9(6):1018–1022.

15. Safar ME, London GM, Plante GE. Arterial stiffness and kidney function. *Hypertension* 2004;43(2):163–168.

16. Oh J, Wunsch R, Turzer M, et al. Advanced coronary and carotid arteriopathy in young adults with childhood-onset chronic renal failure. *Circulation* 2002;106(1): 100–105.

17. Tornig J, Gross ML, Simonaviciene A, et al. Hypertrophy of intramyocardial arteriolar smooth muscle cells in experimental renal failure. *J Am Soc Nephrol* 1999; 10(1):77–83.

18. Vuurmans TJ, Boer P, Koomans HA. Effects of endothelin-1 and endothelin-1 receptor blockade on cardiac output, aortic pressure, and pulse wave velocity in humans. *Hypertension* 2003;41(6):1253–1258.

19. Safar ME, London GM, Plante GE. Arterial stiffness and kidney function. *Hypertension* 2004;43(2):163–168.

20. Schwarz U, Buzello M, Ritz E, et al. Morphology of coronary atherosclerotic lesions in patients with end-stage renal failure. *Nephrol Dial Transplant* 2000;15(2): 218–223.

21. Schrier RW, Abraham WT. Hormones and hemodynamics in heart failure. *N Engl J Med* 1999;341(8):577–585.

22. McAlister FA, Ezekowitz J, Tonelli M, et al. Renal insufficiency and heart failure: prognostic and therapeutic implications from a prospective cohort study. *Circulation* 2004;109(8):1004–1009.

23. Buzello M, Törnig J, Faulhaber J, et al. The apolipoprotein e knockout mouse: a model documenting accelerated atherogenesis in uremia. *J Am Soc Nephrol* 2003;14: 311–316.

24. Griendling KK, Minieri CA, Ollerenshaw JD, et al. Angiotensin II stimulates NADH and NADPH oxidase activity in cultured vascular smooth muscle cells. *Circ Res* 1994;74(6):1141–1148.

25. Bongartz LG, Cramer MJ, Doevendans PA, et al. The severe cardiorenal syndrome: Guyton revisited. *Eur Heart J* 2005;26(1):11–17.

26. Brugts JJ, Knetsch AM, Mattace-Raso F, et al. Renal function and risk of myocardial infarction in an elderly population: the Rotterdam Study. *Arch Intern Med* 2005;165(22):2659–2665.

27. Muntner P, He J, Astor BC, et al. Traditional and nontraditional risk factors predict coronary heart disease in chronic kidney disease: results from the atherosclerosis risk in communities study. *J Am Soc Nephrol* 2005;16(2):529–538.

28. Hansson L, Zanchetti A, Carruthers SG, et al. Effects of intensive blood-pressure lowering and low-dose aspirin in patients with hypertension: Principal results of the Hypertension Optimal Treatment (HOT) randomised trial. *Lancet* 1998;351(9118): 1755–1762.

29. Culleton BF, Larson MG, Wilson PWF, et al. Cardiovascular disease and mortality in a community-based cohort with mild renal insufficiency. *Kidney Int* 1999; 56:2214–2219.

30. Dumaine R, Collet JP, Tanguy ML, et al. SYCOMORE Investigators. Prognostic significance of renal insufficiency in patients presenting with acute coronary syndrome (the Prospective Multicenter SYCOMORE study). *Am J Cardiol* 2004;94(12): 1543–1547.

31. Donal N, Reddan LS, Manjushri VB, et al. Renal function, concomitant medication use and outcomes following acute coronary syndromes. *Nephrol Dial Transplant* 2005;20(10):2105–2112.

32. Lechner BL, Bockenhauer D, Iragorri S, et al. The risk of cardiovascular disease in adults who have had childhood nephrotic syndrome. *Pediatr Nephrol* 2004;19(7): 744–748.

33. Culleton BF, Larson MG, Wilson PW, et al. Cardiovascular disease and mortality in a community-based cohort with mild renal insufficiency. *Kidney Int* 1999;56(6): 2214–2219.

34. Yuyun MF, Khaw KT, Luben R, et al. Microalbuminuria independently predicts all-cause and cardiovascular mortality in a British population: The European Prospective Investigation into Cancer in Norfolk (EPIC-Norfolk) population study. *Int J Epidemiol* 2004;33(1):189–198.

35. Henry RM, Kostense PJ, Bos G, et al. Mild renal insufficiency is associated with increased cardiovascular mortality: The Hoorn Study. *Kidney Int* 2002;62(4): 1402–1407.

36. Hillege HL, Fidler V, Diercks GFH, et al. for the Prevention of Renal and Vascular End Stage Disease (PREVEND) Study Group. Urinary albumin excretion predicts cardiovascular and noncardiovascular mortality in general population. *Circulation* 2002;106:1777–1782.

37. Klausen K, Borch-Johnsen K, Feldt-Rasmussen B. Very low levels of microalbuminuria are associated with increased risk of coronary heart disease and death independently of renal function, hypertension, and diabetes. *Circulation* 2004;110: 32–35.

38. Bosman DR, Winkler AS, Marsden JT, et al. Anemia with erythropoietin deficiency occurs early in diabetic nephropathy. *Diabetes Care* 2001;24(3):495–499.

39. Stenvinkel P, Barany P. Anaemia, rHuEPO resistance, and cardiovascular disease in end-stage renal failure; links to inflammation and oxidative stress. *Nephrol Dial Transplant* 2002;17(Suppl 5):32–37.

40. Singer J, Thompson CR, Ross H, et al. Prevalent left ventricular hypertrophy in the predialysis population: identifying opportunities for intervention. *Am J Kidney Dis* 1996;27(3):347–354.

41. London GM, Pannier B, Guerin AP, et al. Alterations of left ventricular hypertrophy in and survival of patients receiving hemodialysis: follow-up of an interventional study. *J Am Soc Nephrol* 2001;12(12):2759–2767.

42. Pereira AA, Sarnak MJ. Anemia as a risk factor for cardiovascular disease. *Kidney Int Suppl* 2003;(87):S32–S39.

43. Karpati I, Balla J, Szoke G, et al. Frequency of hyperhomocysteinemia in hemodialysis patients with folic acid supplementation. *Orv Hetil* 2002;143(27): 1635–1640.

44. Selhub J, Jacques PF, Rosenberg IH, et al. Serum total homocysteine concentrations in the third National Health and Nutrition Examination Survey (1991–1994): population reference ranges and contribution of vitamin status to high serum concentrations. *Ann Intern Med* 1999;131:331–339.

45. Ducloux D, Ruedin C, Gibey R, et al. Prevalence, determinants, and clinical significance of hyperhomocyst(e)inaemia in renal-transplant recipients. *Nephrol Dial Transplant* 1998;13:2890–2893.

46. Suliman ME, Stenvinkel P, Barany P, et al. Hyperhomocysteinemia and its relationship to cardiovascular disease in ESRD: influence of hypoalbuminemia, malnutrition, inflammation, and diabetes mellitus. *Am J Kidney Dis* 2003;41(3 Suppl 1): S89–S95.

47. Boushey CJ, Beresford SA, Omenn GS, et al. A quantitative assessment of plasma homocysteine as a risk factor for vascular disease. Probable benefits of increasing folic acid intakes. *JAMA* 1995;274:1049–1057.

48. Suliman ME, Lindholm B, Barany P, et al. Hyperhomocysteinemia in chronic renal failure patients: relation to nutritional status and cardiovascular disease. *Clin Chem Lab Med* 2001;39(8):734–348.

49. Bostom AG, Culleton BF. Hyperhomocysteinemia in chronic renal disease. *J Am Soc Nephrol* 1999;10(4):891–900.

50. Kes P. Hyperhomocysteinemia in end-stage renal failure. *Acta Med Croatica* 2000;54(4/5):175–181.

51. De Vriese AS, Verbeke F, Schrijvers BF, et al. Is folate a promising agent in the prevention and treatment of cardiovascular disease in patients with renal failure? *Kidney Int* 2002;61(4):1199–1209.

52. Neves KR, Graciolli FG, dos Reis LM, et al. Adverse effects of hyperphosphatemia on myocardial hypertrophy, renal function, and bone in rats with renal failure. *Kidney Int* 2004;66(6):2237–2244.

53. Basic-Jukic N, Kes P. Hyperphosphatemia and cardiovascular risk in patients on dialysis. *Acta Med Croatica* 2004;58(3):207–213.

54. Qunibi WY. Consequences of hyperphosphatemia in patients with end-stage renal disease (ESRD). *Kidney Int* 2004;(90):S8–S12.

55. Rasic S, Kulenovic I, Uncanin S. Parathormone as a cardiovascular risk factor in uraemic patients on haemodialysis treatment. *Med Arh* 2005;59(4):231–234.

56. Slinin Y, Foley RN, Collins AJ. Calcium, phosphorus, parathyroid hormone, and cardiovascular disease in hemodialysis patients: the USRDS waves 1, 3, and 4 study. *J Am Soc Nephrol* 2005;16(6):1788–1793.

57. Perkovic V, Hewitson TD, Kelynack KJ, et al. Parathyroid hormone has a prosclerotic effect on vascular smooth muscle cells. *Kidney Blood Press Res* 2003;26(1):27–33.

58. Block GA, Klassen PS, Lazarus JM, et al. Mineral metabolism, mortality, and morbidity in maintenance hemodialysis. *J Am Soc Nephrol* 2004;15(8):2208–2218.

59. Ketteler M, Westenfeld R, Schlieper G, et al. Pathogenesis of vascular calcification in dialysis patients. *Clin Exp Nephrol* 2005;9(4):265–270.

60. Brancaccio D, Zoccali C. The continuous challenge of cardiovascular and bone and bone disease in uremic patients: clinical consequences of hyperphosphatemia and advanced therapeutic approaches. *J Nephrol* 2006;19(1):12–20.

61. Block GA, Port FK. Re-evaluation of risks associated with hyperphosphatemia and hyperparathyroidism in dialysis patients: recommendations for a change in management. *Am J Kidney Dis* 2000;35(6):1226–1237.

62. Yamauchi A, Fukuhara Y, Yamamoto S, et al. Oncotic pressure regulates gene transcriptions of albumin and apolipoprotein B in cultured rat hepatoma cells. *Am J Physiol* 1992;263:C397–C404.

63. Vaziri ND, Liang KH. Acyl-coenzyme A:cholesterol acyltransferase inhibition ameliorates proteinuria, hyperlipidemia, lecithin-cholesterol acyltransferase, SRB-1, and low-density lipoprotein receptor deficiencies in nephrotic syndrome. *Circulation* 2004;110(4):419–425.

THE METABOLIC

SYNDROME

Luther T. Clark
Suzette Graham-Hill

The *metabolic syndrome* refers to a specific clustering of cardiovascular risk factors (abdominal obesity, atherogenic dyslipidemia, elevated blood pressure (BP), insulin resistance, a prothrombotic state, and a proinflammatory state) in the same individual.[1-3] Patients with the metabolic syndrome—also known as insulin resistance syndrome, metabolic syndrome X, dysmetabolic syndrome, and cardiometabolic syndrome—are at increased risk for the development of diabetes and cardiovascular disease (CVD).[1-10] Although there is some debate about use of the term "syndrome"[11] for cardiometabolic risk factor clustering, a diagnosis of the metabolic syndrome provides early identification of individuals with accelerated cardiovascular risk, and therefore an earlier opportunity to intervene on all cardiovascular risk factors.

EVOLUTION OF CARDIOMETABOLIC RISK FACTOR CLUSTERING AS A SYNDROME

The propensity for clustering of metabolic and cardiovascular risk factors in the same individual has been recognized for many years. Perhaps the first description of cardiometabolic risk factor clustering appeared in the medical literature in 1923 when Eskil Kylin (1889–1975), a Swedish physician, described a syndrome involving hypertension, hyperglycemia, and hyperuricemia.[12] Sixty-five years later, in 1988, Reaven described a cluster of risk factors for diabetes and CVD (hypertension, hyperglycemia, glucose intolerance, elevated triglycerides [TGs], and low high-density lipoprotein cholesterol [HDL-C]) that he named "Syndrome X,"[13] and introduced the concept of insulin resistance. In 1998, the World Health Organization (WHO) proposed the term metabolic syndrome rather than insulin resistance syndrome, since insulin resistance alone could not explain all components of the syndrome.[14] The WHO defined "metabolic syndrome" as clustering of hypertension, low HDL, hypertriglyceridemia, insulin resistance, glucose intolerance or type 2 diabetes, high waist-to-hip ratio, and microalbuminuria. However, use of the term metabolic syndrome remained relatively uncommon until 2001 when the National Cholesterol Education Program Adult Treatment Panel (NCEP-ATP III) identified the metabolic syndrome as a risk factor for CVD, and as a target for lipid-modifying and other CVD risk reduction therapies.[1]

ETIOLOGY OF THE METABOLIC SYNDROME

The etiology of the metabolic syndrome has not been fully elucidated. However, there appears to be at least three potential etiologic pathways[3]: (1) overweight and obesity; (2) insulin resistance; and (3) certain independent factors (aging, proinflammatory states, and hormonal changes) that mediate specific components of the syndrome.

Obesity, in particular abdominal obesity, increases risk for hypertension, increased total cholesterol, decreased HDL-C, hyperglycemia, and CVD. Furthermore, a proinflammatory state and a prothrombotic state often accompany and may be a consequence of obesity.[3] The strong linkages of obesity and other CHD risk factors led the NCEP-ATP to define the metabolic syndrome primarily as a clustering of metabolic complications of obesity[1–3] and attribute the increasing prevalence of metabolic syndrome in the United States largely to the increasing epidemic of obesity.

A second pathway and etiologic hypothesis for the metabolic syndrome is insulin resistance. Many investigators/clinicians believe that insulin resistance is the primary causative factor[4,13] and some diagnostic criteria include it as an essential feature.[14] Insulin resistance and hyperinsulinemia may enhance output of very low-density lipoprotein (VLDL) TGs (thus raising TGs levels), predisposes to glucose intolerance, and increase BP.[3,4,13] However, abdominal obesity and insulin resistance are closely linked and are associated in a bidirectional cause and effect relationship. Therefore, efforts to dissociate the effects of abdominal obesity and primary insulin resistance, and to attribute a primary causative role for either entity have been difficult and complicated. Most obese individuals (body mass index [BMI] ≥ 30 kg/m^2) have insulin resistance. However, in some populations (e.g., South Asians), primary insulin resistance commonly occurs with only mild to moderate overweight.[15]

In addition to abdominal obesity and insulin resistance, each of the other components of the metabolic syndrome has its own genetic and acquired factors which may contribute to pathogenesis. Advancing age is associated with increased prevalence of the metabolic syndrome and may affect all of the pathogenic factors.

EPIDEMIOLOGY

The prevalence of metabolic syndrome is increasing in the general population in the United States and varies according to the definition of metabolic syndrome used and the population studied. The diagnostic criteria proposed by the NCEP and that proposed by the WHO are currently the most widely used. According to a recent analysis of data from the Third National Health and Nutrition Examination Survey (NHANES III),[16] almost 50 million Americans (23.7% of the population) have the metabolic syndrome (Fig. 14-1). African American women and Hispanic men and women have the highest prevalence of the metabolic syndrome.[16] This is attributable mainly to the disproportionate occurrence of elevated BP, obesity, and diabetes in African Americans, and the high prevalence of obesity and diabetes in Hispanics. In the NHANES III analysis, African American women had an approximately 57% higher prevalence than African American men, and Hispanic women had an approximately 26% higher prevalence than Hispanic men. Susceptibility to the specific risk factors of the metabolic syndrome varies among ethnic groups[16–18] Whites of European ancestry have a greater predisposition to atherogenic dyslipidemia, whereas blacks of African descent are more prone to hypertension, type 2 diabetes, and obesity. Hispanics, Pacific Islanders, and Native

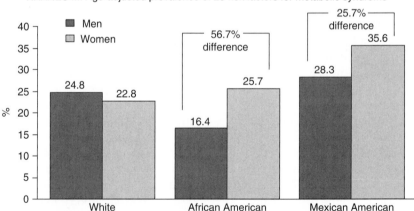

NHANES III: Age-adjusted prevalence of ≥3 risk factors for metabolic syndrome*

NHANES III = third National Heath and Nutrition Examination Survey; ATP = Adult Treatment Panel.
*Criteria based on ATP III; diabetics were included in diagnosis; overall unadjusted prevalence was 21.8%.

Figure 14-1 **Age-adjusted prevalence of ≥3 risk factors for metabolic syndrome. *Criteria based on ATP III; diabetics were included in diagnosis; overall adjusted prevalence was 21.8%.** *(Source: Reproduced with permission from Ford ES, Giles WH, Dietz WH. Prevalence of the metabolic syndrome among US adults: findings from the Third National Health and Nutritional Examination Survey. JAMA 2002;287:356–359.)*

Americans (NA) are less likely to develop hypertension than blacks, but appear to be particularly susceptible to type 2 diabetes. Individuals of Asian descent appear to have a higher than average predisposition to developing the metabolic syndrome at relatively low BMI levels.[15]

CLINICAL DIAGNOSIS OF THE METABOLIC SYNDROME

Several clinical definitions of the metabolic syndrome currently exist. As noted above, the diagnostic criteria proposed by the NCEP[1] and that proposed by the WHO[14] are currently the most widely used. Recently, the American Heart Association and the National Heart Lung and Blood Institute (AHA-NHLBI) provided an updated definition of the metabolic syndrome.[2,3] The joint AHA-NHLBI definition is the same as that in the NCEP-ATP III 2001 guidelines[1,3] with minor revisions, the key revision being the lowering of the threshold for diagnosis of impaired fasting glucose (IFG) from 110 to 100 mg/dL consistent with the recently modified American Diabetes Association (ADA) recommendations.[19] According to this updated criteria, the metabolic syndrome is present when three or more of the following five abnormalities are present (Table 14-1): (1) waist circumference (WC) >102 cm (40 in.) in men or >88 cm (35 in.) in women, (2) serum TG level ≥150 mg/dL, (3) HDL-C level <40 mg/dL in men or <50 mg/dL in women, (4) BP ≥130/85 mmHg, and (5) serum glucose ≥100 mg/dL.[1,3] In the original NCEP-ATP III definition, the criteria for abnormal IFG was ≥110 mg/dL.[1]

In addition to the widely used NCEP-ATP III criteria and the recently released AHA-NHLBI definitions of the metabolic syndrome, several other definitions currently in use (Table 14-2) include (1) the WHO definition[14]

Table 14-1 **Criteria for Clinical Diagnosis of the Metabolic Syndrome***

Risk Factor	Defining Level
Abdominal obesity (WC)	
Men	>102 cm (>40 in.)
Women	>88 cm (>35 in.)
TGs	≥150 mg/dL
HDL-C	
Men	<40 mg/dL
Women	<50 mg/dL
BP	≥130/85 mmHg
Fasting glucose	≥100 mg/dL[†]

*Diagnosis requires presence of three or more criteria.

[†]Revised per the most recent ADA definition.

Source: Modified from Refs. 1 and 3.

Table 14-2 *Criteria Proposed for Clinical Diagnosis of Metabolic Syndrome*

Clinical Measure	WHO (1998)	EGIR	ATP III (2001)	AACE (2003)	IDF (2005)
Insulin resistance	IGT, IFG, T2DM, or lowered insulin sensitivity* plus any 2 of the following	Plasma insulin >75th percentile plus any 2 of the following	None, but any 3 of the following 5 features	IGT or IFG plus any of the following based on clinical judgment	None
Body weight	Men: waist-to-hip ratio >0.90; women: waist-to-hip ratio >0.85 and/or BMI >30 kg/m²	WC ≥94 cm in men or ≥80 cm in women	WC ≥102 cm in men or ≥88 cm in women†	BMI ≥25 kg/m²	Increased WC (population specific) plus any 2 of the following
Lipid	TG ≥150 mg/dL and/or HDL-C <35 mg/dL in men or <39 mg/dL in women	TG ≥150 mg/dL and/ or HDL-C <39 mg/dL in men or women	TG ≥150 mg/dL HDL-C <40 mg/dL in men or <50 mg/dL in women	TG ≥150 mg/dL and HDL-C <40 mg/dL in men or <50 mg/dL in women	TG ≥150 mg/dL or on TG Rx HDL-C <40 mg/dL in in men or <50 mg/dL in women or on HDL-C Rx
Blood pressure	≥140/90 mm Hg	≥140/90 mm Hg or on hypertension Rx	≥130/85 mm Hg	≥130/85 mm Hg	≥130 mm Hg systolic or ≥85 mm Hg diastolic or hypertension Rx
Glucose	IGT, IFG, or T2DM	IGT or IFG (but not diabetes)	>110 mg/dL (includes diabetes)‡	IGT of IFG (but not diabetes)	≥100 mg/dL (includes diabetes)
Other	Microalbuminuria			Other features of insulin resistance§	

T2DM indicates type 2 diabetes mellitus; WC, waist circumference; BMI, body mass index; and TG, triglycerides. All other abbreviations as in text.

*Insulin sensitivity measured under hyperinsulinemic euglycemic conditions, glucose uptake below lowest quartile for background population under investigation.

†Some male patients can develop multiple metabolic risk factors when the waist circumference is only marginally increased (eg, 94 to 102 cm [37 to 39 in]). Such patients may have a strong genetic contribution to insulin resistance. They should benefit from changes in lifestyle habits, similar to men with categorical increases in waist circumference.

‡The 2001 definition identified fasting plasma glucose of ≥110 mg/dL (6.1 mmol/L) as elevated. This was modified in 2004 to be ≥100 mg/dL (5.6 mmol/L), in accordance with the American diabetes Association's updated definition of IFG.[46,47,77]

§Includes family history of type 2 diabetes mellitus, polycystic ovary syndrome, sedentary lifestyle, advancing age, and ethnic groups susceptible to type 2 diabetes mellitus.

Source: Modified from Refs. 3, 42, 43, and 78.

which requires an index of insulin resistance and includes microalbumin-uria, (2) the 2003 American Association of Clinical Endocrinologists (AACE) criteria (a modification of the ATP III criteria to refocus on insulin resistance as the primary cause of metabolic risk factors, uses BMI rather than WC to measure central obesity, introduces ethnicity as a risk factor),[20] and (3) the recently released International Diabetes Federation (IDF) definition,[21] which is also a modification of the NCEP-ATP III criteria, but in addition to taking into account the ADA's lowered fasting glucose cut point for normal glucose tolerance, also makes abdominal obesity a necessary criteria for diagnosis.

For practicing clinicians, there is an *ICD-9-CM (International Classification of Diseases, Ninth Revision, Clinical Modification)* diagnostic code (277.7)[22] that allows clinicians to code for the metabolic syndrome. The introduction of the ICD-9 code in 2001 may become increasingly important as treatments for the metabolic syndrome become available. Although the metabolic syndrome has become widely used and has received increased attention during the past several years, the ADA and the European Association for the Study of Diabetes recently called for a rethinking and re-evaluation of the metabolic syndrome as a discrete entity.[11]

CARDIOVASCULAR RISK AND THE METABOLIC SYNDROME

Each of the components of the metabolic syndrome increases risk for the development of CVD, in particular atherosclerosis and coronary heart disease (CHD). In addition, several recent studies have now demonstrated that the metabolic syndrome—usually defined by ATP III or WHO criteria—increases the risk of developing CVD by as much as fourfold.[1–10,23–32] However, some studies did not demonstrate an increased risk.[33,34]

In the Framingham cohort, the metabolic syndrome predicted approximately 25% of all new CVD.[2,10] The absolute risk for CHD in men ranged from 10 to 20%, less than the threshold required by the NCEP to qualify as a CHD risk equivalent. The NCEP defines CHD risk equivalent as an absolute, 10-year risk for developing a major coronary event (myocardial infarction or CHD death) of >20%, equal to that of persons with established CHD.[1] In Framingham women (who were generally under 50 years of age), the metabolic syndrome increased risk for CVD, but the 10-year risk did not exceed 10%. Most of the risk associated with the metabolic syndrome was attributable to age, BP, total cholesterol, diabetes, and HDL-C. Obesity, TGs, and glucose levels (in the absence of diabetes) contributed little additional risk.

The recently published INTERHEART study evaluated risk factors for acute myocardial infarction in 52 countries.[35] The investigators found a prevalence of 26% for the metabolic syndrome (modified ATP and WHO definitions) and that among traditional risk factors, diabetes, hypertension, and abdominal obesity together account for approximately 50% of the risk of a first myocardial infarction.[35]

Metabolic Syndrome in Patients with Diabetes

Although the prevalence of the metabolic syndrome varies in the general population and among ethnic groups, the prevalence is consistently high, 70–90%, in patients with diabetes regardless of ethnicity or diagnostic criteria used.[9,25,33,36–39] In studies that included only patients initially free of CVD, prevalence was lower but still high, 38–53%.[40]

METABOLIC SYNDROME, PREDIABETES, AND DIABETES

In the Framingham Heart Study Cohort, the presence of metabolic syndrome was highly predictive of new-onset type 2 diabetes mellitus (T2DM) in men and women.[10] The overall relative risk was greater than four, and explained approximately half of the population-attributable risk for diabetes.[10] In other studies, the relative risk for the development of T2DM varied from 3.5 in WOSCOPS,[41] approximately 2 in the Strong Heart Study (SHS),[34] approximately 6 with 3 metabolic syndrome components and 18 with ≥4 metabolic syndrome traits in the Beaver Dam Study,[42] 6.3 in the San Antonio Heart Study,[43] and <1.5 in the Pima Indian Study.[44]

T2DM has historically been defined by the elevation of fasting or postchallenge blood glucose. However, it is now well established that a core metabolic abnormality in T2DM is insulin resistance. Prediabetes refers to IFG (100–125 mg/dL) or impaired glucose tolerance (IGT) (plasma level of 140–199 mg/dL for 2 hours after a 75-g oral glucose challenge). Patients with prediabetes are at very high risk for conversion to frank T2DM (rates of 3–11% per year).[45] These levels of glucose intolerance are common metabolic abnormalities in the metabolic syndrome and a number of other metabolic disorders (Fig. 14-2).[46] Thus, the enormous overlap in these conditions is not surprising. More than 40 million adults in the United States have prediabetes. These individuals usually, but not always, have additional risk factors (hypertension, dyslipidemia) for CVD. While the metabolic syndrome will include the vast majority of persons with prediabetes, the conditions are not the same. One or both conditions may be present in the same individual. Presence of the metabolic syndrome[3] requires the presence of three or more CVD risk factors, one of which can be IFG (or prediabetes). Thus, the two conditions are metabolically distinct, and have quite different criteria for diagnosis and different, albeit overlapping, treatment implications. Although IFG increases cardiovascular risk,[47] it does not do so to the same degree as overt diabetes.

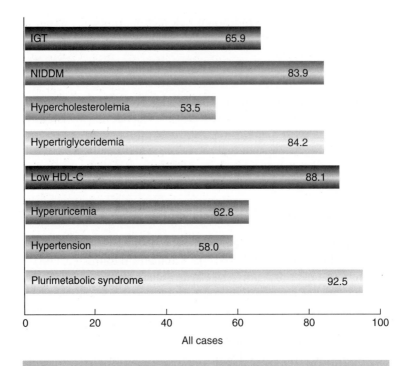

Figure 14-2 **Prevalence rates (%) of insulin resistance in selected metabolic disorders. IGT, Impaired glucose tolerance; NIDDM, non-insulin-dependent diabetes mellitus.** *(Source: Reproduced with permission from Bonora E, Kiechl S, Willeit J, et al. Prevalence of insulin resistance in metabolic disorders: the Bruneck Study. Diabetes 1998;47: 1643–1649.)*

CLINICAL MANAGEMENT OF THE METABOLIC SYNDROME

Overall Clinical Management Goals

The overall clinical management goal in individuals with the metabolic syndrome is the same as for the clinical management of other CVD risk factors—reduction of CVD morbidity and mortality. In addition, prevention of T2DM is another clinical management goal when it is not already present.

Treatment of the metabolic syndrome consists primarily of two strategies (Fig. 14-3): (1) modification or reversal of the root causes, including weight reduction and increased physical activity; and (2) direct treatment of the metabolic risk factors, including atherogenic dyslipidemia, elevated BP, the prothrombotic state, and underlying insulin resistance.[1,2,48,49] Although it is

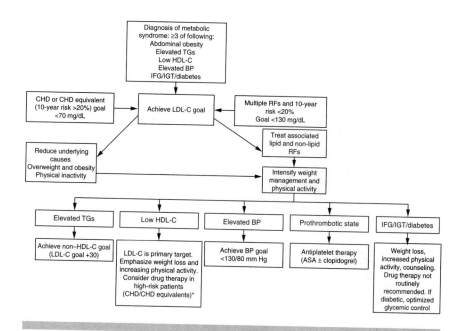

Figure 14-3 **Therapeutic approach to the metabolic syndrome.** *(Source: Reprinted with permission from Clark LT, Ferdinand KC, Ferdinand DP, et al. Contemporary Management of the Metabolic Syndrome 2005: Special Focus: Implications for the Diabetic and Prediabetic Patient. Association of Black Cardiologists, Inc and McMahon Publishing Group, 2005. Available at: www.abcardio.org)*

important that all components of the metabolic syndrome be controlled, a recent analysis by Wong et al. estimated that >80% of cardiovascular events in people with the metabolic syndrome could be prevented by optimal control of BP, HDL-C, and low-density lipoprotein cholesterol (LDL-C).[50] Patients with the metabolic syndrome should increase their physical activity level, lose weight (if overweight), and have their BP and lipid abnormalities treated to recommended goals. Although most of the demonstrated successes in reducing CVD in clinical practice have been achieved through pharmacologic modification of the associated risk factors, the greatest potential benefit from management of the metabolic syndrome lies in reversing its root causes: overweight/obesity and physical inactivity.

OBESITY

Obesity is a major component of the metabolic syndrome and a strong correlate of insulin resistance (Figs. 14-4 and 14-5). Most individuals with

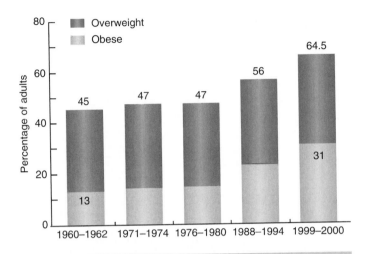

Figure 14-4 **Prevalence of overweight and obesity in the United States (1960–2000).** *(Source: Reproduced with permission from Bonow RQ. Primary prevention of cardiovascular disease: a call to action. Circulation 2002;106:3140–3141.)*

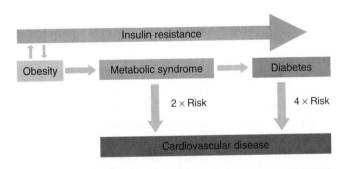

Figure 14-5 **Relationship of obesity, metabolic syndrome, type 2 diabetes, and CVD.** *(Source: Modified with permission from Reilly MP, Rader DJ. The metabolic syndrome; more than the sum of its parts? Circulation 2003;108:1546–1551. Lüscher TF, Creager MA, Beckman JA, et al. Diabetes and vascular disease: pathophysiology, clinical consequences, and medical therapy: part II. Circulation 2003;108:1655–1661.)*

the metabolic syndrome are overweight or obese, and most persons with insulin resistance have abdominal obesity.[1,2,51-57] Obesity and overweight status increases the risk of CHD, stroke, hypertension, and type 2 diabetes in adults, and is associated with insulin resistance in normoglycemic individuals as well as those with type 2 diabetes. Abdominal (central), visceral, or predominantly upper-body distribution of body fat is a stronger risk factor for CVD than is obesity per se. The insulin resistance associated with abdominal/visceral adiposity appears to be, at least in part, due to abnormalities in fatty acid metabolism. Abdominal/visceral adiposity is associated with an increased release of free fatty acids into the portal blood, which, in turn, leads to hepatic overproduction of triglycerides and decreased synthesis of HDL-C, both characteristic of the metabolic syndrome. Interventions that prevent accumulation of abdominal/visceral adiposity decrease age-related increases in insulin resistance and IGT.

Weight reduction and increased physical activity are first-line therapy to improve all components of the metabolic syndrome.[1,3,48,58,59] Dietary therapy and increased physical activity are the cornerstones of therapy for obesity although in some individuals adjunctive pharmacologic therapy might also be an appropriate option. Achieving and sustaining weight loss is often very challenging for patients and providers. However, it is important not to underestimate the impact of a healthy lifestyle, including diet and exercise, for weight reduction as well as on lowering the risks of morbidity and mortality. The initial target for weight loss should be 10% decrease in body weight within 6–12 months.

ATHEROGENIC DYSLIPIDEMIA

Dyslipidemia is an important component of the metabolic syndrome and an important link to increased risk for atherosclerosis. An elevation in LDL-C levels is not a component of the metabolic syndrome, although abnormalities in LDL particle size are. The triad of lipid abnormalities—elevated TG levels, reduced HDL-C levels, and a preponderance of small dense LDL particles—are often referred to as "atherogenic dyslipidemia" and are recommended as a target for therapeutic intervention.[1,48] While it is generally recognized that elevated level of LDL-C is a potent risk factor for atherosclerosis and CAD, it is less well appreciated that all of the three components of the atherogenic dyslipidemia triad are associated with atherogenesis and increased CAD risk.[60-63] TGs are a major source of the atherogenic apoprotein B-100 containing lipoproteins, which include VLDL, intermediate-density lipoprotein (IDL), and LDL. HDL-C modulates atherosclerosis through the reverse cholesterol transport process. Small dense LDL particles have a greater propensity for being oxidized and to penetrate the arterial intima than their larger, more buoyant precursors.

Total and LDL Cholesterol

Although increased total and LDL-C, per se, are not components of the metabolic syndrome, the NCEP-ATP III recommends that in individuals with the metabolic syndrome, as in others, LDL-C should be the primary target of lipid-modifying therapy.[1,3,48] Intensive treatment is recommended for very high-risk, high-risk, and moderately high-risk patients. Very high-risk patients are candidates for an optional LDL-C goal of <70 mg/dL and include individuals with established CVD and the metabolic syndrome, and those with CVD and diabetes. Patients with the metabolic syndrome without CVD are considered to be at moderately high risk for CHD and are candidates for the LDL-C optional goal of <100 mg/dL.

Elevated Triglycerides

Elevated serum TG levels (≥150 mg/dL) are an independent risk factor for CHD. Hypertriglyceridemia can be caused by obesity, physical inactivity, a high-carbohydrate diet (>60% of calories), diabetes mellitus, as well as certain drugs (estrogens, corticosteroids), excessive alcohol intake, and genetic disorders. The goal of therapy in patients with elevated TGs is to achieve a level <150 mg/dL. The treatment strategy for reducing TGs should take into consideration the severity and cause of TG elevation. In patients with borderline high TG levels (150–199 mg/dL), dietary modification, weight reduction, and increased physical activity are the first-line therapies. Drug therapy, in addition to lifestyle changes, may be necessary in individuals with TGs >200 mg/dL. When TG levels are >200 mg/dL, ATP III guidelines recommend that VLDL cholesterol (VLDL-C) should be targeted by using non-HDL-C goals set at 30 mg/dL higher than the LDL-C goal.[1,48] Non-HDL-C refers to the concentration of LDL-C plus VLDL-C, and can be determined by subtracting HDL-C from total cholesterol levels—measurements that can be obtained with fasting and nonfasting determinations. The non-HDL-C goal can be achieved by intensifying the therapy to reduce LDL-C or VLDL-C. In patients requiring drug therapy, cautious addition of fibrate or nicotinic acid to a low-fat diet (≤15% of daily calories) is beneficial in many patients. Patients with very high TG levels (≥500 mg/dL) are at risk for developing acute pancreatitis, and TG-lowering should be the primary objective.

Low HDL Cholesterol

The NCEP-ATP III guidelines define low HDL-C as <40 mg/dL in men and women.[1,48] However, for diagnosis of the metabolic syndrome, HDL <40 mg/dL in men or <50 mg/dL in women is considered abnormal and one of the diagnostic criteria. Low HDL-C is a strong and independent predictor of CHD.[1,48,60,63] Low HDL-C may be caused by factors associated with insulin resistance, such as elevated TGs, type 2 diabetes, excess weight, physical inactivity, high carbohydrate consumption, cigarette smoking, and certain drugs (beta-blockers, anabolic steroids, progesterone). In individuals with low HDL-C levels, the primary therapeutic objective is to achieve the recommended LDL-C goal.[1,48] After this has been achieved, emphasis shifts to weight reduction and increased physical activity. If the TG level is elevated, reduction of non-HDL-C is the secondary target. If the TG level is not elevated (<200 mg/dL), specific therapies to increase HDL-C may be considered (fibrates, nicotinic acid).

HYPERTENSION/ELEVATED BLOOD PRESSURE

Both systolic hypertension and diastolic hypertension are established risk factors for CVD.[64] Systolic BP is a better predictor than diastolic BP of risk for CHD, heart failure, stroke, end-stage renal disease, and overall mortality. Diet and other lifestyle therapies are the essential first steps of therapy for elevations of BP in individuals with or without the metabolic syndrome. However, many patients will require pharmacologic intervention to reach treatment goals. In patients with the metabolic syndrome and elevated BPs (≥130/85 mmHg), application of the Seventh Report of the Joint National Committee on Prevention, Detection, Evaluation, and Treatment of High Blood Pressure (JNC7) guidelines would suggest pharmacologic treatment to achieve the target goal of <130/80 mmHg.[64]

INSULIN RESISTANCE (IMPAIRED FASTING GLUCOSE/IMPAIRED GLUCOSE TOLERANCE)

Impaired fasting glucose (100–125 mg/dL) is a common metabolic abnormality in the metabolic syndrome, and in a number of other metabolic disorders.[1,2,9,10,46,48] The safest, most effective, and preferred means to reduce insulin resistance is weight reduction and increased physical activity in overweight and obese persons. In the ATP III guidelines, although IFG was not recommended as a direct target for drug therapy, its presence signifies the need for more intensive lifestyle therapies that will often correct it. Several drugs, for example, the thiazolidinediones and metformin, are currently available that appear to reduce insulin resistance. However, it has not yet been demonstrated that these drugs provide an associated decrease in CVD morbidity and mortality in patients with the metabolic syndrome. The benefits of the "insulin sensitizers" for glucose intolerance prior to the onset of frank diabetes, and their possible benefits on cardiovascular risk reduction, await the results of ongoing clinical trials.

INFLAMMATION

Vascular inflammation has recently been recognized as an important contributor to the etiology, progression, and complications of atherosclerosis. Levels of the inflammatory marker, high-sensitivity C-reactive protein (Hs-CRP), correspond with the individual components of the metabolic syndrome, and at all levels of severity of the metabolic syndrome (Fig. 14-6).[8] Hs-CRP adds

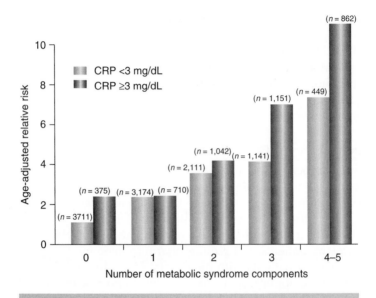

Figure 14-6 **Relative risks of future cardiovascular events, according to the number of components of metabolic syndrome and according to CRP levels ≥ or <3.0 mg/dL.** *(Source: Reproduced with permission from Ridker PM, Buring JE, Cook NR, et al. C-reactive protein, the metabolic syndrome, and risk of incident cardiovascular events: an 8-year follow-up of 14,719 initially healthy American women.* Circulation *2003;107:391–397.)*

important and independent prognostic information on subsequent risk.[1,8,48] However, the potential role of vascular inflammation as a direct target of therapy and the extent to which reducing vascular inflammation will be beneficial in terms of CVD prevention are yet to be determined in clinical trials.

PROTHROMBOTIC STATE

The dyslipidemia and insulin resistance of the metabolic syndrome are associated with a prothrombotic state (increased prothrombotic activity and decreased fibrinolytic activity) reflected in increased concentrations and activity of coagulation factors, and overexpression of plasminogen activator inhibitor (PAI)-1. Therapies designed to improve the metabolic abnormalities of the metabolic syndrome are likely to reduce hyperactivity of platelets, decrease the intensity of the prothrombotic state, and normalize the activity of the fibrinolytic system in the blood and vessel walls. Currently, low-dose aspirin (ASA, 75–160 mg/day) is the only routinely recommended antithrombotic therapy for primary prevention of CVD.[65,66] Clopidogrel may be beneficial in ASA-intolerant patients and those with established peripheral arterial disease or CHD.

SCREENING AND RISK ASSESSMENT

The metabolic syndrome is common—particularly in middle-aged and older adults—and its presence identifies individuals with accelerated cardiovascular risk. Therefore, intensified efforts are needed to screen and adequately treat persons with the metabolic syndrome. Evaluation for presence of cardiometabolic risk factors should be standard in initial patient assessment by primary care providers. Important initial steps would include (1) the widespread incorporation of WC measurements during routine physical examinations, (2) improved compliance with NCEP recommendations to obtain a full fasting lipid profile for all adults, and incorporation of fasting glucose measurement at point-of-care testing stations. This would increase diagnosis of the metabolic syndrome and provide patients immediate feedback regarding these important components of the metabolic syndrome. In particular, if one component of the metabolic syndrome is present, the others should be looked for. Information on obesity, hypertension, the metabolic syndrome as risk factors for CVD, and the benefits of physical activity and nutrition should be widely disseminated. A special campaign to prevent and control childhood obesity should be carried out.

THE METABOLIC SYNDROME IN ETHNIC GROUPS

African Americans

Recognition, diagnosis, and treatment of the metabolic syndrome in African Americans have the potential for reducing cardiovascular morbidity and mortality, and also the potential for contributing to the reduction of health disparities. African Americans have the highest overall mortality rate from CHD of any ethnic group, particularly out-of-hospital deaths, and especially at younger ages.[67,68] Although the reasons for the excess mortality among African Americans have not been fully elucidated, a high prevalence of certain coronary risk factors, patient delays in seeking medical care, and under-treatment of high-risk individuals contribute importantly.

The prevalence of certain CHD risk factors and clustering of risk factors is greater in African Americans than in the general population. Hypertension, left ventricular hypertrophy, T2DM, obesity, cigarette smoking, and physical inactivity occur more frequently in African Americans. Also, African Americans are 1.5 times more likely to have multiple risk factors than whites.[69–71] Since two of the root contributors to the metabolic syndrome (overweight/obesity and physical inactivity) and three of the five components of the metabolic syndrome (obesity, elevated BP, IFG, and diabetes) are more common in African Americans, their increased risk for the development of the metabolic syndrome and its adverse consequences (particularly in black females) make this an especially important issue to address for preventing and reducing CVD risk.

Although the age-adjusted prevalence of the metabolic syndrome in all African Americans in the NHANES III analysis was similar to that in the overall U.S. population, African American women appear to be particularly predisposed to development of the syndrome.[10,16,72,73] This was attributable mainly to the disproportionate occurrence in African Americans of elevated BP, obesity, and diabetes. In the Jackson Heart Study,[74] more than a third (37.2%) of the 5302 men and women in the population-based study of African Americans met the criteria for metabolic syndrome. Of the five components comprising the syndrome, increased WC and high BP were most prevalent (65.3 and 63.7%, respectively).

Hispanic Americans

Hispanics are the largest and fastest growing minority group in the United States. In the 2000 Census, 32.8 million Hispanics (12% of the population) lived in the United States.[75] The Hispanic population is increasing at a rate five times that of the general population and it has been estimated that Hispanics will become the largest minority group in the United States early in the twenty-first century. Hispanics are a heterogeneous population with national origins or ancestry that may include Puerto Ricans, Cubans, Mexicans, Spaniards, and other Latinos. Approximately 66% of the U.S. Hispanics are of Mexican origin, 15% South and Central American, 9% Puerto Rican, and 4% Cuban.[75] In the NHANES III analysis, Mexican American males (28.3%) and females (35.6%) had the highest prevalence of metabolic syndrome (Fig. 14-1).[16] Despite their higher rates of metabolic syndrome, diabetes, obesity, lower HDL-C and higher TG levels, lower socioeconomic status (SES) and barriers to health care, several studies have suggested that Hispanics have lower all-cause and cardiovascular mortality rates than non-Hispanic whites and non-Hispanic blacks.[16,76–78] This observation has been referred to by some as the "Hispanic Paradox,"[77] although a recent study provided evidence against the Hispanic Paradox in a population of diabetic individuals. Even though Hispanics may have lower than expected mortality rates than non-Hispanic blacks and non-Hispanic whites, heart disease and stroke still remain the leading cause of death, both in Hispanic males and in Hispanic females. Thus, one should not conclude that Hispanics are protected from CHD or that they should be treated less aggressively than other groups.

Native Americans (American Indians)

Cardiovascular disease mortality rates vary among the NA communities in the United States. However, NA have the highest prevalence of diabetes in the United States, and CVD in NA communities—unlike for other ethnic groups—is increasing.[34,79,80] Data from the NHANES III which assessed the prevalence of metabolic syndrome in U.S. adults did not include data for NA. The baseline examination of the Strong Heart Study (SHS), a longitudinal, population-based study of CVD and CVD risk factors in 4549 NA, was concurrent with NHANES III. The prevalence of metabolic syndrome in SHS men (43.6%) and women (56.7%) aged 45–49 years was more than twice that among all men and women in NHANES III (a prevalence ratio of 2.18 in men and 2.45 in women, respectively). Efforts to treat the metabolic syndrome, reduce cholesterol, and other CHD risk factors in this population are especially important because of the higher CHD incidence and the higher associated mortality rates.

Asian and Pacific Islanders

Limited information is available about the prevalence and risks of the metabolic syndrome in Asians. In the Honolulu Heart Program, an ongoing prospective study of CHD and stroke in a cohort of Japanese American men living in Hawaii, CHD and CVD mortality rates were lower than in the general U.S. population.[81] A recent analysis of the NCEP criteria for diagnosing metabolic syndrome in Asians suggested that this criteria underestimates the true prevalence and that the criteria for central obesity and the WC cutoff should be modified.[82]

South Asians

According to the 2000 Census, there are approximately 2 million people in the United States who identify themselves as Asian Indians or Indian Americans—first- and second-generation immigrants or those whose ancestors migrated to the United States from India.[83] There has been special interest in this group because they have very high prevalence rates of coronary disease at younger ages in the absence of traditional risk factors.[84] Although the prevalence of obesity is not high in Asian Indians, the higher CHD risk in this population appears to be related, at least in part, to a higher prevalence of insulin resistance, the metabolic syndrome, and diabetes.[15,84] Special attention should be given to detection of CHD risk factors and life style changes in South Asians.

SUMMARY

The metabolic syndrome is highly prevalent in the U.S. population, currently affecting approximately one in four adults, and the prevalence is increasing. African American women, Hispanic men and women, and South Asian Indians appear to be particularly predisposed to development of the metabolic syndrome. Patients with the metabolic syndrome are at high risk for the development of diabetes and accelerated CVD. Obesity, particularly abdominal obesity is strongly related to the metabolic syndrome, and the rising prevalence of obesity in the United States is cause for particular concern. Since the root causes of the metabolic syndrome (overweight/obesity and physical inactivity) are reversible and the individual components of the metabolic syndrome are modifiable, recognition of the metabolic syndrome provides the opportunity for risk reduction in this high-risk group of patients. Since all of the components of the metabolic syndrome may be improved by weight reduction and increased physical activity, this remains the cornerstone of therapy. A diagnosis of the metabolic syndrome provides early identification of individuals at accelerated risk for development of diabetes and CVD, and therefore an earlier opportunity to intervene.

REFERENCES

1. Third Report of the National Cholesterol Education Program (NCEP) Expert Panel on Detection, Evaluation, and Treatment of High Blood Cholesterol in Adults (Adult Treatment Panel III) Final Report. *Circulation* 2002;106:3146–3421.

2. Grundy SM, Cleeman JI, Daniels SR, et al. Diagnosis and management of the metabolic syndrome. An American Heart Association/National Heart, Lung, and Blood Institute Scientific Statement. *Circulation* 2005;112:2735–2752.

3. Grundy SM, Brewer HB Jr, Cleeman JI, et al. for the Conference Participants. Definition of Metabolic Syndrome: Report of the National Heart, Lung, and Blood Institute/American Heart Association Conference on Scientific Issues Related to Definition. *Circulation* 2004;109:433–438.

4. Ferrannini E, Haffner SM, Mitchell BD, et al. Hyperinsulinaemia: the key feature of a cardiovascular and metabolic syndrome. *Diabetologia* 1991;34:416–422.

5. Ford ES. The metabolic syndrome and mortality from cardiovascular disease and all-causes: findings from the National Health and Nutrition Examination Survey II Mortality Study. *Atherosclerosis* 2004;173:309–314.

6. Cameron AJ, Shaw JE, Zimmet PZ. The metabolic syndrome: prevalence in worldwide populations. *Endocrinol Metab Clin North Am* 2004;33:351–375.

7. Lakka HM, Laaksonen DE, Lakka TA, et al. The metabolic syndrome and total and cardiovascular disease mortality in middle-aged men. *JAMA* 2002;288: 2709–2716.

8. Ridker PM, Buring JE, Cook NR, et al. C-reactive protein, the metabolic syndrome, and risk of incident cardiovascular events: an 8-year follow-up of 14,719 initially healthy American women. *Circulation* 2003;107:391–397.

9. Alexander CM, Landsman PB, Teutsch SM, et al. Third National Health and Nutrition Survey (NHANES III); National Cholesterol Education Program (NCEP). NCEP-defined metabolic syndrome, diabetes, and prevalence of coronary heart disease among NHANES III participants age 50 years and older. *Diabetes* 2003;52:1210–1214.

10. Wilson PWF, D'Agostino RB, Parise H, et al. Metabolic syndrome as a precursor of cardiovascular disease and type 2 diabetes mellitus. *Circulation* 2005;112:3066–3072.

11. Kahn R, Buse J, Ferrannini E, et al. The metabolic syndrome: time for a critical reappraisal. Joint statement from the American Diabetes Association and the European Association for the Study of Diabetes. *Diabetes Care* 2005;28:2289–2304.

12. Alberti G. Introduction to the metabolic syndrome. *Eur Heart J* 2005;7(Suppl D): D3–D5.

13. Reaven GM. Banting lecture 1988. Role of insulin resistance in human disease. *Diabetes* 1988;37:1595–1607.

14. World Health Organization: definition, diagnosis and classification of diabetes mellitus and its complications: report of a WHO consultation. Part 1: diagnosis and classification of diabetes mellitus. Geneva: World Health Organization, 1999. Available at: http://www.staff.ncl.ac.uk/philip.home/who_dmg.pdf. Accessed March 7, 2006.

15. Vikram NK, Pandey RM, Misra A, et al. Non-obese (body mass index < 25 kg/m2) Asian Indians with normal waist circumference have high cardiovascular risk. *Nutrition* 200319(6):503–509.

16. Ford ES, Giles WH, Dietz WH. Prevalence of the metabolic syndrome among US adults: findings from the Third National Health and Nutritional Examination Survey. *JAMA* 2002;287:356–359.

17. Hall WD, Clark LT, Wenger NK, et al. The metabolic syndrome in African Americans: a review. *Ethn Dis* 2003;13:414–428.

18. Grundy SM. Obesity, metabolic syndrome, and coronary atherosclerosis. *Circulation* 2002;105:2696–2698.

19. The Expert Committee on the Diagnosis and Classification of Diabetes Mellitus: follow-up report on the diagnosis of diabetes mellitus. *Diabetes Care* 2003;26:3160–3167.

20. Einhorn D, Reaven GM, Cobin RH, et al. American College of Endocrinology position statement on the insulin resistance syndrome. *Endocr Pract* 2003;9:237–252.

21. International Diabetes Federation. Worldwide definition of the metabolic syndrome. Available at: http://www.idf.org/webdata/docs/IDF_Metasyndrome_definition.pdf. February 12, 2006.

22. Ford ES. Rarer than a blue moon: the use of a diagnostic code for the metabolic syndrome in the U.S. *Diabetes Care* 2005;28:1808–1809.

23. Girman CJ, Rhodes T, Mercuri M, et al. for the 4S Group, the AFCAPS/TexCAPS Research Group: the metabolic syndrome and risk of major coronary events in the Scandinavian Simvastatin Survival Study (4S) and the Air Force/Texas Coronary Atherosclerosis Prevention Study (AFCAPS/TexCAPS). *Am J Cardiol* 2004;93:136–141.

24. Hunt KJ, Resendez RG, Williams K, et al. National Cholesterol Education Program versus World Health Organization metabolic syndrome in relation to all-cause and cardiovascular mortality in the San Antonio Heart Study. *Circulation* 2004;110:1251–1257.

25. Isomaa B, Almgren P, Tuomi T, et al. Cardiovascular morbidity and mortality associated with the metabolic syndrome. *Diabetes Care* 2001;24:683–689.

26. Nigam A, Bourassa MG, Fortier A, et al. The metabolic syndrome and its components and the long-term risk of death in patients with coronary heart disease. *Am Heart J* 2006;151:514–521.

27. Kuusisto J, Lempiainen P, Mykkanen L, et al. Insulin resistance syndrome predicts coronary heart disease events in elderly type 2 diabetic men. *Diabetes Care* 2001;24:1629–1633.

28. Lempiainen P, Mykkanen L, Pyorala K, et al. Insulin resistance syndrome predicts coronary heart disease events in elderly non-diabetic men. *Circulation* 1999;100: 123–128.

29. Malik S, Wong ND, Franklin SS, et al. Impact of the metabolic syndrome on mortality from coronary heart disease, cardiovascular disease and on all causes in United States adults. *Circulation* 2004;110:1245–1250.

30. Onat A, Ceyhan K, Basar O, et al. Metabolic syndrome: major impact on coronary risk in a population with low cholesterol levels: a prospective and cross-sectional evaluation. *Atherosclerosis* 2002;165:285–292.

31. Pyorala M, Miettinen H, Halonen P, et al. Insulin resistance syndrome predicts the risk of coronary heart disease and stroke in healthy middle-aged men: the 22-year follow-up results of the Helsinki Policemen Study. *Arterioscler Thromb Vasc Biol* 2000;20:538–544.

32. Scuteri A, Najjar S, Morrell C, et al. The metabolic syndrome in older individuals: prevalence and prediction of cardiovascular events. *Diabetes Care* 2005;28:882–887.

33. Bruno G, Merletti F, Biggeri A, et al. for the Casale Monferrato Study. Metabolic syndrome as a predictor of all-cause and cardiovascular mortality in type 2 diabetes: the Casale Monferrato Study. *Diabetes Care* 2004;27:2689–2694.

34. Resnick HE, Jones K, Ruotolo G, et al. for the Strong Heart Study. Insulin resistance, the metabolic syndrome, and risk of incident cardiovascular disease in non-diabetic American Indians: the Strong Heart Study. *Diabetes Care* 2003;26:861–867.

35. Rosengren A, Hawken S, Ounpuu S, et al. Association of psychosocial risk factors with risk of acute myocardial infarction in 11119 cases and 13648 controls from 52 countries (the INTERHEART study): case-control study. *Lancet* 2004;364: 953–962.

36. Ilanne-Parikka P, Eriksson JG, Lindstrom J, et al. for the Finnish Diabetes Prevention Study Group. Prevalence of the metabolic syndrome and its components: findings from a Finnish general population sample and the Diabetes Prevention Study cohort. *Diabetes Care* 2004;27:2135–2140.

37. Relimpio F, Martinez-Brocca MA, Leal-Cerro A, et al. Variability in the presence of the metabolic syndrome in type 2 diabetic patients attending a diabetes clinic: influences of age and gender. *Diabetes Res Clin Pract* 2004;65:135–142.

38. Bonora E, Targher G, Formentini G, et al. Metabolic syndrome is an independent predictor of cardiovascular disease in type 2 diabetic subjects: prospective data from the Verona Diabetes Complications Study. *Diabet Med* 2004;21: 52–58.

39. Costa LA, Canani LH, Lisboa HR, et al. Aggregation of features of the metabolic syndrome is associated with increased prevalence of chronic complications in type 2 diabetes. *Diabet Med* 2004;21:252–255.

40. Sone H, Mizuno H, Fujii H, et al. Is the diagnosis of metabolic syndrome useful for predicting cardiovascular disease in Asian diabetic patients? Analysis from the Japan diabetes complications study. *Diabetes Care* 2005;28:1463–1471.

41. Sattar N, Gaw A, Scherbakova O, et al. Metabolic syndrome with and without C-reactive protein as a predictor of coronary heart disease and diabetes in the West of Scotland Coronary Prevention Study. *Circulation* 2003;108:414–419.

42. Klein BE, Klein R, Lee KE. Components of the metabolic syndrome and risk of cardiovascular disease and diabetes in Beaver Dam. *Diabetes Care* 2002;25: 1790–1794.

43. Lorenzo C, Okoloise M, Williams K, et al. The metabolic syndrome as predictor of type 2 diabetes: the San Antonio Heart Study. *Diabetes Care* 2003;26: 3153–3159.

44. Hanson RL, Imperatore G, Bennett PH, et al. Components of the "metabolic syndrome" and incidence of type 2 diabetes. *Diabetes* 2002;51:3120–3127.

45. Gabir MM, Hanson RL, Dabelea D, et al. The 1997 American Diabetes Association and 1999 World Health Organization criteria for hyperglycemia in the diagnosis and prediction of diabetes. *Diabetes Care* 2000;23:1108–1112.

46. Bonora E, Kiechl S, Willeit J, et al. Prevalence of insulin resistance in metabolic disorders: the Bruneck Study. *Diabetes* 1998;47:1643–1649.

47. Tominaga M, Eguchi H, Manaka H, et al. Impaired glucose tolerance is a risk factor for cardiovascular disease, but not impaired fasting glucose. The Funagata Diabetes Study. *Diabetes Care* 1999;22:920–924.

48. Grundy SM, Cleeman JI, Bairey Merz CN, et al. Implications of recent clinical trials for the National Cholesterol Education Program Adult Treatment Panel III guidelines. *Circulation* 2004;110:227–239.

49. Clark LT, Ferdinand KC, Ferdinand DP, et al. Contemporary Management of the Metabolic Syndrome 2005: Special Focus: Implications for the Diabetic and Prediabetic Patient. Association of Black Cardiologists, Inc and McMahon Publishing Group, 2005. Available at: www.abcardio.org

50. Wong ND, Pio JR, Franklin SS, et al. Preventing coronary events by optimal control of blood pressure and lipids in patients with the metabolic syndrome. *Am J Cardiol* 2003;91:1421–1426.

51. Pi-Sunyer FX. Pathophysiology and long-term management of the metabolic syndrome. *Obes Res* 2004;12:174S–180S.

52. Despres JP. The insulin resistance–dyslipidemic syndrome of visceral obesity: effect on patient's risk. *Obes Res* 1998;6:8S–17S.

53. Bjorntorp P. Body fat distribution, insulin resistance, and metabolic diseases. *Nutrition* 1997;13:795–803.

54. Brunzell JD, Hokanson JE. Dyslipidemia of central obesity and insulin resistance. *Diabetes Care* 1999;22:C10–C13.

55. Bonow RO. Primary prevention of cardiovascular disease: a call to action. *Circulation* 2002;106:3140–3141.

56. Reilly MP, Rader DJ. The metabolic syndrome: more than the sum of its parts? *Circulation* 2003;108:1546–1551.

57. Lüscher TF, Creager MA, Beckman JA, et al. Diabetes and vascular disease: pathophysiology, clinical consequences, and medical therapy: part II. *Circulation* 2003;108:1655–1661.

58. NHLBI Obesity Education Initiative Expert Panel. Clinical guidelines on the identification, evaluation, and treatment of overweight and obesity in adults: the evidence report. *Obes Res* 1998;6(Suppl 2):51S–209S.

59. Klein S, Burke LE, Bray GA, et al. AHA Scientific Statement. Clinical implications of obesity with specific focus on cardiovascular disease. *Circulation* 2004;110: 2952–2967.

60. Gordon DJ, Probstfield JL, Garrison RJ, et al. High-density lipoprotein cholesterol and cardiovascular disease: four prospective American studies. *Circulation* 1989;79:8–15.

61. Assmann G, Schulte H. Relation of high-density lipoprotein cholesterol and triglycerides to incidence of atherosclerotic coronary artery disease (the PRO-CAM experience). *Am J Cardiol* 1992;70:733–737.

62. Austin MA. Plasma triglyceride as a risk factor for cardiovascular disease. *Can J Cardiol* 1998;14(Suppl B):14B–17B.

63. Boden WE. High-density lipoprotein cholesterol as an independent risk factor in cardiovascular disease: assessing the data from Framingham to the Veterans Affairs High-Density Lipoprotein Intervention Trial. *Am J Cardiol* 2000;86:19L–22L.

64. Chobanian AV, Bakris GL, Black HR, et al. The Seventh Report of the Joint National Committee on Prevention, Detection, Evaluation, and Treatment of High Blood Pressure: the JNC7 Report. *JAMA* 2003;289:2560–2571.

65. Pearson TA, Blair SN, Daniels SR, et al. AHA guidelines for primary prevention of cardiovascular disease and stroke. 2002 Update: consensus panel guide to comprehensive risk reduction for adult patients without coronary or other atherosclerotic vascular diseases. American Heart Association Science Advisory and Coordinating Committee. *Circulation* 2002;106:388–391.

66. Smith SC, Blair SN, Bonow RO, et al. AHA/ACC guidelines for preventing heart attack and death in patients with atherosclerotic cardiovascular disease. 2001 Update: a statement for healthcare professionals from the American Heart Association and the American College of Cardiology. *Circulation* 2001;104:1577–1579.

67. Clark LT. Issues in minority health: atherosclerosis and coronary heart disease in African Americans. *Med Clin North Am* 2005;89:977–1001.

68. Clark LT, Ferdinand KC, Flack JM, et al. Coronary heart disease in African Americans. *Heart Dis* 2001;3:97–108.

69. Rowland ML, Fulwood R. Coronary heart disease risk factor trends in blacks between the First and Second National Health and Nutrition Examination Surveys, United States, 1971–1980. *Am Heart J* 1984;108:771–779.

70. Cutter GR, Burke GL, Dyer AR, et al. Cardiovascular risk factors in young adults. The CARDIA baseline monograph. *Control Clin Trials* 1991;12:1S–77S.

71. Hutchinson RG, Watson RL, Davis CE, et al. Racial differences in risk factors for atherosclerosis. The ARIC study. *Angiology* 1997;48:279–290.

72. Hall WD, Watkins LO, Wright JT, et al. The metabolic syndrome: recognition and management. *Dis Manag* 2006;9(1):16–33.

73. Smith SC Jr, Clark LT, Cooper RS, et al. Discovering the full spectrum of cardiovascular disease: Minority Health Summit 2003: Report of the Obesity, Metabolic Syndrome, and Hypertension Writing Group. *Circulation* 2005;111:e134–e139.

74. Taylor H. Metabolic syndrome in African Americans, elderly. Jackson Heart Study and Metabolic Syndrome. AHA Scientific Sessions, 2005.

75. The Hispanic Population in the United States: March 2000. U.S. Census Bureau, Population Division, Ethnic & Hispanic Statistics Branch. Available at: http://www.census.gov/population/www/socdemo/hispanic/ho00.html. Accessed March 8, 2006.

76. Hunt KJ, Williams K, Resendez RG, et al. All-cause and cardiovascular mortality among diabetic participants in the San Antonio Heart Study: evidence against the Hispanic Paradox. *Diabetes Care* 2002;25(9):1557–1563.

77. Markides KS, Coreil J. The health of Hispanics in the southwestern United States: an epidemiologic paradox. *Public Health Rep* 1986;101:253–265.

78. Liao Y, Cooper RS, Cao G, et al. Mortality from coronary heart disease and cardiovascular disease among adult U.S. Hispanics: findings from the National Health Interview Survey (1986 to 1994). *J Am Coll Cardiol* 1997;30:1200–1205.

79. Lee ET, Howard BV, Savage PJ, et al. Diabetes and impaired glucose tolerance in three American Indian populations aged 45–74 years: the Strong Heart Study. *Diabetes Care* 1995;18:599–610.

80. Howard BV, Lee ET, Cowan LD, et al. Rising tide of cardiovascular disease in American Indians: the Strong Heart Study. *Circulation* 1999;99:2389–2395.

81. Burchfiel CM, Sharp DS, Curb DJ, et al. Hyperinsulinemia and cardiovascular disease in elderly men. *Arterioscler Thromb Vasc Biol* 1998;18:450–457.

82. Tan C, Ma S, Wai D, et al. Can we apply the National Cholesterol Education Program Adult Treatment Panel definition of the metabolic syndrome to Asians? *Diabetes Care* 2004;27:1182–1186.

83. The Asian Population: 2000 (Census 2000 Brief). Issued February 2002. Available at: http://www.census.gov/prod/2002pubs/c2kbr01-16.pdf. Accessed March 8, 2006.

84. Enas EA. Clinical implications: dyslipidemia in the Asian Indian population. Monograph was adapted from material presented at the 20th Annual Convention of the American Association of Physicians of Indian Origin, Chicago, IL, 2002. Available at: http://www.cadiresearch.com/downloads/AAPImonograph.pdf. Accessed March 8, 2006.

CARDIOVASCULAR DISEASE AND HYPERGLYCEMIA: RATIONALE AND APPROACHES TO TREATMENT

Mary Ann Banerji

INTRODUCTION

Diabetes is a multifaceted disorder. Accelerated cardiovascular disease (CVD) is one of the most important complications of diabetes. Although the hallmark of diabetes is hyperglycemia, it has been difficult to separate its contribution to the increased CV risk from the traditional and nontraditional risk factors.

The first part of this chapter presents the evidence for hyperglycemia's key role in increased CV risk, increased inflammation, and oxidative stress. The second part addresses the principles of treating hyperglycemia in the context of CVD. This is the most complex and vexing aspect of diabetes treatment. Although treatment also includes targeting blood pressure, lipids, inflammation, insulin resistance and prothrombotic states as well as good nutrition, appropriate physical activity, and the absence of tobacco smoking, these are beyond the scope of this chapter.

DOES GLYCEMIC CONTROL MATTER IN CORONARY ARTERY DISEASE? THE EVIDENCE

Epidemiologic Studies

Type 2 diabetes is associated with increased CV risk and adverse outcomes associated with myocardial infarction (MI).[1] Overall, approximately 20% of patients with CVD are known to have diabetes; of these, 75% die of CVD.

Population studies have reported that diabetes is associated with a four- to fivefold increase in the prevalence of heart disease compared to individuals without diabetes.[2-6] Lesser degrees of glucose intolerance or impaired glucose tolerance as well as blood glucose values in the upper range of "normal" have also been associated with increased CVD (Fig. 15-1).[7-9] Long-term follow-up of type 2 diabetes patients in the United Kingdom Prospective Diabetes Study (UKPDS) found that higher blood sugars were associated with greater macro- and microvascular complications.[10]

Numerous studies report that hyperglycemia is an independent risk factor for mortality during an acute myocardial infarction (AMI) and a key risk factor for the subsequent development of heart failure.[11,12] Indeed, in the postthrombolytic era, hyperglycemia of 198 mg/dL predicts in-hospital and 12-month mortality, irrespective of a presenting diagnosis of diabetes.[13]

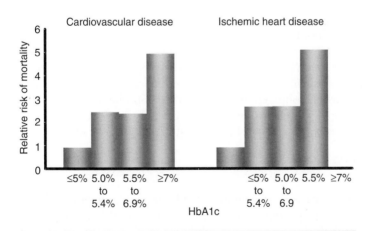

Figure 15-1 **Glycemic control and the risk of mortality as it relates to CVD. *P < 0.001 age-adjusted death rates for linear trend.** (Source: Adapted from Khaw K-T, Wareham N, Luben R, et al. Glycated haemoglobin, diabetes, and mortality in men in the Norfolk cohort of European Prospective Investigation of Cancer and Nutrition (EPIC-Norfolk). Br Med J 2001;322:15–18.)

Similarly, a study of nondiabetic individuals at even lower levels of hyperglycemia, above and below 133 mg/dL, reported significant differences in 2-year survival and reinfarction rates after an AMI.[14] Bolk et al.'s data confirm this: glycemia predicted mortality after a MI at levels of 140 mg/dL.[15] In a North American multicenter study, a history of diabetes alone conferred a twofold higher mortality following an MI and was similar in risk as a history of a prior MI compared with neither; the presence of both was associated with a four- to sixfold increase in mortality compared with neither.[16] This is similar to Whiteley et al.'s data from Scotland and replicates the findings of Haffner et al.[17,18]

Individuals with diabetes have more extensive coronary artery disease (CAD) with one study reporting 42% with three-vessel disease compared with 30% in nondiabetics.[19] With thrombolysis and early revascularization, the endpoints of mortality and MI have improved for diabetics, but not to the same degree as for nondiabetics (decrease in mortality from 30 to 21% in diabetics compared with 12 to 9% for nondiabetics).[20]

The exact glycemic threshold for increased congestive heart failure (CHF) and in-hospital mortality in patients with AMI is not known, although presenting plasma glucoses of 110 mg/dL or greater conferred increased risk with or without diabetes.[21] Some consider elevated blood glucose during an AMI to be an epiphenomenon and therefore not significant. However, using an oral glucose tolerance test (OGTT), Norhammar et al. found that levels of hyperglycemia and glucose intolerance at the time of discharge among patients with AMI and no known history of diabetes were equally divided into normal, impaired, and diabetic and that these groups were virtually unchanged 3 months later.[22] Fully two-thirds of the patients had some form of glucose intolerance underscoring the high prevalence of this phenomenon in patients with AMI. Bartnik et al. went on to highlight that the two-thirds (67%) with abnormal glucose tolerance had a high degree of adverse CV endpoints when followed for 34 months.[23] Similar data were reported by Stranders et al.[24] High frequencies of glucose intolerance (82%) have also been reported among Asian Indians with AMI without known diabetes.[25]

Intervention Studies

DIABETES

If hyperglycemia is associated with adverse CV outcomes, does lowering blood sugar improve outcome? Few good studies address this question using intensive glycemic management while controlling for other known CV risk factors. The Action to Control Cardiovascular Risk in Diabetes (ACCORD) study is a National Institutes of Health (NIH) funded trial currently underway and designed to investigate whether glycemic control in conjunction with blood pressure and lipid control affects CVD outcomes in type 2 diabetes.[26]

The UKPDS, begun in the 1970s, was a large randomized-controlled trial of approximately 15,000 newly identified patients with type 2 diabetes.

Intensive glycemic regulation failed to show improvement in mortality. In hindsight, this is unsurprising, as the level of glycemic control was inadequate; changes in treatment were made only when the fasting plasma glucose (FPG) was >270 mg/dL. Predictably, the epidemiologic analysis of the study showed a strong association of glycemia with macro and microvascular complications.[27] Among type 1 diabetes, long-term follow-up of patients who had intensive compared to conventional glycemic treatment in the Diabetes Control and Complications Trial (DCCT), had 50% fewer CV events.[28] Thus, improved glycemic control can ameliorate CV outcomes in both type 1 and type 2 diabetes.

ACUTE MYOCARDIAL INFARCTION

Does intensive glycemic control matter in an AMI? Several studies shed light on this and raise new questions. In 1962, Sodi-Pallares et al. thought that infusions of glucose, insulin, and potassium (GIK) might stabilize electrical activity of the myocardium, decrease arrhythmias, and improve myocardial metabolism.[29] A subsequent series of small studies, largely in the prethrombolytic era, used this approach with variable success. A meta-analysis of nine of the studies (1900 patients) concluded that GIK compared to placebo significantly reduced in-hospital mortality (21% vs. 16%) and estimated that 49 lives were saved for every 1000 patients treated.[30] Only two were randomized-controlled trials and only one used reperfusion methods. One study in patients with STEMI (ST elevation myocardial infarction) showed a 30% decrease in mortality when the GIK infusion volume was decreased.[31]

In the era of reperfusion, the ECLA (Estudios Cardiologicos Latinoamerica) reported pilot data showing a 66% reduction in AMI mortality in Europeans using GIK in patients who received reperfusion treatment.[32] Based on these data, the large international ECLA-CREATE trial of ~20,000 patients with AMI evolved respectively.[33] In contrast to the pilot data, this larger study showed no beneficial effect of GIK infusions compared to controls (mortality was 10% for both groups). Possible reasons include population differences (80% were Chinese, Indian, or Pakistani), delay in use of GIK infusions (4.7 hours after onset of symptom and 1 hour after reperfusion therapy), and overall high mortality rate of 10%. A possible explanation for this result is that, to be most effective, the GIK infusion should be started within 1 hour of symptom onset. Regional data were not presented in this study, making it difficult to assess whether a European or Asian bias might exist. In its favor is its large size since many smaller negative studies are frequently not published leading to the erroneous impression that the treatment is efficacious.

A Dutch study showed a 71% reduction in mortality when AMI patients without heart failure (80% of AMIs) were given GIK within 2 hours of symptom onset (mortality 1.2% vs. 4.2% for GIK vs. controls).[34]

These data raise the question of differences in study design, population, or "standard care" between the Dutch study, which found GIK treatment to reduce mortality, and the largely Asian ECLA-CREATE study, which did not (1.2% vs. 10.2%) reduce mortality with GIK infusion. A second Dutch study, Glucose-Insulin-Potassium Study 2 (GIPS-2), will prospectively test the efficacy of GIK in patients with AMI, without heart failure.

Results so far imply promise but important clinical questions remain, including the dose of GIK, the amount of fluid infused, the timing of its use (in animals models, GIK is very effective when used within 3–5 minutes of an occlusion), and the optimum population.

The first DIGAMI (Diabetes Mellitus, Insulin Glucose Infusion in Acute Myocardial Infarction) study used insulin infusions in patients with AMI and diabetes who were eligible for thrombolytic and beta-blocker therapy.[35] Following a 24-hour insulin infusion, patients received multidose insulin for 3 months; thereafter treatment was individualized. One and 3 years mortality rates were significantly reduced with insulin (29% relative reduction [18% vs. 26.1%] at 1 year). In patients without prior insulin use and low CV risk (age <70 years, no prior MI or CHF and no use of digoxin), use of the insulin infusion conferred a benefit as early as 3 months with a RR reduction of 52% ($P < 0.02$) at 1 year. Admission glucose was associated with higher mortality in both treatment groups.

In DIGAMI, it was not clear if the benefit of the insulin treatment was due to acute or long-term use. To test this, DIGAMI-2[36] randomized 1253 patients to one of three arms: (i) acute insulin, then long-term insulin-based glycemic control, (ii) insulin and glucose followed by standard glycemic control, and (iii) routine management. In addition, patients received "standard of care" therapies including aspirin, statins, angiotensin-converting enzyme inhibitor (ACEI), beta-blockers, thrombolytic agents, and revascularization. Unexpectedly, there were no significant differences in 2-year mortality among the three groups (23, 21, and 18%, respectively). The results did not support the hypothesis that acute insulin followed by long-term insulin was better than acute insulin therapy alone or that treatment with insulin and glucose was better than conventional treatment. These results are not surprising as in other studies, given the circumstances of the trial: (1) the glycemic treatment strategies did not result in differences in metabolic control as a large number of the conventionally controlled group received insulin, (2) target blood glucose levels were not achieved with intensive insulin treatment, and (3) there was an overall lower than expected mortality in the conventionally treated group (17.9% in 2 years). Importantly, epidemiologic analysis showed that higher glucoses were a predictor of long-term mortality.

CRITICAL CARE

With the role of hyperglycemia as a risk factor for mortality still not definitively decided, the Leuven group studied this question in a surgical intensive care unit (ICU) by randomizing patients to intensive and nonintensive glycemic control. In 2001, they published their landmark, single center study; it tested the effect of intensive glycemic regulation using IV insulin (compared to usual glycemic care) on mortality and morbidity in patients admitted to a surgical ICU.[37] Of the 1400 patients, approximately two-thirds had undergone cardiac surgery and ~16% had diabetes in each of the treatment groups. The insulin treatment strategies created two distinct groups based on blood sugars (mean 103 ± 19 mg/dL vs. 153 ± 33 mg/dL) and achieved a 58% reduction in mortality (4.6% vs. 8%) in the intensive group when compared to the nonintensive group. Interestingly, the most benefit was seen in patients who stayed in the ICU >5 days (Fig. 15-2).

In addition, a variety of secondary endpoints including need for transfusion, dialysis, ventilator support, multiorgan failure, polyneuropathy, and sepsis were markedly improved with intensive insulin treatment by 34–50%. Indeed, these data suggested that there was no threshold below which there was no further benefit; glucose of <6.1 mmol/L had significantly better outcomes than those at 6.1–8.3 mmol/L which were significantly better than those at >8.3 mmol/L.

These data were supported by data in cardiothoracic units where insulin-controlled glycemia resulted in improved outcomes such as sepsis and days spent in the ICU following surgery.[38] The Leuven study quickly became the

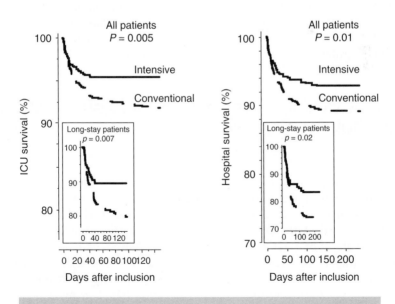

Figure 15-2 **Mortality: Kaplan-Meier plots.** (Source: Adapted from Van den Berghe G, Wouters P, Weekers F, et al. Intensive insulin therapy in critically ill patients. N Engl J Med 2001;345:1359–1367.)

standard-bearer for glycemic control in hospitalized patients, especially in the surgical ICU.

The Leuven group next addressed whether intensive glycemic control was beneficial in the medical ICU, where patients tend to be much sicker.[39] Using the same single center as the first study, patients who were expected to remain in the medical ICU for more than 3 days were randomized to intensive or conventional glycemic treatment using insulin infusions; they maintained one group with a blood sugar of 80–110 mg/dL, while the other group was treated only if they were above 215 mg/dL. Early parenteral nutritional support was provided. The overall hospital mortality was not different (40% vs. 37%) in the two groups. In the two groups, secondary end-points showed that with intensive treatment, morbidity was reduced for mechanical ventilation, acute renal injury, and earlier discharge from the hospital and ICU, especially in those who stayed longer than 5 days. Interestingly, in the two groups, in-hospital mortality was significantly reduced from 51 to 45% as well as morbidity.

Not all aspects of intensive glycemic regulation were beneficial. Patients who stayed less than 3 days actually had *higher* mortality rates if they received intensive insulin treatment. Hypoglycemia was associated with a 66% mortality in the intensive insulin treatment group and a 44% mortality in the conventionally treated group. The authors noted that risk factors for hypoglycemia were hepatic and renal failure and a >3 days ICU stay. Several other smaller studies have shown improved ICU outcomes with intensive glycemic regulation.[40] These data together raise important questions regarding identifying the ICU population most likely to benefit from intensive glycemic regulation, the level of glycemia, and the timing of the intervention.

HOW DOES INSULIN TREATMENT AND TIGHT GLYCEMIC CONTROL HELP SURVIVAL?

Mechanism of Action

Understanding possible mechanisms of action requires consideration of the metabolic effects of stress hormones and metabolism.

Normal myocardial metabolism uses free fatty acids (FFA) as fuel in the fasted state and switches to glucose during the "insulinized" fed state. Under the stress of a MI, catecholamines are released, cause an increase in lipolysis, and hence circulating FFAs. In addition, catecholamines cause a decrease in insulin secretion. Since insulin suppresses lipolysis, the decrease in insulin tends to further increase lipolysis and FFAs. During ischemia, the FFAs increase myocardial oxygen consumption, change calcium channel activity, and promote arrhythmias[41]; glucose uptake is reduced and energy production derives from FFAs. In this situation, the use of insulin would be expected to improve metabolism by decreasing lipolysis and FFA and increasing glucose uptake; this might explain some of the beneficial effects of insulin infusion therapy during acute coronary syndromes (ACS).

FREE FATTY ACIDS

FFAs inhibit glucose transporter 4 (GLUT-4) action and thereby reduce cellular glucose uptake and energy production. This occurs because FFAs phosphorylate serine kinases on insulin-receptor substrate 1 (IRS 1) of the post-insulin receptor cascade, decrease phosphorylation of the appropriate substrate tyrosine kinase, and in turn decrease phosphatidylinositol-3 (PI-3) kinase and GLUT-4 translocation from the intracellular space to the cell surface.[42] Increased FFAs also decrease myocardial energy or adenosine triphosphate (ATP) production through another mechanism. Mitochondrial energy production from glucose depends on glycolysis, with pyruvate being converted to acetyl CoA with oxidative phosphorylation producing ATP. Acetyl CoA is processed through the tricarboxylic acid (TCA) cycle and in the presence of oxygen, oxidative phosphorylation produces ATP. This process relies on a proton gradient across the inner mitochondrial membrane; when this gradient is diminished, ATP synthesis is impaired. Uncoupling proteins uncouple the protons from oxidative phosphorylation, diminishing the gradient and losing the protons to heat rather than generating ATP.[43] Studies in human heart tissue have correlated increased plasma FFAs with a decrease in myocardial uncoupling protein 2 and 3 as well as decrease GLUT-4 transporters supporting the concept that increased FFA levels are associated with decreased myocardial energy production.[44]

GLUCOSE, INSULIN, STRESS, AND INFLAMMATION

Stress hormones increase gluconeogenesis, reduce insulin secretion and cellular glucose uptake. Under normal circumstances, intracellular glucose goes through the Krebs cycle and undergoes oxidative phosphorylation to produce ATP as well as small amounts of superoxide. An important intracellular regulator is nitric oxide (NO). NO is generated by the action of nitric oxide synthase (NOS) on L-arginine. There are several forms of NOS. Constitutively active forms present in low levels are eNOS (endothelial NOS) and nNOS (neuronal NOS). These forms are associated with low levels of NO and are involved with antiapoptosis in some cell types and vasodilatation. Inducible NOS or iNOS can be induced in all cells under certain circumstances and results in high levels of NO which is associated with apoptosis and cytotoxicity.[45] High blood sugars result in higher amounts of superoxide and reactive oxygen species (ROS). This superoxide combines with intracellular NO to produce peroxynitrite which adds nitrites to key proteins in the mitochondrial respiratory chain. This leads to decreased electron transport activity and decreased ATP production.[46] Glucose also increases nuclear factor-kappa B (NF-κB) which increases inflammatory cytokines, markers of endothelial dysfunction (E-selectin and ICAM), and iNOS. Hypoxia and increased cytokines also increase peroxynitrite.

In contrast, insulin has opposite effects: decreases superoxide, cytokines, iNOS, and matrix metalloproteinase-9 (MMP-9) and promoting vasodilatation, and decreased inflammation.[47] By decreasing blood sugar, insulin may have beneficial effects at many different mechanisms. These concepts agree with the Leuven study in which intensive insulin treatment and blood sugar control prevented liver mitochondrial damage as well as morbidity and mortality.[48]

Gao et al. tested the individual components of the GIK infusion to determine what factor preserved myocardium. Using the ischemia-reperfusion model of rat myocardium, they found that insulin was responsible for the beneficial effects.[44] Insulin activated the PI-3 kinase-Akt pathway demonstrating that even in the ischemia-reperfusion model this pathway is preserved. Akt in turn phosphorylated eNOS, increasing NO production. This was associated with decreased apoptosis and increased myocardial survival.

In addition to lowering blood glucose, preventing lipolysis and increased FFAs, insulin may have direct salutary effects. These include improvements in lipids, inflammation, and endothelial function. In the Leuven study, poor outcomes were associated with elevated triglycerides, low high-density lipoprotein (HDL), and low-density lipoprotein (LDL) cholesterol levels. Use of insulin and glycemic regulation resulted in reversal of these findings. Improvement in dyslipidemia accounted for a large part of the beneficial effect of insulin on death and organ failure.[49] The explanation for this is unclear but may involve the role of lipoproteins as scavenger molecules.[50,51]

It is also possible for insulin treatment to be detrimental. This could occur if the PI-3 kinase pathway was inhibited (as in insulin resistance) to the extent that excess insulin stimulated the still responsive mitogen-activated protein (MAP) kinase pathway and might explain increased vascular abnormalities.[49] Clinical data on the use of exogenous insulin use do not support this; it is possible that it occurs in some subgroups. Finally, the beneficial effects of insulin treatment could be abolished in case of excessive hypoglycemia and consequent morbidity.

HYPERGLYCEMIA AND PANCREATIC BETA-CELL DYSFUNCTION IN TYPE 2 DIABETES

Effect of Intensive Insulin Treatment

A recent study reported a high prevalence of abnormal glucose tolerance in patients who had an AMI. OGTT at the time of discharge from the hospital and 3 months later showed that one-third of the patients had impaired glucose tolerance [IGT], one-third had diabetes, and one-third had normal glucose tolerance.[52] Patients identified as type 2 diabetes were more insulin resistant than those who were normal. Importantly, beta-cell function was worse with worsening glucose tolerance and correlated with higher admission blood glucose levels. Just as an improved metabolic milieu is beneficial both for overall survival and for organ function in general, it is likely to be beneficial for pancreatic beta-cell function as well. Hyperglycemia has been shown to be associated with beta-cell apoptosis, inflammation, oxidative stress, and decreased insulin production and secretion.[53] Improved beta-cell function is likely then to decrease CV disease.

REMISSION OF NEW-ONSET DIABETES WITH INTENSIVE INSULIN THERAPY

Normalization of blood sugar reverses beta-cell abnormalities in a rodent model.[53] Data in patients with new-onset hyperglycemia are consistent with the concept that an improved metabolic milieu may ameliorate the beta-cell dysfunction and hyperglycemia found in two-thirds of patients who present with an AMI. Our data show that a period of intensive glycemic control in newly identified African American individuals with type 2 diabetes may induce long-lasting remission of hyperglycemia in 40–50% of patients.[54–56] The remissions last a median of 3 1/2 years. Although glycemic control is most easily achieved with multiple insulin injections it also may occur with oral sulfonylurea or diet therapy.[57] Similar data are reported in whites, Turks, Chinese, and animal models suggesting that remission may be a ubiquitous phenomenon.[53,58–60] Normalization of hyperglycemia appears to reverse beta-cell decline and preserve beta-cell function through reducing beta-cell inflammation and oxidative stress. Importantly however, this reversal of beta-cell decline does not occur in any model if the duration of hyperglycemia has been prolonged.

These data suggest that intensive glycemic control instituted at the time diabetes is identified results in improved pancreatic beta-cell function, overall long-term improved glycemia, and decreased CV morbidity and mortality.

APPROACHES TO TREATMENT OF HYPERGLYCEMIA IN PATIENTS WITH DIABETES AND CARDIOVASCULAR DISEASE

This section will review the diagnosis of diabetes, goals of treatment, and approaches to the management hyperglycemia in diabetes

Diagnosis of Diabetes and Glucose Intolerance

- The diagnosis of diabetes is made in one of three ways:
  1. FPG >126 mg/dL
  2. Random blood glucose >200 mg/dL plus symptoms
  3. Two-hour glucose after 75 g of oral glucose (OGTT) >200 mg/dL

- The diagnosis of impaired glucose tolerance is made by:
  Two-hour glucose after 75 g of oral glucose (OGTT) >140 and <200 mg/dL
- The diagnosis of impaired fasting glucose is made by:
  A FPG >100 mg/dL

The cornerstone of treating hyperglycemia in diabetes involves medical nutrition therapy or diet, increased physical activity, and pharmacologic agents targeting the major physiologic alterations in diabetes. The glycemic target measured is a biologic marker, the glycosylated hemoglobin or A1c level, which reflects an integrated glycemic excursion of both the fasting and postprandial plasma (PP) glucoses.[60] Home monitoring of blood glucose is ideal to optimize glycemic control.

Review of Altered Physiology in Diabetes

Key physiologic abnormalities include insulin resistance and decreased insulin secretion. Insulin resistance is present in both diabetes and obesity and is associated with many of the CV risk factors found in diabetes.

How can insulin deficiency coexist with hyperinsulinemia in type 2 diabetes? Insulin resistance is a state in which a given amount of insulin fails to lower blood sugar. The blood sugar then increases and stimulates the secretion of more insulin; in the presence of this increased insulin, the blood sugar normalizes but at the expense of a higher ambient insulin level. This process may continue indefinitely without the development of hyperglycemia. However, patients who are unable to maintain this compensatory increase in beta-cell secretion have a fall in insulin levels relative to this increased requirement leading to a rise in blood sugar. At this point, the diagnosis of diabetes can be made. Initially, only postprandial glucose becomes elevated but as time goes on, the liver becomes dysregulated and the FPG rises as a result of deranged insulin and glucagon effects. An elevated FPG reflects increased endogenous glucose output, largely from the liver. Normally, insulin suppresses hepatic glucose output; in diabetes, inadequate levels of insulin result in fasting hyperglycemia. Glucagon is a counterregulatory hormone normally secreted to counteract hypoglycemia by increasing hepatic glucose output to raise the blood sugar. Glucagon is increased in diabetes and contributes to increased blood sugar. A recently appreciated component of glucose metabolism involves incretins, such as glucagon-like peptide-1 (GLP-1) and glucose-dependent insulinotropic polypeptide (GIP). Incretins, especially GLP-1, are hormones from the L cells of the intestines, secreted during meals which have pleotrophic effects. GLP-1 increases insulin release in a glucose-dependent manner, decreases glucagon, slows gastric emptying time, increases satiety, and decreases weight. GLP-1 is decreased in diabetes.

The key distinguishing feature of type 2 diabetes is an absolute or relative insulin deficiency. Other abnormalities include elevated glucagon, decreased incretins, and elevated FFA levels (worsens insulin resistance and may decrease insulin secretion).

Any *therapeutic strategy* must address the insulin deficiency of diabetes. This can be accomplished using insulin itself or by increasing pancreatic beta-cell insulin production with secretagogues such as sulfonylureas and meglitinides. Alternatively, the need for insulin can be decreased using insulin sensitizers such as metformin or the thiazolidinediones. Decreasing insulin resistance using these agents will not improve glycemia if the patient does not produce at least a minimum amount of insulin. Newer drugs alter the glucagon excess and involve intestinal hormones.

PHARMACOLOGIC TREATMENT OF DIABETES IN PATIENTS WITH CARDIOVASCULAR DISEASE

This section discusses glycemic management by the type of patient the clinician is likely to encounter: (1) ACS, (2) CVD, and (3) CHF.

Patients with Acute Coronary Syndromes (Including Patients in the ICU)

GLYCEMIC GOALS OF TREATMENT

A guiding principle should be a target glucose level as low as possible without compromising patient safety.

The normal FPG ranges from 70 to 100 mg/dL. The diagnosis of diabetes is made with either a FPG >126 mg/dL or a 2-hour blood glucose >200 mg/dL during an OGTT on two separate occasions. Impaired glucose tolerance is defined as either fasting glucose of >100 mg/dL or a 2-hour blood glucose of 140–200 mg/dL during an OGTT. Within this context, the immediate question concerns the goal for blood sugar in patients with diabetes.

In patients with *ACS and diabetes*, there is no established evidenced-based target for glycemia. The evidence suggests that adverse CV events occur at blood glucose levels which are lower than those causing microvascular complications. A composite of several studies suggest that levels of 80–120 mg/dL would be a reasonable target. It is critical to identify hyperglycemia in individuals who are admitted for ACS. It is no longer acceptable to ignore the blood glucose as simply a response to stress.

Evidence presented earlier argues for intensive glycemic regulation. In the coronary care unit (CCU) or the medical intensive care unit (MICU) this is most consistently accomplished using insulin.

Insulin

If the patient has diagnosed diabetes and is on insulin, the dose should be adjusted to optimize glycemia. Both type 1 or type 2 diabetes patients require increased insulin because of associated stress.

Even without a diagnosis of diabetes if the blood glucose is elevated on more than one occasion, the patient should be treated with insulin. Insulin can be administered either using a basal and prandial approach or a continuous insulin drip. The traditional "sliding scale insulin," although easy, should not be used because of its unacceptably high rates of hypoglycemia and overall poorer outcomes compared to prospectively administered insulin regimes.

Continuous insulin infusion

The advantages of a continuous insulin infusion are ease of adjustment and a rapid response time (Table 15-1).[61] The disadvantage is the need for frequent glycemic monitoring. While they are conceptually straightforward, they do require significant education of staff members on the treatment team since it is more labor intensive. There are many stakeholders to bring together including nurses, technicians, pharmacists, physicians, and other providers as well as administrators. A person assigned to act as a diabetes champion may be an approach to mobilizing and maintaining changes in the culture of diabetes care in the CCU and ICU (as well as on the wards and outpatient settings). There are also cost considerations since insulin infusions are labor intensive. However, better clinical outcomes and shorter ICU stays especially following postcoronary artery bypass grafting may argue for this approach.[38]

Transitioning to subcutaneous insulin from a continuous insulin infusion

Once patients with an ACS have stabilized clinically, continuous insulin should be discontinued and glycemia managed using intermittent subcutaneous insulin injections such as the basal-prandial and other approaches. Patients on insulin pumps should be continued on this.

Basal-prandial insulin approach or basal-bolus

It is an alternative to the continuous insulin infusion *or* the next step after continuous insulin infusion (see Table 15-2 for calculations). The principle behind this approach is that there is a basal glucose need for insulin (largely based on hepatic glucose output) and a prandial need for insulin (to deal with meal-related rises in blood sugar). A basal dose of long-acting insulin (glargine) is used with short-acting insulin (insulin aspart or lys-pro) administered before meals. The basal dose is usually 50% and the prandial doses ~ 0.15% of the total daily insulin requirements. The total daily insulin requirement is calculated as 0.5 weight in kilograms. The objective of the prandial dose of insulin is to take care of the meal-associated rise in blood glucose. The objective of the basal dose of insulin is to take care of the fasting and plasma glucose levels between meals (largely suppressing hepatic glucose production). If the blood glucose before a meal is elevated then a correction dose may be added to the amount calculated for that meal. The advantage is

Table 15-1   **Algorithm to Calculate an Intravenous Insulin Drip Using Regular Insulin**

General Guidelines: **Goal BG** = _____ (Usually 80–180 mg/dL)
- Standard drip: 100 units/100 mL 0.9% NaCl via an infusion device
- Surgical patients who have received an oral diabetes medication within 24 h should start when BG >120 mg/dL. All other patients can start when BG ≥70
- Insulin infusions should be discontinued when a patient is eating AND has received first dose of subcutaneous insulin

Intravenous Fluids:

- Most patients will need 5–10 GM of glucose per hour
  - D_5W or D_5W 1/2 NS at 100–200 mL/h or equivalent (TPN and enteral feeds)

Initiating the Infusion:
- **Algorithm 1:** Start here for most patients.
- **Algorithm 2:** For patients not controlled with Algorithm 1, or start here if s/p CABG, s/p solid organ transplant or islet cell transplant, receiving glucocorticoids, or patient with diabetes receiving >80 units/day of insulin as an outpatient.
- **Algorithm 3:** For patients not controlled on Algorithm 2. NO PATIENTS START HERE without authorization from the endocrine service.
- **Algorithm 4:** For patients not controlled on Algorithm 3. NO PATIENTS START HERE.
- Patients not controlled with the above algorithms need an endocrine consult.

Algorithm 1		Algorithm 2		Algorithm 3		Algorithm 4	
BG	Units/h	BGl	Units/h	BG	Units/h	BG	Units/h
<60 = Hypoglycemia (see below for treatment)							
<70	Off	<70	Off	<70	1	<70	Off
70–109	0.2	70–109	0.5	70–109	2	70–109	1.5
110–119	0.5	110–119	1	110–119	3	110–119	3
120–149	1	120–149	1.5	120–149	4	120–149	5
150–179	1.5	150–179	2	150–179	5	150–179	7
180–209	2	180–209	3	180–209	6	180–209	9
210–239	2	210–239	4	210–239	7	210–239	12
240–269	3	240–269	5	240–269	8	240–269	16
270–299	3	270–299	6	270–299	10	270–299	20
300–329	4	300–329	7	300–329	12	300–329	24
330–359	4	330–359	8	330–359	14	330–359	28
>360	6	>360	12	>360	16	>360	

Table 15-1   **Algorithm to Calculate an Intravenous Insulin Drip Using Regular Insulin (Continued)**

Moving from Algorithm to Algorithm:
- Moving Up: An algorithm failure is defined as blood glucose outside the goal range (see above goal), and the blood glucose does not change by at least 60 mg/dL within 1 h.
- Moving Down: When blood glucose is <70 mg/dL × 2.

Patient Monitoring:
- Check capillary BG every hour until it is within goal range for 4 h, then decrease to every 2 h for 4 h, and if remains stable may decrease to every 4 h.
- Hourly monitoring may be indicated for critically ill patients even if they have stable blood glucose.

Treatment of Hypoglycemia **(BG <60 mg/dL):**
- Discontinue insulin drip AND
- Give $D_{50}W$ IV
  Patient awake: 25 mL (1/2 amp)
  Patient not awake: 50 mL (1 amp)]
- Recheck BG every 20 min and repeat 25 mL of $D_{50}W$ IV if <60 mg/dL. Restart drip once blood glucose is >70 mg/dL × 2 checks. Restart drip with lower algorithm (see moving down)

Notify the Physician:
- For any blood glucose change >100 mg/dL in 1 h.
- For blood glucose >360 mg/dL

For hypoglycemia which has not resolved within 20 min of administering 50 mL of $D_{50}W$ IV and discontinuing the insulin drip.

Adapted from Ref. 61.

that meal times can be flexible, especially if patients have decreased appetites or procedures that make them unable to eat at fixed times. The disadvantage is that too high a basal dose of long-acting insulin may result in hypoglycemia. Table 15-2 lists an approach to calculating basal and prandial doses of insulin as well as correction doses.

Other subcutaneous insulin regimens

(a) Another alternative is the use of *subcutaneous regular insulin* every 6 hours. Its advantage is that it avoids long-acting insulin in situations when the daily requirement may not be known or if the clinical situation is unstable. The disadvantage is the need for on-time meals to coincide with insulin peaks Duration of insulin and their peak times of action are listed in Table 15-3. (b) Finally, regular insulin may be combined with NPH and used

Table 15-2 **Calculating the Basal and Prandial Insulin Dose**

Dose	Example (78-kg Adult)
Basal (~50% of total daily dose [TDD] of insulin) 0.2–0.5 units/kg/day	16–35 units/day
Prandial 0.1 unit/kg/meal	8 units/meal
Correction (add to the prandial dose)	
If blood glucose is 150–199 mg/dL, add 0.015 units/kg	1 unit/meal
If blood glucose is 200–299 mg/dL, add 0.07 units/kg	5 units/meal
If blood glucose is >300 mg/dL, add 0.1 units/kg	8 units/meal
Summary	
Basal insulin once a day	16 glargine once a day
At each meal: If the premeal glucose is <150 mg/dL	8 units aspart or lispro

as a two- or three-dose regimen to achieve glycemic control. While this can work, and for many years was the mainstay of treatment, the peak actions often coincide and make hypoglycemia more frequent. Meals are not flexible with this regimen. Finally, inhaled insulin[71] is a promising new approach to insulin delivery.

OTHER CONSIDERATIONS

It is difficult to predict what will happen to blood glucoses in patients with known diabetes who are admitted for ACS. Stress may worsen glycemia while lack of food intake (patients are often NPO [nothing by mouth]) may improve glycemia. All patients should have their blood sugar assessed for unidentified hyperglycemia. If the blood sugar is elevated on more than one occasion, diabetes should be considered and appropriate treatment initiated. Ideally, at the time of discharge, an OGTT should be performed.

Oral antidiabetic agents are not generally advisable during an ACS or if patients are in critical care. Insulin is preferred to treat the hyperglycemia during a suspected or diagnosed ACS, until the patient is clinically stabilized.

A review of nonglycemic treatment during an ACS is beyond the scope of this chapter and includes beta-blockers, nitrates, antihypertensives, and antilipid and antiplatelet drugs.

Table 15-3 **Insulin Preparations**

Insulin	Trade Name	Onset	Peak	Duration (h)	Comments
Ultrashort acting					
Aspart	NovoLog	10–30 min	30–90 min	3–4	
Lispro	Humalog	10–30 min	30–90 min	3–4	
Glulisine	Apidra	10–30 min	30–90 min	3–4	
Short acting					
Regular	Novolin-R	30–60 min	2–3 h	3–6	
Humulin-R		30–60 min	2–3 h	3–6	
Intermediate acting					
NPH	Novolin-N	2–4 h	6–10 h	10–16	
Humulin-N		2–4 h	6–10 h	10–16	
Long acting					
Glargine	Lantus	3–4 h	None	18–24	Cannot be mixed
Detimer	Leuhis		None	14	
Combinations					
70% NPH-30% regular	70–30	30–60 min	Both	10–16	
50% NPH-50% regular	50–50	30–60 min	Both	10–16	
75% NPL-25% insulin lispro		15–30 min	Both	10–16	
705% NPH-30% insulin aspart		15–30 min	Both	10–16	
Inhaled insulin	Exubera		30–90 min		

Abbreviation: NPL, neutral protamine lispro.

Patients with Coronary Artery Disease and Diabetes

GLYCEMIC GOALS OF TREATMENT

An A1c as low as possible without causing harm:

- American Diabetes Association <7.0%
- European Diabetes Association <6.5%
- American Association of Clinical Endocrinology <6.5%

In patients with diabetes and coronary heart disease or CHF, standard guidelines should be followed. The American Association of Clinical Endocrinology and the European Diabetes Association have established an A1c goal of <6.5% for patients with diabetes. The American Diabetes Association goal is <7.0% and is based on evidence from trials using microvascular endpoints; it is likely that glycemic goals of impacting CV disease will be lower.[9] The weight of the evidence and a rationale concept indicate that the A1c goals should be as low as possible without causing harm. Definitive evidence for glycemic targets will be available when the ACCORD study is completed.[26]

TREATMENT STRATEGY

Patients may be placed on insulin, oral antidiabetic agents, or newer injectables such as exenetide. The precise sequence in which this is done is of less significance than that glycemic goals are met and that patients do not have unacceptable side effects (Fig. 15-3). Data show that clinicians often wait for several years before making meaningful therapeutic changes in the regimen. Importantly, many of these agents may (and must) be combined. In general, patients with type 2 diabetes will require polypharmacy for glycemic control.

Insulin

In type 1 diabetes, insulin is the agent of choice. It may be used as multiple daily subcutaneous injections such as a basal-prandial regimen as described

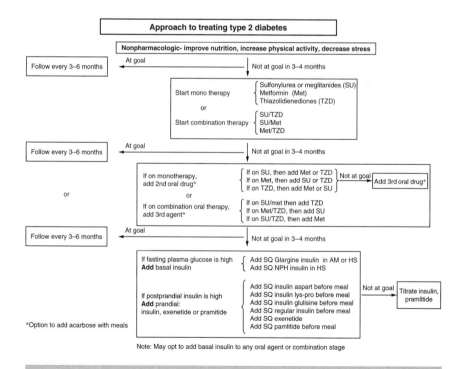

Figure 15-3 **Approach to treating type 2 diabetes.**

above, use of intermediate-acting insulin such as NPH insulin, or as a continuous subcutaneous insulin pump. Approaches to the use of the insulin pump are well described and the reader is referred to these.[62] While they allow for the ultimate in flexibility, they also require continuous monitoring and are not suitable for everyone. There are disposable pen injectors for convenience and even a device with large mechanicals and numbers (the Innolet) to facilitate use by arthritic hands and low vision common comorbidities among elderly patients. There is no indication for use of oral agents in this group. Insulin requirements may decrease if patients loose renal function for any reason.

In type 2 diabetes, insulin may be used as the sole drug or in combination with other oral agents. Frequently, patients are on oral antidiabetic agents without reaching their glycemic goal and require insulin. Poor glycemic control and elevated A1c levels are seen with either elevated fasting or PP glucoses. Each requires a somewhat different strategy.

If the *fasting or basal plasma glucose is elevated*, it is reasonable to add a single dose of long-acting insulin (glargine) once a day or intermediate-acting insulin (NPH) at bedtime.[63] to suppress hepatic glucose output. A reasonable starting dose is 10 units of glargine or NPH. Once the dose of insulin is titrated up to achieve the desired fasting glucose, overall glycemic control will improve. One study of type 2 diabetes patients showed that over 40 units of insulin was required to achieve a target FPG of 100 mg/dL. Despite normal FPG levels, the overall glycemic control may still not be at goal. This is usually because of persistent elevation of the postprandial blood sugar. An approach to increasing glargine insulin (or NPH insulin) is to increase the dose by 2–3 units per day until a fasting glucose of ~100-110 mg/dL is achieved

If the *postprandial blood glucoses are elevated* (determined by home monitoring of capillary blood glucoses) then a short-acting insulin may be added at the time of meals. These insulins (aspart and lyspro) act very rapidly and should be used at the time of a meal and not 30 minutes before. In patients who are unwell with poor appetites, these may even be used after the meal is eaten allowing for an assessment of the amount of food actually ingested and the exact amount of insulin needed. Regular insulin may be used as well. An approach to adding a correction dose to the meal-associated insulin is shown in Table 15-2.

In patients on multiple oral antidiabetic agents as well as multiple doses of insulin, the dose of insulin may either be gradually titrated up.

For new-onset diabetes patients: If the blood glucose is particularly elevated this author's preference is to begin with insulin therapy several times a day for a period of time. This will allow for a rapid correction of blood sugars and an overall improved metabolic status. It may permit development of long-term remission and the subsequent use of a low dose of an oral antidiabetic agent to maintain glycemic control.[54–59]

ORAL ANTIDIABETIC AGENTS

General Considerations

In treating patients with oral agents it is useful to recall that there are numerous pathophysiologic abnormalities in type 2 diabetes and it is rare that target glycemic goals are achieved by any single drug. Thus, it is wise to start a patient on one agent, rapidly titrate to near maximum dose, and then within a short time to add a second (or third) antidiabetic agent. The key is to normalize the blood glucose to the target level. There are several good reviews available.[64,65]

For new-onset diabetes patients: If the blood glucose is particularly elevated or the patient has hyperglycemic symptoms, this author's preference is to begin with insulin therapy several times a day for a period of time for reasons noted above. If the glucoses are not very elevated (<250 mg/dL), patients may be started on oral antidiabetic agents with a rapid titration to achieve glycemic goals.

For previously treated patients: If not at glycemic goal, patients should remain on their medication and first titrate to maximal or submaximal doses and then add one or two oral agents or insulin as needed.

Established oral antidiabetic drugs

See Tables 15-4 and 15-5 for doses, adverse effects, and mechanism of action:

- Sulfonylureas and other K_{ATP} channel blockers raise intracellular calcium and ATP and thus increase insulin secretion. These include glimepiride, glipizide, glyburide, and glibenclamide as well as repaglinide and nateglinide (the latter are short-acting agents used with meals). Side effects of these agents include hypoglycemia. They tend to decrease the A1c by about 1–2%.

- *Biguanides*: Metformin is the only approved agent in the United States and the most commonly prescribed for diabetes. It acts by increasing insulin sensitivity, mainly at the level of the liver (decreasing liver glucose output) and also by increasing peripheral muscle insulin sensitivity. Few common side effects include nausea, diarrhea, and other gastrointestinal (GI) problems. These may be minimized by starting with low doses and titrating up slowly. An important but very uncommon side effect is the development of lactic acidosis; lactic acidosis carries a 50% mortality. The development of lactic acidosis may be minimized by avoiding its use in patients with low glomerular filtration rates (GFR; <60 mL/min), low muscle mass, the elderly, with serum creatinine >1.4 mg/dL for women and 1.6 mg/dL for men, and in situations where hypotension may occur including trauma, ACS, and sepsis. If used alone, hypoglycemia does not occur; however, in combination

Table 15-4 *Oral Antidiabetes Pharmacologic Agents*

	Trade Name	Starting Dose	Usual Dose	Maximum Dose	Tablet Size	Expected Decrease in A1c
Insulin secretagogues						
Sulfonylureas						
Glipizide	Glucotrol (XL)	2.5–5.0 mg/day	10 mg/day	20 mg/day	2.5, 5, 10 mg	1–2%
Glimepiride	Amaryl	1.2 mg with meals	1–4 mg with meals	8 mg	1, 2, 4 mg	1–2%
Glyburide	Micronase, Glynase, Diabeta	2.5 mg/day	10 mg/day	20 mg/day	1.2, 1.5, 2.5, 3, 6, 10 mg	1–2%
Meglitinides						
Repaglinide	Prandin	1 mg with meals	4 mg bid or tid	16 mg/day	0.5, 1.0, 2.0 mg	0.5–1.0%
Nateglinide	Starlix	120 mg with meals	120 mg tid with meals	Same	60, 120 mg	0.5–1.0%
Insulin sensitizers						
Thiazolidinediones						
Rosiglitazone	Avandia	4 mg (2 mg bid)	8 mg (4 mg bid)	Same	2, 4, 8 mg	1–2%
Pioglitazone	Actos	15 mg	45 mg/day	Same	15, 30, 45 mg	1–2%
Biguanides						
Metformin	Glucophage (XR)	500 (250 mg) with meals	1000 mg bid with meals	2550	500, 1000, 850 mg	1–2%
Incretin based GLP-1 receptor agonist						
Exenetide*	Byetta	5 or 10 µg SQ				

DPP-4 inhibitors†						
Vildagliptin						
Sitagliptin	Januvia	100 mg/day	100 mg/day, with or without meals	100 mg/day	25, 50, 100 mg	1%
Saxagliptin						
Alpha glucosidase inhibitors						
Miglitol	Glyset	25 mg tid with meals	100 mg tid with meals	Same		0.5–1.9%
Acarbose	Precose					0.5–0.8%
Amylin analogues						
Pramlitide*	Amylin					
Combinations						
Glyburide-Metformin	Glucovance				1.25–250, 2.5–500, 5–500 mg	
Glipizide-metformin	Metaglip				2.5–250, 2.5–500, 5–500 mg	
Rosiglitazone-metformin	Avandamet				1–500, 2–500, 4–500, 2–1000, 4–1000 mg	

*Subcutaneous injection.

†DPP-4 inhibitors are oral—increased endogenous GLP-1.

Table 15-5 *Antidiabetic Agents—Adverse Effects and Primay Action*

	Caution/ Contraindications	Hypogly-cemia*	Edema/Fluid Retention	CHF	Weight GI	Change	Primary Action
Insulin— all types	Renal/hepatic insufficiency	√	+/–			↑	Adds insulin ↓ FPG and PP glucose
Insulin							
secretagogues							
Sulfonylureas							
Glipizide	Hepatic insufficiency	√				↑	↑ insulin; ↓ FPG and PP glucose
Glimepiride	Hepatic/renal insufficiency	√				↑	↑ insulin; ↓ FPG and PP glucose
Glyburide	Hepatic/renal insufficiency	√				↑	↑ insulin; ↓ FPG and PP glucose
Meglitinides							
Repaglinide	Hepatic/renal insufficiency	√				↑	↑ insulin; ↓ PP glucoses
Nateglinide	Hepatic/renal insufficiency	√				↑	↑ insulin; ↓ PP glucoses
Insulin sensitizers							
Thiazolidinediones							
Rosiglitazone	LFT >2.5 × ULN Class 3 or 4 heart failure		√	√		↑	↑ insulin sensitivity ↓ FPG and PP glucose
Pioglitazone	LFT >2.5 × ULN Class 3 or 4 heart failure		√	√		↑	↑ insulin sensitivity ↓ FPG and PP glucose

Agent	Contraindications		Hypoglycemia*	Mechanism
Biguanides				
Metformin	Renal insufficiency† Class 3 or 4 heart failure	↓/↔	√	↑ insulin sensitivity ↓ FPG and PP glucose
Incretin based				
GLP-1 receptor agonist				
Exenetide‡		→	√	↓ glucagon, ↑ satiety ↑ insulin secretion ↓ PP glucoses
DPP-4 inhibitors§ (vilgagliptin, satagliptin, and saxagliptin)		↔		↓ glucagon, ↑ satiety ↑ insulin secretion; ↑ GLP-1 ↓ PP glucoses
Alpha glucosidase inhibitors				
Miglitol	GI disease	↔	√	↓ CHO absorb. ↓ PP glucoses
Acarbose	GI disease	↔	√	↓ CHO absorb. ↓ PP glucoses
Amylin analogues				
Pramlitide		↔/↓	√	↓ glucagon ↑ insulin secretion, ↓ PP glucoses

Abbreviations: LFT, liver function test; ULN, upper limit of normal.

*Hypoglycemia when used as monotherapy.

†Serum creatinine >1.4 mg/dL for women and 1.6 mg/dL for men. GI side effects include nausea, diarrhea, bloating, and flatulence.

‡Subcutaneous injection.

§DPP-4 inhibitors are oral—increase endogenous GLP-1 not yet approved for use.

with insulin or insulin secretagogues, hypoglycemia may develop. One estimate of GFR is the Cockcroft Gault equation: (140-age) × weight (kg)/(serum creatinine in mg/dL) × 72. For women this is corrected for by multiplying by 0.85.[66] A retrospective Medicare cohort study suggests that metformin use may not be detrimental in patients with diabetes after an AMI.[67] Metformin is contraindicated in class 3 and 4 heart failure.

- *Thiazolidinediones:* Rosiglitazone and pioglitazone are insulin sensitizers which improve glucose transport. In addition, they have been reported to improve HDL-cholesterol in some studies and increase the buoyancy of LDL cholesterol particles as well as having salutary vascular effects.[68] It is logical to use insulin sensitizers if CVD is a result of insulin resistance. The Bypass Angioplasty Revascularization Investigation in Type 2 Diabetics (BARI 2D) trial is an ongoing NIH trial designed to answer the question of whether insulin sensitizers (rosiglitazone) have CV benefits in diabetes patients with CAD. The PROactive study showed a lower recurrence rate of a second MI patients with type 2 diabetes over a 3-year follow-up period (7.2% in controls vs. 5.3% in patients on 45 mg of pioglitazone). By treating 1000 patients with pioglitazone, 22 recurrent MIs were prevented.[69] While it did not achieve its primary endpoint of a reduction of combined parameters, it did achieve its secondary endpoint with a 16% relative risk decrease in death, nonfatal MI, or stroke. Other ongoing studies which address thiazolidinediones in treating vascular disease include Diabetes Resduction Aseessment with Rampiril and/or rosiglitazone Medications (DREAM) and Pericope.[70]

Their slower onset of action make combining this agent with a more rapid-acting agent such as an insulin secretagogue or metformin attractive and such fixed combinations exist. Side effects include fluid retention, dilutional anemia, and infrequent CHF. When used alone, hypoglycemia usually does not occur, however, when used with insulin or insulin secretagogues, hypoglycemia may develop. Thiazolidinediones are contraindicated in class 3 and 4 heart failure.

- *Alpha glucosidase inhibitors:* Miglitol or acarbose block the disaccharidase enzymes in the jejunum and delays the absorption of complex sugars, thus lowering the postprandial glucose rise. Side effect includes increased intestinal gas which may be socially disturbing to patients and may be minimized by gradually titrating the dose upward. Monotherapy is unassociated with hypoglycemia but combined with insulin or secretagogues may cause hypoglycemia. An important practical consideration is the mandatory treatment of hypoglycemia with dextrose and not a disaccharide such as fructose (in fruit juice) or sucrose (table sugar). This is because complex sugars cannot be broken down and absorbed in the presence of alpha glucosidase inhibitors.

Newer injectable antidiabetic drugs

- *Pramlitide*: Amylin is normally produced in the pancreas and is deficient in diabetes. It is injected with meals and causes the blood sugar to decrease; it is associated with some weight loss and early satiety. Nausea is a known side effect but may decrease over time and with slow titration.
- *Exenetide*: This is a GLP-1 analogue and increases meal-associated insulin secretion. The incretin GLP-1 is deficient in diabetes.[71] Exenetide is a synthetic analogue of a protein from a lizard's saliva (*Heloderma suspectum*) and interacts with the GLP-1 receptor. This is administered as a subcutaneous injection and increases endogenous insulin secretion. Other actions include slowing of gastric emptying, improved insulin sensitivity, inhibition of glucagon secretion, and increased satiety and weight loss. Together these effects results in lower blood sugars. When used alone, this drug does not cause hypoglycemia. Exenetide may also increase beta-cell differentiation to produce new beta cells. Nausea may be a significant side effect for some patients but may diminish with time.
- *Inhaled insulin*: Insulin is administered through inhalation and because of this has the potential to be acceptable to a much larger number of patients because it avoids injections. This drug has been approved for use by the U.S. Food and Drug Administration, but has not yet been launched.

Antidiabetic drugs in development

- *GLP-1 or incretin-based treatments*: GLP-1 is an incretin which has a very short half-life in the blood stream and is degraded by an enzyme know as dipeptidyl dipeptidase 4 or DPP-4. Inhibitors of this enzyme, DPP-4 inhibitors are being developed; early studies demonstrate increased circulating plasma GLP-1 levels, decreased glucagon levels, and improved glycemic control without additional weight gain. Three oral drugs currently being developed include sitagliptin, vildagliptin, and saxagliptin. Only sitagliptin is currently approved in the U.S.
- *Peroxisome proliferator-activated receptors (PPAR) alpha and gamma agonists*: These drugs improve carbohydrate as well as lipid metabolism. None have been approved yet for treatment.

Herbals and nontraditional remedies

- *Herbals*: Many patients use complementary and alternative medications (CAM) for diabetes. This is especially true among immigrant groups from Asia, Latin America, the Caribbean, and Africa. These include *Coccinia indica*, *Momordica charantia* (kerela or bitter melon or cersee tea), bitter aloe vera, *Gymnema sylvestre*, *Panax quinquefolius* (ginseng), and

Opuntia streptacantha (nopal or prickly pear). An important clinical consideration is that the physician or provider enquire about their use and document it. There is no evidence that herbal remedies for diabetes should be used during an ACS. This author's preference is to discontinue these during an ACS.

Nontraditional herbal concoctions may include but not identify traditional pharmacologic agents such as chlorpropamide. It is important to know what the patient is using since there may be adverse effects (such as prolonged hypoglycemia or hyponatremia with chlorpropamide). Some antidiabetic agents sold on the street include combinations of phenformin (a biguanide banned from the United States for its association with lactic acidosis) and chlorpropamide.

Patients with Congestive Heart Failure and Diabetes

Overall principles of glycemic treatment include those outlined above for patients with diabetes and CVD. Treatment choices should be in the context of overall CHF considerations of fluid retention and hypoxia.

Notable issues include the use of metformin and thiazolidinediones. These are contraindicated in patients with class 3 and 4 heart failure. The thiazolidinediones tend to accumulate fluid and infrequently patients develop acute CHF. CHF patients (not class 3 or 4) on insulin may develop significant pedal edema when thiazolidinediones are added. While this does not contraindicate their use, it does mean that clinicians should be vigilant. In a retrospective review of Medicare beneficiaries, thiazolidinedione prescription is associated with a higher risk of readmission for heart failure after MI.[67]

Other Therapeutic Considerations for Patients with Diabetes and Cardiovascular Disease

1. Aggressive management of other nonglycemic CV risk factors is mandatory to maximize benefit to the patient. There is strong evidence that these patients should be aggressively treated in terms of hypertension. Clear evidence exists for use of beta-blockers, ACE inhibitors, and angiotensin receptor blockers (ARBs). Aggressive control of lipids and early use of statins as well as use of antiplatelet agents are needed to decrease mortality and morbidity. Discontinuing smoking is an essential aspect of treatment.
2. *Medical nutrition therapy and diet*: This is one of the fundamental aspects of diabetes treatment. Most patients with diabetes are overweight or obese and benefit from dietary modification. To lose 1 pound per week requires a calorie deficit of 500 calories per day, that is, a net deficit 3500 calories equals 1 pound of weight lost. Difficulties in losing weight and maintaining a weight-reduced state are well known and are based on environmental and physiologic reasons. Environmental reasons include

the easy availability of inexpensive, large portions of tasty, calorie-dense food relentlessly advertised and the lack of inexpensive healthy choices.[72] The physiologic reason is the development of biologic changes which counteract weight loss such as decreases in leptin level.[73] Neither of these forces can be easily overcome through individual "will power" and choice; social and political changes must evolve in order to reverse this. Finally, considerable data exist that low carbohydrate diets permit weight loss and maintenance without constant feelings of hunger.[74] Regardless of whether a patient can actually lose weight, it is beneficial to change the composition of the diet.

3. *Physical activity*: Physical activity, when done regularly, provides an excellent basis for glycemic control.[75-77] Again, societal mores mitigate against regular exercise. In patients with CV disease, exercise may require supervision and at the very least a stress test to determine the amount of exercise that can be safely performed. Another difficulty lies in the fact that unless done carefully, exercise may cause injury making patients even more sedentary. There are many programs suitable for patients with diabetes and CV disease such as seated aerobics. Walking is also an excellent form of exercise that many can participate in.

CONCLUSION

Hyperglycemia has adverse CV effects mediated through inflammation and increased oxidative stress. Control of hyperglycemia has been shown to be associated with improved micro- and macrovascular outcomes. Multiple physiologic abnormalities dictate the use of monotherapy or combination therapy using sulfonylureas, meglitinides, metformin, thiazolidinediones, and acarbose. New and promising drugs target the incretin system. Insulin may be used alone or in combination with these agents.

Finally, treatment strategies must address the need for aggressive lipid lowering, blood pressure control, antiplatelet activity, medical nutrition therapy, increased physical activity, and smoking cessation.

REFERENCES

1. Kannel WB, McGee DL. Diabetes and cardiovascular disease: the Framingham study. *JAMA* 1979;241:2035–2038.

2. Malmberg K, Ryden L. Myocardial infarction in patients with diabetes mellitus. *Eur Heart J* 1988;9:259–264.

3. Pyorala K, Savolainen E, Lehtovirta E, et al. Glucose tolerance and coronary heart disease: Helsinki policemen study. *J Chronic Dis* 1979;32:729–745.

4. Fuller JH, Shipley MJ, Rose G, et al. Coronary-heart-disease risk and impaired glucose tolerance: the Whitehall study. *Lancet* 1980;1:1373–1376.

5. Fox CS, Coady S, Sorlie PD, et al. Trends in cardiovascular complications of diabetes. *JAMA* 2004;292:2495–2499.

6. Glucose tolerance and mortality: comparison of WHO and American Diabetes Association diagnostic criteria. The DECODE study group. European Diabetes Epidemiology Group. Diabetes epidemiology: collaborative analysis of diagnostic criteria in Europe. *Lancet* 1999;354:617–621.

7. Coutinho M, Gerstein HC, Wang Y, et al. The relationship between glucose and incident cardiovascular events: a metaregression analysis of published data from 20 studies of 95,783 individuals followed for 12.4 years. *Diabetes Care* 1999;22: 233–240.

8. Tirosh A, Shai I, Tekes-Manova D, et al. Israeli Diabetes Research Group. Normal fasting plasma glucose levels and type 2 diabetes in young men. *N Engl J Med* 2005;353(14):1454–1462.

9. Khaw K-T, Wareham N, Luben R, et al. Glycated haemoglobin, diabetes, and mortality in men in the Norfolk cohort of European Prospective Investigation of Cancer and Nutrition (EPIC-Norfolk). *Br Med J* 2001;322:15–18.

10. Stratton IM, Adler AI, Neil HA, et al. Association of glycaemia with macrovascular and microvascular complications of type 2 diabetes (UKPDS 35): prospective observational study. *BMJ* 2000;321:405–412.

11. Abbud ZA, Shindler DM, Wilson AC, et al. Effect of diabetes mellitus on short- and long-term mortality rates of patients with acute myocardial infarction: a statewide study: Myocardial Infarction Data Acquisition System Study Group. *Am Heart J* 1995;130:51–58.

12. Lewis EF, Moye LA, Rouleau JL, et al. CARE Study. Predictors of late development of heart failure in stable survivors of myocardial infarction: the CARE study. *J Am Coll Cardiol* 2003;42(8):1446–1453.

13. Wahab NN, Cowden EA, Pearce NJ, et al. Is blood glucose an independent predictor of mortality in acute myocardial infarction in the thrombolytic era? *J Am Coll Cardiol* 2002;40:1748–1754.

14. Norhammar AM, Ryden L, Malmberg K. Admission plasma glucose: independent risk factor for long-term prognosis after myocardial infarction even in nondiabetic patients. *Diabetes Care* 1999;22:1827–1831.

15. Bolk J, van der PT, Cornel JH, et al. Impaired glucose metabolism predicts mortality after a myocardial infarction. *Int J Cardiol* 2001;79:207–214.

16. Mukamal KJ, Nesto RW, Cohen MC, et al. Impact of diabetes on long-term survival after acute myocardial infarction: comparability of risk with prior myocardial infarction. *Diabetes Care* 2001;24(8):1422–1427.

17. Whiteley L, Padmanabhan S, Hole D, et al. Should diabetes be considered a coronary heart disease risk equivalent? Results from 25 years of follow-up in the Renfrew and Paisley survey. *Diabetes Care* 2005;28:1588–1593.

18. Haffner SM, Lehto S, Ronnemaa T, et al. Mortality from coronary heart disease in subjects with type 2 diabetes and in non diabetic subjects with and without prior myocardial infarction. *N Engl J Med* 1998;339:229–234.

19. Inzucchi SE, Oral antihyperglycemic therapy for type 2 diabetes; scientific review. *JAMA* 2002;287:360–372.

20. Norhammar A, Malmberg K, Diderholm E, et al. Diabetes mellitus: the major risk factor in unstable coronary artery disease even after consideration of the extent of coronary artery disease and benefits of revascularization. *J Am Coll Cardiol* 2004;43(4):585–591.

21. Capes SE, Hunt D, Malmberg K, et al. Stress hyperglycaemia and increased risk of death after myocardial infarction in patients with and without diabetes: a systematic overview. *Lancet* 2000;355:773–778.

22. Norhammar A, Tenerz A, Nilsson G, et al. Glucose metabolism in patients with acute myocardial infarction and no previous diagnosis of diabetes mellitus: a prospective study. *Lancet* 2002;359:2140–2144.

23. Bartnik M, Malmberg K, Norhammar A, et al. Newly detected abnormal glucose tolerance: an important predictor of long term outcomes after myocardial infarction. *Eur Heart J* 2004;25:1990–1997.

24. Stranders I, Diamant M, van Gelder RE, et al. Admission blood glucose level as a risk indicator of death in myocardial infarction in patients with and without diabetes. *Arch Intern Med* 2004;164:982–988.

25. Ramachandaran A, Snehalatha C, Sathyamurthy I, et al. High incidence of glucose intolerance in Asian Indian subjects with acute coronary syndrome. *Diabetes Care* 2005;28:2492–2496.

26. Available at: www.accordtrial.org

27. Effect of intensive blood-glucose control with metformin on complications in overweight patients with type 2 diabetes (UKPDS 34). UK Prospective Diabetes Study (UKPDS) Group. *Lancet* 1998;352(9131):854-865. Erratum in: *Lancet* 1998;352(9139):1558.

28. Nathan DM, Cleary PA, Backlund JY, et al. Diabetes Control and Complications Trial/Epidemiology of Diabetes Interventions and Complications (DCCT/EDIC) Study Research Group. Intensive diabetes treatment and cardiovascular disease in patients with type 1 diabetes. *N Engl J Med* 2005;353:2643–2653.

29. Sodi-Pallares D, Testelli MR, Fishter B. Effects on an intravenous infusion of potassium-insulin-glucose solution of the electrocardiographic signs of myocardial infarction. A preliminary clinical report. *Am J Cardiol* 1962;9:166–181.

30. Fath-Ordoubadi F, Beatt KJ. Glucose-insulin-potassium therapy for treatment of acute myocardial infarction: an overview of randomized placebo-controlled trials. *Circulation* 1997;96:1152–1156.

31. Krljanac G, Vasiljevic Z, Radovanovic M, et al. Effects of glucose-insulin-potassium infusion on ST-elevation myocardial infarction in patients treated with thrombolytic therapy. *Am J Cardiol* 2005;96:1053–1058. Epub August 24, 2005.

32. Diaz R, Paolasso EA, Piegas LS, et al. Metabolic modulation of acute myocardial infarction. The ECLA (Estudios Cardiologicos Latinoamerica) Collaborative Group. *Circulation* 1998;98:2227–2234.

33. The CREATE-ECLA Trial Group Investigators. Effect of glucose-insulin-potassium infusion on mortality in patients with acute st-segment elevation myocardial infarction: the CREATE-ECLA Randomized Controlled Trial. *JAMA* 2005;293:437–446.

34. van der Horst IC, Zijlstra F, van't Hof AW, et al. Zwolle Infarct Study Group. Glucose-insulin-potassium infusion inpatients treated with primary angioplasty for acute myocardial infarction: the glucose-insulin-potassium study: a randomized trial. *J Am Coll Cardiol* 2003;42(5):784–791.

35. Malmberg K, Ryden L, Efendic S, et al. Randomized trial of insulin-glucose infusion followed by subcutaneous insulin treatment in diabetic patients with acute myocardial infarction (DIGAMI study): effects on mortality at 1 year. *J Am Coll Cardiol* 1995;26:57–65.

36. Malmberg K, Ryden L, Wedel H, et al. DIGAMI 2 Investigators. Intense metabolic control by means of insulin in patients with diabetes mellitus and acute myocardial infarction (DIGAMI 2): effects on mortality and morbidity. *Eur Heart J* 2005;26:650–661.

37. Van den Berghe G, Wouters P, Weekers F, et al. Intensive insulin therapy in critically ill patients. *N Engl J Med* 2001;345:1359–1367.

38. Furnary AP, Gao G, Grunkemeier GL, et al. Continuous insulin infusion reduces mortality in patients with diabetes undergoing coronary artery bypass grafting. *J Thorac Cardiovasc Surg* 2003;125:1007–1021.

39. Van den Berghe G, Wilmer A, Hermans G, et al. Intensive insulin therapy in the medical ICU. *N Engl J Med* 2006;354(5):449–461.

40. Krinsley JS. Effect of an intensive glucose management protocol on the mortality of critically ill adult patients. *Mayo Clin Proc* 2004;79(8):992–1000. Erratum in: *Mayo Clin Proc* 2005;80:1101.

41. Oliver MF, Opie LH. Effects of glucose and fatty acids on myocardial ischaemia and arrythmias. *Lancet* 1994;343:155–158.

42. Dresner A, Laurent D, Marcucci M, et al. Effects of free fatty acids on glucose transport and IRS-1-associated phosphatidylinositol 3-kinase activity. *J Clin Invest* 1999;103:253–259.

43. Lowell B, Shulman G. Mitochondrial dysfunction and type 2 diabetes. *Science* 2005;307:384–378.

44. Gao F, Gao E, Yue T-L, et al. Nitric oxide mediates the antiapoptotic effect of insulin in myocardial ischemia-reperfusion. The roles of PI3-kinase, Akt, and endothelial nitric oxide synthase phosphorylation. *Circulation* 2002;105:1497–1502.

45. Kim YM, Bombeck CA, Billiar TR. Nitric oxide as a bifunctional regulator of apoptosis. *Circ Res* 1999;84:253–256.

46. Aulak K, Koeck T, Crabb JW, et al. Dynamics of protein nitration in cells and mitochondria. *Am J Physiol Circ Physiol* 2004;286:H30–H38.

47. Aljada A, Ghanim H, Mohanty P, et al. Insulin inhibits the pro-inflammatory transcription factor early growth response gene-1 (Egr)-1 expression in mononuclear cells (MNC) and reduces plasma tissue factor (TF) and plasminogen activator inhibitor-1 (PAI-1) concentrations. *J Clin Endocrinol Metab* 2002;87:1419–1422.

48. Vanhorebeek I, De Vos R, Mesotten M, et al. Strict blood glucose control with insulin in critically ill patients protects hepatocytic mitochondrial ultrastructure and function. *Lancet* 2005;365:53–59.

49. Hseuh W, Mesotten D, Swinnen JV, et al. Contribution of circulating lipids to the improved outcome of critical illness by glycemic control with intensive insulin therapy. *J Clin Endocrinol Metab* 2004;89:219–226.

50. Harris HW, Grunfeld C, Feingold KR, et al. Human very low density lipoproteins and chylomicrons can protect against endotoxin-induced death in mice. *J Clin Invest* 1990;86:696–702.

51. Harris HW, Grunfeld C, Feingold KR, et al. Chylomicrons alter the fate of endotoxin, decreasing tumor necrosis factor release and preventing death. *J Clin Invest* 1993;91:1028–1034.

52. Wallander M, Bartnik M, Efendic S, et al. Beta cell dysfunction in patients with acute myocardial infarction but without previously known type 2 diabetes: a report from the GAMI study. *Diabetologia* 2005;48:2229–2235.

53. Leibowitz G, Yuli M, Donath MY, et al. Beta-cell glucotoxicity in the Psammomys obesus model of type 2 diabetes. *Diabetes* 2001;50(Suppl 1):S113-S117.

54. Banerji MA. Diabetes in African Americans: unique pathophysiological features. Review. *Curr Diab Rep* 2004;4:219–223.

55. Banerji MA, Chaiken RL, Lebovitz HE. Long-term remission in NIDDM in Blacks. *Diabetes* 1996;45:337–341.

56. McFarlane SI, Chaiken RL, Hirsch S, et al. Near-normoglycaemic remission in African-Americans with type 2 diabetes mellitus is associated with recovery of beta cell function. *Diabet Med* 2001;18:10–16.

57. Ryan EA, Imes S, Wallace C. Short-term intensive insulin therapy in newly diagnosed type 2 diabetes. *Diabetes Care* 2004;27:1028–1032.

58. Ilkova H, Glaser B, Tunckale A, et al. Induction of long-term glycemic control in newly diagnosed type 2 diabetic patients by transient intensive insulin treatment. *Diabetes Care* 1997;20:1353–1356.

59. Yanbing Li, Wen Xu, Zhihong Liao, et al. Induction of long-term glycemic control in newly diagnosed type 2 diabetic patients is associated with improvement of β-cell function *Diabetes Care* 2004;27:2597–2602.

60. Monnier L, Lapinski H, Colette C. Contributions of fasting and postprandial plasma glucose increments to the overall diurnal hyperglycemia of type 2 diabetic patients: variations with increasing levels of HbA(1c). *Diabetes Care* 2003;26:881–885.

61. Trence DL, Kelly, JL, Hirsch IB. The rationale and management of hyperglycemia for in-patients with cardiovascular disease: time for change. *J Clin Endocrinol Metab* 2003;88:2430–2437.

62. Hoogma RP, Hammond PJ, Gomis R, et al. 5-Nations Study Group. Comparison of the effects of continuous subcutaneous insulin infusion (CSII) and NPH-based multiple daily insulin injections (MDI) on glycaemic control and quality of life: results of the 5-nations trial. *Diabet Med* 2006;23:141–147.

63. Riddle MC, Rosenstock J, Gerich J. Insulin Glargine 4002 Study Investigators. The treat to-target trial: randomized addition of glargine or human NPH insulin to oral therapy of type 2 diabetic patients. *Diabetes Care* 2003;26:3080–3086.

64. Inzucchi SE, Oral antihyperglycemic therapy for type 2 diabetes; scientific review. *JAMA* 2002;287:360–372.

65. Krentz AJ, Bailey CJ. Oral antidiabetic agents: current role in type 2 diabetes mellitus. Drugs 2005;65:385–411.

66. Cockcroft DW, Gault MH. Prediction of creatinine clearance from serum creatinine. *Nephron* 1976;16:31–41.

67. Inzucchi SE, Masoudi FA, Wang Y, et al. Insulin-sensitizing antihyperglycemic drugs and mortality after acute myocardial infarction. *Diabetes Care* 2005;28:1680–1689.

68. Lebovitz HE, Banerji MA. Treatment of insulin resistance in diabetes mellitus. *Eur J Pharmacol* 2004;490:135–146.

69. Dormandy JA, Charbonnel B, Eckland DJ, et al. PROactive investigators. Secondary prevention of macrovascular events in patients with type 2 diabetes in the PROactive Study (PROspective pioglitAzone Clinical Trial In macroVascular Events): a randomised controlled trial. *Lancet* 2005;366:1279–1289.

70. Gerstein HC, Yusuf S, Holman R, et al. The DREAM Trial Investigators. Rationale, design and recruitment characteristics of a large, simple international trial of diabetes prevention: the DREAM trial. *Diabetologia* 2004;47:1519–1527.

71. Heine RJ, Van Gaal LF, Johns D, et al. GWAA Study Group. Exenatide versus insulin glargine in patients with suboptimally controlled type 2 diabetes: a randomized trial. *Ann Intern Med* 2005;143(8):559–569.

72. Available at: www.yaleruddcenter.org.

73. Rosenbaum M, Goldsmith R, Bloomfield D, et al. Low-dose leptin reverses skeletal muscle, autonomic, and neuroendocrine adaptations to maintenance of reduced weight. *J Clin Invest* 2005;115:3579–3586.

74. Atkins RC, Ornish D, Wadden T. Low-carb, low-fat diet gurus face off. Interview by Joan Stephenson. *JAMA* 2003;289:1767–1768, 1773.

75. Jonker JT, De Laet C, Franco OH, et al. Physical activity and life expectancy with and without diabetes. *Diabetes Care* 2006;29:38–43.

76. Ellis SE, Elasy TA, Sigal RJ, et al. Exercise and glycemic control in diabetes. *JAMA* 2001;286:2941–2942.

77. Eriksson KF, Lindgarde F. Poor physical fitness, and impaired early insulin response but late hyperinsulinaemia, as predictors of NIDDM in middle-aged Swedish men. *Diabetologia* 1996;39:573–579.

CARDIOVASCULAR

IMAGING IN DIABETES

Jason M. Lazar
Louis Salciccioli

BACKGROUND

Diabetes is a well-known risk factor for cardiovascular disease (CVD) morbidity and mortality and its prevalence is rising in the United States. Diabetes is a major risk factor for CVD. CVD is a leading cause of mortality and morbidity in diabetic patients. Diabetic patients often experience atypical symptoms including silent ischemia. Accordingly, cardiovascular risk stratification is important but remains challenging. Imaging is playing an increasingly important role in guiding and monitoring medical and revascularization therapies. These factors will undoubtedly increase the demand for CV imaging procedures in this population. In the recent report of the Adult Treatment Panel of the National Cholesterol Education Program (NCEP),[1] type 2 diabetes was accorded a coronary artery disease (CAD) risk-equivalent as the incidence of myocardial infarction (MI) in diabetics without prior MI was found to be similar to that of nondiabetics with prior MI during 7-year follow-up.[2]

Interpretation of studies evaluating various cardiovascular imaging techniques in diabetics is made difficult by the heterogeneity of patients, subgroup analysis of larger studies of unselected patients, multiple clinical settings, variable study methodologies, variable incorporation of disease management programs, and by inclusion in the medical, CV, and endocrinology publications. Variability in combined cardiac endpoints further complicates the matter. The American Diabetes Association (ADA), American Heart Association (AHA), American College of Cardiology (ACC), and other groups have published position papers addressing CV risk in diabetics.[3–7]

The goals of CV imaging include risk stratification and prediction, evaluation of patient response to interventions, and identification of novel genetic, cellular, and molecular determinants of risk. There exist a number of clinical and experimental techniques that assess different aspects of atherogenesis and cardiac function. To accomplish these goals, there exist a number of techniques by which to measure subclinical atherosclerosis and vascular disease including ankle-brachial index, stress testing, carotid ultrasound, echocardiography, applanation tonometry, magnetic resonance imaging (MRI), and computed tomographic angiography. The purpose of this chapter is to review the use of these techniques in the diabetic population.

SCREENING

Clinical Evaluation

The clinical evaluation of all patients requires a careful medical history, which is directed at identifying concomitant CV risk factors and eliciting symptoms of atherosclerotic disease including angina, dyspnea, claudication, or erectile dysfunction. Evaluation of the diabetic patient poses some caveats. Firstly, the symptoms of cardiac disease are often atypical in the diabetic population. A higher prevalence of silent ischemia in the diabetic population renders a history of angina less reliable. In addition, all diabetics fall into the intermediate if not high-risk category and would therefore prompt either noninvasive or invasive testing. Although electrocardiograms are routinely obtained to detect ischemic ST-T changes, these findings are unreliable in screening for clinically significant coronary disease. Perhaps the greatest value of the resting electrocardiogram is the exclusion of left ventricular dysfunction in the absence of major electrocardiographic (ECG) findings. Multiple studies have confirmed the negative predictive value of a normal or near normal electrocardiogram for left ventricular dysfunction. However, none have specifically addressed the diabetic population. A recent study of 965 diabetics in Italy found the prevalence of left ventricular hypertrophy defined by ECG Cornell voltage-duration product to be 17.1%.[8] Moreover, left ventricular hypertrophy is a well-known independent predictor of adverse cardiac events. Although one study found left ventricular mass is associated with urinary albumin excretion levels, body mass index, and systolic blood pressure (SBP) in type 2 diabetics,[9] another study found fasting insulin levels the best predictor of left ventricular mass.[10] In a substudy of 468 patients with diabetes mellitus (DM) and hypertension in the Appropriate Blood Pressure Control in Diabetes (ABCD) trial, change in voltage was an independent predictor of CV events along with treatment assignment (enalapril vs. nisoldipine), the presence of coronary disease at baseline, and the duration of DM.[11] In addition, QT prolongation is a marker of increased CV risk in both the general population and diabetics.[12,13] In a recent study of 1221 subjects from Sweden, a new Q/QS pattern on the resting ECG, regardless of history of MI, was a predictor of total and CV mortality.[14]

Cardiac Diagnostic Testing

Cardiac diagnostic testing is commonly used to improve the accuracy of risk stratification using clinical criteria. There exist a number of methods by which to assess myocardial ischemia and left ventricular function. Despite technologic advances in the diagnosis and treatment of CVDs, the standard treadmill exercise stress test (EST) remains an important modality in the evaluation of CAD. Its widespread availability and high diagnostic yield make the stress test a gatekeeper for more expensive and invasive procedures. There are several existing published guidelines for risk assessment in patients with CVD or those at risk for CVD (Table 16-1). The French Guideline for Detection of Silent Myocardial Ischemia in patients with diabetes suggests that screening for silent myocardial ischemia should be performed in patients with diabetes and one additional factor: peripheral arterial disease, proteinuria, or the presence of major CVD risk factors.[6] They specifically mention the use of exercise treadmill testing or thallium stress testing. The ACC/AHA Guidelines for Exercise Testing give screening by exercise treadmill testing in patients with diabetes a data quality rating of IIb, that is, its usefulness or efficacy is less well established by evidence or opinion. They add that exercise testing "might be useful in people with

Table 16-1 **Risk Stratification**

Guideline	
ACC/AHA Exercise testing	Do not specifically address Consider if "heightened pretest risk" Before starting vigorous activity (if age >35, type 1 DM >15 years, type 2 DM >10 years, suspected CAD, other risk factors, PAD, neuropathy)
ADA/ACC	Typical or atypical symptoms, peripheral arterial disease, cerebrovascular disease, rest ECG changes, the presence of two or more major CVD risk factors, before vigorous activity if age >35 years
French	Diabetes and one additional factor: peripheral arterial disease, proteinuria, or the presence of major CVD risk factors
AHA Prevention IV Conference	Insufficient evidence for recommendation
US Preventive Services Task Force	Insufficient evidence for recommendation

heightened pretest risk." The updated 2002 guidelines, however, gives a rating of IIa for stress testing in diabetics who are to begin vigorous exercise.[15,16] The ADA/ACC Consensus Statement on diabetes and CV risk suggests that noninvasive cardiac testing be performed in patients with diabetes and one additional factor: peripheral arterial disease, cerebrovascular disease, rest ECG changes, or presence of two or more major CVD risk factors.[3] ACC/ AHA currently recommends that they belong in the same high-risk category previously reserved for patients with known CAD. Critics of these guidelines would counter that routine noninvasive testing is unnecessary because it would not change management or lead to improved outcomes.

Treadmill exercise evokes a number of physiologic responses including biochemical, electrophysiologic, and hemodynamic changes which are recorded but often overlooked in the reporting of stress test results.[17] These data provide diagnostic and prognostic importance and should be collectively considered in the interpretation of the EST. Therefore, the EST should not be reported simply as positive or negative on the basis of ECG changes. The following parameters should be considered in the interpretation of any EST according to the mnemonic EDCBA:

- E: The conventional criterion for an abnormal exercise ECG is 1 mm of horizontal or downsloping ST-segment depression at 80 ms after the end of the QRS complex (from the J point). In most series, the sensitivity of an abnormal ECG ranges from 65 to 70% and the specificity ranges from 85 to 90%.[18] ST-segment displacement is more likely in flow limiting (>50% luminal diameter narrowing) epicardial CAD and in multivessel as compared to single vessel coronary disease. ST depressions occur most commonly in the lateral leads and least commonly in the anterior leads. They may be upsloping, horizontal, or downsloping with upsloping changes being less specific and usually indicating lesser degrees of ischemia. Horizontal ST changes are intermediate and a downsloping pattern of ST-segment depression is more specific for myocardial ischemia and often indicates more severe ischemia. The location of ST-segment depressions does not indicate the region of the heart subserved by a stenosed coronary artery. Therefore, it is the presence and not the location of ST depressions that is meaningful. In contrast, ST-segment elevations are much less common, are felt to indicate transmural ischemia, and are referable to a specific region of the left ventricle. False positive ST depressions are commonly seen in patients with baseline ST segment and T-wave changes on resting ECG, left ventricular hypertrophy, patients on digitalis, cardiomyopathies, and premenopausal women.
- D: Is a diagnostic heart rate achieved and what is the duration of exercise? The diagnostic potential of a stress test could be expected to be lowered if a patient were unable to perform a workload substantial enough to induce myocardial ischemia. Because heart rate is the chief determinant

of myocardial oxygen demand, the peak heart rate achieved strongly influences the sensitivity of EST. Historically, a stress test is "diagnostic" when the patient achieves 85% predicted maximal heart rate. The predicted maximal heart rate strongly correlates with age by the following regression equation: 220-age. However, there is considerable scatter around this line with a standard deviation of ±12 bpm. Nonetheless, several studies have shown the sensitivity of the exercise ECG to be decreased with peak heart rates <85% of target. Alternatively, the double product includes SBP as well as heart rate.

The duration of the symptom-limited test carries strong prognostic significance. It is an indirect measure of workload with the number of minutes exercised on a Bruce protocol correlating well with peak ventilatory oxygen consumption in metabolic equivalents (METS). Accordingly, ventilatory 02 consumption (MET level) can be estimated from workload or actually measured by gas exchange analysis during treadmill exercise. Numerous studies have shown long-term prognosis to be related to functional capacity.[19] One study found a 1-year mortality of 1% and a 4-year mortality of 7% in patients able to exercise 12 minutes on a Bruce protocol and exceed a heart rate of 160 bpm regardless of the presence of coronary disease on cardiac catheterization.[18] Other studies have found the inability to complete two stages of a Bruce protocol (6 minutes) to be associated with a poor prognosis.[20]

- C: Chest pain also finds itself amongst the indicators to terminate an exercise test and is more predictive of CAD if combined with the ECG. Weiner et al. reported on 281 consecutive patients studied with treadmill testing and coronary angiography with following responses: 76 patients with ST depression and treadmill test-induced chest pain, 85 patients with ST depression and no chest pain, 40 patients with a treadmill test-induced chest pain who had no ST changes, and 80 patients with neither chest pain nor ST changes.[21] They found that 91% of the first group, 65% of the second group, 72% of the third group, and only 35% of the fourth group had significant angiographically determined CAD. Cole and Ellestad followed 1402 patients with abnormal treadmill tests. Exercise-induced angina identified 85% of true positive tests, while ST depression alone identified only 64%. Men aged 41–50 with angina had a three- to fourfold greater incidence of coronary events.[22] Therefore, the presence of chest pain during exercise stress testing carries diagnostic and prognostic value. Zellweger et al. followed 1737 diabetic patients that had myocardial perfusion imaging (MPI) for a median of 2 years. They found that in asymptomatic diabetics positive tests and critical events were similar to those diabetics with angina (3.4 vs. 5.6, respectively), however, shortness of breath was the best predictor, with the outcome three times worse (13.2%).[23]

- *B*: The normal blood pressure response to dynamic upright exercise consists of a progressive increase in systolic BP with little change or a decrease in diastolic BP resulting in a widened pulse pressure. Although exercise-induced hypotension may be caused by exhaustion, valvular heart disease, cardiomyopathy, or antihypertensive medications, it is generally regarded as a consequence of extensive ischemia resulting from triple vessel or left main coronary disease. Exercise-induced hypotension has been demonstrated in multiple studies to predict a poor prognosis. Exercise-induced hypertension (SBP >220 mmHg) occurs in hypertensives and is also a precursor to hypertension.
- *A*: With regard to arrhythmias, premature ventricular and atrial complexes are the most common rhythm abnormalities during exercise testing. Although the literature on premature ventricular complexes is mixed, their prognostic significance appears more related to underlying conditions including ischemia and ventricular dysfunction, than to the arrhythmias themselves. Exercise-induced ventricular arrhythmias generally increase in prevalence with age. Premature ventricular complexes during recovery may be more significant than those that occur during exercise. Nonsustained ventricular tachycardia is uncommon during routine clinical treadmill testing (prevalence ~ 2%), is well tolerated, and has a prognosis determined by the accompanying ischemia and left ventricular dysfunction.

The utility of the EDCBA approach for EST interpretation is highlighted by the development of a scoring system including some of the aforementioned variables in order to determine mortality risk. The Duke University study prospectively developed a quantitative exercise treadmill score and nomogram for predicting prognosis from patients referred for exercise stress testing.[24] The following parameters were independently associated with prognosis: total exercise time in minutes, maximum ST-segment deviation in millimeters, and treadmill angina index (0 = no angina, 1 = nontypical limiting angina, 2 = limiting angina which causes test termination). The treadmill exercise score was calculated as: exercise time – (5 × ST-segment deviation) – (4 × treadmill angina index). The risk categories based on the calculated exercise treadmill score were: high risk: a treadmill score <10, associated with a 5-year survival rate of 72%, moderate risk: a treadmill score from 10 to +4, associated with a 5-year survival rate of 91%, low risk: a treadmill score ≥ to +5, associated with a 5-year survival rate of 97%. The corresponding cardiac event (MI or sudden death) rates were 63, 86, and 93%, respectively. The Duke investigators subsequently validated the treadmill score in a group of 613 consecutive outpatients with suspected CAD referred for EST and found the treadmill score more useful among outpatients than among inpatients. Four-year survival rates were: 99, 95, and 79% in low, moderate, and high-risk groups, respectively.

Over the last decade, there has been a growing recognition of the prognostic value of additional physiologic parameters including heart rate and blood pressure responses. Heart rate and blood pressure responses are often impaired in diabetic subjects and are unrelated to the presence of autonomic dysfunction.[25,26] In healthy subjects, heart rate typically increases during treadmill exercise and then decelerates within 1 minute of recovery. A number of studies have found delayed heart rate recovery associated with increased CV risk. Among 5190 healthy adults without medically treated diabetes enrolled in the Lipid Research Clinics' Prevalence Study who underwent exercise testing, abnormal heart rate recovery was found in 33% of subjects and was associated with impaired fasting glucose and with diabetes and in turn was predictive of overall mortality. Fasting plasma glucose is strongly and independently associated with abnormal heart rate recovery, even at nondiabetic levels.[27] In another study of 2333 male diabetics, the 5-minute heart rate recovery was independently predictive of CV and all-cause death at 14.9 years follow-up.[28]

In a manner analogous to the heart rate response, SBP normally increases during aerobic exercise and falls rapidly during recovery. Delay in the fall of SBP during recovery is marker of significant coronary stenoses. The SBP ratio is the ratio of the postexercise SBP at 1, 2, or 3 minutes to the peak SBP during exercise. In one study of diabetics referred for cardiac catheterization, a SBP ratio >0.87 was associated with significant stenoses. The sensitivity, specificity, and accuracy of ST changes combined with a SBP ratio >0.87 for detecting stenoses in patients with DM were 68, 82, and 74%, respectively.[29]

Exercise Tolerance Testing

There are significantly fewer data regarding the predictive power of exercise testing in patients with diabetes. Lee et al. studied 1282 male veterans presenting with chest pain and found 38% of diabetics and 38% of nondiabetics to have an abnormal exercise test result.[30] The sensitivity and specificity of the exercise test was 47 and 81% in diabetics and 52 and 80% in nondiabetics. This study showed the standard exercise test has similar diagnostic characteristics in diabetic as in nondiabetic patients.

Limited data nonetheless suggest that whereas symptoms may be unreliable for detection of ischemic heart disease in patients with diabetes, ischemic findings on exercise ECG appear to be at least as predictive of prognosis in patients with diabetes (and possibly indicative of even worse outcome) than in nondiabetic patients. Exercise tolerance is an important predictor of adverse outcomes in diabetics. One study of 68 diabetic males referred for stress testing, diabetic men who were able to exercise for 440 seconds on a treadmill using a Bruce protocol were at low risk of a coronary event during 12- to 18-month follow-up.[31] Although the French guidelines specifically mention the use of exercise treadmill testing or thallium stress testing and exercise stress testing is more cost-effective than stress echocardiography and stress perfusion imaging,[32] exercise tolerance in patients with diabetes is frequently impaired due to noncardiac disease such as claudication and polyneuropathy. In one study, only 68% of patients had a diagnostic test.[33]

To overcome these limitations, other stress modalities including pharmacologic stress testing (dipyridamole, adenosine, dobutamine) coupled with imaging techniques have become increasingly used with high sensitivity and specificity for the noninvasive diagnosis of CAD. While imaging techniques including radionuclide and echocardiography are more expensive, their diagnostic accuracies are generally higher than exercise electrocardiography with sensitivities and specificities ranging from 90 to 95% for both techniques. The superiority of imaging techniques may be explained by the ischemic cascade, which describes the sequence of events occurring at the onset of myocardial ischemia. Although initially observed during coronary angioplasty balloon inflation, the following manifestations are felt to follow stress-induced ischemia as well: diastolic dysfunction followed by segmental systolic dysfunction, ECG changes, and lastly chest pain. ECG changes and chest pain are late and less reliable indicators of ischemia.

Stress Nuclear

Radionuclide MPI is an established and noninvasive imaging technique with diagnostic and prognostic efficacy in the investigation of CAD.[34] MPI carries over a 35-year track record in clinical use and is the only widely available test for assessing myocardial perfusion directly. Although there are variations in the protocols performed in different centers, MPI assesses inhomogeneity of radionuclide uptake as a marker of abnormal regional myocardial perfusion (Fig. 16-1). MPI used as an adjunct to either exercise or pharmacologic stress confers a higher diagnostic accuracy than exercise electrocardiography alone. To date, a number of studies have confirmed that stress single-photon emission computed tomography (SPECT) provides incremental prognostic value and achieves adequate risk stratification in diabetic cohorts.[35-41] Reversible perfusion defects indicating myocardial ischemia occur in 22–58% of diabetics.[42,43] In a study of 133 consecutive diabetic patients with suspected CAD, stress-induced perfusion defects occurred in 31% of the patients regardless of a history of chest pain.[44] In this study, reversible defects were associated with inducible ST-segment depression during myocardial perfusion scintigraphy (MPS) stress (odds ratio [OR] 3.2). In another study of asymptomatic diabetics, the ECG stress test was abnormal in 21% of subjects, whereas myocardial scintigraphy was abnormal in additional 16%.[45] Both the ECG stress test (OR 3.9, $P = 0.008$) and myocardial scintigraphy (OR 3.8, $P = 0.009$) were univariate predictors of cardiac events. The negative predictive value of the ECG stress test was 97%. Among 1427 asymptomatic diabetic patients without known CAD, abnormal stress SPECT imaging scans were associated with Q waves on electrocardiogram

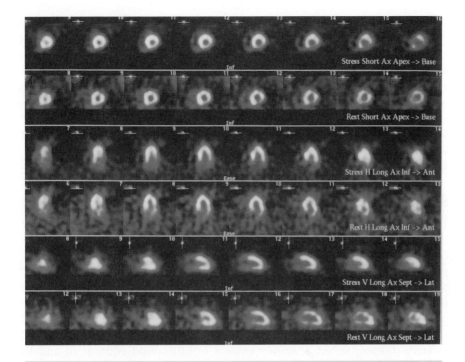

Figure 16-1 **Myocardial perfusion SPECT image. Both stress and rest images are displayed. Lack of radiotracer (or defect) in a particular segment of the left ventricle suggests a hemodynamically significant coronary stenosis. Stress and rest images are compared and these defects are classified as reversible or fixed, indicating ischemia or scar in that segment.**

and peripheral arterial disease.[43] Annual mortality rates for patient subsets categorized by SPECT imaging scans were high risk 5.9%, intermediate risk 5.0%, and low risk 3.6%. In another study of 6173 consecutive patients who underwent rest thallium-201/adenosine technetium-99m sestamibi MPI, Berman et al. found diabetic women and patients with insulin-dependent diabetes mellitus (IDDM) to have greater risk of cardiac death than other patients for any MPS result.[35] The role of stress perfusion imaging was evaluated prospectively in the Detection of Ischemia in Asymptomatic Diabetics (DIAD) study, in which 1123 patients with type 2 diabetes, aged 50–75 years, with no known or suspected CAD, were randomly assigned to either stress testing and 5-year clinical follow-up or to follow-up only.[46] Twenty-two percent had silent ischemia, including 83 with regional myocardial perfusion abnormalities and 30 with normal perfusion but other abnormalities including ST-segment depression, ventricular dilation, or rest ventricular dysfunction. Abnormal Valsalva (OR 5.6), male sex (OR 2.5), and diabetes duration (OR 5.2) were predictors of abnormal tests. Autonomic neuropathy, a common and well-recognized serious complication of DM, is also associated with perfusion abnormalities. After percutaneous coronary intervention, asymptomatic diabetic patients followed by MPI have a high frequency of persistent silent ischemia found and this is associated with a high risk for repeat intervention but not major cardiac events.[47] Although a low-risk MPI scan suggests a low event rate, this window appears to be shorter in diabetics than nondiabetics. Several studies suggest an increased event rate after 2 years, suggesting the need for more frequent testing in diabetics.[48,49]

Stress Echocardiography

The development of digital technology helped foster the era of stress echocardiography, which has grown in popularity over the last 10–15 years and is recommended by the ACC as a valid and clinically useful technique, presenting several advantages over the radionuclide techniques. It is a less expensive test, providing immediate results without radiation exposure and provides additional information regarding left ventricular muscle mass, pulmonary artery pressures, or valvular heart disease. Although echocardiographic image quality is reduced in very obese patients or patients with chronic obstructive pulmonary disease, technical improvements in ultrasound equipment and the use of intravenous contrast agents have made stress echo feasible in the majority of these patients. In patients who are not able to exercise on the treadmill, bicycle exercise or dobutamine stress echocardiography (DSE) may be substituted. Vasodilators are less reliable and are seldom used in conjunction with echocardiography. The specificity of stress echocardiography has been called into question. Among 52 patients with DM, the sensitivity, specificity, positive, and negative predictive values of DSE for detection of CAD were 82, 54, 84, and 50%, respectively.[50] Despite a low reported specificity, stress echocardiography appears more specific in predicting cardiac events as compared to stress perfusion imaging.[51] False positive findings on both stress perfusion and echocardiographic imaging have been attributed to microvascular disease and abnormal endothelial dysfunction, which may be underestimated by conventional coronary angiography. Moreover, exercise and DSE have been shown to predict cardiac events in diabetic patients with known or suspected CAD and add additional prognostic information as compared with the exercise ECG.[52-54]

Transthoracic Echocardiography

In addition to the regional or global left ventricular dysfunction that may occur in patients with CAD or cardiomyopathy, the transthoracic echocardiogram may reveal subclinical diastolic or systolic left ventricular dysfunction that has been associated with underlying CAD or diabetic cardiomyopathy.

Diastolic dysfunction may be demonstrated by the ratio of the early to late mitral valve Doppler inflow pattern (Figs. 16-2 ad 16-3), or more recently by tissue Doppler imaging (Figs. 16-4 ad 16-5) and other techniques such as the left ventricular-mitral color Doppler M-mode flow propagation velocity (Fig. 16-6).[55] Tissue Doppler imaging is felt to be more sensitive and less load dependent than traditional blood velocity Doppler measures. Studies have suggested subclinical disease may be a precursor to overt coronary disease with subsequent increase in mortality.[56,57] Boyer et al. studied 61 normotensive diabetics with normal stress echocardiograms, and found the prevalence of diastolic dysfunction to be 75% when multiple Doppler techniques were used. Tissue Doppler imaging was the most sensitive, alone detecting diastolic dysfunction in 63% of patients.[58] Diastolic dysfunction, especially determined by tissue Doppler imaging, has been reported to result in impaired exercise tolerance.[59-61] Recently, Fang et al. studied with tissue Doppler imaging 219 diabetics with negative stress echocardiograms and without hypertrophy, and found 29% to have subclinical left ventricular systolic or diastolic dysfunction. Systolic dysfunction was associated with poor diabetic control. Diastolic dysfunction was associated with age and hypertension, and metformin treatment had a weak adverse effect on diastolic

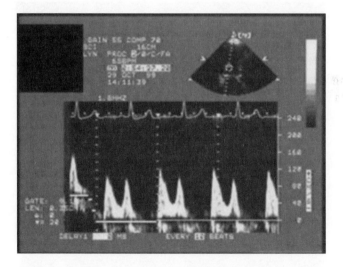

Figure 16-2 **Normal mitral valve Doppler E/A inflow pattern. The mitral valve inflow Doppler E/A pattern is one of the Doppler methods used to evaluate diastolic function of the left ventricle. The velocity of the early diastolic filling wave (E wave) is greater than the late filling wave (A wave). This is usually but not always indicative of normal diastolic function.**

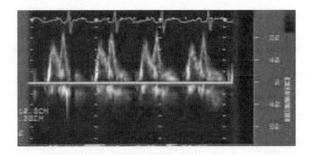

Figure 16-3 **Reversal of the mitral valve Doppler E/A inflow pattern. The A wave has greater velocity than the E wave. This suggests reduced relaxation of the left ventricle and early diastolic dysfunction.**

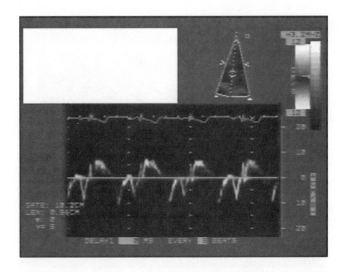

Figure 16-4 **Normal tissue Doppler pattern from the mitral valve annulus. Tissue Doppler can quantify the direction and velocity of myocardial movement, and is a newer method of evaluating both systolic and diastolic function. The early downward diastolic deflection represents the initial velocity of the ventricular septum away from the apex, and is greater than the late diastolic movement. This suggests normal diastolic function.**

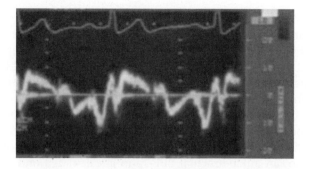

Figure 16-5 **Reversal of the normal tissue Doppler pattern. The late diastolic velocity of the annulus is greater than the early. This suggests reduced left ventricular relaxation and diastolic dysfunction.**

dysfunction. Insulin therapy had a protective effect on systolic function.[62] Despite many studies in the literature, varying techniques to evaluate subclinical diastolic and systolic disease are used with varying populations, thus limiting definitive conclusions. There are also no definitive data to suggest that screening and treatment of subclinical abnormalities resulted in benefit, and so screening is not generally recommended. This awaits further study.

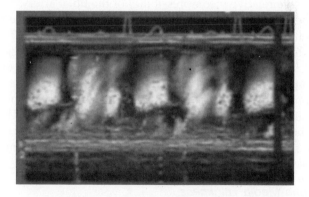

Figure 16-6 *Transmitral color Doppler M-mode imaging (flow propagation velocity). From color Doppler imaging the flow velocity of blood into the left ventricle can be quantified. A reduced slope of the color Doppler jet into the left ventricle suggests reduced flow velocities and therefore delayed filling, indicative of diastolic dysfunction.*

Ankle-Brachial Blood Pressure Index

The ankle-brachial blood pressure index (ABI) is a simple inexpensive method that has been proposed as a marker of subclinical atherosclerosis. It is performed by measuring blood pressure in both upper and lower extremities. Although it is technically feasible to measure blood pressure by sphygmomanometry, it is more commonly measured by recording of the Doppler waveforms, thereby making it a true imaging technique. Doppler recording allows for localization of atherosclerotic disease to the posterior tibial and dorsalis pedis arteries, whereas sphygmomanometry does not. By use of either method, an ankle-brachial SBP ratio is calculated and an ABI <0.90 constitutes a diagnosis of peripheral arterial disease. Numerous studies have demonstrated the predictive value of a low ABI for adverse CV events in the general population and in diabetic subjects.[63,64]

A study from England showed high prevalences of peripheral vascular disease in persons with type 1 (8.7%) and type 2 diabetes (23.5%).[64] Age, cerebrovascular disease, CAD, glucose, body mass index, and cholesterol in type 2 diabetes and age and proteinuria in type 1 diabetes were significant predictors of peripheral vascular disease. In another study of 1087 patients with type 1 diabetes and 1060 patients with type 2 diabetes, low ABI was associated with coronary heart disease (OR 9.3 vs. 3.5), diabetic nephropathy (OR 3.0 vs. 2.8), neuropathy (OR 7.9 vs. 1.8), foot ulceration (OR 8.9 vs. 5.5), increased daily insulin requirement >0.6 $\mu m/kg$ (OR 5.2 vs. 2.9), and diabetes duration of 20–29 years (OR 28.9).[65]

Diabetic patients may also show an abnormally high ABI, which has been attributed to the relative incompressibility of the tibial artery.[66,67] While earlier studies excluded subjects with abnormally high ABI, more recent studies have examined the significance of this finding. Among 4393 American Indians in the Strong Heart Study, 4.9% had low ABI whereas a high ABI occurred in 9.2%.[68] Subjects in the Strong Heart Study are well known to have a high prevalence of diabetes and obesity. Diabetes, albuminuria, and hypertension occurred with greater frequency among persons with low (60.2, 44.4, and 50.1%) and high (67.8, 49.9, and 53%) ABIs. The U-shaped association between ABI and mortality risk suggested that the upper limit of normal ABI should not exceed 1.40. In these patients, toe brachial index has been proposed to be a superior measure.

Carotid Intima-Media Thickness

A number of studies have used B-mode ultrasound to measure carotid intimal-medial thickness as an indicator of the severity of carotid atherosclerosis.[69] Carotid intima-media thickness measurements use B-mode ultrasound to measure the lumen and wall of the carotid artery (Fig. 16-7). Ultrasonography of the arterial wall allows detection of structural changes including thickening and plaque as well as functional changes including stiffness associated with preclinical atherosclerosis. An increased thickness of the

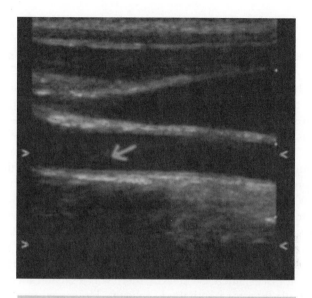

Figure 16-7 **Carotid artery ultrasound image. In addition to visualizing atherosclerotic plaque, the carotid intima-media thickness can be measured. This method may be used to evaluate for early atherosclerotic changes.**

carotid artery wall is thought to be a sign of early atherosclerosis and may be detected by measuring the combined intima-media thickness. Prospective population-based studies have shown that carotid intima-media thickness provides incremental predictive value on CV risk. Carotid intima thickness has been found in a number of studies to be greater in diabetic than in non-diabetic subjects.[70] Among subjects with diabetes, greater carotid intima-media thickness has been associated with a prior diagnosis of diabetes and fasting glucose level,[71] insulin resistance,[70,72] and triglycerides and the total-to-high-density lipoprotein (HDL) cholesterol ratio.[73] Carotid intimal-medial thickness has been correlated with QT prolongation.[74] Diabetics have also been shown to have a greater rate of intima-media thickness progression than nondiabetics.[71]

Electron Beam Computed Tomography

Electron beam computed tomography (EBCT) is a noninvasive procedure that detects CAD by measuring the amount of coronary artery calcium (CAC) within the coronary arteries. There is a strong correlation between the presence of coronary calcium and the amount of atheromatous plaque. The coronary artery calcium score (CCS) score is an independent predictor of coronary heart disease. In general, a score of zero implies no identifiable plaque and a very low CV risk, scores ranging from 1 to 10 imply a minimal plaque burden with low CV risk, scores from 11 to 100 imply a mild or minimal coronary stenosis and moderate CV risk, and CAC scores between 101 and 400 imply a definite plaque burden and high likelihood of obstructive disease, and scores >400 indicates an extensive plaque burden with a high likelihood of significant coronary stenosis.[75] Numerous studies have evaluated the measurement of CAC in type 1 and type 2 diabetics. The relationship between CAC and atheromatous plaque is similar in diabetics as in nondiabetics, although some have suggested CCS should be adjusted higher in diabetics to improve the specificity of scoring for obstructive coronary disease.[76] Among 30,904 asymptomatic individuals, younger diabetic individuals were found to have calcified plaque burden comparable to that of older individuals without diabetes.[77] In another study of 10,377 asymptomatic individuals referred for electron beam tomography imaging, the 903 subjects who were diabetic had higher mean calcium scores.[78] During a mean follow-up of 5 years, for every increase in CCS, there was a greater increase in mortality for diabetic than for nondiabetic subjects. However, patients suffering from diabetes with no CAC demonstrated a survival similar to that of individuals without diabetes and no detectable calcium (98.8 and 99.4%, respectively, $P = 0.5$). One study found CAC scores were positively correlated with glucose, insulin, and homeostasis model assessment (HOMA) insulin resistance,[79] whereas another found higher scores associated with hypertension.[80] In diabetics, calcium scores appear more closely associated with CAD than to clinical symptoms or ECG changes. In type 1 diabetics, CAC scores were an independent correlate of MI or obstructive CAD in both sexes and was the strongest independent correlate in men, but was not independently associated with angina and ischemic ECG changes in either sex.[81] Hosoi et al. studied 282 patients with chest pain (36% diabetics), who were referred for underwent coronary angiography and EBCT and found sensitivity and specificity of EBCT to detect significant coronary stenoses ≥50% were not significantly different between diabetic and nondiabetic patients. In diabetic patients, a CCS ≥90 was associated with 75% sensitivity and 75% specificity, whereas a CCS ≥200 was associated with 64% sensitivity and 83% specificity.[82] However, data regarding coronary calcium scores in diabetics are conflicting. The South Bay Heart Watch study showed that coronary calcium score risk groups were significantly associated with events in nondiabetic subjects (relative risk [RR] ≥2.6, $P < 0.01$), but not in diabetic subjects (RR ≤1.7, $P > 0.05$).[83] Berman et al. reviewed 1195 patients who had both MPS imaging and coronary calcium scoring by CT. They found patients with a calcium scores <100 an ischemic myocardial perfusion study was unlikely, so in patients with low calcium scores noninvasive testing may not be necessary. Normal MPS patients, however, frequently have extensive atherosclerosis by calcium scoring. In patients with scores >400, the frequency of inducible ischemia was significant and so these patients may be candidates for stress perfusion imaging. Scores in the 100–400 range constituted a "grey" zone in which further study was suggested.[84] These findings have lead the AHA to cautiously advocate the use of coronary calcium screening in nondiabetic asymptomatic subjects at intermediate disease risk. Additional studies are needed to determine the predictive value of coronary calcium scores for clinical events in patients with diabetes.

Coronary Computed Tomography Angiography

Coronary computed tomography angiography (CTA) is an accurate and reliable method for performing noninvasive coronary angiography (Fig. 16-8).[85–88]

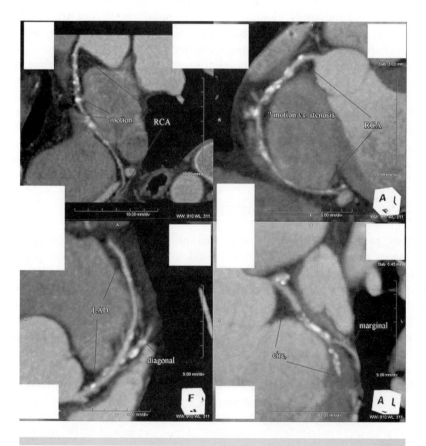

Figure 16-8 **Image obtained from a 64-slice CT scanner. With the use of intravenous contrast and the continued improvement in CT scan technology, the coronary arteries can be imaged and evaluated for atherosclerotic lesions.**

The development of 16, 32, and 64-slice scanners has improved the performance of coronary CTA over prior CT techniques, increasing the average number of assessable coronary segments to approximately 90%. CTA studies have shown a 92–95% sensitivity for detecting stenoses of 50% or greater. The assessment of atherosclerotic plaques by imaging techniques may prove valuable for the identification of vulnerable plaques. There are no data regarding the diagnostic accuracy of CTA for detecting and assessing the extent of CAD specifically in patients with diabetes.

Magnetic Resonance Imaging

While MRI has contributed greatly to the assessment of ventricular structure and function, MR angiography has progressed slowly to visualize the coronary arteries. Cardiac motion interferes with the ability of cardiac magnetic resonance to adequately visualize coronary anatomy. Recent studies have suggested that MRI may be able to reliably quantitate the lipid-rich core and fibrous cap, allowing plaque characterization.[89,90] Although high-resolution MRI can differentiate plaque components, and under some circumstances, it may be able to identify vulnerable plaque, outcome studies to predict future CVD events in diabetic and nondiabetic patients are lacking. MR also has the ability to quantitate blood flow and measure flow reserve. The Multi-Ethnic Study of Atherosclerosis (MESA) study found myocardial blood flow reserve using adenosine-induced hyperemia and MRI reduced in some patients with coronary risk factors, but not in diabetics.[91] Recommendation of this technique for risk assessment awaits further data.

OTHER IMAGING MODALITIES

Cardiac radionuclide imaging with metaiodobenzylguanidine (MIBG), an analog of norepinephrine, has been used to evaluate cardiac sympathetic activity in clinical research studies. MIBG imaging allows the evaluation of receptor density and sympathetic tone. The regional distribution and extent of denervation may be assessed. Diabetic autonomic neuropathy increases both morbidity and mortality rates in diabetic patients.[92] Patients with diabetic autonomic neuropathy tend to have greater MIBG abnormalities. Abnormalities of cardiac sympathetic activity may contribute to arrhythmias. QT interval prolongation and QT dispersion have been associated with sudden death in diabetic patients, but most studies have not shown a relationship between QT abnormalities and degree of MIBG uptake.[93] Also, in some studies autonomic neuropathy and MIBG abnormality have been associated with left ventricular dysfunction.[94] The exact role of MIBG imaging in diabetic patients awaits further studies.

Arterial Stiffness

Arterial stiffness is the major determinant of systolic pressure and has been shown to be predictive of CV events in a variety of patient populations. At present, there exist a variety of methods by which to measure stiffness including carotid artery and aortic ultrasound, and arterial tonometry.[95] Pulse wave analysis (PWA) is a technique that allows the accurate recording of peripheral pressure waveforms and generation of the corresponding central waveform via a mathematical transfer function. The central aortic pressure tracing can be analyzed and separated into two components including the initial portion of the upstroke due to ejection of blood and a secondary component due to wave reflection. A stiffer arterial system will result in more rapid wave reflection and therefore an augmented systolic pressure. Stiffness may therefore be calculated from a number of parameters that quantify reflection including the augmentation pressure and index (Fig. 16-9). This technique has grown in popularity over the last several years and has been used in a few studies to evaluate CAD in diabetics. The results vary depending on the specific parameters evaluated. One study found that among 385 postmenopausal women, aged 50–74 years, PWV associated with body mass index, fasting glucose, DM, and triglycerides after adjustment for age, mean arterial blood pressure, and heart rate. Height and HDL cholesterol were inversely related to PWA.[96] In another study, diabetics were found to have higher pulse pressure and pulse wave velocity values but not augmentation index than controls.[97] Gender appears to be an important determinant of stiffness among type 2 diabetics as greater age-related stiffening of the aorta was found in women as compared with men.[98] In 102 asymptomatic type 2 diabetic patients, arterial stiffness assessed by brachial-ankle pulse wave velocity was associated with carotid intima-media thickness, independent of age and other risk factors.[99]

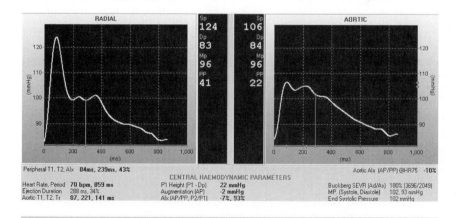

Figure 16-9 **Radial artery and aortic waveforms obtained by radial artery tonometry. Peripheral radial artery waveforms are easily obtained, and central aortic waveforms are generated with the use of a transfer function. Arterial tonometry allows measurement of central aortic pressures and indices of vascular stiffness.**

SUMMARY

Coronary artery disease in patients with diabetes is frequently silent, further advanced at the time of diagnosis, and associated with an unfavorable prognosis compared with CAD in patients without diabetes. The reduction of CV risk in the diabetic often requires a multidisciplinary approach to optimize risk assessment and monitoring of therapy. After clinical evaluation, refinement of risk stratification frequently relies on noninvasive imaging techniques. The information provided by noninvasive diagnostic testing is essential in those patients with an intermediate clinical risk for cardiac events. Noninvasive testing may include routine treadmill exercise testing, echocardiographic stress testing with dobutamine or exercise, and/or thallium perfusion imaging. Additional methods include determination of ankle-brachial index, carotid intimal-medial thickness, determination of arterial stiffness, computed tomography calcium scoring and coronary angiography, and MRI. In general, therapies are tailored individually depending on the severity of abnormalities. In addition, the severity of the risk assessment may influence the timing of intervention. Stress myocardial perfusion and echocardiographic imaging have been shown to have significant value in the diagnosis and prognosis of CAD in women. Stress imaging has been shown to add incremental value to the use of clinical variables or exercise electrocardiogram stress testing alone in the risk stratification of diabetic patients. Although normal stress imaging studies are generally associated with a low risk <1% annual risk of cardiac death or MI, patients with diabetes are at significantly greater risk than nondiabetics with normal studies, especially after 2 years. In the setting of an abnormal stress imaging study, the risk conferred by any given extent and severity of perfusion abnormality is greater in patients with diabetes than in nondiabetics. The risk is greater for insulin-dependent versus non-insulin-dependent diabetes. Clinical information adds incremental prognostic value over perfusion results and can further adjust risk based on imaging studies. Both clinical information and results of imaging studies should be used together to risk stratify and plan intervention in the diabetic patient.

REFERENCES

1. National Cholesterol Education Program (NCEP) Expert Panel on Detection, Evaluation, and Treatment of High Blood Cholesterol in Adults. Third report of the National Cholesterol Education Program (NCEP) Expert Panel on Detection, Evaluation, and Treatment of High Blood Cholesterol in Adults (Adult Treatment Panel III): final report. *Circulation* 2002;106:3143–3421.

2. Haffner SN, Lehto S, Ronnemma T, et al. Mortality from coronary heart disease in subjects with type 2 diabetes and in nondiabetic subjects with and without myocardial infarction. *N Engl J Med* 1998;339:229–234.

3. American Diabetes Association. Consensus development conference on the diagnosis of coronary heart disease in people with diabetes. *Diabetes Care* 1998;21:1551–1559.

4. Redberg RF, Greenland P, Fuster V, et al. Prevention Conference VI: Diabetes and Cardiovascular Disease Writing Group III: risk assessment in persons with diabetes. *Circulation* 2002;105:E144–E152.

5. Grundy SM, Howared B, Smith S, et al. Prevention Conference VI: Diabetes and Cardiovascular Disease: executive summary. *Circulation* 2002;105:2231–2239.

6. Puel J, Valensi P, Vanzetto G, et al. Societe francaise de cardiologie (SFC). Association de langue francaise pour l'etude du diabete et des maladies metaboliques (ALFEDIAM). Identifying myocardial ischaemia in diabetics. SFC/ALFEDIAM joint recommendations. *Arch Mal Coeur Vaiss* 2004;97(4):338–357.

7. US Preventative Services Task Force. Screening for coronary heart disease: recommendation statement. *Ann Intern Med* 2004;140:569–572.

8. Bruno G, Giunti S, Bargero G, et al. Sex differences in prevalence of electrocardiographic left ventricular hypertrophy in Type 2 diabetes: the Casale Monferrato Study. *Diabet Med* 2004;21(8):823–828.

9. Suzuki K, Kato K, Hanyu O, et al. Left ventricular mass index increases in proportion to the progression of diabetic nephropathy in Type 2 diabetic patients. *Diabetes Res Clin Pract* 2001;54(3):173–180.

10. de Kreutzenberg SV, Avogaro A, Tiengo A, et al. Left ventricular mass in type 2 diabetes mellitus. A study employing a simple ECG index: the Cornell voltage. *J Endocrinol Invest* 2000;23(3):139–144.

11. Havranek EP, Esler A, Estacio RO, et al. Differential effects of antihypertensive agents on electrocardiographic voltage: results from the Appropriate Blood Pressure Control in Diabetes (ABCD) trial. *Am Heart J* 2003;145(6):993–998.

12. Cardoso CR, Salles GF, Deccache W. Prognostic value of QT interval parameters in type 2 diabetes mellitus: results of a long-term follow-up prospective study. *J Diabetes Complicat* 2003;17(4):169–178.

13. Veglio M, Chinaglia A, Cavallo-Perin P. QT interval, cardiovascular risk factors and risk of death in diabetes. *J Endocrinol Invest* 2004;27(2):175–181.

14. Dunder K, Lind L, Zethelius B, et al. A new Q/QS pattern on the resting electrocardiogram is associated with impaired insulin secretion and a poor prognosis in elderly men independently of history of myocardial infarction. *J Intern Med* 2004;255(2):221–228.

15. Gibbons RJ, Balady GJ, Beasley JW, et al. ACC/AHA Guidelines for Exercise Testing: a report of the American College of Cardiology/American Heart Association Task Force on Practice Guidelines (Committee on Exercise Testing). *J Am Coll Cardiol* 1997;30:260–315.

16. Gibbons RJ, Balady GJ, Bricker JT, et al. ACC/AHA 2002 guideline update for exercise testing: a report of the American College of Cardiology/American Heart Association Task Force on Practice Guidelines (Committee on Exercise Testing). *J Am Coll Cardiol* 2002;40:1531–1540.

17. McNeer JF, Margolis JR, Lee KL, et al. The role of the exercise test in the evaluation of patients for ischemic heart disease. *Circulation* 1978;57:64–70.

18. Gianrossi R, Detrano R, Mulvihill D, et al. Exercise-induced ST depression in the diagnosis of coronary artery disease: a meta-analysis. *Circulation* 1989;80:87–98.

19. Blair SN, Kampert JB, Kohl HW III, et al. Influences of cardiorespiratory fitness and other precursors on cardiovascular disease and all-cause mortality in men and women. *JAMA* 1996;276:205–210.

20. Bruce RA, DeRouen TA, Hossack KF. Value of maximal exercise tests in risk assessment of primary coronary heart disease events in healthy men: five years' experience of the Seattle heart watch study. *Am J Cardiol* 1980;46:371–378.

21. Weiner DA, Ryan TJ, Parsons L, et al. Long-term prognostic value of exercise testing in men and women from the Coronary Artery Surgery Study (CASS) Registry. *Am J Cardiol* 1995;75:865–870.

22. Cole JP, Ellestad MH. Significance of chest pain during treadmill exercise: correlation with coronary events. *Am J Cardiol* 1978;41(2):227–232.

23. Zellweger MJ, Hachamovitch R, Kang X, et al. Prognostic relevance of symptoms versus objective evidence of coronary artery disease in diabetic patients. *Eur Heart J* 2004;25:543–550.

24. Mark DB, Shaw L, Harrell FE Jr, et al. Prognostic value of a treadmill exercise score in outpatients with suspected coronary artery disease. *N Engl J Med* 1991;325:849–853.

25. Radice M, Rocca A, Bedon E, et al. Abnormal response to exercise in middle-aged NIDDM patients with and without autonomic neuropathy. *Diabet Med* 1996;13(3):259–265.

26. Bottini P, Tantucci C, Scionti L, et al. Cardiovascular response to exercise in diabetic patients: influence of autonomic neuropathy of different severity. *Diabetologia* 1995;38(2):244–250.

27. Panzer C, Lauer MS, Brieke A, et al. Association of fasting plasma glucose with heart rate recovery in healthy adults: a population-based study. *Diabetes* 2002;51(3):803–807.

28. Cheng YJ, Lauer MS, Earnest CP, et al. Heart rate recovery following maximal exercise testing as a predictor of cardiovascular disease and all-cause mortality in men with diabetes. *Diabetes Care* 2003;26(7):2052–2057.

29. Yamaguchi M, Shimizu M, Ino H, et al. Diagnostic usefulness of the post-exercise systolic blood pressure response for the detection of coronary artery disease in patients with diabetes mellitus. *Jpn Circ J* 2000;64(12):949–952.

30. Lee DP, Fearon WF, Froelicher VF. Clinical utility of the exercise ECG in patients with diabetes and chest pain. *Chest* 2001;119(5):1576–1581.

31. Rubler S, Gerber D, Reitano J, et al. Predictive value of clinical and exercise variables for detection of coronary artery disease in men with diabetes mellitus. *Am J Cardiol* 1987;59(15):1310–1313.

32. Hayashino Y, Nagata-Kobayashi S, Morimoto T, et al. Cost-effectiveness of screening for coronary artery disease in asymptomatic patients with Type 2 diabetes and additional atherogenic risk factors. *J Gen Intern Med* 2004;19(12): 1181–1191.

33. Bacci S, Villella M, Villella A, et al. Screening for silent myocardial ischaemia in type 2 diabetic patients with additional atherogenic risk factors: applicability and accuracy of the exercise stress test. *Eur J Endocrinol* 2002;147(5):649–654.

34. Klocke FJ, Baird MG, Bateman TM, et al. ACC/AHA/ASNC guidelines for the clinical use of cardiac radionuclide imaging: a report of the American 1995 guidelines for the clinical use of radionuclide imaging. *J Am Coll Cardiol* 2003;42: 1318–1333.

35. Berman DS, Kang X, Hayes SW, et al. Adenosine myocardial perfusion single-photon emission computed tomography in women compared with men: impact of diabetes mellitus on incremental prognostic value and effect on patient management. *J Am Coll Cardiol* 2003;41:1125–1133.

36. Giri S, Shaw LJ, Murthy DR, et al. Impact of diabetes on the risk stratification using stress single-photon emission computed tomography myocardial perfusion imaging in patients with symptoms suggestive of coronary artery disease. *Circulation* 2002;105:32–40.

37. Kang X, Berman DS, Lewin HC, et al. Incremental prognostic value of myocardial perfusion single photon emission computed tomography in patients with diabetes mellitus. *Am Heart J* 1999;138:1025–1032.

38. Charvat J, Michalova K, Taborska K, et al. Comparison of the exercise ECG and stress myocardial SPECT in detection of the significant coronary artery disease in the asymptomatic patients with diabetes mellitus type 2. *Bratisl Lek Listy* 2004;105(2):56–61.

39. Khaleeli E, Peters SR, Bobrowsky K, et al. Diabetes and the associated incidence of subclinical atherosclerosis and coronary artery disease: implications for management. *Am Heart J* 2001;141:637–644.

40. Nesto RW, Watson FS, Kowalchuk GJ, et al. Silent myocardial ischemia and infarction in diabetics with peripheral vascular disease: assessment by dipyridamole thallium-201 scintigraphy. *Am Heart J* 1990;120:1073–1077.

41. Kang X, Berman DS, Lewin H, et al. Comparative ability of myocardial perfusion single-photon emission computed tomography to detect coronary artery disease in patients with and without diabetes mellitus. *Am Heart J* 1999;137(5):949–957.

42. Miller TD, Rajagopalan N, Hodge DO, et al. Yield of stress single-photon emission computed tomography in asymptomatic patients with diabetes. *Am Heart J* 2004;147(5):890–896.

43. Rajagopalan N, Miller TD, Hodge DO, et al. Identifying high-risk asymptomatic diabetic patients who are candidates for screening stress single-photon emission computed tomography imaging. *J Am Coll Cardiol* 2005;45(1):43–49.

44. Prior JO, Monbaron D, Koehli M, et al. Prevalence of symptomatic and silent stress-induced perfusion defects in diabetic patients with suspected coronary artery disease referred for myocardial perfusion scintigraphy. *Eur J Nucl Med Mol Imaging* 2005;32(1):60–69.

45. Cosson E, Paycha F, Paries J, et al. Detecting silent coronary stenoses and stratifying cardiac risk in patients with diabetes: ECG stress test or exercise myocardial scintigraphy? *Diabet Med* 2004;21(4):342–348.

46. Wackers FJ, Young LH, Inzucchi SE, et al. Detection of Ischemia in Asymptomatic Diabetics Investigators. Detection of silent myocardial ischemia in asymptomatic diabetic subjects: the DIAD study. *Diabetes Care* 2004;27(8):1954–1961.

47. L'Huillier I, Cottin Y, Touzery C, et al. Predictive value of myocardial tomoscintigraphy in asymptomatic diabetic patients after percutaneous coronary intervention. *Int J Cardiol* 2003;90(2/3):165–173.

48. Hachamovitch R, Hayes S, Friedman JD, et al. Determinants of risk and its temporal variation in patients with normal stress myocardial perfusion scans: what is the warranty period of a normal scan? *J Am Coll Cardiol* 2003;41:1329–1340.

49. Kamalesh M, Feigenbaum H, Sawada S. Challenge of identifying patients with diabetes mellitus who are at low risk for coronary events by use of cardiac stress imaging. *Am Heart J* 2004;147:561–563.

50. Hennessy TG, Codd MB, Kane G, et al. Evaluation of patients with diabetes mellitus for coronary artery disease using dobutamine stress echocardiography. *Coron Artery Dis* 1997;8(3/4):171–174.

51. Penfornis A, Zimmermann C, Boumal D, et al. Use of dobutamine stress echocardiography in detecting silent myocardial ischaemia in asymptomatic diabetic patients: a comparison with thallium scintigraphy and exercise testing. *Diabet Med* 2001;18(11):900–905.

52. Marwick TH, Case C, Sawada S, et al. Use of stress echocardiography to predict mortality in patients with diabetes and known or suspected coronary artery disease. *Diabetes Care* 2002;25(6):1042–1048.

53. Bigi R, Desideri A, Cortigiani L, et al. Stress echocardiography for risk stratification of diabetic patients with known or suspected coronary artery disease. *Diabetes Care* 2001;24(9):1596–1601.

54. Schinkel AF, Elhendy A, van Domburg RT, et al. Prognostic value of dobutamine-atropine stress myocardial perfusion imaging in patients with diabetes. *Diabetes Care.* 2002;25(9):1637–1643.

55. Appleton CP, Firstenberg MS, Garcia MJ, et al. The echo-Doppler evaluation of left ventricular diastolic function: a current perspective [review]. *Cardiol Clin* 2000;18:513–546.

56. Kuller LH, Shemanski L, Psaty BM, et al. Subclinical disease as an independent risk factor for cardiovascular disease. *Circulation* 1995;92:720–726.

57. Kuller LH, Velentgas P, Barzilay J, et al. Savage diabetes mellitus: subclinical cardiovascular disease and risk of incident cardiovascular disease and all-cause mortality. *Arterioscler Thromb Vasc Biol* 2000;20(3):823–829.

58. Boyer JK, Thanigaraj S, Schechtman KB, et al. Prevalence of ventricular diastolic dysfunction in asymptomatic, normotensive patients with diabetes mellitus. *Am J Cardiol* 2004;93:870–875.

59. Saraiva RM, Duarte DM, Duarte MP, et al. Tissue Doppler imaging identifies asymptomatic normotensive diabetics with diastolic dysfunction and reduced exercise tolerance. *Echocardiography* 2005;22(7):561–570.

60. Poirier P, Garneau C, Bogaty P, et al. Impact of left ventricular diastolic dysfunction on maximal treadmill performance in normotensive subjects with well-controlled type 2 diabetes mellitus. *Am J Cardiol* 2000;85(4):473–477.

61. Fang ZY, Sharman J, Prins JB, et al. Determinants of exercise capacity in patients with type 2 diabetes. *Diabetes Care* 2005;28(7):1643–1648.

62. Fang ZY, Schull-Meade R, Downey M, et al. Determinants of subclinical diabetic heart disease. *Diabetologia* 2005;48(2):394–402.

63. Vogt MT, McKenna M, Wolfson SK, et al. The relationship between ankle brachial index, other atherosclerotic disease, diabetes, smoking and mortality in older men and women. *Atherosclerosis* 1993;101(2):191–202.

64. Walters DP, Gatling W, Mullee MA, et al. The prevalence, detection, and epidemiological correlates of peripheral vascular disease: a comparison of diabetic and non-diabetic subjects in an English community. *Diabet Med* 1992;9(8):710–715.

65. Zander E, Heinke P, Reindel J, et al. Peripheral arterial disease in diabetes mellitus type 1 and type 2: are there different risk factors? *Vasa* 2002;31(4):249–254.

66. Goss DE, de Trafford J, Roberts VC, et al. Raised ankle/brachial pressure index in insulin-treated diabetic patients. *Diabet Med* 1989;6(7):576–578.

67. Goss DE, Stevens M, Watkins PJ, et al. Falsely raised ankle/brachial pressure index: a method to determine tibial artery compressibility. *Eur J Vasc Surg* 1991;5(1):23–26.

68. Resnick HE, Lindsay RS, McDermott MM, et al. Relationship of high and low ankle brachial index to all-cause and cardiovascular disease mortality: the Strong Heart Study. *Circulation* 2004;109(6):733–739.

69. Mukherjee D, Yadav JS. Carotid artery intimal-medial thickness: indicator of atherosclerotic burden and response to risk factor modification. *Am Heart J* 2002;144(5):753–759.

70. Bonora E, Tessari R, Micciolo R, et al. Intimal-medial thickness of the carotid artery in nondiabetic and NIDDM patients. Relationship with insulin resistance. *Diabetes Care* 1997;20(4):627–631.

71. Wagenknecht LE, D'Agostino R Jr, Savage PJ, et al. Duration of diabetes and carotid wall thickness. The Insulin Resistance Atherosclerosis Study (IRAS). *Stroke* 1997;28(5):999–1005.

72. Teno S, Uto Y, Nagashima H, et al. Association of postprandial hypertriglyceridemia and carotid intima-media thickness in patients with type 2 diabetes. *Diabetes Care* 2000;23(9):1401–1406.

73. Temelkova-Kurktschiev TS, Koehler C, Leonhardt W, et al. Increased intimalmedial thickness in newly detected type 2 diabetes: risk factors. *Diabetes Care* 1999;22(2):333–338.

74. Takebayashi K, Aso Y, Matsutomo R, et al. Association between the corrected QT intervals and combined intimal-medial thickness of the carotid artery in patients with type 2 diabetes. *Metabolism* 2004;53(9):1152–1157.

75. Agatston JAS, Janowitz WR, Hildner Z, et al. Quantification of coronary artery calcium using ultrafast computed tomography. *J Am Coll Cardiol* 1990;15(4):827–832.

76. Khaleeli E, Peters SR, Bobrowsky K, et al. The use of electron beam computed tomography in diabetics. *Am Heart J* 2001;141:637–644.

77. Hoff JA, Quinn L, Sevrukov A, et al. The prevalence of coronary artery calcium among diabetic individuals without known coronary artery disease. *J Am Coll Cardiol* 2003;41(6):1008–1012.

78. Raggi P, Shaw LJ, Berman DS, et al. Prognostic value of coronary artery calcium screening in subjects with and without diabetes. *J Am Coll Cardiol* 2004;43(9): 1663–1669.

79. Arad Y, Newstein D, Cadet F, et al. Association of multiple risk factors and insulin resistance with increased prevalence of asymptomatic coronary artery disease by an electron-beam computed tomographic study. *Arterioscler Thromb Vasc Biol* 2001;21(12):2051–2058.

80. Elkeles RS, Feher MD, Flather MD, et al. PREDICT Study Group. The association of coronary calcium score and conventional cardiovascular risk factors in type 2 diabetic subjects asymptomatic for coronary heart disease (The PREDICT Study). *Diabet Med* 2004;21(10):1129–1134.

81. Olson JC, Edmundowicz D, Becker DJ, et al. Coronary calcium in adults with type 1 diabetes: a stronger correlate of clinical coronary artery disease in men than in women. *Diabetes* 2000;49(9):1571–1578.

82. Hosoi M, Sato T, Yamagami K, et al. Impact of diabetes on coronary stenosis and coronary artery calcification detected by electron-beam computed tomography in symptomatic patients. *Diabetes Care* 2002;25(4):696–701.

83. Qu W, Le TT, Azen SP, et al. Value of coronary artery calcium scanning by computed tomography for predicting coronary heart disease in diabetic subjects. *Diabetes Care* 2003;26(3):905–910.

84. Berman DS, Wong ND, Gransar H, et al. Relationship between stress-induced myocardial ischemia and atherosclerosis measured by coronary calcium tomography. *J Am Coll Cardiol* 2004;44:923–930.

85. Leschka S, Alkadhi H, Plass A, et al. Accuracy of MSCT coronary angiography with 64-slice technology: first experience. *Eur Heart J* 2005;26:1482–1487.

86. Mollet NR, Cademartiri N, van Mieghem CAG, et al. High-resolution spiral computed tomography coronary angiography in patients referred for diagnostic conventional coronary angiography. *Circulation* 2005;112:2318–2323.

87. Leber AW, Knez A, von Ziegler F, et al. Quantification of obstructive and nonobstructive coronary lesions by 64-slice computed tomography: a comparative study with quantitative coronary angiography and intravascular ultrasound. *J Am Coll Cardiol* 2005;46:147–154.

88. Raff GL, Gallagher MJ, O'Neill WW, et al. Diagnostic accuracy of noninvasive coronary angiography using 64-slice spiral computed tomography. *J Am Coll Cardiol* 2005;46:552–557.

89. Cai J, Hatsukami TS, Ferguon MS, et al. In vivo quantitative measurement of intact fibrous cap and lipid-rich necrotic core size in atherosclerotic carotid plaque: comparison of high-resolution, contrast-enhanced magnetic resonance imaging and histology. *Circulation* 2005;112(22):3437–3444.

90. Larose E, Yeghiazarians Y, Libby P, et al. Characterization of human atherosclerotic plaques by intravascular magnetic resonance imaging. *Circulation* 2005;112(15): 2324–2331.

91. Wang L, Jerosch-Herold M, Jacobs DR Jr, et al. Coronary risk factors and myocardial perfusion in asymptomatic adults: the Multi-Ethnic Study of Atherosclerosis (MESA). *J Am Coll Cardiol* 2006;47(3):565–572.

92. Rathmann W, Ziegler D, Jahnke M, et al. Mortality in diabetic patients with cardiovascular autonomic neuropathy. *Diabet Med* 1993;10:820–824.

93. Patel AD, Iskandrian AE. MIBG imaging. *J Nucl Cardiol* 2002;9:75–94.

94. Scognamiglio R, Avogaro A, Casara D, et al. Myocardial dysfunction and adrenergic cardiac innervation in patients with insulin-dependent diabetes mellitus. *J Am Coll Cardiol* 1998;31(2):404–412.

95. O'Rourke MF, Adji A. An updated clinical primer on large artery mechanics: implications of pulse waveform analysis and arterial tonometry. *Curr Opin Cardiol* 2005;20(4):275–281.

96. Lebrun CE, van der Schouw YT, Bak AA, et al. Arterial stiffness in postmenopausal women: determinants of pulse wave velocity. *J Hypertens* 2002;20(11):2165–2172.

97. Lacy PS, O'Brien DG, Stanley AG, et al. Increased pulse wave velocity is not associated with elevated augmentation index in patients with diabetes. *J Hypertens* 2004;22(10):1937–1944.

98. De Angelis L, Millasseau SC, Smith A, et al. Sex differences in age-related stiffening of the aorta in subjects with type 2 diabetes. *Hypertension* 2004;44(1):67–71.

99. Westerbacka J, Leinonen E, Salonen JT, et al. Increased augmentation of central blood pressure is associated with increases in carotid intima-media thickness in type 2 diabetic patients. *Diabetologia* 2005;48(8):1654–1662.

HEMOSTATIC ABNORMALITIES IN DIABETES: HEMATOLOGY FOR THE CARDIOLOGIST

Manish Lakhani
Spyros Kokolis
Erdal Cavusoglu
Gerald Soff
Jonathan Marmur

PLATELET PHYSIOLOGY AND HEMOSTASIS

Diabetes disrupts hemostatic processes by a variety of mechanisms at many different levels. Not only platelets but also other components of the hemostatic process such as vascular endothelial cells, coagulation factors, as well as regulatory mechanisms are altered in diabetes. To understand these abnormalities, it is crucial to have knowledge of the physiology of hemostasis which is highlighted in the first part of this chapter followed by an overview of the pathophysiologic disturbances in hemostasis in patients with diabetes.

Hemostasis

The fine balance between clot formation and lysis is maintained by coordination of multiple delicate processes. When there is breach in the endothelium of the vascular wall, hemostasis, the process of blood clot formation, takes place immediately in a well-organized manner. Disruption at any stage of this multistep process can result in either excessive bleeding or thrombosis. To understand the mechanisms of action of various antiplatelet and antithrombotic drugs, it is essential to understand basic physiologic aspects of the hemostatic process. Platelets, vascular endothelium, and different coagulation factors are major players of hemostasis which are described in this chapter and Fig. 17-1.

Platelets and Cardiovascular Disease

Platelets play a pivotal role in the process of hemostasis. Platelets are formed from fragmentation of megakaryocytes (large multinucleated cells) and have a life span of 8–10 days in peripheral blood. Platelets are anucleate, 2–4 μm in diameter. The normal platelet count is 150000–400000/μL. Platelet cytoplasm contains dense granules and alpha granules which are important in the coagulation process. The endothelium of the vessel wall provides a barrier against circulating platelets adhering to subendothelial matrix proteins

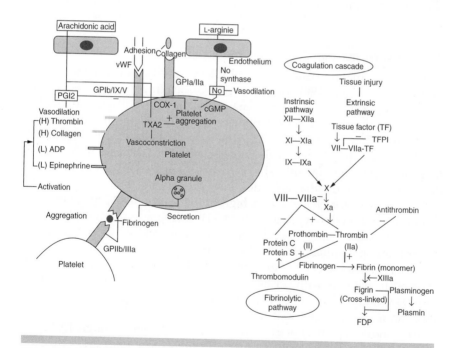

Figure 17-1 **Summary of hemostasis and its regulation by various control mechanisms: platelet functions (adhesion, activation, secretion, and aggregation), coagulation cascade (extrinsic and intrinsic pathways), and fibrinolysis. Abbreviations: (H) means potent and (L) means weak platelet stimulator; cGMP, cyclic guanylate cyclase.**

and also synthesizes prostaglandin I2 (PGI2) and nitric oxide (NO). Major platelet functions responsible for hemostasis are adhesion, activation and secretion, aggregation, and platelet plug formation.

ADHESION

Endothelial cells produce NO and prostacyclin (PGI2) which prevent platelets from adhering to normal endothelial cells. Endothelial trauma results in disruption of these mechanisms. Endothelial trauma also expresses collagen (IV, V, VI), fibronectin, laminin, von Willebrand Factor (vWF), tissue factor (TF), vitronectin, thrombospondin, and fibrin/fibrinogen. Glycoprotein (GP) receptors are located on the surface of platelets and mediate the action of platelets to adhere to surfaces and aggregate.

The binding of vWF to GPIb is the initial step for platelet adhesion and it does not require platelet activation, as seen in Fig. 17-1. The shear stress is an important factor in GPIb-mediated adhesion. In the absence of GPIb, platelets adhere poorly at all shear rates, whereas in the absence of vWF adhesion at high shear rates is affected. The GPIIb/IIIa receptors are involved in mediating platelet aggregation. The receptor undergoes a conformational change after platelet activation and subsequently forms a bridge between platelets.

PLATELET ACTIVATION AND SECRETION

Normally, circulating platelets do not interact with vascular endothelial or smooth muscle cells. Whenever there is a breach in the endothelial cell lining of the vessel wall, platelets come in contact with collagen of the blood vessel wall which is a potent platelet activator. Adenosine diphosphate (ADP) and thromboxane A2 (TXA2) are other platelet stimulators. Platelet activation results in increased cytosolic calcium, decreased electrostatic repulsion, and subsequently shape change of the cell: spiny sphere with filopodia. The filopodia also decrease the electrostatic repulsion. The GPIIb/IIIa receptor changes to a high affinity state. TXA2 is mainly produced through cyclooxygenase 1 (COX-1) in response to multiple stimuli. TXA2 mediates platelet-dependent vasoconstriction. COX-1 exists in platelets and inflammatory cells. TXA2 can be produced even with full inhibition of platelet COX-1. Abnormally high levels of TXA2 have been reported in patients with unstable angina (UA). Activation also results in phosphorylation of select proteins, release of alpha granules and dense granules, and release of lysosomal contents.

ADP induces platelet activation independently and through TXA2 production. ADP is particularly important in high shear rate/stress rheologic conditions, which may explain the greater importance of platelets in arterial rather than venous thrombosis. Various stimuli for activating platelets are shown in Fig. 17-1. Platelet adhesion and platelet activation are also summarized in Fig. 17-1.

PLATELET AGGREGATION

After platelet activation, the next step is platelet aggregation which results in further release of alpha granules, dense granules, lysosomal contents, and surface expression of proteins contained on lysosomal membranes and on alpha-granule membranes. The GPIIb/IIIa complex is the pivotal receptor for platelet aggregation (Fig. 17-1). It is the most abundant receptor on the platelet surface (up to 80,000 receptors per platelet). The receptors have a baseline number on platelets. The number expressed during platelet activation increases. During platelet aggregation the number increases exponentially and becomes a dynamic process over time with continuing internalization and surfacing of receptors.

GPIIb/IIIa is restricted to platelets and megakaryocytes and is found in both primates and nonprimates. Absence of functional GPIIb/IIIa in Glanzmann thrombasthenia leads to recurrent mucocutaneous bleeding and extremely rare visceral bleeding.

Platelet adhesion and activation leads to conformational changes in the GPIIb/IIIa allowing ligand binding. Various ligands which can bind include fibrinogen and vWF. The ability of binding depends on the concentration of the ligands. Recognition specificity is defined by Arg-Gly-Asp (RGD) sequence in all ligands and Lys-Glu-Ala-Gly-Asp-Val sequence in fibrinogen gamma chains. Fibrinogen is the most potent GPIIb/IIIa ligand. Inhibition of platelet aggregation and dissociation of already formed aggregates are two entirely different treatment goals.

PLATELET THROMBUS FORMATION

Both platelet adhesion and activation are necessary for thrombus formation. The GPIIb/IIIa receptor activation is the final common pathway. Fibrinogen and vWF are essential factors. A thin layer of adhesion molecules is the basis of platelet vessel wall contact. Platelet aggregation facilitates thrombus generation and thrombin further activates the platelets (positive feedback). Thrombin also initiates platelet contraction (clot consolidation).

Regulation of Platelet Activation

The most important regulating factor is the effect of flowing blood. Vessel angulation and decreased velocity promote thrombosis. Endothelial cells have prostaglandins (PGs) and NO which prevent platelet activation.

CLOTTING CASCADE

The well-organized and sequential activation of proenzymes or inactive zymogens to active enzymes finally results in fibrin mesh and clot formation, by extrinsic and intrinsic pathways of coagulation. All procoagulants but vWF (which is synthesized in megakaryocytes and endothelial cells) are synthesized in the liver. The coagulation cascade is summarized in Fig. 17-1.

Extrinsic Pathway

Tissue injury results in expression of TF (tissue thromboplastin). TF acts as the cofactor and binds activated factor VII (FVIIa). The TF-FVIIa complex activates factors X and IX. Factor IXa in complex with its cofactor VIIIa also activates factor X. Activation of factor X directly and indirectly via activation of factor IX is important for sustained thrombin generation because of limited TF production in vivo and presence of TF pathway inhibitor.

Intrinsic Pathway

Factor XII (Hageman factor), prekallikrein, and high molecular weight kininogen (HMWK) are plasma proteins which are activated by contact with negatively charged surfaces. Activated factor XII, combined with HMWK, activates factor IX (IXa). Factor IXa in conjunction with factor VIIIa activates factor Xa. Factor VIII is activated by both factor Xa and thrombin. The remainder of the intrinsic pathway uses the same cascade as the extrinsic pathway (the common pathway) involving factors V, prothrombin, and fibrinogen.

Control Mechanism of Coagulation Cascade

Antithrombin (AT) is a circulating plasma protease inhibitor which neutralizes thrombin, factors Xa, IXa, XIIa, and XIa. Tissue factor pathway inhibitor (TFPI) is synthesized by vascular endothelium, circulates in plasma which inhibits factor X by direct inhibition of factor Xa. It also complexes with factor Xa and the complex inhibits TF/FVIIa. The plasma concentration of TFPI is greatly increased following intravenous heparin administration which may contribute to the antithrombotic efficacy of heparin and low molecular weight heparin (LMWH).

Protein C and S

Thrombin binds to thrombomodulin (TM) to form a thrombin-TM complex which activates protein C. Activated protein C in association with protein S, proteolytically inactivates factors Va and VIIIa.

Fibrinolysis

This is a process of clot lysis to restore vessel patency following hemostasis which occurs in conjunction with wound healing and tissue remodeling. Plasminogen binds fibrin and tissue plasminogen activator (tPA) leading to conversion of inactive plasminogen to active, proteolytic plasmin.

Plasmin cleaves the polymerized fibrin strand at multiple sites and releases fibrin degradation products (FDPs). Plasmin also cleaves fibrinogen and a variety of plasma proteins and clotting factors. The process of fibrinolysis runs parallel to the coagulation cascade (Fig. 17-1). Plasmin activity is regulated by plasminogen activators and plasminogen activator inhibitors (PAI-1 and PAI-2) secreted by vessel wall endothelium.

HEMOSTATIC ABNORMALITIES IN DIABETES

Diabetes is a major risk factor for coronary artery disease (CAD) and is considered a CAD risk equivalent. Low-grade inflammation, oxidative stress, impaired fibrinolysis, abnormal levels, and activity of coagulation factors and platelet activation are involved in the pathogenesis of type 2 diabetes mellitus (DM-2) and its complications. Insulin resistance (IR), a precursor to DM-2, correlates with accelerated atherosclerosis and leads to a prothrombotic state. The common metabolic disturbances noted in patients with IR are dyslipidemic lipid triad (elevated very low-density lipoprotein [VLDL], small low-density lipoprotein [LDL] particles, and decreased high-density lipoprotein [HDL] levels), hypertension (HTN), glucose intolerance, and a prothrombotic state (Fig. 17-2).[1] Development of micro- and macrovascular complications and prothrombotic state in diabetes result not only from the effects of hyperglycemia but by many other means.[2] In DM-2, IR is associated with vascular dysfunction/damage, impaired fibrinolysis, and low-grade inflammation independently of obesity, and poor glycemic control. These patients frequently have alterations in coagulation mechanisms which include increased fibrinogen levels, increased PAI-1, and platelet abnormalities,[3-5] that predispose them to arterial thrombosis.

Platelets

Platelet function is disturbed at many levels in diabetes. More or less, all major platelet functions responsible for hemostasis are adversely affected in diabetic patients.

ADHESION

Platelets in patients with diabetes are more reactive; and have greater expression of GPIb/IX/V complex and increased level as well as activity of

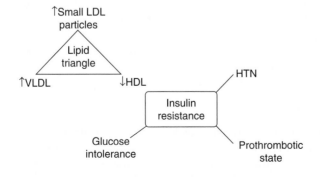

Figure 17-2 **Metabolic abnormalities in patients with IR.**

vWF in blood which makes them more adhesive.[6,7] Platelet reactivity can be increased by direct effect of hyperglycemia[8] or secondary to reduced vascular endothelial production of prostacyclin and NO in patients with IR.[9]

ACTIVATION AND AGGREGATION

The CD40-CD40 ligand system was originally found on CD4+ T lymphocytes and later also found in leukocytic and nonleukocytic cells such as endothelial cells, smooth muscle cells, and on activated platelets. This system plays an important role in progression of atherosclerosis, atherothrombotic complications in cardiovascular disease, and plaque destabilization.[10–12] It is found in two forms: membrane-bound and soluble, both of which may interact with CD40 expressed vascular cells and result in inflammatory response. The soluble, biologically active form of CD40 ligand, soluble CD40 ligand (sCD40L) is released from activated platelets.[13] The CD40-CD40L interactions result in proinflammatory and prothrombotic responses.[14]

Hyperinsulinemia and hyperglycemia but particularly the combination of both create a prothrombotic state and in addition may be proinflammatory and proatherogenic because of the proinflammatory actions of CD40 ligand and TF.[1] Schonbeck et al. have shown that elevated plasma levels of sCD40L was predictive of future cardiovascular event rates in apparently healthy women.[15] Also, a higher level of sCD40L was found in patients with UA.[8] Persistent platelet activation is responsible for increased levels of the soluble form of CD40 ligand in DM-2.[2] Also, a strong correlation between sCD40L and interleukin-6 as well as TF has been demonstrated.[16]

SECRETION

P-selectin

P-selectin is a component of the alpha-granule membrane of the resting platelet. It is expressed after secretion of alpha granules. P-selectin mediates initial adhesion of activated platelets to monocytes and neutrophils. P-selectin is considered the "gold standard" marker of platelet activation. Increased levels of soluble P-selectin are seen in Asian-Indian subjects with impaired glucose tolerance (IGT), DM-2, and IR.[17] Measurement of soluble P-selectin may be a helpful marker of impending coronary artery insult in diabetic patients.[18] However, it is suggested that monocyte-platelet aggregates are a more sensitive marker of in vivo platelet activation than P-selectin.[19]

Coagulation Factors

People with diabetes have higher levels of TF in blood even without overt cardiovascular disease,[16,20] which may be reduced with improving glycemic control.[21] High glucose concentrations increase thrombin-induced TF expression in human endothelial cells.[22] Also, various other coagulation factor abnormalities (VII, IX, VIII, XII, vWF) are found in patients with IR or DM-2.[23–26]

Endothelial Cells

When the endothelium is disrupted, the surrounding intact endothelial cells release arachidonic acid which is converted by COX-1 into TXA2 in platelets and prostacyclin (PGI2) in endothelial cells. TXA2 stimulates platelet aggregation and causes vasoconstriction. PGI2 activates adenylate cyclase, blocks platelet aggregation, and antagonizes TXA2-mediated vasoconstriction.

NO is the endothelium-derived relaxing factor. Its release also mediates smooth muscle growth and migration as well as function of platelets, leucocytes, fibroblast, and parenchymal cells. NO diffuses directly across the platelet membrane and activates guanylate cyclase, which modulates vascular tone in smooth muscle. It causes vasodilation, and inhibits platelet adhesion and aggregation.

There have been reports of decreased synthesis of PGI2 and NO in experimental diabetic models.[27-29] A recent study also reported reduced expression of both endothelial NO synthase and cyclooxygenase 2 (COX-2) proteins, as well as decreased prostacyclin production, in unstimulated human endothelial cells from insulin-dependent diabetic mothers when compared to cells from nondiabetic, control subjects.[30] In diabetic patients, there is increased formation of reactive oxidative species. A damaging molecule, peroxynitrite is generated which inactivates prostacyclin synthase leading to increased formation of vasoconstrictor eicosanoids, which accelerates progression of vascular disease.[31]

Fibrinolysis

Fibrinolysis is an essential process of lysis and organization of clot to restore vessel patency after hemostasis is achieved. The inactive precursor molecule plasminogen binds fibrin and tPA and converts to active, proteolytic plasmin which cleaves polymerized fibrin strands and releases FDPs. Plasmin activity is regulated by plasminogen activator and PAIs released by endothelial cells.

Increased levels of PAI-1 and to a lesser extent levels of fibrinogen, vWF, and factor VIII, were correlated with higher insulin concentrations in 1500 patients with angina.[32] Also, insulin and its precursors correlate with PAI-1 and fibrinogen levels.[33] High levels of PAI-1 result in decreased fibrinolytic activity.[34] The impairment of the fibrinolytic process in diabetic patients is mediated via a number of different mechanisms; these may be a consequence of posttranslational modifications to fibrinogen molecules, resulting from their exposure to the abnormal metabolic milieu associated with diabetes.[35-37] The structure of the fibrin clot is denser, less porous which is more resistant to fibrinolysis in diabetics than nondiabetics.[38-40] These result from decreased binding of tissue-type plasminogen activator and plasminogen to fibrin, increased plasmin inhibitor (α2-antiplasmin) cross-linking, and reduced plasmin generation at the clot surface.[35] In a recently published study, measurement of fibrinolytic capacity with a new method, Euglobulin Clot Lysis Time (ECLT) correlated with the

Framingham risk score and was significantly influenced by the number of clinical cardiovascular risk factors.[41]

Conclusion

There are abnormalities at multiple levels in patients with DM. Platelet dysfunction (resulting from defective adhesion, hypersensitivity to proaggregants, and hyporeactivity to antiaggregants), endothelial dysfunction leading to decreased NO and PGI2 formation, decreased fibrinolysis, oxidative stress, low-grade inflammation, and abnormalities in coagulation factors; all result in amplification of risk of cardiovascular disease in diabetic patients and places diabetes in a special risk category.

ANTIPLATELET AGENTS

Our conception of the pathophysiology of the acute coronary syndromes (ACS) was mainly focused on the degree of stenosis of coronary arteries until recently when the attention shifted toward the theory of plaque rupture and thrombi formation. Inflammation, platelet aggregation in response to plaque rupture, and altered behavior of vascular endothelium play major roles in the pathophysiology of ACS. Thus, in the last decade novel therapies targeted at these levels have emerged. Platelets play a very important role in pathogenesis of ACS. Antiplatelet agents can interfere with platelet function by different mechanisms as seen in Fig. 17-3. They can be categorized as (a) COX-1 inhibitors, (b) ADP inhibitors, (c) GPIIb/IIIa receptor antagonists, and (d) phosphodiesterase and adenosine deaminase inhibitors.

Cox-Dependent Inhibitors

Aspirin irreversibly inhibits platelet COX-dependent aggregability.[42] COX is necessary for production of TXA2 which is responsible for platelet aggregation. The use of aspirin thus reduces the risk of thrombotic vascular events. Aspirin has been shown in various studies to decrease the risk of overall cardiovascular events (myocardial infarction [MI], stroke, and peripheral vascular events). Aspirin is recommended for both primary and secondary prevention of CAD.[43,44]

It is low doses of aspirin that have been shown to selectively inhibit the synthesis of TX while maintaining endothelial cell synthesis of prostacyclin. Prostacyclin is a vasodilator and an inhibitor of platelet aggregation.

The ISIS-2 (Second International Study of Infarction Survival) study was a large randomized study of patients with acute myocardial infarction (AMI) randomized to either aspirin alone, streptokinase alone, or both.[43] This study is considered one of the landmark studies, as it was the first to demonstrate the clinical efficacy of aspirin to decrease mortality during AMI. The reduction in mortality with aspirin alone was similar to that with streptokinase

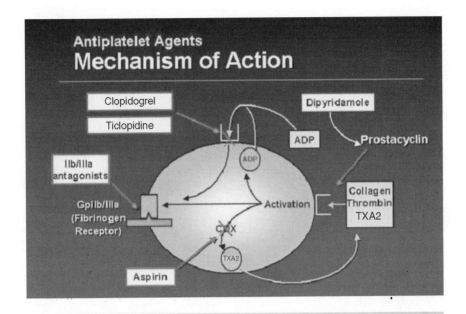

*Figure 17-3 **Mechanisms of action of various antiplatelet agents.** (Source: Adapted from Schafer AL. Antiplatelet therapy.* Am J Med *1996;101:199–209.)*

alone. However, a synergistic effect was noted with the combination of aspirin and streptokinase. Figure 17-4 shows the effect of aspirin alone, placebo, streptokinase alone, and combination of aspirin and streptokinase.

PRIMARY PREVENTION

Primary prevention trials have been done to assess the benefit of prophylactic aspirin use in patients without history of cardiovascular disease. The United States Physician Study is one of the large primary prevention trials which showed that the use of aspirin (325 mg) in low-risk patients was associated with a significant reduction in their risk of first MI, and subsequent follow-up revealed a reduction in overall mortality with aspirin use.

Another British trial[45] was done with a larger population at high risk for coronary events. These patients were randomized to receive low-dose aspirin 75 mg, warfarin (to keep International normalized ratio [INR] 1.5), or a combination of both. The results of this trial, as shown in Fig. 17-5, indicate that with aspirin use there was a significant reduction in primary endpoints (total ischemic heart disease). The combination of the two drugs was associated with increased bleeding episodes.

The Hypertension Optimal Treatment (HOT) study[46] was a large trial looking at patients specifically with HTN. The patients were randomized to

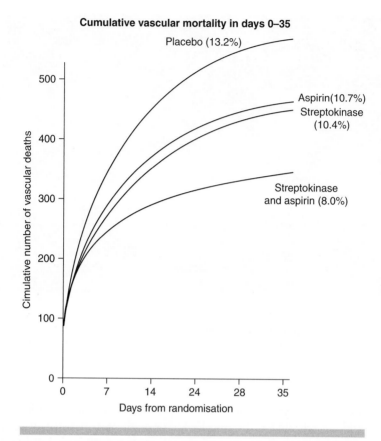

Figure 17-4   **ISIS-2 trial, one of the landmark trials, showed significant survival benefit with early aspirin therapy in MI which was comparable to that with streptokinase (23 and 25% reduction in vascular mortality, respectively). Combination of the two showed additive effect (42% reduction).**

receive either aspirin or placebo but both groups had their blood pressure optimized similarly. The study demonstrated a decrease in the number of cardiovascular events including MI in the aspirin-treated group.

In a primary prevention project, patients with at least one risk factor for CAD were randomized to receive either aspirin or placebo.[47] The study, however, was terminated early due to a significant reduction in primary endpoints (CAD death, nonfatal MI, or nonfatal stroke) in the aspirin-treated group.

A meta-analysis of the randomized trials has found aspirin use to be effective for primary prevention of MI.[48–50] It is also found to have an increased risk of hemorrhagic stroke in patients with aspirin use but the

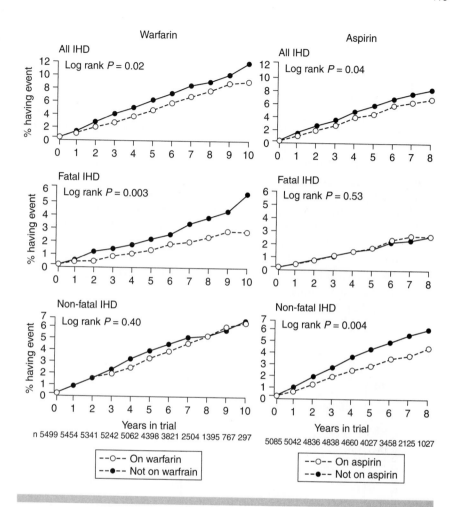

Figure 17-5 **Reduction of incidence of coronary heart disease (CHD) by 20 and 21% with low-dose aspirin and low-intensity warfarin, respectively, in 5499 men.** *(Source: Adapted from The Medical Research Council's General Practice Research Framework: thrombosis prevention trial. Lancet 1998;351 (9098):233–241.)*

benefits outweighed the risk. These studies together have been crucial in establishing guidelines for aspirin use in patients for primary prevention.

SECONDARY PREVENTION

A number of secondary prevention trials have also been done to evaluate the benefit of aspirin use in patients after their first cardiac event to prevent subsequent events. The Antithrombotic Trialist Collaboration reviewed a number of antiplatelet trials.[51] They concluded that the use of antiplatelet therapy was associated with a reduced risk of subsequent vascular events (including MI and stroke) by approximately 22%. The dose of aspirin used in major clinical trials has varied from 75 to 1300 mg/day. The American College of Cardiology (ACC)/American Heart Association (AHA) guidelines recommend initial minimum of 160 mg/day in patients with ACS (this dose was used in the ISIS-2 trial and showed mortality benefit) followed by maintenance dose of 75–80 mg/day.

The Multicenter Myocardial Ischemia Research Group completed a trial looking at aspirin use in patients 1–6 months after MI or episode of UA.[52] Patients taking aspirin were shown to have a decrease rate of all-cause mortality (cardiac death, nonfatal MI) at 23 months as noted in Fig. 17-6.

The VA Cooperative Study was a multicenter double-blind trial of patients after a non-ST-segment elevation MI (NSTEMI) comparing aspirin use versus placebo.[53] The study concluded that the use of aspirin was associated with a reduced rate of death/MI. This was noted to be true even if treatment was discontinued after 12 months.

The Canadian Multicenter Trial was a similar trial in terms of patient selection. The study however had four arms: aspirin alone, sulfinpyrazone

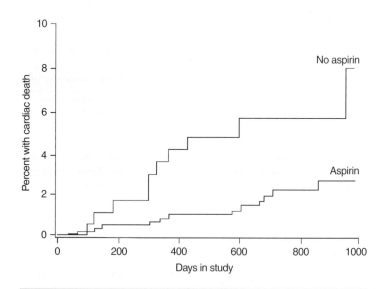

Figure 17-6 **Kaplan-Meier plot of cardiovascular mortality in 936 patients enrolled to 1–6 months after acute coronary event.** *(Source: Adapted from Goldstein RE, Andrews M, Hall WJ, et al. Marked reduction in long-term cardiac deaths with aspirin after a coronary event. J Am Coll Cardiol 1996;28(2):326–330.)*

alone, combination of the two, or placebo.[54] The therapy was started 8 days after admission to the hospital and was continued for 18 months. The results indicated a decrease in mortality and combined endpoints of death and non-fatal MI in the aspirin alone group. Sulfinpyrazone was not associated with any benefit (see Fig. 17-7).

Another secondary prevention trial was the Risk Informed Standards Consensus (RISC) trial 8 which had a similar study population but was randomized to either low-dose aspirin (75 mg/day), heparin (5 days of intermittent infusion), or placebo.[55] This study also found a decrease in the combined primary endpoint in the aspirin-treated group at 5, 30, and 90 days compared to placebo. This benefit was maintained after up to 1 year of therapy. Based on these studies aspirin is recommended for secondary prevention in all patients with coronary events.

ADP-Dependent Inhibitors

There are at least two drugs in clinical use which block the platelets via ADP-dependent mechanisms: clopidogrel (Plavix) and ticlopidine (Ticlid). These drugs block the binding of ADP to the platelet P2Y12 receptor that activates Gi, thereby inhibiting adenylyl cyclase and platelet aggregation. In current practice, clopidogrel is most commonly used. The use of ticlopidine has decreased significantly secondary to major hematologic adverse effects.[56]

The CURE (Clopidogrel in Unstable Angina to Prevent Recurrent Events) trial was a randomized trial of greater than 12,000 patients presenting with

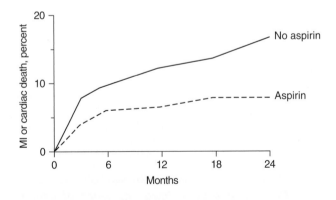

Figure 17-7 **Fifty-one percent reduction in cardiovascular events with use of aspirin in 555 patients with unstable angina.** *(Source: Adapted from Cairns JA, Gent M, Singer J, et al. Aspirin, sulfinpyrazone or both in unstable angina. N Engl J Med 1985;313(22):1369–1375.)*

NSTEMI.[57,58] The results of this trial have lead to the routine use of clopidogrel in patients with ACS. Patients were randomized to receive either aspirin alone or aspirin and clopidogrel. At 9 months, the results indicated a decrease in the primary endpoint (in-hospital ischemia, failure or need for revascularization) with aspirin and clopidogrel combination treatment. Figure 17-8 shows the results of the CURE trial.

The PCI-CURE was a study of a subset of patients from the CURE trial who underwent percutaneous coronary interventions (PCI).[59,61] These patients were randomized to be pretreated with aspirin in combination with either clopidogrel or placebo for 6 days preintervention and continued up to 4 weeks postintervention. The results indicate a reduction in primary endpoints as seen in Fig. 17-9.

CAPRIE (Clopidogrel vs. Aspirin in Patients at Risk of Ischemic Events) was a secondary prevention trial of clopidogrel use in patients with recent stroke, MI, or vascular disease.[61] It was a large trial of greater than 19,000 patients

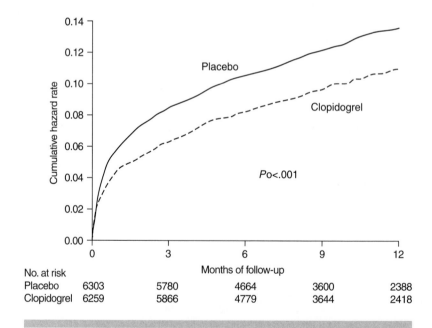

No. at risk					
Placebo	6303	5780	4664	3600	2388
Clopidogrel	6259	5866	4779	3644	2418

Figure 17-8 **CURE trial showed lower incidence of cardiovascular death, nonfatal MI, or stroke (9.3 vs. 11.4) in patients assigned to clopidogrel plus aspirin as compared to placebo plus aspirin (benefit was largely driven by reduction in nonfatal MI).** *(Source: Adapted from The CURE trial: effects of clopidogrel in addition to aspirin in patients with acute coronary syndromes without ST-segment elevation. N Engl J Med 2001;345(7):494–502.)*

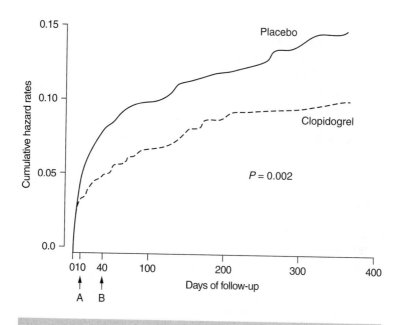

Figure 17-9 **PCI-CURE trial: Clopidogrel pretreatment followed by long-term therapy resulted in significant reduction in cardiovascular death, MI, and urgent target-vessel revascularization in patients with ACS undergoing percutaneous coronary intervention.** *(Source: Adapted from Mehta SR, Yusuf S, Peters RJ, et al. Effects of pretreatment with clopidogrel and aspirin followed by long term therapy in patients undergoing percutaneous coronary interventions. Lancet 2001;358(9281):527–533.)*

with recent vascular event. The results indicate a modest advantage of clopidogrel over aspirin in prevention of events (stroke, MI, and vascular disease) with an annual rate of 5.3% versus 5.8% ($P = 0.043$).

CLARITY-TIMI 28 (Clopidogrel as Adjunctive Reperfusion Therapy-Thrombolysis in Myocardial Infarction 28) and COMMIT/CCS-2 (Clopidogrel and Metoprolol in Myocardial Infarction Trial/Second Chinese Cardiac Study) trials demonstrated the benefit of clopidogrel in the setting of ST-segment elevation MI. CLARITY-TIMI 28 showed that among patients with ST-segment elevation MI treated with an early medical management strategy, use of clopidogrel (300 mg loading followed by 75 mg daily) was associated with a reduction in the primary composite endpoint compared with placebo, driven by the reduction in infarct-artery occlusion.[62,63] In COMMIT/CCS-2, treatment with clopidogrel was associated with a reduction in mortality and in the composite of death, MI, or stroke compared with placebo in patients with ST-segment elevation MI.

The CHARISMA (Clopidogrel for High Atherothrombotic Risk and Ischemic Stabilization, Management, and Avoidance) trial showed no difference in the primary composite endpoint of cardiovascular death, MI, or stroke, in patients with stable cardiovascular disease or with multiple risk factors, with dual antiplatelet therapy consisting of aspirin plus clopidogrel compared to aspirin alone.[64] The subgroup of patients with documented cardiovascular disease showed some benefit with clopidogrel, while patients without cardiovascular disease had no benefit in the primary endpoint and actually had a higher mortality with clopidogrel. These divergent findings suggest that dual antiplatelet therapy may not be beneficial in all patients at risk for cardiovascular disease, but that in patients with established cardiovascular disease, dual therapy may be effective in reducing subsequent events.

Glycoprotein IIB/IIIA Receptor Blockers

There are three GPIIb/IIIa receptor inhibitors in clinical use at present. These are used in the setting of either UA or NSTEMI, or during PCI. The three receptor inhibitors available are: tirofiban (Aggrastat), abciximab (ReoPro), and eptifibatide (Integrelin). More detail regarding the GPIIb/IIIa receptor blockers is described in the Section IV.

Phosphodiesterase and Adenosine Deaminase Inhibitor

Dipyridamole is the only drug in this class that is used in the clinical setting of cardiovascular disease. Inhibition of adenosine deaminase and phosphodiesterase results in accumulation of adenosine, adenine nucleotides, and cyclic adenosine monophosphate (AMP); accumulation causes inhibition of platelet aggregation. It also causes stimulation of prostacyclin or PGD2 which may lead to coronary vasodilation. Clinical trials have not demonstrated any clear benefit in ACS and thus it is not recommended routinely.

Conclusion

Aspirin therapy for primary prevention of cardiovascular events is recommended for apparently healthy men and women whose 10-year risk of first cardiovascular event is 10% or more over a 10-year period as calculated by the Framingham risk score. In patients with ACS, an initial dose of 162–325 mg (chewed to achieve rapid action) followed by 75–162 mg daily should be given. Low-dose aspirin should be continued indefinitely unless contraindicated (in which instance, clopidogrel is a recommended alternative). Addition of clopidogrel in patients with risk factors for CAD but no established CAD is not recommended.

GLYCOPROTEIN IIB/IIIA INHIBITORS

Glycoprotein IIb/IIIa inhibitors are widely used in the setting of ACS and PCI. The three different GPIIb/IIIa inhibitors in clinical use are: abciximab, tirofiban, and eptifibatide.

As described in the previous section, the GPIIb/IIIa receptor plays a crucial role in platelet aggregation. Fibrinogen binds to activated GPIIb/IIIa receptors of two activated platelets and links them together (Fig. 17-2). Each platelet can express up to 80,000 GPIIb/IIIa receptors and thus activated platelets can bind to many other platelets which results in thrombus formation. GPIIb/IIIa inhibitors bind to the IIb/IIIa receptor and this results in inhibition of platelet aggregation and thrombus formation.

Abciximab is a Fab fragment of a monoclonal antibody against the GPIIb/IIIa receptor. Following intravenous administration, its concentration falls rapidly because of binding to the GPIIb/IIIa receptor (the half-life is 30 minutes). The effect of abciximab is dose-dependent and readily reversible with platelet transfusion. Platelet function recovers over 48 hours.

Tirofiban, a nonpeptide molecule and eptifibatide, a synthetic heptapeptide, by molecular structural mimicry, bind to the GPIIb/IIIa receptor. They are reversible antagonists of fibrinogen, with half-lives of 2 and 2.5 hours, respectively. They inhibit platelets in a dose- and concentration-dependent manner.

As per the ACC/AHA practice guidelines, use of GPIIb/IIIa antagonist in patients with ACS (UA or NSTEMI) who are planned to undergo cardiac catheterization and PCI is a class I indication (it may also be used just prior to PCI). The use of eptifibatide or tirofiban in patients with ongoing ischemia, elevated troponins, or with other high-risk features in whom intervention is not planned is a class IIa indication. The use of eptifibatide or tirofiban in patients without continuing ischemia who have no high-risk features and in whom intervention is not planned is a class IIb indication (Fig. 17-10). In addition to the above, use or abciximab in patients in whom PCI is not planned is a class III indication. Figure 17-11 summarized recommendation for use of GPIIb/IIIa in ST-segment elevation MI.

PRISM (Platelet Receptor Inhibition in Ischemic Syndrome Management) was a trial of 3232 patients with either UA or NSTEMI.[65,66] All patients received aspirin and then were randomized to receive either heparin or tirofiban. The trial showed that at 48 hours there was a decrease in the primary composite endpoint of death, MI, or refractory angina in the group receiving tirofiban (3.8% vs. 5.6% with heparin) as seen in Fig. 17-12. This study was followed by the PRISM-PLUS (Platelet Receptor Inhibition in Ischemic Syndrome Management in Patients Limited by Unstable Signs and Symptoms) trial in which 1915 patients were randomized to three different arms: heparin alone, tirofiban alone, or the combination of heparin and tirofiban.[67] The trial was terminated prematurely secondary to the increased mortality in the patients receiving tirofiban only. The results showed a significant reduction in composite primary endpoint at 7 days in the tirofiban and heparin arm. This reduction was maintained at 30 days and 6 months as shown in Fig. 17-13.

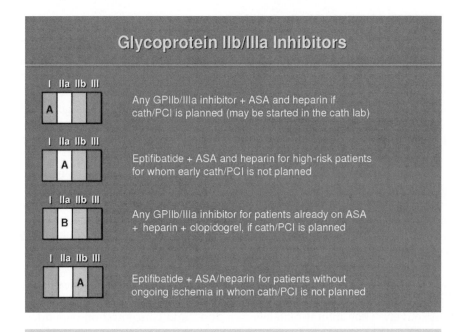

Figure 17-10 **ACC/AHA 2002 UA/NSTEMI guidelines, platelet GPIIb/IIIa inhibitors.** (Source: Adapted from Braunwald, et al. ACC/AHA 2002 guidelines updates for the management of patients with unstable angina and NSTEMI. Circulation 2002;106:1893–1900.)

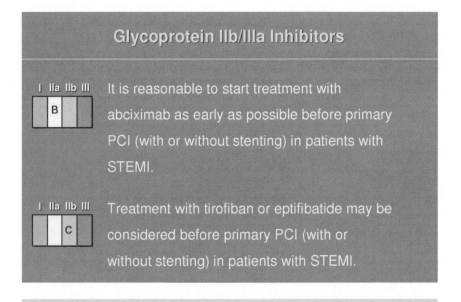

Figure 17-11 **ACC/AHA 2004 guidelines for GPIIb/IIIa inhibitor use in ST-segment elevation MI.** (Source: Adapted from Antman EM, Braunwald E, Beasley JW, et al. ACC/AHA Guidelines. J Am Coll Cardiol 2004;44:671–719.)

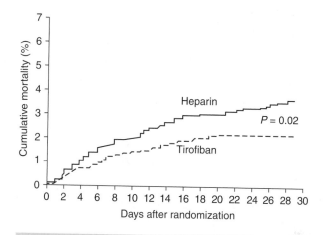

Figure 17-12 **PRISM study showed significant reduction in 30-day mortality in tirofiban arm compared to
heparin arm in patients with UA.** *(Source: Adapted
from: PRISM Study Investigators. Comparison of
aspirin plus tirofiban with aspirin plus heparin for
patients with unstable angina.* N Engl J Med *1998;
338(21):1498–1505.)*

Table 17-1 summarizes major GPIIb/IIIa trials. The EPIC trial was a trial
of 2099 patients with AMI already on aspirin and heparin treatment who
were assigned to receive either abciximab or placebo prior to and during PCI
(Fig. 17-14).[68] The study demonstrated a significant decrease in death, MI, or
need for urgent repeat intervention in the abciximab arm at 30 days post-
PCI. It also demonstrated similar results at 6 months and 3 years follow-up
as seen in Fig. 17-16.

The ADMIRAL (Abciximab Before Direct Angioplasty and Stenting in
Myocardial Infarction Regarding Acute and Long-term Follow-up) study
was a randomized trial of 300 patients, looking at the use of abciximab or
placebo in patients undergoing either percutaneous balloon angioplasty
(PTCA) or stent in the setting of an AMI. Different parameters were measured immediately following the procedure and again at 6 months including
TIMI 3 flow rates, ejection fraction, and need for revascularization.[69] The
results indicated a significant benefit with the use of abciximab. CADILLAC
(Fig. 17-5) was a larger study of 2082 patients with AMI that were randomized
to four arms: PTCA alone, PTCA plus abciximab, STENT alone, or STENT
plus abciximab. The results demonstrated stent to be superior to PTCA
irrespective of abciximab use as seen in Fig. 17-15.

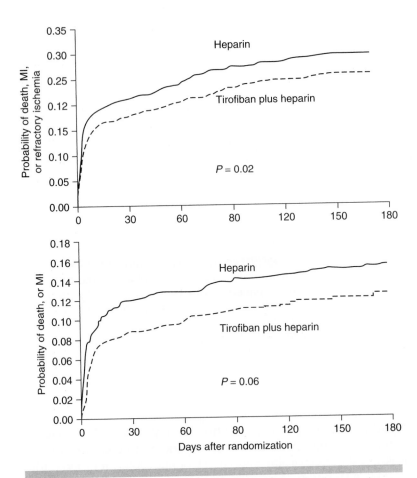

Figure 17-13 **Combination of tirofiban plus heparin resulted in significant reduction in death, MI, or refractory ischemia compared to heparin alone in UA in PRISM-PLUS trial.**

EPILOG was a similar trial in which 2792 patients undergoing PCI were randomized to abciximab with standard-dose heparin, abciximab with low-dose heparin, or placebo with standard-dose heparin. The study was terminated early as it demonstrated a composite event rate at 30 days of 5.4, 5.2, and 11.7%, respectively.[70]

The clinical efficacy of tirofiban and abciximab in patients undergoing PCI was evaluated in TARGET (The Do Tirofiban and ReoPro Give Similar Efficacy Outcomes Trial).[71,72] In this case, 5308 patients undergoing nonemergent PCI were randomized to receive either tirofiban or abciximab prior to the intervention. The results (shown in Fig. 17-16) indicated abciximab to have a greater benefit at 30 days by a reduction in the composite endpoints

Table 17-1 *Design Characteristics of Trials on GPIIb/IIIa Inhibitors in ACS without Persistent ST-Segment Elevation*

	PRISM[7]	PRISM-PLUS[8]	PARAGON-A[9]	PURSUIT[10]	PARAGON-B[11]	GUSTO-IV ACS[12]
Enrolment period	1994–1996	1994–1996	1995–1996	1995–1997	1998–1999	1998–2000
Number of patients	3232	1915	2282	10,948	5225	7800
Last episode of chest pain	≤24 h	≤12 h	≤12 h	≤24 h	≤12 h	≤24h
Indicator of Myocardial Ischemia						
ST depression or ST elevation or	≥1.0 mm ≥1.0 mm (<20 min duration)	≥1.0 mm ≥1.0 mm(<20 min duration)	≥0.5 mm ≥0.5 mm (<30 min duration)	>0.5 mm >0.5 mm (duration not specified)	>0.5 mm >0.5 mm (<30 min duration)	≥0.5 mm >0.5 mm (<30 min duration)
T-wave inversion or	Yes; extent not specified	≥(3.0 mm	Yes; extent not specified	>1 mm	Yes; extent not specified	No
Creatine kinase MB elevation and/or	Yes; extent not specified	Yes; extent not specified	No	Above local ULN	Above local ULN	No
Other conditions	Evidence of CAD based on cardiac history, stress test, or CAG	No	No	No	Troponin T/I elevation above local ULN	Troponin T/I elevation above local ULN

Table 17-1 *Design Characteristics of Trials on GPIIb/IIIa Inhibitors in ACS without Persistent ST-Segment Elevation (Continued)*

	PRISM[7]	PRISM-PLUS[8]	PARAGON-A[9]	PURSUIT[10]	PARAGON-B[11]	GUSTO-IV ACS[12]
Study Medication						
GPIIb/IIIa inhibitor Regimen	Tirofiban a. 0.6 µg/kg bolus + 0.15 µg/kg/min infusion + placebo heparin	Tirofiban a. 0.4 µg/kg bolus + 0.1 µg/kg/min infusion + heparin b. 0.6 µg/kg bolus + 0.15 µg/kg/min infusion + placebo heparin	Lamifiban a. 300 µg bolus + 1 µg/min infusion + random assignment to heparin or heparin-placebo b. 750 µg bolus + 5 µg/min infusion + random assignment to heparin or heparin-placebo c. Placebo + heparin	Eptifibatide a. 180 µg/kg bolus + 1.3 µg/kg/min infusion b. 180 µg/kg/min infusion c. Placebo	Lamifiban a. 500 µg bolus + 1.0–2.0 µg/min infusion (depending on creatinine clearance) b. Placebo	Abciximab a. 250 µg/kg bolus + 0.125 µg/kg/min infusion (maximum 0.10 µg/min) for 24 h b. 250 µg/kg bolus + 0.125 µg/kg/min infusion (maximum 0.10 µg/min) for 48 h c. Placebo
Infusion duration	48 h	48–96 h	72–120 h	72–96 h	72–120 h	24 or 48 h

Additional Management

CAG	Discouraged <48 h after randomization	Recommended 48–96 h after randomization	Discouraged <24 h after randomization	On discretion of treating physician	On discretion of treating physician	Discouraged <48 h after randomization
PCI	Not scheduled	If indicated by angiography	On discretion of treating physician	On discretion of treating physician	On discretion of treating physician	Not scheduled
Aspirin	300–325 mg	325 mg	75–325 mg	80–325 mg	150–325 mg	150–325 mg
Heparin	Heparin part of study regimen; initial dose 5000 U bolus + 1000 U/h infusion	Heparin part of study regimen; initial dose 5000 U bolus + 1000 U/h infusion	Heparin part of study regimen; initial dose weight-adjusted: maximum 5000 U bolus + 1000 U/h infusion	Initial dose 5000 U bolus + 1000 U/h infusion, aiming for aPTT of 50–70 s	Initial dose weight-adjusted: maximum 5000 U bolus + 1000 U/h infusion, aiming for aPTT of 50–70s;	Initial dose weight-adjusted: maximum 5000 U bolus + 800 U/h infusion, aiming for aPTT of 50–70 s; dalteparin maximum 10000 U

Efficacy Endpoints

Primary	Death, MI, or refractory ischemia at 48 h	Death, MI, or refractory ischemia at 7 days	Death or MI at 30 days	Death or MI at 30 days	Death, MI, or severe recurrent ischemia at 30 days	Death or MI at 30 days

Table 17-1 **Design Characteristics of Trials on GPIIb/IIIa Inhibitors in ACS Without Persistent ST-Segment Elevation (Continued)**

	PRISM[7]	PRISM-PLUS[8]	PARAGON-A[9]	PURSUIT[10]	PARAGON-B[11]	GUSTO-IV ACS[12]
Required level of creatine kinase or creatine kinase MB elevation in MI definition	2 × ULN	2 × ULN; in relation to PCI: 3 × ULN	2 × ULN	1 × ULN: in relation to PCI: 3 × ULN; in relation to CABG: 5 × ULN	2 × ULN; in relation to PCI: 3 × ULN; in relation to CABG: 5 × ULN	3 × ULN
Safety Endpoints						
Major bleeding complications	Intracranial hemorrhage; bleeding leading to decrease in hemoglobin concentration of at least 50 g/L; or cardiac tamponade	Intracranial hemorrhage; bleeding leading to decrease in hemoglobin concentration of at least 40 g/L; bleeding requiring transfusion of at least 2 units blood; or bleeding requiring corrective surgery	Intracranial hemorrhage; or bleeding leading to hemodynamic compromise requiring intervention	Intracranial hemorrhage; or bleeding leading to hemodynamic compromise requiring intervention	Intracranial hemorrhage; or bleeding leading to hemodynamic compromise requiring intervention	Intracranial hemorrhage; or bleeding leading to a decrease in hemoglobin concentration of at least 50 g/L

Abbreviations: CAG, coronary angiography; CABG, coronary artery bypass graft, ULN, upper limit of normal.

Adapted from Ref. 90.

426

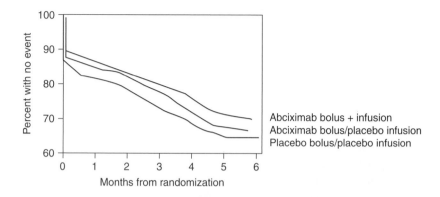

Figure 17-14 **Patients receiving abciximab bolus plus infusion had the lowest restenosis rate at 6 months in EPIC trial.** *(Source: Adapted from Topol EJ, Califf RM, Weisman HF, et al. Randomized trial of coronary intervention with antibody against platelet IIb/IIIa integrin for reduction of clinical stenosis. Lancet 1994;343(8902):881–886.).*

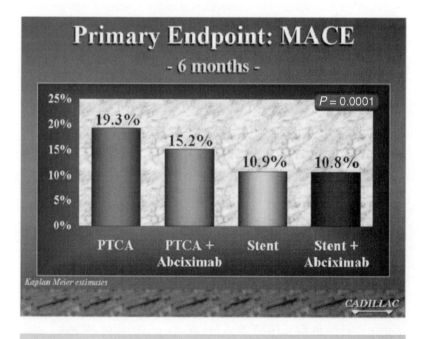

Figure 17-15 **In CADILLAC trial use of stent showed better results irrespective of use of abciximab. P = log rank comparison across all four groups.** *(Source: Adapted from: Stone G. CADILLAC trial. N Engl J Med 2002;346:957–966.)*

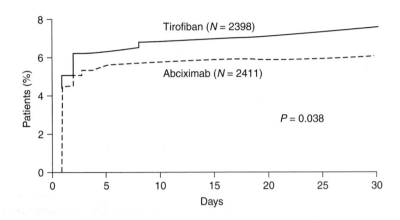

Figure 17-16 **TARGET trial demonstrated superiority of abciximab over tirofiban in patients undergoing stenting (lower death, nonfatal MI, or urgent target-vessel revascularization at 30 days), benefit was limited to patients with ACS.** *(Source: Adapted from Topol EJ, Moliterno DJ, Herrmann HC, et al. Comparison of two platelet glycoprotein IIb/IIIa inhibitors for prevention of ischemic events with percutaneous coronary intervention. N Engl J Med 2001;344(25): 1888–1894.)*

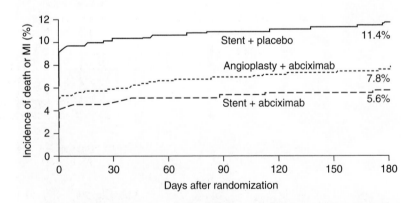

Figure 17-17 **In EPISTENT trial, incidence of death or MI was lower in patients treated with abciximab after stenting compared to angioplasty plus abciximab arm.** *(Source: Adapted from Lincoff AM, Califf RM, Moliterno DJ, et al. Complimentary clinical benefits of coronary artery stenting and blockade of GPIIbIIIa receptors. N Engl J Med 1999;341(5): 319–327.)*

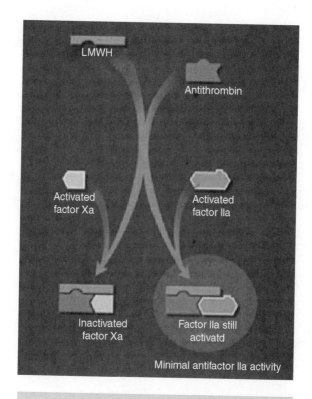

Figure 17-18 **The anticoagulant effects of LMWHs are a result of inhibition of factor Xa and thrombin.**

(6% in abciximab vs. 7.6% tirofiban). This reduction in composite endpoints was not seen at 6 months follow-up.

Another trial looking at the effectiveness of abciximab use in patients undergoing PCI was EPISTENT (Evaluation of IIb/IIIa Platelet Inhibitor for Stenting), which was a randomized trial of 2399 patients. In the study patients undergoing elective or emergent PCI were randomized to stent alone, stent plus abciximab, or PTCA plus abciximab.[73,74,75] The patients were followed for up to 6 months. The study showed that there was a significant reduction of primary endpoints (death, MI, need for urgent revascularization) with abciximab use as seen in Fig. 17-17.

The question whether treatment benefit with abciximab in patients with NSTEMI given prior to PCI in patients with refractory UA was addressed in the CAPTURE trial. The trial was a study of more than 1200 patients randomized to either abciximab or placebo. Treatment was given at least 18–24 hours prior to angioplasty and continued for 1 hour after completion of the procedure. This study was terminated prematurely secondary to a

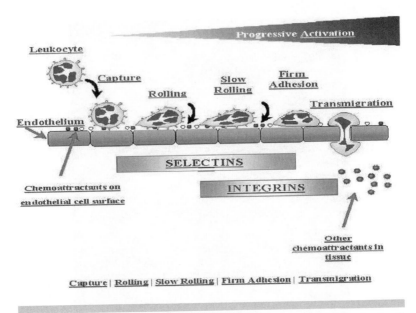

Figure 17-19 **Biochemical action of heparin causing inhibition of cell extravasation.**

decrease in primary endpoints (death, MI, urgent revascularization) at 30 days from 15.9% in placebo to 11.3% in abciximab-treated group.

GUSTO IV was a trial of 7800 patients with UA who were not planned for any intervention. Participants were randomized to receive abciximab bolus with 24-hour infusion, abciximab bolus with 48-hour infusion, or placebo.[76] The trial showed a lack of benefit with abciximab treatment that persisted up to 1 year.

PURSUIT was a multicenter randomized trial of eptifibatide (n = 1487 low dose; n = 4722 high dose) versus placebo (n = 4739) in patients with ACS without persistent ST-segment elevation. The patients were treated with aspirin and heparin and randomly assigned to eptifibatide 180 µg/kg bolus plus 1.3 µg/kg/min infusion, 180 µg/kg bolus plus 2.0 µg/kg/min infusion, or placebo for up to 3 days. Eptifibatide therapy was associated with a significantly lower 30-day event rate of death or nonfatal MI (14.2% vs. 15.7% with placebo).[77]

ESPIRIT (European/Australasian Stroke Prevention in Reversible Ischemia Trial) was a trial randomizing 2064 patients to either placebo or eptifibatide immediately prior to PCI.[78] The dose of eptifibatide used was two boluses followed by maintenance infusion. The study was terminated early secondary to a decrease in primary endpoints (death, MI, urgent revascularization, and switch to IIb/IIIa) in the eptifibatide-treated group (10.5% vs. 6.8%). The benefit remained at 30 days and 6 months follow-up.

The ISAR-REACT (Intracoronary Stenting and Antithrombotic Regimen-Rapid Early Action for Coronary Treatment) trial demonstrated that in patients at low-to-intermediate risk who undergo elective PCI after pretreatment with a high loading dose of clopidogrel (600 mg), abciximab was associated with no clinically measurable benefit within the first 30 days.[85]

The efficacy of GPIIb/IIIa inhibitors in the setting of ACS prompted the studies to evaluate their long-term efficacy in the oral formulation. One such trial, OPUS-TIMI 16 (Orbofiban in Patients with Unstable Coronary Syndromes-Thrombolysis in Myocardial Infarction) evaluated 10,288 patients with ACS, randomized to orbofiban (oral GPIIb/IIIa inhibitor) or placebo.[86] The results of the trial were not promising as it failed to show a decrease in cardiovascular events with orofiban. It showed an increase in mortality in patients receiving active drug.

Another trial, the SYMPHONY trial, randomized 9233 patients with ACS to aspirin, high-dose sibrafiban, or low-dose sibrafiban (oral GPIIb/IIIa inhibitor).[87] The study showed that sibrafiban had no advantage over aspirin in the prevention of major ischemic events and was in fact associated with a higher bleeding rate.

A meta-analysis of all major GPIIb/IIIa inhibitor trials showed that survival benefit was strongly demonstrated in patients with ACS undergoing PCI. In patients managed with medical therapy and not routinely undergoing PCI, modest benefit was shown.[88] Another meta-analysis of diabetic population ($n = 6458$) in six major GPIIb/IIIa inhibitor trials showed a survival benefit among these patients whether managed medically or with PCI, and benefit was most pronounced in diabetic patients undergoing PCI. There was no survival benefit in the nondiabetic group managed medically.[89] GPIIb/IIIa inhibitor use should be targeted to patients undergoing PCI (even more in diabetic patients) or in patients with high-risk for intracoronary thrombotic complications such as troponin positive patients, ongoing ischemia, and patients with dynamic ST changes.

INDIRECT THROMBIN INHIBITORS

Low Molecular Weight Heparin

Low molecular weight heparin is derived from unfractionated heparin (UFH) through a chemical or enzymatic depolymerization process.[90,91] LMWHs have a mean molecular weight of 4000–5000 Da, and like UFH, are heterogeneous in anticoagulant activity and molecular size, ranging from 1000 to 10,000 Da.[92]

LMWHs are considered indirect thrombin inhibitors (DTIs) since their inhibitory activity requires binding to AT via the same pentasaccharide sequence found in UFH (Fig. 17-18).[93] LMWHs have less inhibitory activity against thrombin than against factor Xa since only 25–50% of the LMWH chains are long enough to bridge AT to thrombin. Since factor Xa inhibition does not require bridging between factor Xa and AT, the smaller pentasaccharide-containing chains in LMWH retain their ability to catalyze factor Xa inhibition as can be seen in Fig. 17-18.[93–97,107]

Clinical Data for the use of LMWH in Acute Coronary Syndromes and Percutaneous Coronary Interventions

Large clinical trials evaluating LMWH in the management of patients with UA and non-Q-wave MIs comparing the LMWH enoxaparin to UFH demonstrated reductions in ischemic events with LMWH versus UFH.[98–100] However, there appeared to be a moderate nonsignificant increase in major and minor bleeding with LMWH compared to UFH.[101] The evidence supporting the use of LMWH in PCI is much less clear than that for ACS. There are a number of studies reporting the use of LMWH in PCI (Table 17-2).[102,103–105,112,113,123]

Excretion of LMWH

Low molecular weight heparins are cleared predominantly by the renal system.[93] The plasma half-life of LMWH ranges from 2 to 4 hours after intravenous

Table 17-2 **LMWH Comparative Studies in PCI**

Trial/Study	N	Study Population	Outcomes (%), LMWH Vs. UFH
REDUCE[104] (reviparin)	612	Elective PCI; single lesion	Acute coronary events at 24 h: 3.9 vs. 8.2 Major bleed: 2.3 vs. 2.6
CRUISE[105] (enoxaparin)	261	Elective or urgent PCI	D/MI/Revasc at 30 days: 10.1 vs. 7.6 TIMI major: 2.5 vs. 1.6 TIMI minor: 4.1 vs. 10.5
Legalery et al. (2001) (enoxaparin)[106]	584 enoxaparin vs. 581 UFH (historical control)	Unselected PCI	D/MI/R: 1.3 vs. 2.0 Major bleed: 1.0 vs. 0 Hematoma: 2.6 vs. 1.7

Abbreviations: CRUISE, Coronary Revascularization Using Integrelin and Single Bolus Enoxaparin; D, death; REDUCE, Reduction of Restenosis After PTCA, Early Administration of Reviparin in a Double-Blind Unfractionated Heparin and Placebo-Controlled Evaluation; Revasc, revascularization.

injection and 3 to 6 hours following a subcutaneous injection. The half-life of LMWH increases in patients with renal failure. The LMWH dose should be reduced by 64% in patients with severe renal impairment (creatinine clearance <30 mL/min) due to risk of accumulation that may lead to major bleeding.[93]

Limitations of LMWH

One of the limitations of LMWH is their inability to completely inhibit fibrin-bound thrombin, thus leaving the bound thrombin molecule free and active. This may allow thrombin to regenerate and act as a potent platelet activator.[108] Only 25% of LMWH molecules are large enough to inactivate thrombin, some LMWH agents do not significantly prolong activated clotting time (ACT) or activated partial thromboplastin time (aPTT) tests. Therefore, it becomes difficult to monitor LMWH with these tests in the clinical setting such as an ACS, or PCI.[108,109] LMWH can cross-react with heparin-induced thrombocytopenia (HIT) antibodies and has been reported to cause thrombocytopenia in a small percentage of patients.[110] Unlike UFH, protamine sulfate does not completely inhibit the anticoagulant activity of LMWH to reverse the potential side effects of these anticoagulants.[111] Table 17-3 demonstrates the complications of bleeding from various trials with LMWH.

Indirect Thrombin Inhibitors

Antithrombin is a hematologic factor in the human body in a low concentration. AT inhibits the serine protease coagulation factors (e.g., factor II also

Table 17-3 **LMWH Studies in PCI**

Trial/Study	N	Study Population	Outcomes (%)
Kereiakes et al. (2001) (dalteparin) 40 IU/kg and 60 IU/kg[111]	103	Elective PCI	D/MI/Revasc: 3.7 Major bleed: 2.8 Minor bleed: 10.3 Transfusion: 2.8
Choussat et al. (2002) (enoxaparin) 0.5 mg/kg IV[112]	180	Elective PCI	D/MI/Revasc: 3.9 Major bleed: 0.6 Minor bleed: 2.2
Collet et al. (2001) (enoxaparin) 1 mg/kg every 12 h[146]	132/451	Unselected population of ACS patients undergoing PCI	Death/MI: 3.0 Major bleed: 0.8 Minor bleed: 2.4

Abbreviations: D, death; Revasc, revascularization.

known as thrombin, factors Xa, IXa, and XIa). When the presence of heparin is pharmacologically added, this will increase the effect of AT 1000 times. Heparin does not exist normally in the human body. There is a heparin-like substance that is responsible for the enhancement of the AT. This is called heparin sulfate and has been identified on the surface of endothelial cells. Heparin has the ability to interfere with the leukocyte-endothelial adhesion, diapedesis, and extravasation. It performs these tasks by interacting with various leukocytes and binds to their surfaces. After it binds to the CD11b/CD18 (also known as MAC1), L-selectin, and P-selectin, it may inhibit the various cell adhesion interactions between the leukocytes and the endothelial surface of the arteries. Therefore, diapedesis is inhibited through the endothelium of the vasculature as can be seen in Fig. 17-19.[93–97,108,114]

Cell-derived heparinase enzymes on the endothelial heparin sulfate are involved in basement membrane degradation and digestion of matrix heparin sulfate. Heparin inhibits these enzymes which affects the movement of extravasated cells to various tissue sites. This may therefore cause tissue remodeling in the intimal endothelial architecture of the vessels.

Heparin is a large sulfated polysaccharide polymer as can be seen in Fig. 17-20. Heparin is about 15,000 Da. The drug is given parenterally (intravenously or subcutaneously). The drug is extracted from porcine intestine or bovine lung. Heparin is fast acting and used acutely to decrease the formation of thrombi. (Fig. 17-21).

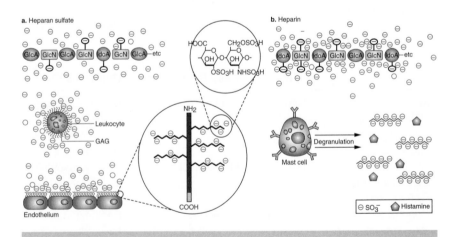

Figure 17-20 **UnFractionated heparin. Heparin is a large sulfated polysaccharide polymer as can be seen in Fig. 17-3. Heparin is about 15,000 Da. The drug is given parenterally (intravenously or subcutaneously). The drug is extracted from porcine intestine or bovine lung.**

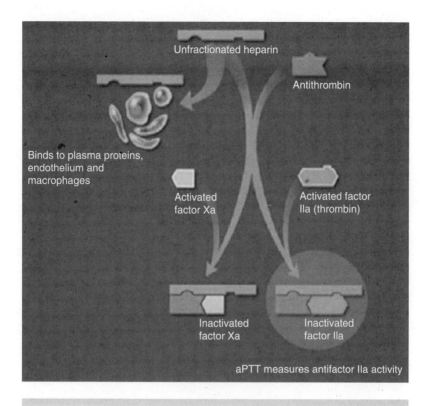

Figure 17-21 **Heparin is fast acting and used acutely to decrease the formation of thrombi, as seen in Fig. 17-4.**

AT is an alpha globulin that inhibits factor II (thrombin, as shown in the Fig. 17-25). This occurs normally in the body over a few hours.[27–29,115–117] Heparin will bind to AT and indirectly create an anticoagulant effect within a few minutes after it is given intravenously. Once heparin binds to AT, a molecular change occurs in the complex which accelerates the ability to bind to factor II (thrombin).[92,115–118]

Factor X is also inhibited by the binding of this complex to UFH with AT as can be seen in Fig. 17-22. However, this binding occurs less often because UFH has a smaller affinity with factor X in comparison to LMWH. Therefore, UFH decreases the organization of thrombi and fibrin formation which prevents clot from further organizing and expanding.[92,115–118]

Excretion of Heparin

Heparin is degraded into inactive compounds by the reticuloendothelial system of the body. The degraded heparin is excreted via the kidneys. Liver failure and renal insufficiency prolong the half-life of UFH.

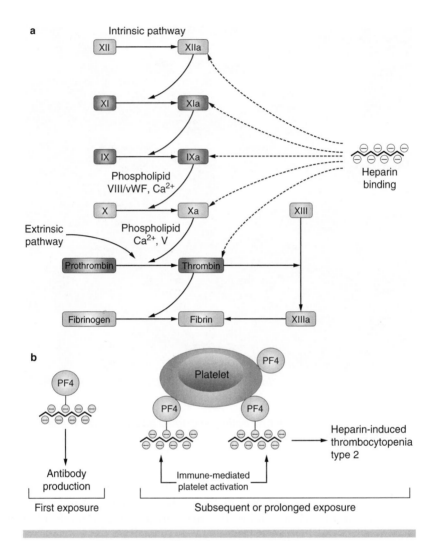

Figure 17-22 **Inhibition of factor X by binding of unfractionated heparin and AT complex, decrease in organization of thrombi and fibrin formation which prevents clot from further organizing and expanding.**

Advantages of Heparin

Heparin is an acidic molecule because of the presence of sulfate and carboxylic acid groups. This allows this molecule to become neutralized by protamine, a basic molecule in nature. Therefore, the reversal agent of UFH is protamine. Heparin is a large molecule that cannot cross the placenta barrier and is the drug of choice for an anticoagulant that can be given in pregnancy.[119]

Table 17-4 **Limitations of UFH**

Limitation	Consequence
Nonspecific binding to plasma proteins and endothelial cells[7,28]	Variability in anticoagulant effect, especially in seriously ill patients[34]
Release of platelet factor 4 and vWF from platelets during clotting	Results in heparin resistance and a need for higher levels of heparin[35]
Inability of heparin to inactivate fibrin-bound thrombin[21]	Thrombin remains active when bound to fibrin and continues to activate platelets[22]
Heparin induces platelet activation[36]	Further activates the clotting cascade and release of heparin-binding proteins
Forms heparin antibodies	Can result in heparin-induced thrombocytopenia-thrombosis syndrome[37]
Dose-dependent half-life[21]	Nonlinear increase in half-life as dose increases
Ill defined dose to achieve target ACT level in PCI	Supra anticoagulation resulting in increased bleeding risk or suboptimal anticoagulation resulting in increased risk of ischemic complications[38]

Limitations of Unfractionated Heparin

Heparin needs to be monitored every day with blood phlebotomization to maintain a therapeutic window 2–2.5 times the normal partial thromboplastin time (PTT) or aPTT levels. The limitations of UFH are further summarized in Table 17-4. Heparin increases the potential for hemorrhagic complications. Therefore, close monitoring of the coagulation factors, hematocrit, and vital signs of the patient need to be performed. Heparin has the potential of inducing an anaphylactic shock because it may be antigenic since it is manufactured from animals.

Heparin can cause HIT or heparin-induced thrombocytopenia-thrombosis syndrome. HIT may occur following the formation of platelet antibodies. There is a decrease in the number of platelets 6–10 days after the initiation of therapy. Therefore, the drug must be immediately discontinued.[110]

Heparin-Induced Thrombocytopenia

There are two types of HIT:

1. HIT type I: This is considered a mild reduction of platelets which is from nonimmunologic mechanisms. This is considered a mild form of HIT.

2. HIT type II: This HIT involves immunologically induced thrombo-
    cytopathologies that may present as mild forms and escalating to
    severe thrombocytopenias with platelets decreasing by 50% or more.
    This phenomenon can potentiate thromboembolic complications
    (Fig. 17-23).[120]

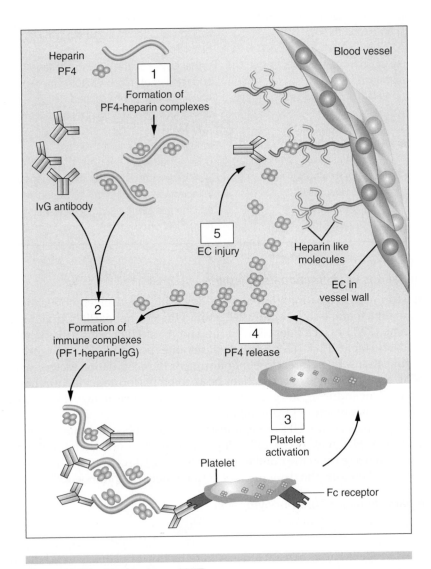

Figure 17-23 **Mechanism of HIT.**

The heparin-induced thrombocytopenia-thrombosis syndrome can occur with the formation of decreased circulating platelets and thrombosis in the vasculature. The chronic use of UFH can decrease the production and activity of AT which increases the risk of thrombosis (Fig. 17-24).

If either of these two disorders occurs, heparin may be substituted with a drug based on the clinical situation: medication that decreases platelet aggregation (.g., aspirin and clopidogrel), oral anticoagulants (e.g., coumarin anticoagulants), or DTIs (e.g., bivalirudin).[121]

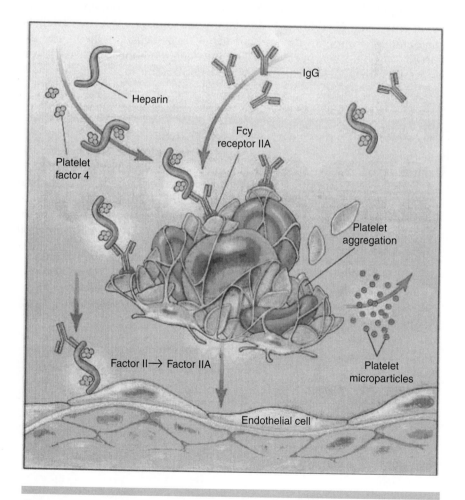

Figure 17-24 **Reduced production and activity of AT and increased risk of thrombosis with chronic use of UFH.**

DIRECT THROMBIN INHIBITORS

Direct thrombin inhibitors (e.g., bivalirudin, argatroban, and hirudin) are able to inhibit thrombin directly. They do not need the cofactor AT and are able to inhibit both fibrin-bound and soluble thrombin. Because of their relatively small size, the interaction of the DTIs with the active site of thrombin is not affected after the binding of thrombin to fibrin at exosite 1.[123] Thus, they are able to inactivate both free thrombin and thrombin bound to fibrin or FDPs. This may be due to a greater affinity of thrombin for exosite 1 (Table 17-5).

Bivalirudin, lepirudin, and hirudin are bivalent DTIs that bind to thrombin at exosite 1 (the substrate recognition site) and at the active site (Figs. 17-25 and 17-26).[124–126] The univalent DTI argatroban binds thrombin only at its active site (Fig. 17-27).[127] In the Direct Thrombin Inhibitor Trialists' Collaborative Group, hirudin and heparin were associated with an increase in major bleeding complications. The bivalent inhibitor, bivalirudin was associated with a lower major bleeding complication rate. This may have been because of its shorter half-life. Bivalirudin was associated with a lower death rate when compared to univalent inhibitors (Fig. 17-28).[128]

Bivalirudin

Bivalirudin is a synthetic 20 amino acid polypeptide modeled after hirudin and is comprised of an active site-directed peptide linked via a tetraglycine spacer to a dodecapeptide analog of the carboxy-terminal of hirudin.[126] Bivalirudin binds thrombin with high affinity at both the active site and exosite 1. Once bound, thrombin slowly cleaves bivalirudin at the active site, resulting in recovery of the function of thrombin's active site.[126] The carboxy-terminal dodecapeptide portion of the bivalirudin molecule remains bound to exosite 1

Table 17-5 **Binding Characteristics of DTIs**

	Binding Characteristics of Direct Thrombin Inhibitors		
Drug	**Molecular Weight**	**Mode of Binding**	**Thrombin Binding Site**
Bivalirudin	~2.2 kDa (20 amino acids)	Reversible bivalent	Active site, exosite 1
r-Hirudin (lepirudin, desirudin)	~7.0 kDa (65 amino acids)	Irreversible, bivalent	Active site, exosite 1
Argatroban	~527 Da	Reversible, univalent	Adjacent to active site

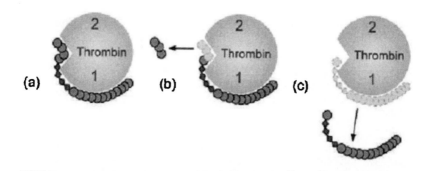

Figure 17-25 **Molecular interactions between the bivalent DTI bivalirudin and thrombin. (a) Bivalirudin binds to two sites on the thrombin molecule: its active site and exosite 1. (b) Bivalirudin is cleaved by thrombin at the active site. (c) The bond between thrombin and the remaining portion of bivalirudin is now weaker, allowing thrombin to resume its hemostatic function.**

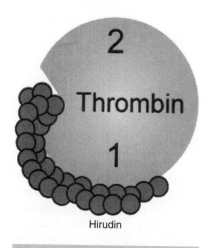

Figure 17-26 **The bivalent binding of hirudin, a DTI. Hirudin binding is highly specific and almost irreversible. Like hirudin, lepirudin is also a bivalent DTI, and also demonstrates nearly irreversible binding to thrombin.**

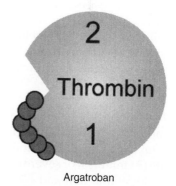

Figure 17-27 **The univalent binding of argatroban. Argatroban reversibly binds only near the active site on thrombin and is characterized by a short half-life.**

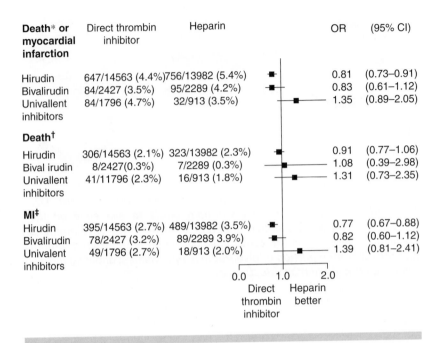

Death* or myocardial infarction	Direct thrombin inhibitor	Heparin		OR	(95% CI)
Hirudin	647/14563 (4.4%)	756/13982 (5.4%)		0.81	(0.73–0.91)
Bivalirudin	84/2427 (3.5%)	95/2289 (4.2%)		0.83	(0.61–1.12)
Univallent inhibitors	84/1796 (4.7%)	32/913 (3.5%)		1.35	(0.89–2.05)
Death†					
Hirudin	306/14563 (2.1%)	323/13982 (2.3%)		0.91	(0.77–1.06)
Bival irudin	8/2427(0.3%)	7/2289 (0.3%)		1.08	(0.39–2.98)
Univallent inhibitors	41/11796 (2.3%)	16/913 (1.8%)		1.31	(0.73–2.35)
MI‡					
Hirudin	395/14563 (2.7%)	489/13982 (3.5%)		0.77	(0.67–0.88)
Bivalirudin	78/2427 (3.2%)	89/2289 3.9%)		0.82	(0.60–1.12)
Univalent inhibitors	49/1796 (2.7%)	18/913 (2.0%)		1.39	(0.81–2.41)

0.0 1.0 2.0
Direct thrombin inhibitor Heparin better

Figure 17-28 **Direct thrombin inhibitor in ACS meta-analysis.** *(Source: Adapted from Direct Thrombin Inhibitor Trialists' Collaborative Group. Direct thrombin inhibitors in acute coronary syndromes: principal results of a meta-analysis based on individual patient's data. Lancet 2002;359:294–302.)*

with low affinity. Therefore, bivalirudin initially acts as a noncompetitive inhibitor of thrombin, but then becomes a competitive inhibitor, enabling thrombin to subsequently participate in hemostatic reactions (Fig. 17-25).

PHARMACODYNAMICS

Bivalirudin is cleared by a combination of proteolytic cleavage and renal mechanisms.[129] Bivalirudin has a half-life of about 25 minutes[130] in patients with normal renal function, with prolongation seen in patients with moderate (34 minutes) or severe (57 minutes) renal impairment (creatinine clearance of 30–59 mL/min and <30 mL/min, respectively). Dose adjustments of the bivalirudin infusion may be required for patients with severe renal impairment and for dialysis-dependent patients.[129] The short half-life of bivalirudin distinguishes it from lepirudin (recombinant hirudin) and may contribute to a more favorable safety profile. Bivalirudin demonstrates linear dose-proportional plasma concentration between dose and anticoagulant effect. The anticoagulant effect of bivalirudin is readily measured by both the ACT and the aPTT. This allows this agent to be administered easily in the catheterization laboratory. Bivalirudin has not demonstrated any cross-reactivity with heparin-induced antibodies in the serum of patients with HIT.

Lepirudin

The recombinant agent lepirudin (hirudin), initially isolated from the salivary glands of the medicinal leech (Hirudo medicinalis), is a 65 amino acid polypeptide.[131] Lepirudin has a high affinity to specifically bind to thrombin. Therefore, the lepirudin/thrombin complex is considered irreversible. There is no antidote to reverse its anticoagulant activity, causing this agent to have a potential disadvantage in clinical use.[125] Lepirudin is cleared primarily via renal mechanisms.[132] After IV injection, the half-life is approximately 50–60 minutes. This may be increased depending on any comorbid diseases.[133] The drug may have an increased concentration in the plasma in patients with renal insufficiency. Therefore, the bolus and infusion dose must be reduced in patients with renal impairment (creatinine clearance <60 mL/min), and the agent is not recommended for use in patients with creatinine clearance <15 mL/min.[133–135] There is a direct linear proportional relationship between the plasma concentrations of lepirudin and the dose administered. The standard ACT assay method cannot be used for routine monitoring of the anticoagulant effects of lepirudin. In general, an aPTT ratio (the patient's aPTT value at any given time divided by an aPTT reference value) is a method employed to monitor the anticoagulation of lepirudin.

PHARMACODYNAMICS

Lepirudin antibodies have been detected in approximately 40% of treated patients.[133,136] These antibodies appear to have an effect on anticoagulant status. These antibodies bind to lepirudin and prolong its half-life causing drug accumulation and possible hemorrhagic complications. There are also different antibodies that appear to neutralize lepirudin's anticoagulant effect.[137]

Argatroban

Argatroban is a synthetic derivative of arginine that binds reversibly to the catalytic site of thrombin.[127] Argatroban does not inhibit other serine proteases, but 54% of the argatroban dose binds to human serum proteins, albumin, and 1-acid GP.[138]

PHARMACODYNAMICS

The primary route of clearance for argatroban is via liver metabolism, with a half-life approximately 54 minutes after IV administration. Hepatic impairment significantly decreases argatroban clearance (approximately fourfold). This will increase its half-life to approximately 181 minutes. Argatroban's anticoagulation effect can be measured using the ACT or the aPTT. The plasma concentrations, dose, and anticoagulant effects are well correlated. There is no cross-reactivity to heparin-induced antibodies with argatroban.

Univalent versus Bivalent Direct Thrombin Inhibitors

In a recent meta-analysis of 11 randomized trials comparing DTIs to UFH in the management of patients with ACS, the authors found a 15% reduction in death/MI in patients treated with a DTI, compared to treatment with UFH.[128] There was a 0.8% absolute risk reduction, maintained at 30 days according to the study. There were similar benefits seen with the DTIs hirudin and bivalirudin, but not with the univalent DTI argatroban. Other trials have also found univalent DTIs (argatroban and two other univalent agents, efegatran and inogatran) to be less effective than the bivalent DTIs (hirudin, bivalirudin) in preventing ischemic events. The bivalent DTI hirudin was associated with a higher cost and increased risk of bleeding compared with UFH.[128] There was an increased risk of major bleeding with hirudin in patients presenting with ST-segment elevation MI. However, bivalirudin was associated with a 50% reduction in major bleeding in patients with ACS. There was a benefit in DTIs, in a small subgroup analysis, on death or MI in trials of both ACS and PCI. However, the univalent DTIs showed a less robust decrease in major bleeding.[128]

Direct Thrombin Inhibitors (Clinical Use in ACS and PCI)

Bivalirudin, lepirudin, and argatroban are the only DTIs approved in the United States. Lepirudin and argatroban are approved for treatment and management of patients with HIT. Argatroban is also approved for use in patients with HIT or at risk for HIT undergoing PCI. Bivalirudin is indicated for use in a broader population of patients with UA undergoing PCI.

BIVALIRUDIN

Of all the available DTIs, bivalirudin appears to offer an alternative to UFH in PCI. In the Bivalirudin Angioplasty Trial (BAT), 4312 patients with UA or post-MI, requiring PCI were randomized in a double-blind fashion to receive bivalirudin or heparin during the procedure.[139] This trial demonstrated a 22% relative risk reduction with bivalirudin in the rate of the composite endpoint of death/MI/repeat revascularization at 7 days (6.2% vs. 7.9%, $P < 0.039$) when compared to heparin. However, the BAT trial was conducted before the widespread use of stents and GPIIb/IIIa inhibitors. The results provided information and suggestions of improved outcomes with the use of bivalirudin over heparin. To assess bivalirudin in the modern interventional setting, several pilot trials have been conducted.

There are three randomized studies that evaluate the safety of bivalirudin and GPIIb/IIIa inhibitors versus UFH and GPIIb/IIIa inhibitors. Although the number of patients in these studies is small, bivalirudin plus abciximab ($n = 60$), eptifibatide ($n = 42$), and tirofiban ($n = 33$) all provide positive safety data consistent with the results seen in BAT for combining bivalirudin with GPIIb/IIIa inhibitors.[140-142] The CACHET B/C and

REPLACE-1 (randomized evaluation of PCI linking angiomax to reduced clinical events) trials[143,144] provide additional preliminary results with bivalirudin in the setting of stents and GPIIb/IIIa inhibition. The CACHET B/C demonstrated a 64% relative risk reduction of death/MI/revascularization for bivalirudin compared with UFH plus abciximab (n = 64; 2.8% vs. 7.8%). Similarly, bivalirudin treatment resulted in a 74% relative risk reduction of major bleeding (1.4% vs. 6.3%). This small trial provided preliminary evidence of a unique reduction in both ischemic and hemorrhagic events associated with the use of bivalirudin.

REPLACE-1, a trial of 1056 patients, provided continued evidence of reduced ischemic and hemorrhagic complications in patients undergoing elective or urgent PCI. Similar to prior investigations, this large pilot study demonstrated a simultaneous reduction in both ischemic and bleeding complications with bivalirudin. There was a relative risk reduction of 19% for the composite 48-hour endpoint death/MI/revascularization and a 22% reduction in major bleeding events observed.[144]

The REPLACE-2 trial[145] was a randomized, double-blind trial of bivalirudin conducted in 6010 patients. The use of bivalirudin plus provisional administration of GPIIb/IIIa inhibitors was compared to UFH with planned GPIIb/IIIa inhibition in patients undergoing PCI. Bivalirudin with provisional GPIIb/IIIa inhibitor use demonstrated a numerically reduced incidence of the composite endpoint (death, MI, revascularization, major bleeding) compared with heparin and GPIIb/IIIa inhibitors. The incidence of death and revascularization was lower for the bivalirudin-treated patients. The incidence of non-Q-wave MIs in this group was numerically, but not significantly higher. In contrast, the incidences of bleeding, transfusions, and thrombocytopenia, however, were significantly lower in patients receiving bivalirudin compared with heparin and provisional GPIIb/IIIa arm (Table 17-6). The 6-month follow-up data from the REPLACE-2 trial demonstrated that patients randomized to heparin with GPIIb/IIIa inhibitor and bivalirudin showed similar rates of MI (1.5%) and revascularization (9.0%). Even though this did not reach statistical significance, the death rate at 6 months and 1 year was numerically lower in the bivalirudin arm compared to UFH and GPIIb/IIIa inhibitors. Therefore, bivalirudin plus a GPIIb/IIIa inhibitor administered on a provisional basis may be an appropriate anticoagulation strategy in a large portion of PCI patients.

In a meta-analysis of 35,970 patients in comparative trials of DTIs versus heparin in patients with ACS or undergoing PCI, the reductions in death or MI with hirudin or bivalirudin were observed. However, similar findings were not observed with univalent agents such as argatroban.[128] This may be because of the statistical power of the studies, but no comparative studies between DTIs exist to establish clear superiority for one agent over the other.

Table 17-6 **Bivalirudin Comparative PCI Trials**

| | | **Bivalirudin Comparative PCI Trials** | | |
| | | | | |
Trial/Study	*N*	*Population*	*Outcomes (%)*	*Bivalirudin Vs. UFH*
BAT (2001)[62]	4312	PCI	D/MI/R at 7 days	6.2 vs. 7.9
			Major bleeding	3.5 vs. 9.3
CACHET (2002)[68]	288	PCI	D/MI/R at 7 days	2.8 vs. 7.8
			Major bleeding	1.4 vs. 6.3
REPLACE-1 (2002)[144]	1056	PCI	D/MI/R at 48 h	6.6 vs. 6.9
			Major bleeding	2.2 vs. 2.7
REPLACE-2 (2003)[69]	6029	PCI	D/MI/R/in-hospital major bleed at 30 days	9.2 vs. 10.0
			D/M/R at 30 days	7.6 vs. 7.1
			Major bleeding	2.4 vs. 4.1

Abbreviations: D, death; R, revascularization.

REFERENCES

1. Grundy SM. Hypertriglyceridemia, atherogenic dyslipidemia, and the metabolic syndrome. *Am J Cardiol* 1998;81:18B–25B.

2. Brownlee M. Biochemistry and molecular cell biology of diabetic complications. *Nature* 2001;414:813–820.

3. Imperatore G, Riccardi G, Iovine C, et al. Plasma fibrinogen: a new factor of the metabolic syndrome: a population-based study. *Diabetes Care* 1998;21:649–654.

4. Byberg L, Siegbahn A, Berglund L, et al. Plasminogen activator inhibitor-1 activity is independently related to both insulin sensitivity and serum triglycerides in 70-year-old men. *Arterioscler Thromb Vasc Biol* 1998;18:258–264.

5. Trovati M, Anfossi G. Insulin, insulin resistance and platelet function: similarities with insulin effects on cultured vascular smooth muscle cells. *Diabetologia* 1998;41:609–622.

6. Tschoepe D, Roesen P, Kaufmann L, et al. Evidence for abnormal platelet glycoprotein expression in diabetes mellitus. *Eur J Clin Invest* 1990;20:166–170.

7. Keating FK, Whitaker DA, Kabbani SS, et al. Relation of augmented platelet reactivity to the magnitude of distribution of atherosclerosis. *Am J Cardiol* 2004;94:725–728.

8. Aukrust P, Muller F, Ueland T, et al. Enhanced levels of soluble and membrane bound CD40 ligand in patients with unstable angina: possible reflection of T

lymphocyte and platelet involvement in the pathogenesis of acute coronary syndromes. *Circulation* 1999;100:614–620.

9. Keating FK, Sobel BE, Schneider DJ. Effects of increased concentrations of glucose on platelet reactivity in healthy subjects and in patients with and without diabetes mellitus. *Am J Cardiol* 2003;92:1362–1365.

10. Mach F, Schonbeck U, Sukhova GK, et al. Reduction of atherosclerosis in mice by inhibition of CD40 signalling. *Nature* 1998;394:200–203.

11. Lutgens E, Gorelik L, Daemen MJ, et al. Requirement for CD 154 in the progression of atherosclerosis. *Nat Med* 1999;5:1313–1316.

12. Grewal IS, Flavell RA. CD40 and CD154 in cell-mediated immunity. *Annu Rev Immunol* 1998;16:111–135.

13. Lee Y, Lee WH, Lee SC, et al. CD40L activation in circulating platelets in patients with acute coronary syndrome. *Cardiology* 1999;92:11–16.

14. Mach F, Schonbeck U, Bonnefoy JY, et al. Activation of monocyte/macrophage functions related to acute atheroma complication by ligation of CD40: induction of collagenase, stromelysin, and tissue factor. *Circulation* 1997;96:396–399.

15. Schonbeck U, Varo N, Libby P, et al. Soluble CD40L and cardiovascular risk in women. *Circulation* 2001;104:2266–2268.

16. Lim HS, Blann AD, Lip GY. Soluble CD40 ligand, soluble P-selectin, interleukin-6, and tissue factor in diabetes mellitus: relationships to cardiovascular disease and risk factor intervention. *Circulation* 2004;109:2524–2528.

17. Gokulakrishnan K, Deepa R, Mohan V, et al. Soluble P-selectin and CD40L levels in subjects with prediabetes, diabetes mellitus, and metabolic syndrome: the Chennai Urban Rural Epidemiology Study. *Metabolism* 2006;55(2):237–242.

18. Aref S, Sakrana M, Hafez AA, et al. Soluble P-selectin levels in diabetes mellitus patients with coronary artery disease. Hematology 2005;10(3):183–187.

19. Michelson AD, Barnard MR, Krueger LA, et al. Circulating monocyte-platelet aggregates are a more sensitive marker of in vivo platelet activation than platelet surface P-selectin: studies in baboons, human coronary intervention, and human acute myocardial infarction. *Circulation* 2001;104(13):1533–1537.

20. Zumbach M, Hofmann M, Borcea V, et al. Tissue factor antigen is elevated in patients with microvascular complications of diabetes mellitus. *Exp Clin Endocrinol Diabetes* 1997;105:206–212.

21. Sambola A, Osende J, Hathcock J, et al. Role of risk factors in the modulation of tissue factor activity and blood thrombogenicity. *Circulation* 2003;107:973–977.

22. Boeri D, Almus FE, Maiello M, et al. Modification of tissue-factor mRNA and protein response to thrombin and interleukin 1 by high glucose in cultured human endothelial cells. *Diabetes* 1989;38:212–218.

23. Wannamethee SG, Lowe GD, Shaper AG, et al. The metabolic syndrome and insulin resistance: relationship to haemostatic and inflammatory markers in older non-diabetic men. *Atherosclerosis* 2005;181:101–108.

24. Haffner S, Temprosa M, Crandall J, et al. Diabetes Prevention Program Research Group. Intensive lifestyle intervention or metformin on inflammation and coagulation in participants with impaired glucose tolerance. *Diabetes* 2005;54:1566–1572.

25. Kain K, Catto AJ, Grant PJ. Associations between insulin resistance and thrombotic risk factors in high-risk South Asian subjects. *Diabet Med* 2003;20:651–655.

26. Freeman MS, Mansfield MW, Barrett JH, et al. Insulin resistance: an atherothrombotic syndrome. The Leeds Family Study. *Thromb Haemost* 2003;89:161–168.

27. Gerrard JM, Stuart MJ, Rao GHR, et al. Alteration in the balance of prostaglandin and thromboxane synthesis in diabetic rats. *J Lab Clin Med* 1980;95:950–958.

28. Johnson M, Harrison HE, Raftery AT, et al. Vascular prostacyclin may be reduced in diabetes in man (Letter). *Lancet* 1979;1:325–326.

29. Bucala R, Tracey KJ, Cerami A. Advanced glycosylation products quench nitric oxide and mediate defective endothelium-dependent vasodilation in experimental diabetes. *J Clin Invest* 1991;87:432–438.

30. Bolego C, Buccellati C, Radaelli T, et al. eNOS, COX-2, and prostacyclin production are impaired in endothelial cells from diabetics. Biochem Biophys Res Commun 2006;339(1):188–190.

31. Richard A. Cohen role of nitric oxide in diabetic complications. *Am J Ther* 2005;12:499–502.

32. Juhan-Vague I, Thompson SG, Jespersen J. Involvement of the hemostatic system in the insulin resistance syndrome: a study of 1,500 patients with angina pectoris: The ECAT Angina Pectoris Study Group. *Arterioscler Thromb* 1993;13(12):1865–1873.

33. Festa A, D'Agostino R, Mykkanen L, et al. Relative contribution of insulin and its precursors to fibrinogen and PAI-1 in a large population with different states of glucose tolerance: The Insulin Resistance Atherosclerosis Study (IRAS). *Arterioscler Thromb Vasc Biol* 1999;19(3):562–568.

34. Juhan-Vague I, Roul C, Alessi MC, et al. Increased plasminogen activator inhibitor activity in non-insulin-dependent diabetic patients: relationship with plasma insulin. *Thromb Haemost* 1989;61:370–373.

35. Dunn EJ, Philippou H, Ariens RA, et al. Molecular mechanisms involved in the resistance of fibrin to clot lysis by plasmin in subjects with type 2 diabetes mellitus. Diabetologia 2006 [Epub ahead of print].

36. Diabetes Control and Complications Trial Research Group. The effect of intensive treatment of diabetes on the development and progression of long-term complications in insulin-dependent diabetes mellitus. *N Engl J Med* 1993;329: 977–986.

37. UK Prospective Diabetes Study Group. Intensive blood glucose control with sulphonylureas or insulin compared with conventional treatment and risk of complications in patients with type 2 diabetes (UKPDS 33). *Lancet* 1998;352:837–853.

38. Jorneskog G, Egberg N, Fagrell B, et al. Altered properties of the fibrin gel structure in patients with IDDM. *Diabetologia* 1996;39:1519–1523.

39. Carr M, Alving B. Effect of fibrin structure on plasmin mediated dissolution of plasma clots. *Blood Coagul Fibrinolysis* 1995;6:567–573.

40. Gabriel D, Muga K, Boothroyd E. The effect of fibrin structure on fibrinolysis. *J Biol Chem* 1992;267:24259–24263.

41. Zouaoui Boudjeltia K, Guillaume M, Henuzet C, et al. Fibrinolysis and cardiovascular risk factors: association with fibrinogen, lipids, and monocyte count. *Eur J Intern Med* 2006;17(2):102–108.

42. Braunwald E *Heart Disease*, 6th ed. WB Saunders Co. 2001:2105–2114.

43. ISIS-2 Collaborative Group. Benefits of aspirin in cardiovascular disease. *Lancet* 1988;2(8607):349–360.

44. Hennekens CH, Jonas MA, Buring JE. Benefits of aspirin in acute myocardial infarction. *Arch Intern Med* 1994;154(1):37–39.

45. The Medical Research Council's General Practice Research Framework: thrombosis prevention trial. *Lancet* 1998;351(9098):233–241.

46. Hansson L, Zanchetti A, Carruthers SJ, et al. Effects of intensive blood pressure lowering and low dose aspirin in patients with hypertension. *Lancet* 1998;351(9118): 1755–1762.

47. Collaborative Group of Primary Prevention Project: Low dose aspirin and vit E in patients at cardiovascular risk. *Lancet* 2001;357(9250):89–95.

48. Hart RG, Halperin JL, McBride R, et al. Aspirin for primary prevention of stroke and other major vascular events. *Arch Neurol* 2000;57(3):326–332.

49. Sanmuganathan PS, Ghahramani PR, Jackson PR, et al. Aspirin for primary prevention of coronary heart disease. *Heart* 2001;85(3):265–271.

50. Hebert PR, Hennekens CH. An overview of the four randomized trials of aspirin therapy in primary prevention of vascular disease. *Arch Intern Med* 2000;160(20):3123–3127.

51. Collaborative meta analysis: Collaborative meta analysis of randomized trials of anti-platelet therapy for prevention of death, myocardial infarction and stroke in high risk patients. *BMJ* 2002;324:(7329):71–86.

52. Goldstein RE, Andrews M, Hall WJ, et al. Marked reduction in long-term cardiac deaths with aspirin after a coronary event. *J Am Coll Cardiol* 1996;28(2): 326–330.

53. Lewis HD Jr, Davis JW, Archibald DG, et al. Protective effects of aspirin against acute myocardial infarction and death in men with unstable angina. *N Engl J Med* 1983;309(7):396–403.

54. Cairns JA, Gent M, Singer J, et al. Aspirin, sulfinpyrazone or both in unstable angina. *N Engl J Med* 1985;313(22):1369–1375.

55. The RISC Group. Risk of myocardial infarction and death during treatment with low dose aspirin and intravenous heparin in men with USA. *Lancet* 1990;336(8719): 827–830.

56. Hurst's. *The Heart*, 10th ed. McGraw-Hill professional, NY. 2001:1240,1377–1380.

57. The CURE trial: effects of clopidogrel in addition to aspirin in patients with acute coronary syndromes without ST-segment elevation. *N Engl J Med* 2001;345(7): 494–502.

58. Budaj A, Yusuf S, Mehta SR, et al. Benefit of clopidogrel in patients with acute coronary syndrome without ST-segment elevation in various risk groups. *Circulation* 2002;106(13):1622–126.

59. Yusuf S, Mehta SR, Zhao F, et al. Early and late effects of clopidogrel in patients with acute coronary syndromes. *Circulation* 2003;107(7):966–972.

60. Mehta SR, Yusuf S, Peters RJ, et al. Effects of pretreatment with clopidogrel and aspirin followed by long term therapy in patients undergoing percutaneous coronary interventions. *Lancet* 2001;358(9281):527–533.

61. CAPRIE Steering Committee. Randomized blinded trial of clopidogrel versus aspirin in patients at risk of ischemic events. *Lancet* 1996;348(9038):1329–1339.

62. Sabatine MS, Cannon CP, Gibson CM. Addition of clopidogrel to aspirin and fibrinolytic therapy for myocardial infarction with ST-segment elevation. *N Engl J Med* 2005;352:1179–1189.

63. COMMITT Collaborative Group. Addition of clopidogrel to aspirin in 45,852 patients with acute myocardial infarction: randomised placebo-controlled trial. *Lancet* 2005;366:1607–1621.

64. Bhatt DL, Fox KA, Hacke W, et al. Clopidogrel and aspirin versus aspirin alone for the prevention of atherothrombotic events. *N Engl J Med* 2006;354(16): 1706–1717.

65. PRISM Study Investigators. Comparison of aspirin plus tirofiban with aspirin plus heparin for patients with unstable angina. *N Engl J Med* 1998;338(21): 1498–1505.

66. Heeschen C, Hamm CW, Goldman B, et al. Troponin concentration for stratification of patients with acute coronary syndrome with therapeutic efficacy of tirofiban. *Lancet* 1999;354:1757–1762.

67. PRISM-PLUS Study Investigators. Inhibition of platelet glycoprotein IIb/IIIa receptor with tirofiban in patients with unstable angina and non Q wave myocardial infarction. *N Engl J Med* 1998;338(21):1488–1497.

68. Topol EJ, Califf RM, Weisman HF, et al. Randomized trial of coronary intervention with antibody against platelet IIb/IIIa integrin for reduction of clinical stenosis. *Lancet* 1994;343(8902):881–886.

69. Montalescot G, Barragan P, Wittenberg O, et al. Platelet glycoprotein IIb/IIIa inhibitin with coronary stenting for acute myocardial infarction. *N Engl J Med* 2001;344(25):1895–1903.

70. EPILOG Investigators. Platelet glycoprotein IIb/IIIa receptor blockade and low dose heparin during percutaneous coronary revascularization. *N Engl J Med* 1997;336(24):1689–1696.

71. Topol EJ, Moliterno DJ, Herrman HC, et al. Comparison of two GPIIb/IIIa inhibitors for prevention of ischemic events with precutaneous coronary revascularization. *N Engl J Med* 2001;344(25):1888–1894.

72. Moliterno DJ, Yakubov S, DiBattiste, et al. Outcomes at 6 months for the direct comparison of tirofiban and abciximab during precutaneous coronary intervention. *Lancet* 2002;360(9330):355–360.

73. EPISTENT Investigators. Randomized placebo-controlled and balloon angioplasty controlled trial to assess safety of coronary stenting with use of GPIIbIIIa inhibitor use. *Lancet* 1998;352(9122):87–92.

74. Randomized placebo-cotrolled trial of abciximab before and during coronary intervention n refractory unstable angina: the CAPTURE stydy. *Lancet* 1997; 349(17):1429–1435.

75. Topol EJ, Mark DB,Lincoff AM, et al. Outcomes at 1 year and economic implications of GPIIbIIIa blockade in patients undergoing coronary revascularization. *Lancet* 1999;354(9195):2019–2024.

76. Simmons ML. Effect of glycoprotein IIb/IIIa receptor blocker abciximab in outcomes of patients with acute coronary syndromes without early coronary revascularization. *Lancet* 2001;357(9272):1915–1924.

77. The PURSUIT Trial Investigators. Platelet glycoprotein IIb/IIIa in unstable angina: receptor suppression using Integrilin (PURSUIT). *N Engl J Med* 1998;339: 436–443.

78. EPSIRIT Investigators. Novel dosing regimen of eptifibatide in planned coronary stent implantation. *Lancet* 2000;356(9247):2037–2044.

79. Blankenship JC,Tasissa G, O'Shea JC, et al. Effects of GPIIbIIIa receptor inhibition on angiographic complications during precutaneous coronary intervention. *J Am Coll Cardiol* 2001;38(3):653–658.

80. O'Shea JC, Buller CE, Cantor WJ. Long-term efficacy of platelet GPIIbIIIa integrin blockade with eptifibatide in coronary stent intervention. *JAMA* 2002;287(5): 618–621.

81. van den Brand M, Laarman GJ, Steg PJ, et al. Assessment of coronary angiograms prior to and after treatment with abciximab and the outcomes of angioplasty in unstable angina patients. *Eur Heart J* 1999;20(21):1572–1578.

82. Klootwijk P, Meij S, Melkert R, et al. Reduction of recurrent ischemia with abciximab during continuous ECG-ischemia monitoring in patients with unstable angina refractory to standard treatment. *Circulation* 1998;98(14):1358–1364.

83. Hamm CW, Heeschen C, Goldmann B, et al. Benefits of abciximab in patients with refractory unstable angina in relation to troponin T levels. *N Engl J Med* 1999;340(21)1623–1629.

84. Braunwald E, Antman EM, Beasley JW, et al. ACC/AHA 2002 guidelines updates for the management of patients with unstable angina and NSTEMI. *Circulation* 2002;106:1893–1900.

85. Adnan K, Julinda M, Helmut S, et al. A clinical trial of abciximab in elective percutaneous coronary intervention after pretreatment with clopidogrel. *N Engl J Med* 2004;350(3):232–238.

86. Cannon CP, McCabe CH, Wilcox RG, et al. Oral glycoprotein IIb/IIIa inhibition with orbofiban in patients with unstable coronary syndrome. *Circulation* 2000;102(2):149–156.

87. SYMPHONY Investigators. Comparison of sirafiban with aspirin for prevention of cardiovascular events after acute coronary syndromes. *Lancet* 2000;355(9201): 335–345.

88. Boersma E, Harrington RA, Moliterno DJ, et al. Platelet glycoprotein IIb/IIIa inhibitors in acute coronary syndromes: a meta-analysis of all major randomized clinical trials. *Lancet* 2002;359:189–198.

89. Marco R, Derek CP, Debabrata M, et al. Platelet glycoprotein IIb/IIIa inhibitors reduce mortality in diabetic patients with non–ST-segment-elevation acute coronary syndromes. *Circulation* 2001;104:2767–2771.

90. Ofosu FA, Barrowcliffe TW. Mechanisms of action of low molecular weight heparins and heparinoids. In: Hirsh J, ed., *Antithrombotic Therapy, Baillieres Clinical Haematology*. London: Bailliere Tindall, Vol. 3, 1990:505–529.

91. Hirsh J, Warkentin TE, Raschke R, et al. Heparin and low molecular weight heparin. Mechanisms of action, pharmacokinetics, dosing considerations, monitoring, efficacy and safety. *Chest* 1998;114(5 Suppl):489S–510S.

92. Weitz JI. Low-molecular-weight heparins. *N Engl J Med* 1997;337:688–698.

93. Anderson W, Harthill JE. Molecular weight dependence of heparin anti-factor Xa activity: Influence of method. *Thromb Res* 1981;21:557–564.

94. Danielsson A, Raub E, Lindahl U, et al. Role of ternary complexes, in which heparin binds both antithrombin and proteinase, in the acceleration of the reactions between antithrombin and thrombin or factor Xa. *J Biol Chem* 1986;261: 15467–15473.

95. Rosenberg RD, Jordan RE, Favreau LV, et al. Highly active heparin species with multiple binding sites for antithrombin. *Biochem Biophys Res Commun* 1979;86: 1319–1324.

96. Jordan RE, Favreau LV, Braswell EH, et al. Heparin with two binding sites for antithrombin or platelet factor 4. *J Biol Chem* 1982;257:400–406.

97. Antman EM, McCabe CH, Gurfinkel EP, et al. Enoxaparin prevents death and cardiac ischemic events in unstable angina/non-Q-wave myocardial infarction. Results of the thrombolysis in myocardial infarction (TIMI) 11B trial. *Circulation* 1999;100:1593–1601.

98. Cohen M, Demers C, Gurfinkel EP, et al. Low-molecular-weight heparins in non-ST-segment elevation ischemia: The ESSENCE trial. Efficacy and safety of subcutaneous enoxaparin versus intravenous unfractionated heparin, in non-Q-wave coronary events. *Am J Cardiol* 1998;82:9L–24L.

99. Wallentin L, Bergstrand L, Dellborg M, et al. Low molecular weight heparin (dalteparin) compared to unfractionated heparin as an adjunct to rt-PA (alteplase) for improvement of coronary artery patency in acute myocardial infarction: The ASSENT Plus study. *Eur Heart J* 2003;24:897–908.

100. Cohen M, Demers C, Gurfinkel EP, et al. A comparison of low-molecular-weight heparin with unfractionated heparin for unstable coronary artery disease. Efficacy and safety of subcutaneous enoxaparin in non-Q-wave coronary events study group. *N Engl J Med* 1997;337:447–452.

101. Collet JP, Montalescot G, Lison L, et al. Percutaneous coronary intervention after subcutaneous enoxaparin pretreatment in patients with unstable angina pectoris. *Circulation* 2001;103:658–663.

102. Ferguson JJ, Antman EM, Bates ER, et al. The use of enoxaparin and GPIIb/IIIa antagonists in acute coronary syndromes. Final results of the NICE 3 study. *J Am Coll Cardiol* 2001;37(2 Suppl A):1253–1297 [abstract].

103. Kereiakes DJ, Grines C, Fry E, et al. The NICE 1 and NICE 4 Investigators, National Investigators Collaborating on Enoxaparin. Enoxaparin and abciximab adjunctive pharmacotherapy during percutaneous coronary intervention. *J Invasive Cardiol* 2001;13:272–278.

104. Bhatt DL, Lee BI, Casterella PJ, et al. Safety of concomitant therapy with eptifibatide and enoxaparin in patients undergoing percutaneous coronary intervention: results of the Coronary Revascularization Using Integrilin and Single Bolus Enoxaparin Study. *J Am Coll Cardiol* 2003;41:20–25.

105. Karsch KR, Preisack MB, Baildon R, et al. Low molecular weight heparin (reviparin) in percutaneous transluminal coronary angioplasty. Results of a randomized, double-blind, unfractionated heparin and placebo-controlled, multicenter trial (REDUCE trial). Reduction of restenosis after PTCA, early administration of reviparin in a double-blind unfractionated heparin and placebo-controlled evaluation. *J Am Coll Cardiol* 1996;28:1437–1443.

106. Legalery P, Seronde MF, Schiele F, et al. Enoxaparin as antithrombotic treatment in patients subject to percutaneous coronary interventions: comparison with unfractionated heparin. *Am J Cardiol* 2002;90(Suppl 6A):163H [abstract].

107. Weitz JI, Leslie B, Hudoba M. Thrombin binds to soluble fibrin degradation products where it is protected from inhibition by heparin-antithrombin but susceptible to inactivation by antithrombin-independent inhibitors. *Circulation* 1998;97:544–552.

108. Duplaga BA, Rivers CW, Nutescu E. Dosing and monitoring of low-molecular-weight heparins in special populations. *Pharmacotherapy* 2001;21:218–234.

109. Lovenox, Aventis Pharmaceuticals, Inc, Bridgewater, NJ (enoxaparin sodium injection) [package insert], 2003.

110. Crowther MA, Berry LR, Monagle PT, et al. Mechanisms responsible for the failure of protamine to inactivate low-molecular-weight heparin. *Br J Haematol* 2002;116:178–186.

111. Kereiakes DJ, Kleiman NS, Fry E, et al. Dalteparin in combination with abciximab during percutaneous coronary intervention. *Am Heart J* 2001;141: 348–352.

112. Choussat R, Montalescot G, Collet JP, et al. A unique, low dose of intravenous enoxaparin in elective percutaneous coronary intervention. *J Am Coll Cardiol* 2002;40:1943–1950.

113. Marmur JD, Anand SX, Bagga RS, et al. The activated clotting time can be used to monitor the low molecular weight heparin dalteparin after intravenous administration. *J Am Coll Cardiol* 2003;41:394–402.

114. Warkentin TE, Crowther MA. Reversing anticoagulants both old and new. *Can J Anaesth* 2002;49:S11–S25.

115. Linhardt RJ, Gunay NS. Production and chemical processing of low molecular weight heparins. *Semin Thromb Hemost* 1999;25(Suppl 3):5–16.

116. Tulinsky A. Molecular interactions of thrombin. *Semin Thromb Hemost* 1996;22:117–124.

117. Rosenberg RD, Oosta GM, Jordan RE, et al. The interaction of heparin with thrombin and antithrombin. *Biochem Biophys Res Commun* 1980;96:1200–1208.

118. Brill-Edwards P, Ginsberg JS, Gent M, et al. Safety of withholding heparin in pregnant women with a history of venous thromboembolism. The recurrence of clot in this Pregnancy Study Group. *N Engl J Med* 2000;343:1439–1444.

119. Aird WC, Eugene MJ. Case 15-2002: a 53-year-old man with a myocardial infarct and thromboses after coronary-artery bypass grafting. *N Engl J Med* 2002;346: 1562–1570.

120. Warkentin TE, Levine MN, Hirsh J, et al. Heparin-induced thrombocytopenia in patients treated with low-molecular weight heparin or unfractionated heparin. *N Engl J Med* 1995;332:1330–1336.

121. Palm M, Mattsson C. Pharmacokinetics of heparin and low molecular weight heparin fragment (Fragmin) in rabbits with impaired renal or metabolic clearance. *Thromb Haemost* 1987;58:932–935.

122. Collet JP, Montalescot G, Choussat R, et al. Enoxaparin in unstable angina patients with renal failure. *Int J Cardiol* 2001;80:81–82.

123. Bates SM, Weitz JI. Direct thrombin inhibitors for treatment of arterial thrombosis: potential differences between bivalirudin and hirudin. *Am J Cardiol* 1998;82:12P–18P.

124. Fenton JW, Villanueva GB, Ofosu FA, et al. Thrombin inhibition by hirudin: how hirudin inhibits thrombin. *Haemostasis* 1991;21(Suppl 1):27–31.

125. Stone SR, Hofsteenge J. Kinetics of the inhibition of thrombin by hirudin. *Biochemistry* 1986;25:4622–4628.

126. Maraganore JM, Bourdon P, Jablonski J, et al. Design and characterization of hirulogs: a novel class of bivalent peptide inhibitors of thrombin. *Biochemistry* 1990;29:7095–7101.

127. Hursting MJ, Alford KL, Becker JC, et al. Novastan (brand of argatroban): a small-molecule direct thrombin inhibitor. *Semin Thromb Hemost* 1997;23:503–516.

128. Direct Thrombin Inhibitor Trialists' Collaborative Group. Direct thrombin inhibitors in acute coronary syndromes: principal results of a meta-analysis based on individual patient's data. *Lancet* 2002;359:294–302.

129. Robson R, White H, Aylward P, et al. Bivalirudin pharmacokinetics and pharmacodynamics: effect of renal function, dose, and gender. *Clin Pharmacol Ther* 2002;71:433–439.

130. Maraganore JM, Adelman BA, Hirulog A. Direct thrombin inhibitor for management of acute coronary syndromes. *Coron Artery Dis* 1996;7:438–448.

131. Maraganore JM. Hirudin, hirulog: advances in antithrombotic therapy. *Perspect Drug Discov Design* 1993;1:461–478.

132. Greinacher A, Lubenow N. Recombinant hirudin in clinical practice: focus on lepirudin. *Circulation* 2001;103:1479–1484.

133. Eikelboom JW, Anand SS, Mehta SR, et al. Prognostic significance of thrombocytopenia during hirudin and heparin therapy in acute coronary syndrome without ST elevation: Organization to Assess Strategies for Ischemic Syndromes (OASIS-2) study. *Circulation* 2001;103:643–650.

134. Greinacher A. Recombinant hirudin for treatment of heparin-induced thrombocytopenia. In: Warkentin TE, Greinacher A, eds., *Heparin-induced Thrombocytopenia*. New York: Marcel Dekker, 2000:313–338.

135. Stringer K, Lindenfield J, Hirudins. Antithrombin anticoagulants. *Ann Pharmacother* 1992;26:1535–1540.

136. Schiele F, Vuillemenot A, Kramarz P, et al. Use of recombinant hirudin as antithrombotic treatment in patients with heparin-induced thrombocytopenia. *Am J Hematol* 1995;50:20–25.

137. Song X, Huhle G, Wang L, et al. Generation of Anti-hirudin antibodies in heparin-induced thrombocytopenic patients treated with r-hirudin. *Circulation* 1999;100:1528–1532.

138. Agatroban injection, GlaxoSmithKline, Research Triangle Park, NC [package insert], 2003.

139. Bittl JA, Chaitman BR, Feit F, et al. Bivalirudin versus heparin during coronary angioplasty for unstable or postinfarction angina: Final report reanalysis of the Bivalirudin Angioplasty Study. *Am Heart J* 2001;142:952–959.

140. Reed MD. Bell, clinical pharmacology of bivalirudin. *Pharmacotherapy* 2002;22:105S–111S.

141. Kleiman NS, Klem J, Fernandes LS, et al. Pharmacodynamic profile of the direct thrombin antagonist bivalirudin given in combination with the glycoprotein IIb/IIIa antagonist eptifibatide. *Am Heart J* 2002;143:585–593.

142. Kleiman NS, Lincoff AM, Sapp SK, et al. Pharmacodynamics of a direct thrombin inhibitor combined with a GP IIb-IIIa antagonist: first experience in humans. *Circulation* 1999;100(Suppl 18):I328 [abstract].

143. Kleiman NS, Lincoff AM, Harrington RA, et al. Antithrombin, antiplatelet therapy or both during PCI: a preliminary randomized trial. *J Am Coll Cardiol* 2001;37(2 Suppl A):1293–1242 [abstract].

144. Lincoff AM, Bittl JA, Kleiman NS, et al. REPLACE Investigators. The REPLACE 1 trial: a pilot study of bivalirudin versus heparin during percutaneous coronary intervention with stenting and GP IIb/IIIa blockade. *J Am Coll Cardiol* 2002; 39(5 Suppl A):16A [abstract].

145. Lincoff AM, Bittl JA, Harrington RA, et al. Bivalirudin and provisional glycoprotein IIb/IIIa blockade compared with heparin and planned glycoprotein IIb/IIIa blockade during percutaneous coronary intervention: REPLACE-2 randomized trial. *JAMA* 2003;289:853–863.

146. Collet JP, Montalescot G, Lison L, et al. Percutaneous coronary intervention after subcutaneous enoxaparin pretreatment in patients with unstable angina pectoris. *Circulation* 2001;103(5):658–663.

CARDIOMETABOLIC

RISK FACTORS AND

CVD IN WOMEN

Judith H. LaRosa
John C. LaRosa

INTRODUCTION

Cardiovascular disease (CVD) is the leading cause of death worldwide[1] with 3.8 million men and 3.4 million women dying of coronary heart disease (CHD) alone each year. However, in the United States, 51% of those who died from CVD were women.[2] Figure 18-1 presents the percentage of CVD deaths by sex[3]; Figure 18-2 presents the percentage of life years lost to disability and Table 18-1 presents the rank order and number of CVD deaths broken down into the two major components of CVD: diseases of the heart and cerebrovascular disease.[4]

CVD morbidity is of equal concern. As demonstrated in Fig. 18-2, both women and men, across the world, suffer from the disabilities imposed by CVD.

Until recently however, CVD, especially CHD, has received less attention in women than in men. In the early 1990s, federal governmental regulations, coupled with national advocacy, focused attention on the need for the inclusion of women and minorities into research studies. As a result, new research findings and their clinical applications, have steadily emerged enhancing knowledge and women's health. Yet, women of all racial and ethnic groups remain at high risk for CVD as they age. An understanding of those risk factors that place women at risk is imperative.

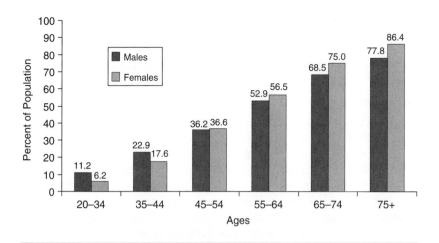

Figure 18-1 **Prevalence of CVDs in Americans aged 20+ by age and sex.** *(Source: Adapted from NHANES 1999–2002)*

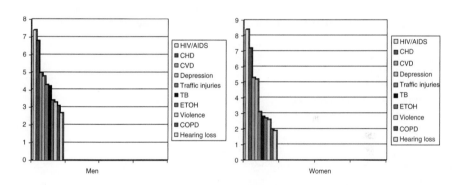

Figure 18-2 **Percentage of disability-adjusted life years (DALY) lost due to top 10 diseases 15+ years internationally.** *(Source: Adapted from http://www. who.int/cardiovascular_diseases/en/cvd_atlas_14_deathHD.pdf (accessed 2002))*[5]

Table 18-1 **Leading Causes of Death: Rank Order and Number by Sex, 2002**

Disease	Male	Female
Diseases of the heart	1 (340,933)	1 (356,014)
Malignant neoplasms	2 (288,768)	2 (268,503)
Cerebrovascular disease	4 (62,622)	3 (100,050)

Source: Adapted from Ref. 4.

CARDIOMETABOLIC RISK FACTORS IN WOMEN

Tobacco Use

Tobacco use has been known for decades as a major risk factor for CVD. Yet, aggressive marketing and relatively cheap prices have kept tobacco, especially cigarettes, in use. Although women did not take up smoking much before the 1920s, they rapidly made up for it during the ensuing decades. By 1965, 34% of American women smoked which represents the highest percentage of women who smoked. Since that time, smoking rates have decreased to about 18% overall.[6] As Table 18-2 demonstrates, there are women who are at much greater risk because of their smoking: American

Table 18-2 **Percentage of Women Smokers Aged ≤18 Years by Selected Characteristics (National Health Interview Survey, United States, 2004)**

Characteristic	Percentage (95% CI)
Race	
American Indian/Alaska Native	28.5 (±11.4)
Asian	4.8 (±2.8)
Black	17.2 (±2.1)
White	20.4 (±0.9)
Hispanic	10.9 (±1.3)
Education	
GED (no diploma)	36.6 (±5.9)
High school graduate	21.1 (±1.4)
Associate degree	18.0 (±2.1)
Some college	20.3 (±1.3)
Undergraduate degree	10.1 (±1.4)
Graduate degree	8.1 (±1.5)
Age group	
18–24	21.5 (±2.3)
25–44	21.4 (±1.2)
45–64	19.8 (±1.2)
≥65	8.1 (±1.0)
Poverty status	
At or above	17.7 (±0.9)
Below	27.1 (±2.2)

Abbreviation: CI, confidence interval.

Source: Adapted from Ref. 6.

Indian/Alaska Native, white, and black women. Those with less education and living in poverty are threatened. Finally, younger women continue to smoke at higher rates.

Smoking among women of childbearing age is of particular concern. Women who take oral contraceptives and who smoke, greatly increase their chance of CVD. While the rates of smoking among younger pregnant women have declined, a troubling 12% continue to smoke.[7]

Smoking is addictive and thus stopping can be a challenge. Within the past two decades, substantial changes have occurred that assist a woman in her attempts to quit. The environment has changed. Many cities are now banning smoking in public places. Antismoking medications are available. Yet too many women, especially young women, continue this practice.

Hypertension

Hypertension increases with age but rises more dramatically after age 45 in both sexes. Among women, the prevalence is highest among black women followed by white and Hispanic women (Fig. 18-3).[8]

One of the most challenging issues is that of hypertension control. While 69% of women are aware of their hypertension, only 56.1% are in treatment and only 35.5% have the disease under control[9] (Table 18-3).

In addition to the racial/ethnic differences, studies have demonstrated that the highest rates of high blood pressure occur among those who are older, overweight, or obese and those who are poor or near poor.[10,11] The death rate from high blood pressure in Black women was 40% compared with 14% for white women. Finally, particular concern must be focused on

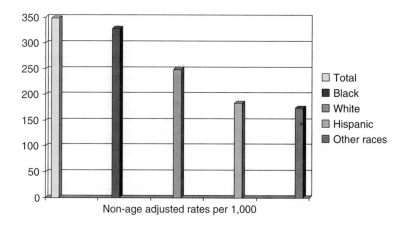

Figure 18-3 **Prevalence of hypertension in women ≥18+ by race Non-age-adjusted rates per 1000.** *(Source: Adapted from National Health Interview Survey, 2002.)*[8]

Table 18-3 **Percentage of Women with Hypertension and among Those with Hypertension, Estimated Percent of Those Who Are Aware, Treated for, and in Control of Their Condition**

HBP Prevalence % (95% CI)	*Awareness % (95% CI)*	*Under Current Rx % (95 CI)*	*Condition Controlled % (95% CI)*
20.0 (27.3–30.8)	69.3 (61.7–77.0)	56.1 (29.2–63.1)	35.5 (28.4–42.7)

Source: Adapted from Ref. 9.

any woman who is obese and taking oral contraceptives. In such women, the risks of high blood pressure rise markedly.[3]

Lipoproteins

Hypercholesterolemia is another significant risk factor for the development of CVD in women. Nationally, 17% of women 20–74 years have high serum cholesterol levels of >240 mg/dL (Table 18-4).[12] The good news is that there has been an 18% reduction in the past 14 years. However, elevated serum levels remain too high among women.

Interestingly, women were more likely to be screened for cholesterol levels but less likely to be aware of their high blood cholesterol level (Tables 18-4 and 18-5).[13]

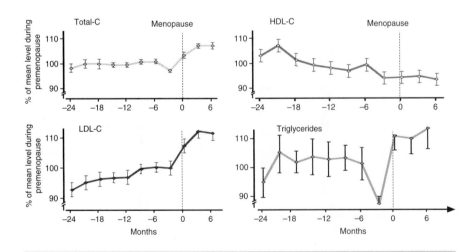

Figure 18-4 **Change in lipids after menopause.** (*Source: Reproduced with permission from Jensen J, Nilas L, Christiansen C, et al. Influence of menopause on serum lipids and lipoproteins. Maturitas 1990;12:321–331.)*

Table 18-4 **Percentage of Women 20+ Years With High Serum Cholesterol Levels (≥240 mg/dL) by Race, 1988–1994 and 1999–2002***

Race/Ethnicity	1988–1994	1999–2002	% Drop
Black	19.9	16.6	17
White	20.7	17.4	16
Mexican	17.7	12.7	28

*Percent of the population, age-adjusted.
Source: Adapted from Ref. 12.

A particular issue in women is the change in total cholesterol composition over the lifespan.[14] In childhood, high-density lipoprotein cholesterol (HDL-C) and low-density lipoprotein cholesterol (LDL-C) levels between males and females are similar. Beginning in puberty, however, HDL-C levels fall in boys while LDL-C levels are maintained. Girls and women, however, maintain higher HDL-C levels and lower LDL-C levels premenopausally. After menopause, LDL-C levels are higher in women than in men of the same age.[15] As in men, circulating cholesterol subfractions are important predictors of CHD risk in women. As total and LDL-C levels rise in women, so does CHD risk. Conversely, as HDL-C levels rise, CHD risk falls.[16]

Table 18-5 **Percentage of Women (20+ Years Positive for Hyperlipidemia**

Screened Within Past 5 Years	Positive for Elevated Blood Cholesterol	Positive for Elevated Blood Cholesterol or Using Cholesterol Lowering Medication	Aware of Elevated Cholesterol Levels
% (95% CI)	% (95% CI)	% (95% CI)	% (95% CI)
64.9	17.9	24.2	61.6
(62.1–67.4)	(16.3–19.4)	(22.6–25.7)	(57.5–65.7)

Source: Adapted from Ref. 13.

Evolving research indicates that lipoprotein subclasses affect women and men differently. In several observational studies, HDL-C is a more potent predictor of risk in women compared to men. Not only are total HDL-C levels higher in women, there is a greater difference in CHD risk per milligram in HDL-C in women. Alternately, LDL-C may not be as strong a predictor of risk in women. Studies in female primates, moreover, indicate that the presence of circulating estrogen interferes with LDL-C uptake in the arterial wall.[17] Thus, at a given level, LDL-C may be less atherogenic in women than men.

The role of triglyceride in the development of CHD is still subject to debate. Triglycerides are not strong statistically independent predictors of CHD when HDL and LDL are considered in multivariate analysis.[18] In older postmenopausal women, however, triglycerides do independently predict CHD risk.[19] Because triglycerides themselves are easily broken down by most tissues and do not accumulate in atherosclerotic plaques, it is unlikely that they themselves are a proximate cause of atherogenesis. Triglycerides in older women, however, may be markers for the presence of other atherogenic lipoproteins. It has been noted, for example, that as women age, the percentage of smaller, more dense LDL rises.[20] Small dense LDL is more susceptible to oxidation and probably more atherogenic.[21] Triglyceride elevations are also associated with lower levels of HDL and higher levels of some key clotting factors. These associations may help to explain the predictive power of triglycerides in some older women.

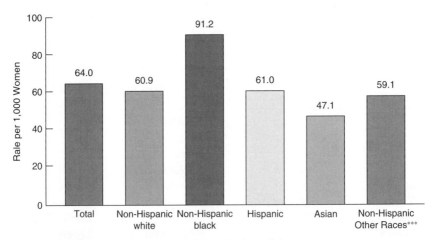

*Reported a health professional has ever told them they have diabetes
**Rates reported are not age-adjusted
***Includes American Indian Native African and those of more than one race

Figure 18-5 **Age-Adjusted Prevalence of Physician-Diagnosed Diabetes in Americans Aged 20 and Older by Race/Ethnicity and Sex, NHANES:1999–2002.**

Table 18-6 **Prevalence of Heart Disease and Stroke Among Women, Age ≥35 Years with and without Diabetes, 1999–2001***

Disease	With Diabetes	Without Diabetes
Coronary heart diseases	18.5 (16.8–20.3)	5.3 (5.0–5.5)
Stroke	7.8 (6.8–8.8)	2.6 (2.5–2.8)

*Percent (95% CI).

Source: Adapted from Ref. 22.

Diabetes

The prevalence of diabetes is rising in the United States, in large part due to the rising rates of obesity. From 1994 to 2002, the prevalence of diabetes among adults in the United States rose 54%. Figure 18-3 indicates the substantial differences in diabetes prevalence among women of different racial and ethnic groups.[8]

Examining CHD risk data, it is evident that women, in general, are at less risk for disease than men until about the time of menopause; that is, unless they have diabetes. Diabetes in women raises the risk of CHD mortality by as much as 3- to 10-fold (Table 18-6).[22,23]

That insulin may have a different effect in women and men is evident not only from studies of body fat distribution, but also by the strength of diabetes as a CHD risk factor in women. Although nondiabetic women and men, as noted, have different CHD rates, these rates remain almost identical in diabetic women and men.[24] Barrett-Connor et al. using Framingham Heart Disease study data showed that "With the diagnosis of diabetes, the relative risk of CVD increases more in women than in men. For instance, the risk of acute myocardial infarction (MI, or heart attack) is 150% greater in diabetic than in nondiabetic women but only 50% greater in diabetic than in nondiabetic men."[25]

The reason for this is uncertain. One explanation may be the greater impact that diabetes has in raising LDL-C and triglyceride levels in diabetic women.[26] Clearly, coronary risk is more strongly associated with high triglyceride and low HDL-C levels in diabetic women, than in diabetic men.[27] Again, how these differences may be related to endogenous gonadal hormone differences in women versus men is yet to be determined.

Fat Distribution

Overweight and obesity begin early. Students in grades 9 through 12 clearly show a prevalence of overweight between the sexes and among racial and ethnic groups (Fig. 18-6).

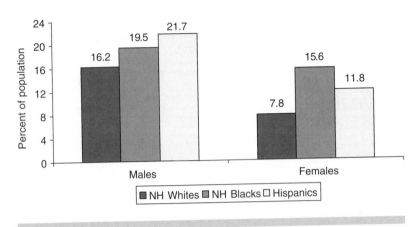

Figure 18-6 **Prevalence of overweight among students in grades 9 through 12 by race/ethnicity and sex, 2003.**

As women grow older, rates of overweight and obesity rise and with it, the risk of CVD. Among women 20 years of age and older, 61.6% are overweight.[3]

In both females and males there is an interesting correlation between the amount of truncal fat and peripheral insulin resistance and the occurrence of other metabolic risk factors. This has led to the hypothesis that truncal fat may somehow raise insulin resistance and cause hyperinsulinemia, hyper-triglyceridemia, low HDL-C, and elevated LDL-C levels.[28] In women, as in men, increased truncal fat is correlated with elevated LDL-C and depressed HDL-C, but in women with elevated testosterone levels,[29,30] it is not. What is clear is that an increase in abdominal fat raises the risk of CHD (Fig. 18-7).

This is further illustrated in a study examining body fat distribution and carotid intima medial thickness. Investigators examined 800 men and women and found that in both there was a strong association between truncal fat and intima media thickness. Overall, men had higher waist-to-hip ratio (WHR) than women and thus greater risk. However, with both men and women, there was a strong association with greater WHI and elevated triglycerides, glycated hemoglobin, and an inverse association with HDL-C.[32]

Metabolic Syndrome

In the past two decades, metabolic syndrome (MetS), or syndrome X, has emerged as a significant predictor of CVD. While the individual factors making up MetS are not new, when combined they represent an even stronger risk than they do alone. Note that while there is no consensus on definition of this syndrome, two sources are generally cited: the World Health Organization (WHO)[33] and the National Cholesterol Education Program Adult Treatment Panel Guidelines III (ATP III).[34] For the purposes of this

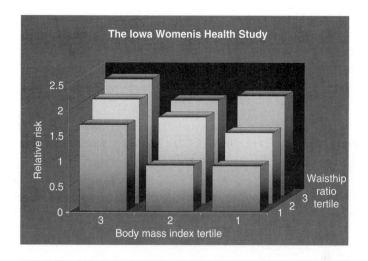

Figure 18-7 **Abdominal fat distribution increases the risk of CHD.** (Source: Reproduced with permission from Folsom AR, Kushi LH, Anderson KE, et al. Associations of general and abdominal obesity with multiple health outcomes in older women. Arch Intern Med 2000;160:2117–2128.)[31]

chapter, the ATP III criteria will be used. These guidelines require three or more of the following symptoms for MetS:

- Large waist circumference (>88 cm in women and >102 cm in men)
- Elevated triglyceride levels >150 mg/dL
- Low HDL-C (men <40 mg/dL and women <50 mg/dL)
- Elevated fasting glucose (110–125 mg/dL)
- Elevated systolic or diastolic blood pressure (>130/85) or self-reported use of antihypertension medications

Initial studies, largely composed of men or those with a family history of type 2 diabetes, confirmed the relationship with CVD morbidity and mortality.[35–37] A more recent study[38] showed that those with MetS, regardless of type 2 diabetes or CVD, were at greater risk for CVD. The study further demonstrated that women with MetS, even those without diabetes, were at greater risk for CHD compared with men. In short, it appears that an individual with MetS has up to a twofold greater risk of developing CVD (Tables 18-7 and 18-8).[38–39]

The presence of two or more CVD risk factors compounds the risk. For example, women who are obese and smoke lose about 7 years of life expectancy compared with nonobese nonsmokers.[40] Black and American Indian/Alaskan Native women had the highest rates for multiple risk factors.[41]

Table 18-7 **Age-Adjusted Prevalence of Individual Metabolic Abnormalities of the Metabolic Syndrome as Defined by ATP III Among 8608 U.S. Adults Aged ≤20 years (NHANES III, 1988–1994)**

Category	Abdominal Obesity	Hypertrigly-ceridemia	Low HDL	HBP or Med Use	High Glucose or Med Use
Men	30.4 ± 1.2	35.0 ± 1.7	35.1 ± 1.5	38.2 ± 0.8	15.6 ± 0.8
Women	46.7 ± 1.2	24.6 ± 1.0	39.1 ± 1.5	29.4 ± 0.8	9.9 ± 0.6
Men					
White	31.3 ± 1.2	36.8 ± 2.0	36.6 ± 1.7	37.3 ± 1.7	15.6 ± 1.0
	23.5 ± 1.3	21.3 ± 1.2	22.6 ± 1.8	49.6 ± 1.6	14.5 ± 1.0
African American					
Mexican	30.0 ± 1.9	40.2 ± 1.5	34.1 ± 2.2	39.8 ± 1.8	21.1 ± 1.4
American	28.6 ± 7.5	29.1 ± 4.0	33.2 ± 5.2	34.3 ± 4.0	14.9 ± 3.4
Other					
Women					
White	43.8 ± 1.4	24.8 ± 1.1	39.1 ± 1.9	27.8 ± 0.9	8.4 ± 0.6
African American	62.3 ± 1.8	35.8 ± 1.5	46.6 ± 1.6	32.9 ± 1.2	18.9 ± 1.3
Mexican American Other	63.2 ± 1.8	35.8 ± 1.5	46.6 ± 1.6	32.9 ± 1.2	18.9 ± 1.3

Source: Adapted from Ref. 39.

Table 18-8 **Adjusted* HRs and 9.5% CIs of CHD for Each Component of the Metabolic Syndrome**

	Women (n = 6881)	Men (n = 5208)
Elevated blood pressure	2.89 (2.18–3.80)	1.55 (1.32–1.83)
Low HDL-C	1.70 (1.30–2.22)	1.59 (1.34–1.88)
High triglycerides	1.22 (0.84–1.50)	1.00 (0.84–1.19)
Elevated fasting glucose	0.99 (0.69–1.42)	1.13 (0.91–1.39)
Large waist circumference	1.05 (0.79–1.39)	0.93 (0.78–1.11)

*Data are means ± SD. Adjusted for age, race/ARIC center, LDL-C, and smoking.

Source: Adapted from Ref. 38.

OTHER FACTORS IN THE CONSIDERATION OF CARDIOVASCULAR DISEASE IN WOMEN

Sex/Gender Differences in Cardiovascular Disease

When asked the leading cause of death in women, many women still respond "breast cancer." Part of the reason may stem from the fact that women often present with CVD about 10–15 years later than do men. Indeed, between the ages of 25 and 34, CVD is twice as prevalent in men as in women. By 45–54, the two sexes are equal. After that women take over as leaders in CVD prevalence.[3]

One reason for the differences may stem from estrogen loss in women as they age. Prevalence rates clearly show that as a woman approaches menopause, her rates of CVD begin to climb. Data from the Pathologic Determinants of Atherosclerosis in Youth (PDAY), autopsies, as well as electron beam tomography have provided strong evidence of the disease progression.[42] As early as 35 years of age, up to 70% of women have fatty streaks with about 30% having atherosclerotic plaques. As women age and approach menopause, plaques continue to expand with the subsequent development of fibrous plaques. At age 65 and beyond, clinical atherosclerosis is apparent and common.[43,44]

Racial/Ethnic Differences in Cardiovascular Disease

Not only do differences exist between the sexes but also they exist among racial and ethnic groups (Table 18-9).[45] Clearly, black women have the highest rates of heart disease and stroke followed by white women.[45] However, the rates of these diseases among all the racial and ethnic groups strongly suggest that more effort is required.

The reasons for such disparity are not fully understood. Examination of CVD risk factors shows that black women have the highest rates for high

Table 18-9 **Death Rates for Diseases of the Heart and Cerebrovascular Disease in Women by Race, 2002***

Race/Ethnicity	Diseases of the Heart	Cerebrovascular Disease
American Indian/Alaskan Native (AI/AA)	123.6	38.0
Asian/Pacific Islander (A/PI)	108.1	45.4
Black	263.2	71.8
White	193.7	53.4
Hispanic	149.7	38.6

*Age-adjusted rates per 100,000 population.

Source: Adapted from Ref. 45.

blood pressure, obesity, and diabetes. These risk factors are also interrelated. Obesity, in itself an important risk factor for CVD, also leads to high blood pressure and diabetes—each an important risk factors for CVD.

Additional factors play an important role in the development of CVD in women of different racial and ethnic groups. When examining comparable socioeconomic status, Winkelby et al.[46] showed that even controlling for socioeconomic status, black and Mexican-American women still have higher rates of risk factors for CVD. Yet, another study[47] showed that at younger ages, women of lower socioeconomic status had higher rates of CVD. However, by 60 years of age, those differences had disappeared.

Another factor that has not been fully studied but which appears to have an important impact is that of culture and neighborhood environments. The force of a community culture can have an important effect on how a woman sees herself: fat, thin, just right; what she eats; and how she maintains her health.[48,49]

SUMMARY

What stands out in study after study is that specific factors elevate the risk for CVD alone and in combination. Furthermore, risk factor prevalence is rising in both women and men globally such that CVD is now the leading cause of death worldwide. While each of the risk factors discussed is important in the development of CVD, type 2 diabetes is of particular concern. This disease eradicates the CVD protection many women enjoy prior to menopause. Type 2 diabetes combined with other risk factors—MetS—further enhances and complicates the danger.

The good news is that these risk factors can be prevented or addressed. Trends over time clearly demonstrate that the prevalence of many of the risk factors has declined in women of all racial and ethnic groups. Yet, ambient threats persist. Poor diet, lack of exercise, and continuing lack of awareness combined with cultural and community perceptions and habits endanger women. As such, women, their health care providers, and the communities in which they live must become more aware and proactive in dealing with these risks. Cultural views must be understood and integrated into changing attitudes and action.

REFERENCES

1. Available at: http://www.who.int/cardiovascular_diseases/en/cvd_atlas_14_deathHD.pdf (accessed 2002).

2. Available at: http://www.cdc.gov/nchs/hus.htm (accessed May 10, 2006).

3. American Heart Association. Heart Disease and Stroke Statistics—2006 Update. Dallas, TX: American Heart Association, 2006. Available at: http://www.americanheart.org/downloadable/heart/1140534985281Statsupdate06book.pdf (accessed 2006).

4. National Center for Health Statistics. Table 31. Health United States, 2005.

5. Available at: http://www.who.int/cardiovascular_diseases/en/cvd_atlas_13_coronaryHD.pdf (accessed May 10, 2006).

6. Centers for Disease Control and Prevention. Cigarette smoking among adults, United States. MMWR 2004;54(44):1121–1126. Available at: http://www.cdc.gov/mmwr/preview/mmwrhtml/mm5420a3.htm (accessed 2005).

7. United States Public Health Service. Surgeon General's Report on Women and Smoking, 2001. Available at: http://www.cdc.gov/tobacco/sgr/sgr_forwomen/factsheet_tobaccouse.htm (accessed 2001).

8. Centers for Disease Control and Prevention, National Center for Health Statistics, National Health Interview Survey. Available at: http://www.cdc.gov/nchs/nhis.htm (accessed May 10, 2006).

9. Centers for Disease Control and Prevention. Racial/ethnic disparities in prevalence, treatment, and control of hypertension—United States, 1999–2002. MMWR 2005. Available at: http://www.cdc.gov/mmwr/preview/mmwrhtml/mm5401a3.htm (accessed 2005).

10. American Heart Association. Statistical Fact Sheet—Populations, Women and Cardiovascular Disease, 2005. Available at: www.americanheart.org (accessed 2005).

11. National Center for Health Statistics. Health United States. Table 69: hypertension (elevated blood pressure) among persons 20 years of age and older, according to sex, age, race, and Hispanic origin, and poverty status 1999–2002, 2005.

12. National Center for Health Statistics. Table 70. Health United States, 2005.

13. Centers for Disease Control and Prevention. Disparities in screening for and awareness of high blood cholesterol—United States, 1999–2002. MMWR 2005. Available at: http://www.cdc.gov/mmwr/preview/mmwrhtml/mm5405a2.htm

14. Jensen J, Nilas L, Christiansen C, et al. Influence of menopause on serum lipids and lipoproteins. Maturitas 1990;12:321–331.

15. Rifkind BM, Segal P. Lipid resource clinics reference values for hyperlipidemia and hypolipidemia. JAMA 1983;250:1869–1872.

16. Manolio T, Pearson TA, Wenger N, et al. Cholesterol and heart disease in older persons and women: review of NHLBI Workshop. Ann Epidemiol 1992;2:161–176.

17. Wagner JD, Clarkson TB, St. Clair RW, et al. Estrogen replacement therapy (ERT) and coronary artery (CA) atherogenesis in surgically postmenopausal cynomolgus monkeys (Abstract). Circulation 1989;80(Suppl):II-31.

18. Austin MA, Hokanson JE, Brunzell JD. Characterization of low-density lipoprotein subclasses: methodologic approaches and clinical relevance. Curr Opin Lipidol 1994;5:395–403.

19. LaRosa JC. Triglycerides and coronary risk in women and the elderly. Arch Intern Med 1997;157:961–969.

20. Campos H, McNamara JR, Wilson PW, et al. Differences in low-density lipoprotein subfractions and apolipoproteins in premenopausal and postmenopausal women. J Clin Endocrinol Metab 1988;67:30–35.

21. De Graaf J, Hak-Lemmers HLM, Hectors MPC, et al. Enhanced susceptibility to in vitro oxidation of the dense low density lipoprotein n subfraction in healthy subjects. Arteriosclerosis 1991;11:298–306.

22. Centers for Disease Control and Prevention. Self-reported heart disease and stroke among adults with and without diabetes—United States, 1999–2001. 2003;52;1065–1070.

23. Hu G, Group DS. Gender differences in all-cause and cardiovascular mortality related to hyperglycemia and newly diagnoses diabetes. *Diabetologia* 2003;46: 608–617.

24. Krolewski AS, Warram JH, Valsania P, et al. Evolving natural history of coronary artery diseases in diabetes mellitus. *Am J Med* 1991;90(Suppl 2A):56S–61S.

25. Barrett-Connor E, Giardina ECV, Gitt AK, et al. The role of diabetes and hyperglycemia. *Arch Intern Med* 2004;164:934–942.

26. Walden CE, Knopp RH, Wahl PW, et al. Sex differences in the effect of diabetes mellitus on lipoprotein triglyceride and cholesterol concentrations. *N Engl J Med* 1984;311:953–959.

27. Goldschmid MG, Barrett-Connor E, Edelstein SL, et al. Dyslipidemia and ischemic heart disease mortality among men and women with diabetes. *Circulation* 1994;89: 991–997.

28. Soler JT, Folsom AR, Kushi LH, et al. Association of body fat distribution with plasma lipids, lipoproteins, apolipoproteins A1 and B in postmenopausal women. *J Clin Epidemiol* 1988;41:75–81.

29. Hauner H, Ditschuneit HH, Pal SB, et al. Fat distribution, endocrine and metabolic profile in obese women with and without hirsutism. *Metabolism* 1988;37:281–286.

30. Daniels SR, Morrison JA, Sprecher DL, et al. Association of body fat distribution and cardiovascular risk factors in children and adolescents. *Circulation* 1999;99:541–545.

31. Folsom AR, Kushi LG, Anderson KE, et al. Associations of general and abdominal obesity with multiple health outcomes in older women. *Arch Intern Med* 2000;160:2117–2128.

32. Lawlor DA, Ebrahim S, Whincup P, et al. Sex differences in body fat distribution and carotid intima media thickness: cross-sectional survey using data from the British regional heart study. *J Epidemiol Community Health* 2004;58:700–704.

33. World Health Organization. Definition, diagnosis, and classification of diabetes mellitus and its complications. *Report of a WHO Consultation. Part I: Diagnosis and Classification of Diabetes Mellitus.* Geneva: World Health Organization, 1999.

34. Expert Panel on the Detection, Evaluation and Treatment of High Blood Cholesterol in Adults: Executive Summary of the Third Report on the National Cholesterol Education Program (NCEP). Expert Panel on the Detection, Evaluation and Treatment of High Blood Cholesterol in Adults (Adult Treatment Panel III). *JAMA* 2001;285:2486–2497.

35. Lakka HM, Laaksonen DE, Lakka TA, et al. The metabolic syndrome and cardiovascular disease mortality in middle-aged men. *JAMA* 2002;288:2709–2716.

36. Isomaa B, Almgren P, Tuomi T, et al. Cardiovascular morbidity and mortality associated with the metabolic syndrome. *Diabetes Care* 2001;24:683–689.

37. Malik S, Wong ND, Franklin SS, et al. Impact of the metabolic syndrome on mortality from coronary heart disease, cardiovascular disease, and all causes in United States adults. *Circulation* 2004;110:1245–1250.

38. McNeill AM, Rosamond WD, Girman CG, et al. The metabolic syndrome and 11-year risk of incident cardiovascular disease in the Atherosclerosis Risk in Communities Study. *Diabetes Care* 2005;28:385–390.

39. Ford ES, Giles WH. Comparison of the prevalence of the metabolic syndrome using two proposed definitions. *Diabetes Care* 2003;26:575–581.

40. Peeters A, Barendregt JJ, Willekens F, et al. Obesity in adulthood and its consequences for life expectancy: a life-table analysis. *Ann Intern Med* 2003;138:24–32.

41. *MMWR* 2005;54(5).

42. McGill HC, CA McMahan, Zieske AW, et al. Effects of nonlipid factors on atherogenesis in youth with a favorable lipid profile. *Circulation* 2001;103:1546–1550.

43. Tejada C, Strong JP, Montenegro MR, et al. Distribution of coronary and aortic atherosclerosis by geographic location, race, and sex. *Lab Invest* 1968;18:509–526.

44. Raggi P, Callister TQ, Cooil B, et al. Identification of patients at increased risk of first unheralded acute myocardial infarction by electron-beam computed tomography. *Circulation* 2000;101:850–855.

45. National Center for Health Statistics. Tables 36 and 37. Health United States, 2005.

46. Winkelby MA, Kramer HC, Ahn DK, et al. Ethnic and socioeconomic differences in cardiovascular disease risk factors: findings for women from the Third National Health and Nutrition Examination Survey: 1988–1994. *JAMA* 1988;280:356–362.

47. Lee JR, Paultre F, Mosca L. The association between educational level and risk of cardiovascular disease fatality among women with cardiovascular disease. *Womens Health Issues* 2005;15:80–88.

48. Finkelstein EA, Khavjou OA, Mobley LR, et al. Racial/ethnic disparities in coronary heart disease risk factors among WISEWOMAN enrollees. *J Womens Health* 2004;13:503–518.

49. Sharma SM, Malacher AM, Giles WH, et al. Racial, ethnic and socioeconomic disparities in the clustering of cardiovascular disease risk factors. *Ethn Dis* 2004;14:43–48.

ASSOCIATIONS OF SLEEP APNEA TO CARDIOVASCULAR DISEASES

ROLE OF DIABETES AND METABOLIC SYNDROME

Girardin Jean-Louis

Ferdinand Zizi

Luther T. Clark

John Kassotis

Cardiovascular diseases are the leading cause of death among adults in developed countries. Health organizations worldwide have become alarmed by recent increases in cardiovascular risk factors (e.g., obesity, hypertension, and diabetes). This has led to a concerted effort to raise awareness among health professionals of those risk factors, as they endeavor to help patients at risk of developing cardiovascular diseases and to reduce the likelihood of having a stroke. In the field of sleep medicine, decades of research have provided evidence supporting the associations of sleep apnea to cardiovascular morbidity and mortality. In the early 1980s, investigators demonstrated that subsequent to tracheostomy patients with sleep apnea experienced decrease in systemic blood pressure (BP) and diminution of cardiac arrhythmia. With the presentation of many case-control studies, replicating similar findings, a concern arose that initial studies may have been confounded by factors, such as age, sex, and body habitus.

Adequate response to address this concern required the performance of several large-scale epidemiologic studies to assess the influence of suspected confounders on the associations between sleep apnea and cardiovascular diseases. Despite adequate methodological and statistical control for known covariates, relationships between these two conditions have persisted. Notwithstanding the significance of these findings, presently there is a growing concern that associations between sleep apnea and cardiovascular diseases might be mediated by the metabolic syndrome. The metabolic syndrome is an emerging public health problem, characterized by central obesity, hypertension, diabetes, and dyslipidemia. Of particular interest is the role played by diabetes, as insulin resistance might be a precursor in the development of metabolic syndrome. It is equally plausible that sleep apnea and metabolic syndrome might have synergistic health risks, since both conditions are predictive of cardiovascular morbidity and mortality.

In this chapter, we present evidence for the associations between sleep apnea and cardiovascular morbidity and proposed underlying anatomic and physiologic mechanisms. Issues pertaining to definition, prevalence, diagnosis, and treatment of sleep apnea are also discussed. We also present evidence supporting the potential mediating effects of the metabolic syndrome and respective intermediate mechanisms involved in proposed causal pathways. The role of each of the component disease entity of the metabolic syndrome is delineated, and pertinent clinical management issues are discussed.

SLEEP APNEA: DEFINITION AND PREVALENCE

Sleep apnea is a serious, potentially life-threatening condition, which was independently introduced into the medical literature by French and German investigators in 1965. It is characterized by repeated cessation of breathing while sleeping, mostly due to complete or partial pharyngeal obstruction. Most sleep apnea cases present with elements of both obstructive and central sleep apnea. Notwithstanding, much of the literature focuses on obstructive sleep apnea, as it is the most prevalent of the sleep-disordered breathing constellation. Objectively, sleep apnea is recognized by a combination of symptoms and laboratory results. These include repetitive apneas and hypopneas, which are accompanied by hypoxia, sleep arousals, and hemo-dynamic changes.[1,2] Moreover, activation of the sympathetic nervous system (SNS) during respiratory events potentiates vasoconstriction and often triggers increases in blood pressure (BP) and heart rate.[3]

Sleep apnea causes significant sleep disturbances, leading to excessive daytime sleepiness and fatigue, which in turn may cause vehicular and industrial accidents.[4-6] Rates of such accidents may be seven times greater than observed in the general population. Research has shown that when left untreated sleep apnea gradually induces cognitive deficits and poor performance.[7] According to a chart audit of 4 million beneficiaries of the Veterans Health Administration, numerous psychiatric comorbid diagnoses accompany sleep apnea including depression (21.8%), anxiety (16.7%), posttraumatic stress disorder (11.9%), psychosis (5.1), and bipolar disorders (3.3%).[8] Sleep apnea is also associated with several cardiorespiratory features (e.g., loud snoring, loud gasps, and daytime breathlessness). Furthermore, most of the risk factors (e.g., age, sex, ethnicity, body habitus, familial predisposition, alcohol, and chronic rhinitis) for sleep apnea can be recognized with appropriate training and education. Other risk factors (e.g., hypertension, diabetes, and dyslipidemia) are also implicated. Yet, most individuals with sleep apnea have not received a comprehensive sleep assessment.

Signs and Symptoms of Sleep Apnea

Loud snoring
Frequent cessation of breathing during sleep
Choking and gasping during sleep
Waking up sweating during the night
Feeling unrefreshed in the morning after a night's sleep
Morning headaches
Daytime sleepiness
Lethargy
Rapid weight gain
Cognitive deficits
Depression

Interestingly, while afflicted patients may wake up hundreds of times during the night, they are often unaware of it. This might explain low complaint rates in clinical histories.[9] In fact, according to the National Commission on Sleep Disorders Research, which reviewed about a million patient records, only 17 positive diagnoses for sleep disorders were found.[10] Thus, the majority of patients with sleep apnea have yet to receive a diagnosis. It has been estimated that 82% of men and 93% of women with moderate to severe sleep apnea remain undiagnosed.[11] Therefore, individuals suffering from comorbid conditions (e.g., hypertension, diabetes, and cardiovascular disease), and who, therefore, are at greater risks for early mortality don't benefit from current treatment regimens.

It is estimated that 2% of middle-aged women and 4% of middle-aged men have five or more apnea/hypopnea episodes per hour of sleep and meet criteria for obstructive sleep apnea.[11,12] Using a respiratory disturbance index (RDI)* of 10 or greater, the Wisconsin Sleep Cohort Study, an epidemiologic study surveying the U.S. adult population, estimated that sleep apnea affects as much as 15% of men and 5% of women between the ages of 30 and 60 years.[13] Prevalence rates are even higher in this age group when laboratory polysomnographic criteria are used. The largest population-based polysomnographic study conducted in the United States revealed that 24% of men and 9% of women had significant sleep apnea.[14] In the clinical setting, the proportion of sleep apnea cases rises to 68%.[15]

Sleep apnea affects individuals of all ages, but prevalence data suggest that it is more common among middle-aged adults between 40 and 60 years old. Notwithstanding, health consequences of sleep apnea tend to decline with age. Arguably, sleep apnea represents a greater threat to individuals' health before their 45th birthday. According to one estimate, 1.6–10.3% of children meet criteria for the condition.[16,17] The prevalence of sleep apnea tends to be higher among older adults. In one study, it was estimated that up to 60% of community-residing older adults have significant sleep apnea.[18] Specifically, 24% of adults older than 65 years had an AHI ≥5 and 62% had an AHI ≥10. Sleep researchers and public health advocates have become concerned over the lack of attention paid to ethnic disparities in seep apnea, as several important epidemiologic and clinical findings have shown greater rates among minority groups.

Typically, the public health literature has tended to list being male, overweight, and over the age of 40, as risk markers for sleep apnea.[11,19] However, recent data strongly suggest that ethnicity should also be considered as an important risk marker. Indeed, hypertension and cardiovascular diseases, which are two of the most important comorbid conditions of sleep apnea, are more prevalent among African Americans.[20,21] Despite these alarming data, the vast majority of suspected cases in minority communities remain undiagnosed and therefore untreated because of the lack of awareness by the public and health care professionals.

---

*The apnea-hypopnea index (AHI) or RDI refers to the total number of apneas (complete cessation of breathing lasting ≥10 seconds) and hypopneas (50% reduction in airflow lasting ≥10 seconds, followed by SaO_2 desaturations) divided by the patient's total sleep time. The AHI or RDI provides a measure of the severity of sleep apnea. AHI <5 is considered normal; AHI values ≥5 and <15 are viewed as mild; AHI values ≥15 and ≤30 are moderate; and AHI values >30 indicate severe sleep apnea.

One population-based study of adult Americans, aged 40–60 years, found that rates of sleep apnea were much higher among members of minority groups, with estimates indicating that 16.3% of ethnic minorities have greater than 20 events per hour as compared to 4.9% of non-Hispanic Whites.[22-24] This ethnic disparity is not solely observable among adults who are 40 years old or older. In effect, in a case-control family study of sleep apnea comparing 225 African Americans and 622 Whites, aged 2–86 years, 31% of African Americans versus 10% of Whites had RDI >10.[22] Also important in that study was the observation that young African Americans may be at increased risk for sleep apnea.

Observed race/ethnic differences in age of onset and anatomic risk factors for sleep apnea prompted the investigation of a possible racial difference in the genetic underpinnings of this condition. One study comparing African Americans and White families found evidence for segregation of a codominant gene with an allele frequency of 0.14 after adjusting for effects of body mass index (BMI) and age. This accounted for 35% of the total variance in sleep apnea severity.[25] Thus, both sleep apnea and cardiovascular disease are highly prevalent among African Americans, and younger African Americans in particular are at increased risks.

PATHOPHYSIOLOGY OF SLEEP APNEA

In the early 1960s, it was becoming evident that upper airway obstruction was fundamental in the pathogenesis of sleep apnea. This notion was supported by studies showing that tracheostomy can reverse the clinical manifestations of sleep apnea.[26] Patients with obstructive sleep apnea have decreased maximal pharyngeal area and greater airway pressure compared to healthy individuals. It was, therefore, proposed that sleep apnea might be caused by upper airway resistance; patients with upper airway resistance have inspiratory flow limitation.[27] Sleep apnea could also be caused by recurrent pharyngeal occlusion, causing partial or complete cessation of airflow. It is known that during sleep upper airway neuromuscular activity diminishes, but reduced neuromuscular activity tends to be more pronounced among patients with obstructive sleep apnea. The reduction in ventilatory effort is the most notable initial event cascading into upper airway obstruction.

Most sleep apnea patients have upper airway obstruction, either in the nasopharynx or the oropharynx.[28] Evidence suggests that both anatomic and physiologic factors combine to cause pharyngeal collapse.[29] Anatomic factors predisposing the upper airway to collapse include enlarged tonsils, macroglossia, micrognathia, retrognathia, and adenotonsillar hypertrophy. It should be noted that only a handful of patients have narrow upper airway due to those anatomic predispositions. Most patients have narrowed airways because of enlarged pharyngeal tissues resulting from obesity. More specifically, increased fat deposits produce enlarged soft palate and uvula. Other factors involved in airway obstruction include a large tongue, vascular congestion, and pulse edema of the pharyngeal mucosa.[30,31] Edema of the pharyngeal wall associated with central venous pressure elevation can produce luminal narrowing and predispose at-risk individuals to airway collapse.

During periods of wakefulness, individuals counteract the effects of upper airway narrowing by compensatory increase in the activity of upper airway dilator muscles. However, efforts to compensate for this narrowing among patients with sleep apnea are virtually ineffective during sleep. Failure to provide compensatory responses leads to imbalance between rival forces promoting collapse of the pharynx and those maintaining upper airway patency.[3,28] The end product of this imbalance is upper airway closure, and the ensuing decrease in ventilation causes hypoxia and hypercapnia. This sets in motion a cascade of events beginning with increased ventilatory efforts leading to labored breathing, which often disturbs the bed partner. Subsequently, afflicted individuals experience cortical arousals and/or abrupt awakenings as they endeavor to breathe. On awakening, the upper airway dilator muscles are reactivated, and airway patency and ventilation are restored. With adequate ventilation, individuals can return to sleep. Unfortunately, in cases of severe sleep apnea this cycle can repeat itself hundreds of times.

DIAGNOSIS OF SLEEP APNEA

No single subjective rating test exists that would allow effective screening of a large number of individuals in the field for sleep apnea. No single device has been recommended that displays optimal sensitivity and specificity for detecting sleep apnea when compared to laboratory polysomnography, the "gold standard."[32] Standard of care for sleep apnea screening typically entails a detailed sleep history, which is performed by a sleep clinician in a structured setting. Whenever possible family members should be queried regarding the patient's sleep patterns, since often times the patient is unaware that he or she is experiencing disordered sleep. Patients with positive screening results are routinely referred to a sleep clinic for a comprehensive assessment of sleep apnea using laboratory polysomnographic studies. In some instances, investigators rely on home recordings or oxymetry to render a sleep apnea diagnosis. This has often complicated the ability to establish head-to-head comparison of rates and/or severity of sleep apnea in published studies.

A nocturnal polysomnographic study incorporates assessment of sleep architecture, airflow and ventilatory effort, arterial blood saturation, electrocardiogram, body position, and periodic limb movement.[33,34] Consistent with the need to arrive at an accurate diagnosis, a sleep specialist typically interprets the results of the study. Although less common, the diagnosis of central sleep apnea, which is a type of sleep-disordered breathing is rendered when a lack of airflow in the absence of ventilatory effort is observed using predetermined criteria.[33] The other type of sleep-disordered breathing, obstructive sleep apnea, is by all account more prevalent and is characterized by closure of the upper airway, causing cessation of airflow despite persistent ventilatory effort.

TREATMENT OF SLEEP APNEA

The most effective, noninvasive treatment for sleep apnea requires the use of continuous positive airway pressure (CPAP). This therapy requires the patient to wear a sealed mask over the nose, or in certain cases both the nose and mouth while sleeping. The patient receives forced room air via the mask (that has been fitted by a technician), increasing the pressure in the oropharyngeal airway, which helps to maintain airway patency. Oral-dental devices may also be used in mild cases or for patients requiring treatment for primary snoring. These are intended to reposition the mandible, thereby maximizing the diameter of the oropharyngeal airway. Yet, in other cases surgical procedures (e.g., uvulopalatopharyngoplasty [UPPP] and laser-assisted uvulopalatoplasty [LAUP]) remain a viable option, albeit the least desired treatment because of their invasiveness and complexity.

The use of CPAP as a therapeutic modality for obstructive sleep apnea is often coupled with some form of behavior modification.[35,36] Thus, the objectives of treatment are to eradicate not only physiologic abnormalities including sleep fragmentation, apneic episodes, and oxygen desaturations but also symptoms such as snoring and daytime sleepiness and to reduce risks for comorbid conditions. Ultimately, weight loss interventions, aiming to reduce total body weight by 7–10%, seems to be the most effective lifestyle modification encouraged by sleep clinicians. Although it is often difficult for patients with sleep apnea to initiate or maintain a weight management program, even modest weight loss may yield significant reduction in symptom severity.[37] This constitutes the standard of care, according to published practice parameters established by the American Academy of Sleep Medicine.[38] In severe cases of sleep apnea, especially in those patients with significant episodes of brady- or tachyarrhythmias gastric bypass surgery should be considered.

SLEEP APNEA: ASSOCIATIONS WITH CARDIOVASCULAR DISEASES

Sleep apnea is thought to be as prevalent as adult diabetes and might affect more than 12 million Americans, according to reports from the National Institutes of Health.[39] Public health advocates view it as big a public health hazard as smoking.[40,41] The National Commission on Sleep Disorders Research estimated that sleep apnea is probably responsible for 38,000 cardiovascular deaths yearly, with an associated 42 million dollars spent on related hospitalizations.[42]

An important review of 54 epidemiologic studies highlights the negative impacts of sleep apnea. Accordingly, sleep apnea is associated with hypertension (18 studies), cardiac arrhythmias (8 studies), coronary heart disease and left ventricular failure (6 studies), pulmonary hypertension (6 studies), stroke (3 studies), road traffic accidents (7 studies), and mortality (6 studies).[43] Furthermore, data obtained from over 6000 middle-aged adults in the Sleep Heart Health Study, a National Heart, Lung, and Blood Institute (NHLBI)-sponsored project, indicate that sleep apnea increases the risk of heart failure by 140%; the risk of stroke is increased by 60% and the risk of coronary heart disease 30%. Patients with severe sleep apnea may have a two- to fourfold greater odds for complex arrhythmias.[44]

Clinical and Epidemiologic Evidence

About three decades ago, two research groups began to study the relationships between sleep apnea and cardiovascular diseases. These studies were largely observational, but results were very impressive. In both laboratories, investigators performed tracheostomy to alleviate comorbid conditions among patients with a diagnosis of sleep apnea. Subsequent to tracheostomy, Coccagna et al. observed complete disappearance of a severe atrial flutter and a postoperative decrease in systemic BP.[1,2] Independently, Guilleminault et al. observed normalization of BP in two hypertensive children with severe sleep apnea within 24 hours after surgery.[29] In another study, Partinen and Guilleminault demonstrated a 10% difference in mortality over a 10-year period, comparing sleep apnea patients who accepted to undergo tracheostomy with those favoring conservative treatment.[45]

A plethora of experimental and clinical studies have been conducted to establish the link of sleep apnea to cardiovascular diseases. Of note, an important study involving 400 patients with sleep apnea showed that 48% of them had cardiac arrhythmias,[46] which often accompany severe nocturnal hypoxemia.[47,48] Remarkably, through follow-up studies tracheostomy eliminated arrhythmias in a subset of those patients. It should be noted that among patients with sleep apnea who experience episodes of prolonged ventricular asystole, invasive electrophysiologic evaluation has failed to establish any anatomic abnormalities or irreversible sinus or AV nodal disease. It is currently recommended that bradyarrhythmias be treated with oxygen therapy or CPAP in patients with sleep apnea, since it is enhanced vagal tone during the hypoxemic episodes that results in bradycardia.

Importance of Confounding Factors

Several epidemiologic and clinical studies have explored the associations between sleep apnea and cardiovascular morbidity. Some of the early studies showing associations between sleep apnea and cardiovascular diseases were questioned, as some could not account for the influence of confounding factors since samples were too small. Critics pointed out that sleep apnea and cardiovascular diseases have common risk factors including age, gender, race/ethnicity, and obesity,[49] which could confound the observed associations. Studies also needed to take into account the fact that patients with sleep apnea were generally unhealthy. One analysis indicated that the 10-year risk of coronary heart disease and stroke, for instance, was approximately 30% among patients with sleep apnea.[50]

More recent large-scale epidemiologic studies have confirmed associations between these two conditions, with adequate statistical control for known confounding factors. In one of those studies, sleep apnea significantly increased the risk for stroke independently of other risk factors (i.e., age, sex, race, smoking, alcohol consumption, BMI, and the presence or absence of diabetes mellitus, dyslipidemia, atrial fibrillation, and hypertension).[15] With adequate adjustment for confounding factors, a cross-sectional study showed that patients with an AHI of 20 or greater had significantly greater odds for stroke (odds ratio, 4.33; 95% confidence interval, 1.32–14.24) relative to individuals without sleep apnea (AHI <5).[51]

The idea of independent associations of sleep apnea with cardiovascular morbidity was further supported using evidence from animal studies. Investigators have demonstrated sleep apnea can be induced in dogs by orchestrating intermittent airway occlusion.[52] This line of experiments led to the observation of sustained daytime hypertension. Other researchers have studied sleep apnea patients presenting without other known medical conditions in order to rule out the influence of confounding factors. Those studies have indicated that patients with sleep apnea were characterized by higher levels of SNS activity during wakefulness as well as during sleep, relative to healthy controls.[53,54] During apnea events, oxygen levels decreased and carbon dioxide levels increased commensurately, which activated the SNS. Higher level of SNS activity induced blood vessel constriction, with BP rising up to 250/150 mmHg. Those patients also exhibited faster heart rates during wakefulness, although heart rates are often less variable.

One of the largest epidemiologic studies conducted to date, the Sleep Heart Health Study sampling 6424 free-living individuals who underwent home polysomnography, has revealed increased risk of coronary artery disease, congestive heart failure, and stroke among patients with severe sleep apnea.[55] Some studies have shown rates of sleep apnea among patients with cardiovascular diseases approximating 51%.[56,57] Others have documented high rates of cardiovascular morbidity among patients with sleep apnea.[58] One study showed that rates of congestive heart failure among patients with sleep apnea rise up to 40%.[55,56,59] For a comprehensive review of the supporting evidence for an independent association between sleep apnea and cardiovascular morbidity, the reader is referred to Lavie et al.'s work.[60–63] We should note that these associations have been convincingly demonstrated using large cohorts in the sleep laboratory as well as in the general population.

Proposed Mechanisms Explaining Link of Sleep Apnea to Cardiovascular Diseases

The underlying mechanisms explaining the associations between sleep apnea and cardiovascular diseases are not entirely understood, although several mechanisms have been proposed. They include sustained sympathetic activation,[64,65] swings in intrathoracic pressure,[66] and oxidative stress and consequently vascular inflammation resulting from the nocturnal hypoxia and reoxygenation cycles.[60,61] With regard to the role of sympathetic activation,

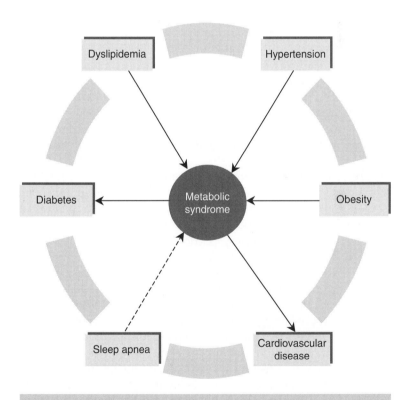

Figure 19-1 **Interrelationships between metabolic diseases comprising the metabolic syndrome and sleep apnea, which has been proposed as a component of the syndrome. Together, these diseases are referred to as the "Syndrome Z." Available epidemiologic and clinical evidence suggest that all of those conditions interact with each other through complex, yet undifferentiated pathophysiologic pathways, thereby increasing cardiovascular risks.** (Source: Ref 80)

investigators have posited that repetitive apneic/hypopneic events along with ensuing arterial desaturation and hypercapnia cause activation of the SNS. This then results in frequent increases in systolic BP that might ultimately lead to hypertension or exacerbation of this condition. Among individuals with moderate to severe sleep apnea systolic and diastolic pressure can rise up to 25% of baseline values.[67,68] Some have advanced that a similar mechanism might explain the link between sleep apnea and tachyarrhythmias, on the one hand.[69] On the other hand, bradyarrhythmias, which are more common than tachyarrhythmias occurring in 20% of patients with sleep apnea,[46–48] might be the resulting effect of an increase in vagal tone due to stimulation of receptor sites in the upper airway.[70]

Other abnormalities observed among patients with sleep apnea might also be involved in the pathogenesis of cardiovascular diseases. These include disorders in coagulation factors, endothelial damage, platelet activation, and an increase in inflammatory mediators.[71] Patients with sleep apnea have characteristically greater levels of endothelin and lower levels of nitric oxide than healthy sleepers. Thus, they often experience greater blood vessel constriction. Afflicted patients may have levels of endothelin rising up to 50%. With CPAP treatment, however, levels of endothelin and circulating nitric oxide invariably return to normal.[72] This elevated endothelin is believed to impair BP regulation as well. Oxidative stress is another factor that can trigger a cascade of events leading to atherogenesis and cardiovascular morbidity.

Recently, research interests have centered on the relative contribution of oxidative stress in explaining the associations between sleep apnea and cardiovascular morbidity.[61,73,74] These investigators have proposed that hypoxia, which is commonly observed in sleep apnea, promotes the formation of reactive oxygen species, particularly during the reoxygenation period; this is believed to be deleterious to cells and tissues. With increased production of reactive oxygen species, a consequential increase in circulating levels of adenosine and urinary uric acid is observed. Reactive oxygen species, however, regulate the activation of critical transcription factors that are redox sensitive, resulting in increased expression of genes, which encode proteins that promote adaptation to hypoxia. It has also been suggested that redox-sensitive transcription factors that elicit inflammatory pathways are also activated, thereby affecting inflammatory and immune responses by promoting activation of endothelial cells, leukocytes, and platelets.[61] Once activated, those cells express adhesion molecules and proinflammatory cytokines that may lead to endothelial injury and dysfunction; this series of events inevitably lead to the development of cardiovascular morbidity.

Observing this chain of events, these investigators surmise that atherogenesis apparently starts soon after the onset of sleep apnea. It is likely that substantial atherosclerotic insults are incurred by the time a diagnosis is rendered, since symptoms become apparent often around the age of 45 years.[61,74]

It is believed that diagnosis at this age may be too late for some patients, given that some of these insults are irreversible. Although such atherogenic damages cannot be reversed, treatment can retard their progress, if not abort them entirely. In part, this provides some explanation as to why many patients with sleep apnea present with cardiovascular morbidity in the clinic. Therefore, in order to prevent cardiovascular morbidity, sleep apnea diagnosis and treatment should be made as early as possible. Evidently, methods that can improve the likelihood of detecting the syndrome earlier are needed. In addition, behavioral strategies to help improve adherence to treatment regimens should be conceived and tested in large-scale studies before final implementation in the clinical setting.

Evidence from CPAP Studies

The link between sleep apnea and cardiovascular disease has been further demonstrated through treatment studies of sleep apnea with nasal CPAP. Those studies have shown remarkable results, which include reduced diurnal and nocturnal BP.[75,76] Among patients with heart failure and congestive heart failure, for instance, treatment of coexisting sleep apnea with CPAP reduces systolic BP and improves left ventricular systolic function.[77] CPAP therapy has been found to eliminate apneic episodes and associated hemodynamic changes occurring during sleep.[54,78] Thus, the adverse effect of sleep apnea on the heart can be halted successfully with CPAP.

The foregoing discussion offers some idea about proposed mechanisms purporting to explain how sleep apnea could cause cardiovascular diseases and the benefits of CPAP therapy. This presentation would be incomplete without considering the potential role of comorbid conditions. In the next section, we present evidence supporting the importance of metabolic syndrome in delineating the link of sleep apnea to cardiovascular morbidity.

COMPLEX RELATIONSHIPS BETWEEN SLEEP APNEA AND CARDIOVASCULAR DISEASES: ROLE OF THE METABOLIC SYNDROME

No conclusive evidence exists for a cause-and-effect relationship between sleep apnea and cardiovascular diseases, although it is believed that various physiologic factors produced by sleep apnea may play a significant role in the pathogenesis of cardiovascular diseases. Sleep apnea is widely recognized for its adverse vascular sequelae: acute myocardial infarction and/or nocturnal angina caused by arterial vasospasm.[75] The relationships between sleep apnea and cardiovascular diseases are rather complex, and several systematic studies are necessary to explicate fully the nature of those relations. These complexities are further compounded by findings suggesting that conditions comprising the metabolic syndrome might mediate effects of sleep apnea on cardiovascular diseases.

Unfortunately, a direct link between the metabolic syndrome and sleep apnea could not be established, as previous research has considered linkage analysis only for individual components of the metabolic syndrome. In the following sections, we consider the role of each component of the metabolic syndrome namely obesity, hypertension, diabetes, and dyslipidemia. First, we discuss issues pertaining to definition and prevalence of metabolic syndrome.

The Metabolic Syndrome: Definition and Prevalence

As early as 1923, Kylin, a Swedish physician, observed a cluster of co-occurring medical conditions namely hyperglycemia, hypertension, obesity, and hyperuricemia.[79] With new evidence, this cluster of metabolic diseases has been renamed numerously culminating in what is currently termed the metabolic syndrome. This has become a growing area of clinical and basic research as well as one that has provided the impetus for new and innovative clinical care. This definition, often used in the cardiovascular field, has been in widespread use beginning in the late 1970s to describe varying associations of health risk factors with diabetes. In the sleep literature, some have coined yet another term "Syndrome Z" to explain such interrelated diseases. This incorporates the typical features of "Syndrome X" namely central obesity, hypertension, diabetes, and dyslipidemia, with the addition of sleep apnea.[80]

While sleep scientists acknowledge the importance of metabolic diseases in assessing cardiovascular risks, they are also interested in understanding the circadian rhythms of BP patterns (dippers vs. nondippers). There is preliminary evidence that the temporal distribution of BP could be used to predict vascular events. Evidence shows that abnormal patterns of BP variation correlate with advanced target organ damage and poor cardiovascular prognosis.[81-83] Important work is underway to elucidate the contribution of circadian patterns of tumor necrosis factor-alpha (TNF-α) and interleukin-6 (IL-6) in BP variations among sleep apnea patients.

The metabolic syndrome is an emerging public health concern.[84] It constitutes a collection of interrelated risk factors of metabolic origin that increase chances of developing heart disease, stroke, and diabetes. It increases the risk for coronary heart disease at any low-density lipoprotein cholesterol (LDL-C) level, and it is associated with prothrombotic and proinflammatory states, two common risk factors for coronary heart disease and diabetes mellitus.[73,85-87] The metabolic syndrome is now recognized as an important contributor to the development of atherosclerosis and cardiovascular diseases. Individuals presenting with characteristics of the metabolic syndrome are at increased risks of developing type 2 diabetes,[87,88] and those with diabetes are at increased risks of developing cardiovascular diseases.[89]

Individuals with metabolic syndrome have several co-occurring disorders of the body's metabolism: obesity, hypertension, dyslipidemia, and hypercholesterolemia. The causes of this condition are rather complex, and empirical data are in the beginning stages in shedding light on these complexities. To date, the most consistent observation has been that most patients who meet criteria for metabolic syndrome are older and obese; they also tend to exhibit insulin resistance. However, it remains unclear whether obesity or insulin resistance is the cause of metabolic syndrome or a byproduct of a more extensive metabolic disorder. One theory that has been advanced postulates that insulin resistance might be the principal determinant of the metabolic syndrome.[90-92] This explains, in part, why recent research has focused on the role of insulin resistance and glucose intolerance.

According to the third National Health and Nutrition Examination Survey (1988–1994) of 8814 adults (aged ≥20 years), the age-adjusted prevalence of the metabolic syndrome was 23.7%.[93] We also note that metabolic syndrome affects 25% of overweight adult Americans, according to a 2002 report from the Centers for Disease Control (CDC). Of note, the age-adjusted prevalence was similar for men (24.0%) and women (23.4%), but African American women had approximately a 57% higher prevalence than did African American men.

Since the first observation of the first cluster of metabolic diseases, many definitions have been offered by different research groups. As the metabolic syndrome is now recognized as a worldwide health concern a more formal definition has been proposed by several organizations, including the World Health Organization (WHO), the National Cholesterol Education Program (NCEP), and the American Association of Clinical Endocrinologists. In Table 19-1, we compare criteria provided by the WHO and the NCEP. These have been set forth to allow consensus agreement in recognizing the components of the metabolic syndrome as well as in identifying high-risk individuals.[85,90,94] It should be noted that other criteria have been proposed by the American Heart Association (AHA)/NHLBI and the European Group for Study of Insulin Resistance (see AHA/NHLBI Scientific Statement).[95] In sum, they all share similar definitional criteria, although they differ somewhat regarding etiology of the metabolic syndrome and degree of importance assigned to each of its components.

Sleep Apnea and Cardiovascular Diseases: Role of Obesity

According to the National Institutes of Health/National Institutes of Diabetes & Digestive & Kidney Diseases (NIDDK), approximately two-thirds of American adults are either overweight (BMI >25; 33%) or obese (BMI >30; 31%). These findings are consistent with CDCs data from the National Health and Nutrition Examination Survey, suggesting that 20.9% of Americans are obese. African Americans are at greater risks because they are disproportionately more obese compared to Whites (see Table 19-2).

Table 19-1 **WHO and NCEP ATP III Definition of the Metabolic Syndrome***

Characteristic	WHO	NCEP ATP III
Hypertension	Current antihypertensive therapy and/or BP >140/90	BP medication or BP >130/85
Dyslipidemia	Plasma triglycerides >1.7 mmol/L (150 mg/dL) and/or HDL <0.9 mmol/L (35 mg/dL) in men and <1.0 mmol/L (<40 mg/dL) in women	Plasma triglycerides >150 mg/dL, HDL-C <40 mg/dL in men and <50 mg/dL in women
Obesity	BMI >30 and/or waist/hip ratio >0.90 in men and >0.85 in women	Waist circumference >40 cm in men and >50 cm in women
Diabetes	Type 2 diabetes or IGT	Fasting blood sugar >110 mg/dL
Other	Microalbuminuria = overnight urinary albumin excretion rate >20 μg/min (30 mg/g Cr)	
Requirements for diagnosis	Type 2 diabetes or IGT and any two of the above criteria. If normal glucose tolerance is found, three other disorders must be present	Any three of the above disorders

*Information in the table was obtained from guidelines provided by the WHO and the NCEP.

Table 19-2 **Trends in Obesity by Race/Ethnicity***

Race/Ethnicity	1991	1995	1998	1999	2000	2001
African American	19.3	22.6	26.9	27.3	29.3	31.1
White	11.3	14.5	16.6	17.7	18.5	19.6

*Data obtained from CDC; values represent percent of cases.

The age-adjusted prevalence of overweight/obesity in racial/ethnic minorities, especially minority women, is higher than in Whites in the United States, reaching a critical level of greater than two-thirds of the female minority population.[96,97]

It has long been recognized that obesity plays a pivotal role in the development of sleep apnea. Indeed, research has shown that it constitutes the most significant predictor of sleep apnea.[98,99] A recent study of obese men (BMI $\geq$ 30 kg/m^2) without major medical illnesses indicated that 60% of them met criteria for sleep-disordered breathing and 27% had obstructive sleep apnea.[100] It is estimated that 60–90% of patients with sleep apnea are obese (defined as BMI >28 kg/m^2), and that a BMI of 28 kg/m^2 has a sensitivity of 93% and a specificity of 74% for sleep apnea.[99] The risk of having moderate to severe sleep apnea over a 4-year period increases sixfold among persons gaining 10% excess weight.[101] Thus, it has been assumed that the high incidence of cardiovascular morbidity among patients with sleep apnea is explained by the presence of obesity.[102,103]

Most of the initial reports wrestled with the idea that associations of sleep apnea with cardiovascular morbidity were confounded by underlying obesity. Since both sleep apnea and cardiovascular morbidity are linked to obesity, some investigators have conjectured a viable hypothesis, which suggested that both conditions are caused by a defect in a common pathway potentially resulting from central (visceral) obesity. Plausibly, with the onset of sleep apnea individuals develop leptin resistance, which in turn contributes to further weight gain. Leptin is an adipocyte-derived hormone that regulates weight by controlling appetite and energy expenditure. We should also consider that inflammatory cytokines TNF-α and IL-6, which are associated with daytime sleepiness, might also be involved in the causal pathway as they are elevated among obese patients with sleep apnea.[104] Hence, confronted with new empirical evidence the debate has recently evolved, and currently the comorbid relationship of sleep apnea to cardiovascular diseases is seen as manifestations of the metabolic syndrome.

Sleep Apnea and Cardiovascular Diseases: Role of Hypertension

One of the complexities permeating relations between sleep apnea and cardiovascular diseases relates to the fact that both conditions are potentially characterized by similar pathogenetic mechanisms.[105] Both sleep apnea and cardiovascular diseases are linked to hypertension.[13,106–108] Results of several multivariate analytical models have indicated that sleep apnea represents an independent risk factor for hypertension,[13,62,109] and hypertension constitutes a significant predictor of cardiopulmonary deaths among patients with sleep apnea.[62]

Regarding the link between sleep apnea and hypertension, there are data suggesting that approximately 40% of patients with sleep apnea suffer from hypertension, whereas 30% of hypertensive patients have occult sleep apnea.[106]

Data from the Wisconsin Sleep Cohort Study, sampling 1060 women and men aged 30–60 years, showed that at a BMI of 30 kg/m^2 and an AHI of 15 was associated with BP increases of 3.6 mmHg for systolic (95% confidence interval, 1.3–6.0) and 1.8 mmHg for diastolic (95% confidence interval, 0.3–3.3). Further analyses indicated a dose-response relationship between sleep apnea and BP, independent of confounding factors.[13]

Data from the same study exploring the relationship between sleep apnea and hypertension indicated that the severity of sleep apnea based on initial sleep studies could predict the development of new hypertension during the subsequent 4 years. Even with control for known confounders, analyses suggested the odds ratios for the presence of hypertension at follow-up were 1.42 (95% confidence interval, 1.13–1.78) with an AHI of 0.1–4.9 at base line relative to none, 2.03 (95% confidence interval, 1.29–3.17) with an AHI of 5.0–14.9, and 2.89 (95% confidence interval, 1.46–5.64) with an AHI of 15.0 or more.[101,110] These data are consistent with findings of the Sleep Heart Health Study, a community-based multicenter study involving 6132 patients.[111] Investigators found that mean systolic and diastolic BP and prevalence of hypertension increased significantly with increasing severity of sleep apnea. Sleep apnea severity constitutes an independent risk factor for hypertension. Notably, this observation held even at relatively low AHI levels (AHI = 10). Furthermore, clinical evidence suggests that treatment of sleep apnea results in a diminution of daytime systemic BP,[107] although it has not been conclusively demonstrated that CPAP treatment lowers BP on a long-term basis.

The link between hypertension and sleep apnea has been convincingly demonstrated, and the fact that these two conditions are more prevalent among African Americans renders this population at increased risks for mortality.[20,63,112] Results of several multivariate analytical models have indicated that sleep apnea represents an independent risk factor for hypertension in Caucasians and African Americans.[13,62,109] Although the pathophysiologic mechanisms involved in the expression of hypertension among patients with sleep apnea have yet to be fully elucidated, there are suggestions that autonomic mechanisms are involved.[113–115] We also note that emerging evidence demonstrates that the link between these two conditions might be independent of other known comorbidities,[13,62,109] but family history might play a role.

Previous studies have shown that BP level is significantly higher among normotensive individuals with a family history of hypertension compared to those without a positive history.[116–120] Similarly, these individuals are characterized by a greater BMI.[116,120] These findings led to the hypothesis that a family history of hypertension might have a similar influence on sleep apnea. To test this hypothesis, we performed a study including 162 African American patients that were referred to a sleep clinic in Brooklyn, NY for a nocturnal polysomnographic sleep study.[121] Results of that study indicated that hypertensive African American patients reporting a family history of hypertension did not have significantly greater rate of sleep apnea, relative to those with no family history, although trends favored greater rates for the former. However, hypertensives with a positive family history exhibited a significantly greater number of oxygen desaturations and apnea hypopnea indices than their counterparts. As expected, hypertensive patients showed worse oxygenation and respiratory characteristics than did normotensive patients, but those characteristics were demonstrably worse among hypertensive patients with a positive family history.

Sleep Apnea and Cardiovascular Diseases: Role of Diabetes

The obesity pandemic over the last decade has accompanied a rise in the prevalence of type 2 diabetes mellitus, which begins with impaired glucose tolerance (IGT) affecting 11–15.6% of the U.S. population.[122] According to data from the Third National Health and Nutrition Examination Survey, 5.1% of the U.S. adults have an existing diagnosis for diabetes; an additional 2.7% met criteria for the diagnosis, but have yet to receive one.[122] Analysis from the same research group indicated that 15.6% of adult Americans exhibit glucose intolerance (140 mg/dL) and 6.9% showed impaired fasting glucose levels ($\geq$110 mg/dL).[122]

On a parallel tract, there is a growing body of evidence suggesting that sleep apnea is involved in the pathogenesis of altered glucose metabolism. A number of epidemiologic and experimental studies have shown that patients with sleep apnea have increased glucose levels and increased insulin resistance,[100,123–125] which might predispose afflicted individuals to developing type 2 diabetes mellitus. Cross-sectional data suggest that associations of sleep apnea with greater glucose levels and increased insulin resistance might be independent of the presence of obesity.[100,104,123,126] It is known that both obese and nonobese patients with sleep apnea are insulin resistant, whereas not all apnea patients are obese. More specifically, investigators have proposed the following likely scenario. Sleep apnea causes an increase in sympathetic activity,[78,127] and increased sympathetic activity impairs glucose homeostasis by enhancing glycogen breakdown and gluconeogenesis.[128] Hence, recurrent hypoxemia along with abnormal sympathetic activity, commonly observed among patients with sleep apnea, might mediate the relationships between insulin resistance and sleep apnea (see Fig. 19-2).

Data from the Sleep Heart Health Study, which enrolled 2000 patients, indicated that the prevalence of diabetic 2-hour glucose tolerance values increased from 9.3% among patients with an AHI <5 to 15% among those with an AHI >15.[124] The odds ratio for having an abnormal glucose tolerance was 1.44 among patients with an AHI $\geq$15. Results of that study also indicated that insulin resistance was also greatest among the latter group. This study provided evidence that apnea-induced hypoxemia is associated with glucose intolerance and insulin resistance.[124] Moreover, data from the Nurse's Health Study suggest that curtailed sleep duration resulting from

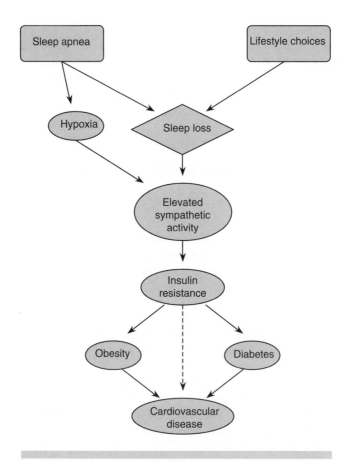

Figure 19-2 **Proposed pathway linking sleep loss to insulin resistance and cardiovascular disease. Of note, in most cases obesity triggers the onset of sleep apnea.**

sleep fragmentation induced by sleep apnea may also lead to the development or exacerbation of type 2 diabetes mellitus.[129,130] This is corroborated by analysis of data from the Sleep Heart Health Study.[131] Compared with individuals sleeping 7–8 hours per night, individuals sleeping ≤5 hours or <6 hours per night had adjusted odds ratios for diabetes of 2.51 (95% confidence interval, 1.57–4.02) and 1.66 (95% confidence interval, 1.15–2.39), respectively. On balance, there are data suggesting that the associations between sleep apnea and diabetes might be mediated through obesity, a common risk factor,[132] although the prevalence of periodic breathing itself remained significantly higher among diabetic individuals, even after control for covariates. Thus, more definitive explanation of these relations awaits further empirical studies.

Given the potential effects of reduced sleep on glucose metabolism, one wonders about the overall, long-term health impact of curtailed sleep time on American adults. Converging data indicate that the U.S. population has been sleeping less and less.[133–135] Interestingly, although sleep duration is a strong predictor of morbidity and mortality, among American adults we found that the quality of one's well-being hinged on the quality, rather than on the quantity of one's sleep.[136] Based on the most recent report by investigators from the University of California, San Diego who studied over 1 million men and women aged 30–102 years, the greatest longevity was observed among individuals sleeping 7 hours per night. Those who slept 8 hours or more experienced significantly increased mortality risks, as did participants who reported sleeping 6 hours or less. The increased risk of mortality exceeded 15% for individuals who reportedly slept >8.5 hours or <3.5 or 4.5 hours.[137,138] It would be interesting to examine whether excess mortality was associated with IGT/insulin resistance or type 2 diabetes mellitus in that study. Controlled studies seem necessary to answer the question as to the correct sleep time for optimal survival.

If in fact it can be demonstrated that there is an independent association of sleep apnea to impaired glucose metabolism, this might offer another mechanism to explain increased cardiovascular morbidity. Evidently, this will require better delineation of the contribution of cytokines and leptin. In support of such hypotheses, investigators have pointed out that CPAP studies produced significant improvement in insulin sensitivity and left ventricular function with a corresponding decrease in BP.[125,139] CPAP therapy can also normalize leptin levels, thereby reducing central obesity. It should be noted, however, that some studies have not shown significant improvement in metabolic disorders subsequent to CPAP treatment, but those clinical studies had several limitations. These include limited treatment compliance, inadequate duration of treatment, and some may have been underpowered to detect statistical effects. In light of such evidence, therapeutic approaches might integrate methods to increase sleep time both via reduction of sleep apnea severity as well as through lifestyle modifications. Synergistically, these would confer significant benefits in the management of cardiovascular complications, resulting from uncontrolled diabetes and/or untreated sleep apnea.

Sleep Apnea and Cardiovascular Diseases: Role of Dyslipidemia

Dyslipidemia is yet another condition characterizing the metabolic syndrome. It is primarily a disorder of lipoprotein metabolism, usually caused by excessively high cholesterol levels. It is a known risk factor in the development of coronary artery disease,[140] and is highly prevalent among hypertensive adults. Data from the Multi-Ethnic Study of Atherosclerosis, a multicenter study of 6814 persons aged 45–84 years, indicated that 29.3% met criteria for dyslipidemia.[141] In that study, the prevalence of dyslipidemia was similar among ethnic groups, although a disproportionate number of

African Americans and Hispanics, relative to Whites, did not receive treatment to control their dyslipidemia.[141] These findings were inconsistent with data obtained from the Genetic Obesity Associations (GENOA) study, indicating that the prevalence of dyslipidemia was significantly greater among Whites than among African Americans. Among women, rates were 64.7 and 49.5%; $P < 0.001$, respectively; whereas for men, rates were 78.4 and 56.7%; $P < 0.001$, respectively.[142] Patterns of treatment were nonetheless similar, favoring better treatment for Whites.

Both factors involved in developing dyslipidemia (i.e., high triglyceride levels and low high-density lipoprotein [HDL]) are affected by obesity, a common predictor of sleep apnea and cardiovascular morbidity. With increased adiposity, a commensurate increase in triglyceride levels is observed, whereas HDL levels decrease.[103,143,144] Given that most of the available evidence comes from cross-sectional data, it remains a daunting task to establish directional causality. In that regard, it cannot be said that dyslipidemia causes sleep apnea or that sleep apnea causes dyslipidemia, although the two conditions tend to aggregate among patients with increased adiposity. It would certainly help to view these associations in the context of data pointing to a direct correlation between lipid profile and cortical arousals, as often observed among patients with sleep apnea. Patients with sleep apnea exhibit greater HDL dysfunction and oxidized LDL levels compared to matched control persons.[145] Of note, AHI explained 30% of the variance in HDL dysfunction in sleep apnea.

Moreover, clinical evidence indicates that patients with abnormal serum lipid/lipoprotein levels improved significantly with CPAP or bilevel positive airway pressure (BiPAP) therapy.[146] In that follow-up (6 months) study of 127 patients, investigators observed that the mean HDL-C serum level increased significantly by 5.8%. Such therapeutic interventions are consistent with the Third Report of the Expert Panel on Detection, Evaluation, and Treatment of High Blood Cholesterol in Adults (ATP III).[147] Accordingly, reduction of dyslipidemia is a potential secondary target of risk-reduction therapy, which could improve management of the metabolic syndrome.

CONCLUSION

The aforementioned associations do not seem to be fortuitous, judging from the consistency across studies. The epidemiologic and clinical evidence summarized in this chapter constitutes a growing body of literature demonstrating relationships between sleep apnea and diverse systemic abnormalities. The epidemiologic evidence is abundant, but data explaining causal pathways are lacking. It may be that the associations noted among those metabolic disorders point to a maladaptive autonomic response of chemoreceptors, reacting to hypoxia, hypercapnia, and acidosis commonly found in sleep apnea.[148] Activation of the SNS through hypoxia and hypercapnia triggers an inflammatory response cascading in several downstream consequences including hypertension, diabetes, and dyslipedemia.[64] It seems prudent, therefore, that patients with a suspicion of sleep apnea and meeting criteria for metabolic syndrome be properly screened. A detailed sleep evaluation should be performed for individuals with positive screening results and CPAP therapy should be considered in the management of individuals with sleep apnea to help reduce associated cardiovascular risks.

Clinical trials involving the use of CPAP/BiPAP therapy have delineated its positive benefits (see Fig. 19-3). This therapeutic modality is very effective in improving left ventricular ejection fraction and quality of life, lowers BP

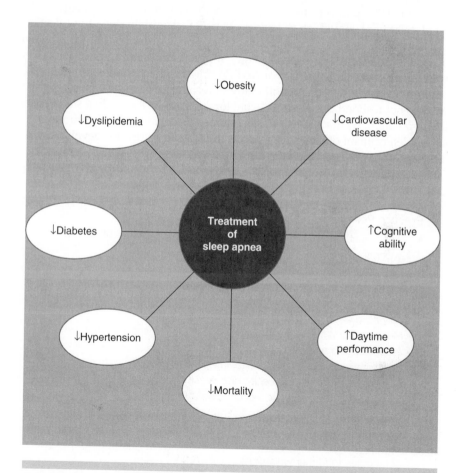

Figure 19-3 **Benefits of sleep apnea treatment, which may include CPAP/BiPAP therapy (sometimes used in combination with behavior modification), use of oral-dental devices, or surgical procedures (e.g., UPPP and LAUP).**

and sympathetic activity, and reduces mortality among patients with congestive heart failure.[76,149] Among patients with coronary artery disease, CPAP treatment significantly reduces risks of cardiovascular death, acute coronary syndrome, and hospitalization for heart failure.[150] Utilization of CPAP lowers BP and improved mood of patients with a dual diagnosis of sleep apnea and stroke.[151] Moreover, CPAP therapy has significant effects on lipid levels.[146] CPAP studies show significant improvement in insulin sensitivity and left ventricular function with a corresponding decrease in BP.[139]

The Third Report of the Expert Panel on Detection, Evaluation, and Treatment of High Blood Cholesterol in Adults (ATP III) identifies the metabolic syndrome as a potential secondary target of risk-reduction therapy.[147] It is recommended that patients meeting criteria for the syndrome receive adequate, tailored treatment aimed at reducing obesity through lifestyle modifications including increased physical activity and improved dietary habits. Indeed, evidence from randomized controlled trials suggests that weight loss among overweight and obese individuals reduces BP, improves lipid profiles, and improves blood glucose levels. Pharmacotherapy is recommended only for individuals who do not respond positively to behavioral therapies. As gradual sleep loss in the population, be it a sequela of sleep apnea or behaviorally determined, is a strong determinant of insulin resistance, individuals at risk for developing cardiovascular diseases should be encouraged to sleep efficiently.

Practice Points

- Sleep apnea is associated with diabetes independently of obesity and hypertension.
- Treatment of sleep apnea improves diabetes.
- Sleep apnea is associated with insulin resistance independently of obesity.
- Sleep apnea contributes to stroke, as over 80% of stroke victims reportedly have sleep apnea.
- Sleep apnea is more prevalent among African Americans; young African Americans are at increased risks.
- Sleep apnea should be a key factor in the fight to reduce health disparities in cardiovascular diseases, obesity, diabetes, hypertension, and dyslipidemia.
- Sleep apnea contributes to visceral obesity by increasing nocturnal cortisol and insulin that promote visceral adiposity, metabolic abnormalities, and cardiovascular dysfunction.
- Individuals with sleep apnea develop leptin resistance, which in turn contributes to further weight gain.
- Assessment of sleep apnea is recommended for patients with hypertension, diabetes, obesity, and dyslipidemia.
- Assessment of sleep apnea is recommended for patients with congestive heart failure, acute coronary syndrome, cardiac arrhythmias, and stroke.

FUTURE DIRECTIONS AND CLINICAL IMPLICATIONS

The epidemiologic and clinical studies summarized in this chapter have no doubt provided the framework for future research in the underpinnings of the metabolic syndrome and related morbidities. It would appear that available data have raised many important issues that require empirical testing, although initial questions regarding relationships between sleep apnea and cardiovascular morbidity or between sleep apnea and metabolic syndrome have been addressed to some extent. Whether the metabolic syndrome represents a mediating factor in the link of sleep apnea to cardiovascular diseases remains to be determined. Alternatively, the metabolic syndrome itself might potentiate the effects of sleep apnea on cardiovascular diseases.

Available data have not yielded evidence to support which factor is the root cause of the co-occurrence of those interrelated metabolic conditions, but insulin resistance and obesity have been offered as potential candidates. This gives rise to the need for empirical studies testing causal models to explain links among sleep apnea, cardiovascular morbidity, and metabolic syndrome. One could imagine the difficulties inherent in performing experimental tests of cause-and-effect relationships of those factors. Such linkage analyses could benefit from the application of path analysis, which would require large-scale recruitment. Such analyses should be considered in future studies.

Future research is necessary to rank individuals with regards to their risk of sudden cardiac death and target them for educational and medical intervention. Research is also needed to establish noninvasive markers with adequate sensitivity and specificity in predicting which patients are at greater risk. For example, patients with sleep apnea showing depressed left ventricular function should be considered at greater risk from ventricular arrhythmias and other cardiovascular events. Identification and treatment of patients with overlapping syndromes (e.g., congestive heart failure and chronic obstructive pulmonary disease [COPD] with sleep apnea) is paramount in the fight to reduce cardiovascular morbidity.

While we wait for answers to those important questions, many interventions can be envisaged to improve the management of existing metabolic disorders. First, as sleep apnea is highly prevalent among patients with diabetes, hypertension, and dyslipidemia, it seems prudent that a sleep apnea screening questionnaire be administered to those at-risk patients. Likewise, such questionnaires should be given to patients with increased adiposity in the neck area and/or who present with abdominal (visceral) obesity. Second, patients meeting criteria for sleep apnea should be referred to a sleep clinic for a detailed laboratory study. Third, tailored behavioral interventions should be developed to ensure adherence to CPAP/BiPAP treatment recommendation. Four, weight management programs should be designed to assist patients in their effort to reduce their body weight, as weight reduction helps diminish the severity of sleep apnea, thereby improving overall health, daytime performance, cognitive ability, and quality of well-being.

Brief Sleep Apnea Screening Questionnaire

Do you snore on a regular basis?
Do you ever wake up suddenly, gasping or choking for air?
Do you experience excessive sleepiness during the day?
Do you experience headaches, sore throat, or dry mouth in the morning
  after waking up?
Do you have difficulty remembering things or concentrating on routine tasks?

It is evident that the recent rise in metabolic disorders comprising the metabolic syndrome affects persons of differing age groups, of both gender, and across geographic regions. However, public health advocates have been particularly concerned about individuals living in at-risk, underserved communities that are traditionally underrepresented in the health care industry. In the African American community, for instance, cardiovascular risk factors enumerated in this chapter are disproportionately higher. In the public health literature, many have argued in favor of greater access to health care, reasoning that with greater access there will be a commensurate decline in morbidity and mortality. There are data indicating that even when African Americans have adequate insurance coverage they are not as likely as their White counterparts to utilize available services.[152] This suggests that community physicians have to develop novel strategies to encourage participation in health care practices.

In the extant literature, there is ample evidence demonstrating minority disparities. However, there is little research on intervention to reduce such disparities. There is an emerging consensus that health care practices must take into account patients' attitudes and belief systems as well as their ethnic origin and degrees of acculturation. Preliminary results of a collaborative study at Long Island University have indicated that patients with breast cancer often rely on their spiritual leaders and/or religious leaders to make important health decisions.[153] Often, these individuals are more influential than primary care physicians in affecting health care decision-making processes. Using a tailored behavioral education program, we have observed that when such factors are incorporated in intervention strategies to help minority women with breast cancer and when adequate care is dispensed by culturally competent health professionals, adherence to health care practices increases substantially (unpublished data).

It is of interest to determine the efficacy of similar intervention programs geared toward helping patients with metabolic risk factors for cardiovascular diseases. Consistent with the evidence presented in this chapter, it is hoped that sleep apnea will be included in the list of metabolic disorders disproportionately affecting African Americans. The recognition of sleep apnea as a minority health disparity issue would provide the impetus for more clinical studies aiming at attenuating cardiovascular morbidity among African Americans via a reduction in the incidence of sleep apnea.

REFERENCES

1. Coccagna G, Mantovani M, Brignani F, et al. Tracheostomy in hypersomnia with periodic breathing. *Bull Physiopathol Respir (Nancy)* 1972;8:1217–1227.

2. Coccagna G, Mantovani M, Brignani F, et al. Continuous recording of the pulmonary and systemic arterial pressure during sleep in syndromes of hypersomnia with periodic breathing. *Bull Physiopathol Respir (Nancy)* 1972;8:1159–1172.

3. Hedner J, Ejnell H, Sellgren J, et al. Is high and fluctuating muscle nerve sympathetic activity in the sleep apnoea syndrome of pathogenetic importance for the development of hypertension? *J Hypertens Suppl* 1988;6:S529–S531.

4. Narkiewicz K, Montano N, Cogliati C, et al. Altered cardiovascular variability in obstructive sleep apnea. *Circulation* 1998;98:1071–1077.

5. Findley LJ, Weiss JW, Jabour ER. Drivers with untreated sleep apnea. A cause of death and serious injury. *Arch Intern Med* 1991;151:1451–1452.

6. Stoohs RA, Guilleminault C, Itoi A, et al. Traffic accidents in commercial long-haul truck drivers: the influence of sleep-disordered breathing and obesity. *Sleep* 1994;17:619–623.

7. El Ad B, Lavie P. Effect of sleep apnea on cognition and mood. *Int Rev Psychiatry* 2005;17:277–282.

8. Sharafkhaneh A, Giray N, Richardson P, et al. Association of psychiatric disorders and sleep apnea in a large cohort. *Sleep* 2005;28:1405–1411.

9. Rosen RC, Zozula R, Jahn EG, et al. Low rates of recognition of sleep disorders in primary care: comparison of a community-based versus clinical academic setting. *Sleep Med* 2001;2:47–55.

10. The National Commission on Sleep Disorders Research. Available at: http://www.stanford.edu/~dement/overview-ncsdr.html (Accessed on 8-20-02, 2002).

11. Young T, Finn L. Epidemiological insights into the public health burden of sleep disordered breathing: sex differences in survival among sleep clinic patients. *Thorax* 1988;53(Suppl 3):S16–S19.

12. Young T, Peppard P. Sleep-disordered breathing and cardiovascular disease: epidemiologic evidence for a relationship. *Sleep* 2000;23(Suppl 4):S122–S126.

13. Young T, Peppard P, Palta M, et al. Population-based study of sleep-disordered breathing as a risk factor for hypertension. *Arch Intern Med* 1997;157:1746–1752.

14. Young T, Palta M, Dempsey J, et al. The occurrence of sleep-disordered breathing among middle-aged adults [see comments]. *N Engl J Med* 1993;328:1230–1235.

15. Yaggi HK, Concato J, Kernan WN, et al. Obstructive sleep apnea as a risk factor for stroke and death. *N Engl J Med* 2005;353:2034–2041.

16. Brunetti L, Rana S, Lospalluti ML, et al. Prevalence of obstructive sleep apnea syndrome in a cohort of 1,207 children of southern Italy. *Chest* 2001;120:1930–1935.

17. Schechter MS. Technical report: diagnosis and management of childhood obstructive sleep apnea syndrome. *Pediatrics* 2002;109:e69.

18. Ancoli-Israel S, Kripke DF, Klauber MR, et al. Sleep-disordered breathing in community-dwelling elderly. *Sleep* 1991;14:496–500.

19. Gottlieb DJ, Whitney CW, Bonekat WH, et al. Relation of sleepiness to respiratory disturbance index: the Sleep Heart Health Study. *Am J Respir Crit Care Med* 1999;159:502–507.

20. Silverberg DS, Oksenberg A, Iaina A. Sleep-related breathing disorders as a major cause of essential hypertension: fact or fiction? *Curr Opin Nephrol Hypertens* 1998;7:353–357.

21. Meetze K, Gillespie MB, Lee FS. Obstructive sleep apnea: a comparison of black and white subjects. *Laryngoscope* 2002;112:1271–1274.

22. Redline S, Tishler P, Hans M, et al. Racial differences in sleep-disordered breathing in African-Americans and Caucasians. *Am J Respir Crit Care Med* 1997;155: 186–192.

23. Kripke DF, Ancoli-Israel S, Klauber MR, et al. Prevalence of sleep disordered breathing in ages 40–64 years: a population-based survey. *Sleep* 1997;20:65–76.

24. Ancoli-Israel S, Klauber MR, Stepnowsky C, et al. Sleep-disordered breathing in African-American elderly. *J Gerontol* 1989;44:M18–M21.

25. Buxbaum SG, Elston RC, Tishler PV, et al. Genetics of the apnea hypopnea index in Caucasians and African Americans: I. Segregation analysis. *Genet Epidemiol* 2002;22:243–253.

26. Jung R. Physiology and pathophysiology of sleep. *Med Welt* 1965;24:1358–1359.

27. Badr MS, Kawak A, Skatrud JB, et al. Effect of induced hypocapnic hypopnea on upper airway patency in humans during NREM sleep. *Respir Physiol* 1997;110: 33–45.

28. Remmers JE, Launois S, Feroah T, et al. Mechanics of the pharynx in patients with obstructive sleep apnea. *Prog Clin Biol Res* 1990;345:261–268.

29. Guilleminault C, Tilkian A, Dement WC. The sleep apnea syndromes. *Annu Rev Med* 1976;27:465–484.

30. Chaban R, Cole P, Hoffstein V. Site of upper airway obstruction in patients with idiopathic obstructive sleep apnea. *Laryngoscope* 1988;98:641–647.

31. Smith PL, Gold AR, Meyers DA, et al. Weight loss in mildly to moderately obese patients with obstructive sleep apnea. *Ann Intern Med* 1985;103:850–855.

32. Rechtshaffen A, Kales A. *A Manual of Standardized Terminology, Techniques, and Scoring Systems of Sleep Stages of Human Subjects.* Los Angeles: UCLA Brain Information Service/Brain Research Institute, 1968:10.

33. Kryger M, Roth T, Dement W, (eds., *Principles and Practice of Sleep Medicine.* New York: W.B. Saunders, 2002:1–1336.

34. Chesson AL Jr, Ferber RA, Fry JM, et al. The indications for polysomnography and related procedures. *Sleep* 1997;20:423–487.

35. Edinger JD, Hoelscher TJ, Marsh GR, et al. A cognitive-behavioral therapy for sleep-maintenance insomnia in older adults. *Psychol Aging* 1992;7:282–289.

36. Edinger JD, Carwile S, Miller P, et al. Psychological status, syndromatic measures, and compliance with nasal CPAP therapy for sleep apnea. *Percept Mot Skills* 1994;78:1116–1118.

37. Strobel RJ, Rosen RC. Obesity and weight loss in obstructive sleep apnea: a critical review. *Sleep* 1996;19:104–115.

38. The American Academy of Sleep Medicine (Practice Parameters). Available at: http://www.aasmnet.org/practiceparameters.htm (Accessed 8-24-02, 2002).

39. The National Heart Lung and Blood Institute (NHLBI). Available at: http://www.nhlbi.nih.gov/resources/docs/plandisp.htm (Accessed on 8-20-02, 2002).

40. Phillipson EA. Sleep apnea: a major public health problem. *N Engl J Med* 1993;328:1271–1273.

41. Report of the Scientific Committee on Tobacco and Health. Available at: http://www.doh.gov.uk/public/scoth.htm (Accessed on 8-05-02, 2002).

42. The National Commission on Sleep Disorders Research. *Wake Up America: A National Sleep Alert*. Washington, DC: US Government Printing Office, 1993, 2002.

43. Wright J, Johns R, Watt I, et al. Health effects of obstructive sleep apnea and the effectiveness of continuous positive airways pressure: a systematic review of the research evidence. *BMJ* 1997;314:851–860.

44. Mehra R, Benjamin EJ, Shahar E, et al. Association of nocturnal arrhythmias with sleep-disordered breathing: the Sleep Heart Health Study. *Am J Respir Crit Care Med* 2006;173:910–916.

45. Partinen M, Guilleminault C. Evolution of obstructive sleep apnea syndrome. In: Partinen M, Guilleminault C, eds., *Obstructive Sleep Apnea Syndrome*. New York: Raven Press, 1990:15–23.

46. Guilleminault C, Connolly SJ, Winkle RA. Cardiac arrhythmia and conduction disturbances during sleep in 400 patients with sleep apnea syndrome. *Am J Cardiol* 1983;52:490–494.

47. Hoffstein V. Blood pressure, snoring, obesity, and nocturnal hypoxaemia. *Lancet* 1994;344:643–645.

48. Hoffstein V, Mateika S. Cardiac arrhythmias, snoring, and sleep apnea. *Chest* 1994;106:466–471.

49. Stradling J. Sleep apnea does not cause cardiovascular disease. *Am J Respir Crit Care Med* 2004;169:148–149.

50. Kiely JL, McNicholas WT, Zgierska A, et al. Cardiovascular risk factors in patients with obstructive sleep apnoea syndrome. Obstructive sleep apnea and risk factors for coronary artery disease. *Eur Respir J* 2000;16:128–133.

51. Aartz M, Young T, Finn L, et al. Association of sleep-disordered breathing and the occurence of stroke. *Am J Respir Crit Care Med* 2005;172:1447–1451.

52. Brooks D, Horner RL, Render-Teixeira CL, et al. Obstructive sleep apnea as a cause of systemic hypertension: evidence from a canine model. *J Clin Invest* 1997;99:106–109.

53. Somers VK, Gami AS, Olson LJ. Treating sleep apnea in heart failure patients: promises but still no prizes. *J Am Coll Cardiol* 2005;45:2012–2014.

54. Somers VK. Sleep: a new cardiovascular frontier. *N Engl J Med* 2005;353: 2070–2073.

55. Shahar E, Whitney CW, Redline S, et al. Sleep-disordered breathing and cardiovascular disease: cross-sectional results of the Sleep Heart Health Study. *Am J Respir Crit Care Med* 2001;163:19–25.

56. Javaheri S, Parker TJ, Liming JD, et al. Sleep apnea in 81 ambulatory male patients with stable heart failure. Types and their prevalences, consequences, and presentations. *Circulation* 1998;97:2154–2159.

57. Javaheri S, Corbett WS. Association of low PaCO2 with central sleep apnea and ventricular arrhythmias in ambulatory patients with stable heart failure. *Ann Intern Med* 1998;128:204–207.

58. Pepperell JC, Davies RJ, Stradling JR. Systemic hypertension and obstructive sleep apnoea. *Sleep Med Rev* 2002;6:157–173.

59. Sin DD, Fitzgerald F, Parker JD, et al. Risk factors for central and obstructive sleep apnea in 450 men and women with congestive heart failure. *Am J Respir Crit Care Med* 1999;160:1101–1106.

60. Lavie L, Lotan R, Hochberg I, et al. Haptoglobin polymorphism is a risk factor for cardiovascular disease in patients with obstructive sleep apnea syndrome. *Sleep* 2003;26:592–595.

61. Lavie L. Obstructive sleep apnoea syndrome: an oxidative stress disorder. *Sleep Med Rev* 2003;7:35–51.

62. Lavie P, Herer P, Hoffstein V. Obstructive sleep apnoea syndrome as a risk factor for hypertension: population study. *BMJ* 2000;320:479–482.

63. Lavie P, Herer P, Peled R, et al. Mortality in sleep apnea patients: a multivariate analysis of risk factors. *Sleep* 1995;18:149–157.

64. Fletcher EC. Cardiovascular disease associated with obstructive sleep apnea. *Monaldi Arch Chest Dis* 2003;59:254–261.

65. Fletcher EC. Sympathetic over activity in the etiology of hypertension of obstructive sleep apnea. *Sleep* 2003;26:15–19.

66. Parker JD, Brooks D, Kozar LF, et al. Acute and chronic effects of airway obstruction on canine left ventricular performance. *Am J Respir Crit Care Med* 1999;160: 1888–1896.

67. Shepard JW Jr, Garrison MW, Grither DA, et al. Relationship of ventricular ectopy to oxyhemoglobin desaturation in patients with obstructive sleep apnea. *Chest* 1985;88:335–340.

68. Shepard JW Jr, Garrison MW, Grither DA, et al. Relationship of ventricular ectopy to nocturnal oxygen desaturation in patients with chronic obstructive pulmonary disease. *Am J Med* 1985;78:28–34.

69. Gami AS, Pressman G, Caples SM. Association of atrial fibrillation and obstructive sleep apnea. *Circulation* 2004;110:364–367.

70. Zwillich C, Devlin T, White D, et al. Bradycardia during sleep apnea. Characteristics and mechanism. *J Clin Invest* 1982;69:1286–1292.

71. Dyken ME, Somers VK, Yamada T, et al. Investigating the relationship between stroke and obstructive sleep apnea. *Stroke* 1996;27:401–407.

72. Ip MS, Lam B, Chan LY, et al. Circulating nitric oxide is suppressed in obstructive sleep apnea and is reversed by nasal continuous positive airway pressure. *Am J Respir Crit Care Med* 2000;162:2166–2171.

73. Kasasbeh E, Chi DS, Krishnaswamy G. Inflammatory aspects of sleep apnea and their cardiovascular consequences. *South Med J* 2006;99:58–67.

74. Lavie L. Sleep-disordered breathing and cerebrovascular disease: a mechanistic approach. *Neurol Clin* 2005;23:1059–1075.

75. Fletcher EC. Cardiovascular effects of continuous positive airway pressure in obstructive sleep apnea. *Sleep* 2000;23(Suppl 4):S154–S157.

76. Kaneko Y, Floras JS, Usui K, et al. Cardiovascular effects of continuous positive airway pressure in patients with heart failure and obstructive sleep apnea. *N Engl J Med* 2003;348:1233–1241.

77. Malone S, Liu PP, Holloway R, et al. Obstructive sleep apnoea in patients with dilated cardiomyopathy: effects of continuous positive airway pressure. *Lancet* 1991;338:1480–1484.

78. Somers VK, Dyken ME, Clary MP, et al. Sympathetic neural mechanisms in obstructive sleep apnea. *J Clin Invest* 1995;96:1897–1904.

79. Kylin E. Studien uber das Hypertonie-Hyperglykamie-Hyperurikamiesyndrome. *Zentralblatt fur innere Medizin* 1923;44:105–127.

80. Wilcox I, McNamara SG, Collins FL, et al. Syndrome Z: the interaction of sleep apnoea, vascular risk factors and heart disease. *Thorax* 1998;53(Suppl 3):S25–S28.

81. Kario K, Shimada K, Pickering TG. Abnormal nocturnal blood pressure falls in elderly hypertension: clinical significance and determinants. *J Cardiovasc Pharmacol* 2003;41(Suppl 1):S61–S66.

82. Kario K, Pickering TG, Matsuo T, et al. Stroke prognosis and abnormal nocturnal blood pressure falls in older hypertensives. *Hypertension* 2001;38:852–857.

83. Wilcox I, Grunstein RR, Collins FL, et al. Circadian rhythm of blood pressure in patients with obstructive sleep apnea. *Blood Press* 1992;1:219–222.

84. Zimmet P, Magliano D, Matsuzawa Y, et al. The metabolic syndrome: a global public health problem and a new definition. *J Atheroscler Thromb* 2005;12:295–300.

85. Grundy SM. Metabolic syndrome scientific statement by the American Heart Association and the National Heart, Lung, and Blood Institute. *Arterioscler Thromb Vasc Biol* 2005;25:2243–2244.

86. Grundy SM, Cleeman JI, Daniels SR, et al. Diagnosis and management of the metabolic syndrome: an American Heart Association/National Heart, Lung, and Blood Institute scientific statement. *Curr Opin Cardiol* 2006;21:1–6.

87. Grundy SM. Metabolic syndrome: therapeutic considerations. *Handb Exp Pharmacol* 2005;(170):107–133.

88. Grundy SM. A constellation of complications: the metabolic syndrome. *Clin Cornerstone* 2005;7:36–45.

89. Alexander CM. The coming of age of the metabolic syndrome. *Diabetes Care* 2003;26:3180–3181.

90. Reaven G. The metabolic syndrome or the insulin resistance syndrome? Different names, different concepts, and different goals. *Endocrinol Metab Clin North Am* 2004;33:283–303.

91. Reaven GM. Insulin resistance, cardiovascular disease, and the metabolic syndrome: how well do the emperor's clothes fit? *Diabetes Care* 2004;27:1011–1012.

92. Reaven G, Abbasi F, McLaughlin T. Obesity, insulin resistance, and cardiovascular disease. *Recent Prog Horm Res* 2004;59:207–223.

93. Ford ES, Giles WH, Dietz WH. Prevalence of the metabolic syndrome among US adults: findings from the third National Health and Nutrition Examination Survey. *JAMA* 2002;287:356–359.

94. Alberti KG. The costs of non-insulin-dependent diabetes mellitus. *Diabet Med* 1997;14:7–9.

95. Grundy SM, Cleeman JI, Daniels SR, et al. Diagnosis and management of the metabolic syndrome: an American Heart Association/National Heart, Lung, and Blood Institute Scientific Statement. *Circulation* 2005;112:2735–2752.

96. Margolis ML, Christie JD, Silvestri GA, et al. Racial differences pertaining to a belief about lung cancer surgery: results of a multicenter survey. *Ann Intern Med* 2003;139:558–563.

97. Blackstock AW, Herndon JE, Paskett ED, et al. Outcomes among African-American/non-African-American patients with advanced non-small-cell lung carcinoma: report from the Cancer and Leukemia Group B Racial and ethnic disparities in the receipt of cancer treatment. *J Natl Cancer Inst* 2002;94:284–290.

98. Grunstein R, Wilcox I, Yang TS, et al. Snoring and sleep apnoea in men: association with central obesity and hypertension. *Int J Obes Relat Metab Disord* 1993;17:533–540.

99. Kushida CA, Efron B, Guilleminault C. A predictive morphometric model for the obstructive sleep apnea syndrome. *Ann Intern Med* 1997;127:581–587.

100. Punjabi NM, Sorkin JD, Katzel LI, et al. Sleep-disordered breathing and insulin resistance in middle-aged and overweight men. *Am J Respir Crit Care Med* 2002;165:677–682.

101. Peppard PE, Young T, Palta M, et al. Longitudinal study of moderate weight change and sleep-disordered breathing. *JAMA* 2000;284:3015–3021.

102. Coughlin SS, Calle EE, Teras LR, et al. Diabetes mellitus as a predictor of cancer mortality in a large cohort of US adults. *Am J Epidemiol* 2004;159:1160–1167.

103. Coughlin SR, Mawdsley L, Mugarza JA, et al. Obstructive sleep apnoea is independently associated with an increased prevalence of metabolic syndrome. *Eur Heart J* 2004;25:735–741.

104. Vgontzas AN, Papanicolaou DA, Bixler EO, et al. Sleep apnea and daytime sleepiness and fatigue: relation to visceral obesity, insulin resistance, and hypercytokinemia. *J Clin Endocrinol Metab* 2000;85:1151–1158.

105. Marcus DM, Lynn J, Miller JJ, et al. Sleep disorders: a risk factor for pseudotumor cerebri? *J Neuroophthalmol* 2001;21:121–123.

106. Fletcher EC. The relationship between systemic hypertension and obstructive sleep apnea: facts and theory. *Am J Med* 1995;98:118–128.

107. Mayer J, Becker H, Brandenburg U, et al. Blood pressure and sleep apnea: results of long-term nasal continuous positive airway pressure therapy. *Cardiology* 1991;79:84–92.

108. Hoffstein V, Chan CK, Slutsky AS. Sleep apnea and systemic hypertension: a causal association review. *Am J Med* 1991;91:190–196.

109. Ohayon MM, Guilleminault C, Priest RG, et al. Is sleep-disordered breathing an independent risk factor for hypertension in the general population (13,057 subjects)? *J Psychosom Res* 2000;48:593–601.

110. Peppard PE, Young T, Palta M, et al. Prospective study of the association between sleep-disordered breathing and hypertension. *N Engl J Med* 2000;342:1378–1384.

111. Nieto FJ, Young TB, Lind BK, et al. Association of sleep-disordered breathing, sleep apnea, and hypertension in a large community-based study. Sleep Heart Health Study. *JAMA* 2000;283:1829–1836.

112. Harding SM. Complications and consequences of obstructive sleep apnea. *Curr Opin Pulm Med* 2000;6:485–489.

113. Phillips BG, Somers VK. Hypertension and obstructive sleep apnea. *Curr Hypertens Rep* 2003;5:380–385.

114. Wolk R, Shamsuzzaman AS, Somers VK. Obesity, sleep apnea, and hypertension. *Hypertension* 2003;42:1067–1074.

115. Loredo JS, Clausen JL, Nelesen RA, et al. Obstructive sleep apnea and hypertension: are peripheral chemoreceptors involved? *Med Hypotheses* 2001;56:17–19.

116. Kawabe H, Saito I, Nagano S, et al. Relation of home blood pressure to body weight in young normotensive men with or without family history of hypertension. *Am J Hypertens* 1994;7:498–502.

117. Czarkowski M, Chojnowski K, Osikowska-Loksztejn M, et al. Blood pressure in young men with a family history of primary hypertension: traditional and 24-hour blood pressure measurements. *Pol Tyg Lek* 1994;49:221–224.

118. Balwierz P, Grzeszczak W. Influence of family history of hypertension on blood pressure in young healthy men. *Pol Arch Med Wewn* 2003;109:7–14.

119. Ibsen KK. Blood-pressures in offspring of hypertensive parents. *Acta Paediatr Scand* 1984;73:842–847.

120. Narkiewicz K, Gatti P, Garavelli G, et al. Relation between family history of hypertension, overweight and ambulatory blood pressure: the HARVEST study. *J Hum Hypertens* 1995;9:527–533.

121. Jean-Louis G, Zizi F, Casimir G, et al. Sleep-disordered breathing and hypertension among African Americans. *J Hum Hypertens* 2005;19:485–490.

122. Harris MI. Diabetes in America: epidemiology and scope of the problem. *Diabetes Care* 1998;21(Suppl 3):C11–C14.

123. Ip MS, Lam B, Ng MM, et al. Obstructive sleep apnea is independently associated with insulin resistance. *Am J Respir Crit Care Med* 2002;165:670–676.

124. Punjabi NM, Shahar E, Redline S, et al. Sleep-disordered breathing, glucose intolerance, and insulin resistance: the Sleep Heart Health Study. *Am J Epidemiol* 2004;160:521–530.

125. Punjabi NM, Polotsky VY. Disorders of glucose metabolism in sleep apnea. *J Appl Physiol* 2005;99:1998–2007.

126. Spiegel R, Knudtson K, Leproult R, et al. Sleep loss: a novel risk factor for insulin resistance and Type 2 diabetes. *J Appl Physiol* 2005;99:2008–2019.

127. Fletcher GF. How to implement physical activity in primary and secondary prevention. A statement for healthcare-professionals from the Task Force on Risk-reduction, American Heart Association. *Circulation* 1997;96:355–357.

128. Punjabi NM, Ahmed MM, Polotsky VY, et al. Sleep-disordered breathing, glucose intolerance, and insulin resistance. *Respir Physiol Neurobiol* 2003;136:167–178.

129. Ayas NT, White DP, Manson JE, et al. A prospective study of sleep duration and coronary heart disease in women. *Arch Intern Med* 2003;163:205–209.

130. Ayas NT, White DP, Al Delaimy WK, et al. A prospective study of self-reported sleep duration and incident diabetes in women. *Diabetes Care* 2003;26:380–384.

131. Gottlieb DJ, Punjabi NM, Newman AB, et al. Association of sleep time with diabetes mellitus and impaired glucose tolerance. *Arch Intern Med* 2005;165:863–867.

132. Sanders MH, Givelber R. Sleep disordered breathing may not be an independent risk factor for diabetes, but diabetes may contribute to the occurrence of periodic breathing in sleep. *Sleep Med* 2003;4:349–350.

133. Jean-Louis G, Kripke DF, Ancoli-Israel S, et al. Sleep duration, illumination, and activity patterns in a population sample: effects of gender and ethnicity. *Biol Psychiatry* 2000;47:921–927.

134. 2005 Omnibus Sleep in America Poll. National Sleep Foundation, 2005.

135. Patel SR, Ayas NT, Malhotra MR, et al. A prospective study of sleep duration and mortality risk in women. *Sleep* 2004;27:440–444.

136. Jean-Louis G, Kripke DF, Ancoli-Israel S. Sleep and quality of well-being. *Sleep* 2000;23:1115–1121.

137. Kripke DF, Simons RN, Garfinkel L, et al. Short and long sleep and sleeping pills. Is increased mortality associated? *Arch Gen Psychiatry* 1979;36:103–116.

138. Kripke DF, Garfinkel L, Wingard DL, et al. Mortality associated with sleep duration and insomnia. *Arch Gen Psychiatry* 2002;59:131–136.

139. Harsch IA, Hahn EG, Konturek PC. Insulin resistance and other metabolic aspects of the obstructive sleep apnea syndrome. *Med Sci Monit* 2005;11: RA70–RA75.

140. Stamler J, Wentworth D, Neaton JD. Is relationship between serum cholesterol and risk of premature death from coronary heart disease continuous and graded? Findings in 356,222 primary screenees of the Multiple Risk Factor Intervention Trial (MRFIT). *JAMA* 1986;256:2823–2828.

141. Goff DC Jr, D'Agostino RB Jr, Haffner SM, et al. Insulin resistance and adiposity influence lipoprotein size and subclass concentrations. Results from the Insulin Resistance Atherosclerosis Study. *Metabolism* 2005;54:264–270.

142. O'Meara JG, Kardia SL, Armon JJ, et al. Ethnic and sex differences in the prevalence, treatment, and control of dyslipidemia among hypertensive adults in the GENOA study. *Arch Intern Med* 2004;164:1313–1318.

143. Kiely JL, McNicholas WT. Cardiovascular risk factors in patients with obstructive sleep apnoea syndrome. *Eur Respir J* 2000;16:128–133.

144. Zgierska A, Gorecka D, Radzikowska M, et al. Obstructive sleep apnea and risk factors for coronary artery disease. *Pneumonol Alergol Pol* 2000;68:238–246.

145. Tan KC, Chow WS, Lam JC, et al. HDL dysfunction in obstructive sleep apnea. *Atherosclerosis* 2006;184:377–382.

146. Borgel J, Sanner BM, Bittlinsky A, et al. Obstructive sleep apnoea and its therapy influence high-density lipoprotein cholesterol serum levels. *Eur Respir J* 2006;27:121–127.

147. Expert Panel on Detection, Evaluation, and Treatment of High Blood Cholesterol in Adults. Executive summary of the third report of the National Cholesterol Education Program (NCEP) expert panel on detection, evaluation and treatment of high blood cholesterol in adults (Adult Treatment Panel III). *JAMA* 2001;285:2486–2497.

148. Lee PY, Yun AJ, Bazar KA. Acute coronary syndromes and heart failure may reflect maladaptations of trauma physiology that was shaped during premodern evolution. *Med Hypotheses* 2004;62:861–867.

149. Mansfield DR, Gollogly NC, Kaye DM, et al. Controlled trial of continuous positive airway pressure in obstructive sleep apnea and heart failure. *Am J Respir Crit Care Med* 2004;169:361–366.

150. Milleron O, Pilliere R, Foucher A, et al. Benefits of obstructive sleep apnoea treatment in coronary artery disease: a long-term follow-up study. *Eur Heart J* 2004;25:728–734.

151. Sajkov D, Wang T, Saunders NA, et al. Daytime pulmonary hemodynamics in patients with obstructive sleep apnea without lung disease. *Am J Respir Crit Care Med* 1999;159:1518–1526.

152. Wang F, Javitt JC, Tielsch JM. Racial variations in treatment for glaucoma and cataract among Medicare recipients. *Ophthalmic Epidemiol* 1997;4:89–100.

153. Jean-Louis G, Magai C, Pierre-Louis J, et al. Insomnia complaints and repressive coping among Black and White Americans. *Sleep* 2005;28:232 Abstract.

HEALTH DISPARITIES AND

CARDIOVASCULAR

DISEASE

Luther T. Clark
Ruth C. Browne
Ronald Kokolis
Marilyn White
Susana Morales

INTRODUCTION

Cardiovascular disease (CVD), and in particular, ischemic heart disease is the leading cause of death in the United States for Americans of both genders and of all racial and ethnic backgrounds.[1-5] African Americans (non-Hispanic U.S. blacks) have the highest overall coronary heart disease (CHD) mortality rate and the highest out-of-hospital coronary death rate of any ethnic group in the United Sates, particularly at younger ages.[6-11] Furthermore, while the mortality rate for heart disease has been declining during the past several decades, the rate of decline has been less in the black community. Indeed, non-Hispanic blacks are the only ethnic group in the United Sates whose CHD mortality rate is in excess of the established national 2010 target (Fig. 20-1).[12]

The reasons for the earlier onset and excess CVD deaths among African Americans have not been fully elucidated. However, it is clear that there is a high prevalence of diabetes and other coronary risk factors, patient delays in seeking medical care, delays in diagnosis and treatment of high-risk individuals, and limited access to cardiovascular care (preventive, maintenance, and procedures such as cardiac catheterization, coronary interventions, and bypass surgery).

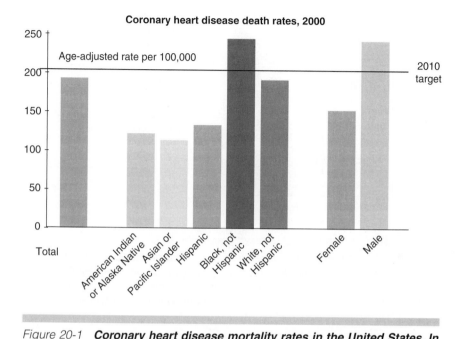

Figure 20-1 **Coronary heart disease mortality rates in the United States. In 2000, the only ethnic group whose CHD death rate exceeded the 2010 target was non-Hispanic blacks, accounting for the entire national mortality overage.** *(Source: Adapted from http://www.cdc.gov/nchshome.htm.)*

In this chapter, the terms "African American," "black," and "non-Hispanic black" are used synonymously and interchangeably.

HISTORICAL PERSPECTIVE

According to the National Institutes of Health (NIH), "Health disparities are differences in the incidence, prevalence, mortality, and burden of diseases and other adverse health conditions that exist among specific population groups in the United States."[13] The Institute of Medicine (IOM) defines health care disparities as "racial or ethnic differences in the quality of health care that are not due to access-related factors or clinical needs, preferences, and appropriateness of intervention" (Fig. 20-2).[14] Both these definitions mean that African Americans, Hispanics, Native Americans, and some Asian subgroups—populations in which health disparities exist—suffer more illness, die younger, and receive suboptimal health care when compared to whites.

Disparities in outcomes from various diseases between blacks—for whom there are more data than for other minority groups—and whites have

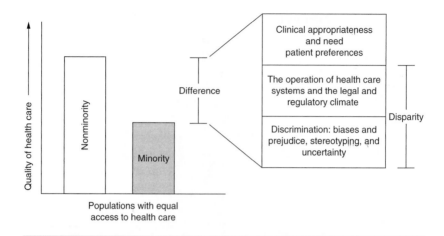

Figure 20-2 **Differences, disparities, and discrimination: populations with equal access to health care.** *(Source: Adapted from Smedley BD, Stith AY, Nelson AR, eds. Committee on Understanding and Eliminating Racial and Ethnic Disparities in Health Care Unequal Treatment: Confronting Racial and Ethnic Disparities in Health Care. Washington, DC: The National Academies Press, 2003.)*

been documented for as long as records have been kept. The recent heightened interest in disparities began in 2002 following publication of the IOM's report, *Unequal Treatment: Confronting Racial and Ethnic Disparities in Health care,*[14] which added to the already growing body of literature documenting the continuing existence of health disparities in the United States. The IOM report concluded that racial and ethnic minorities receive lower quality health care than whites, even when they are insured to the same degree and when other health care access-related factors, such as the ability to pay for care, are the same. The IOM Committee reviewed evidence of disparities in care for a range of illnesses, and discovered the most glaring to be in treatment for CVD, particularly for African American patients.

Seventeen years previously, in 1985, the U.S. Department of Health and Human Services (DHHS) released a comprehensive and groundbreaking report—*Secretary of Health and Human Services Report on Black and Minority Health*—which found that African Americans, Hispanics, Native Americans, and some Asian and Pacific Islander benefited less from recent advances in scientific knowledge and medical care than their white counterparts.[15] The report raised particular attention to the finding that blacks suffered an annual excess of approximately 60,000 preventable deaths, most of which were due to CVDs.[15] The release of this DHHS report increased awareness and heightened interest in minority health issues, particularly disparities in health status, access to health care, quality of health care, and outcomes.

Prior to the 1985 DHHS report, several studies and reports had underscored the need to address the disparity in the burden of death and illness experienced by African Americans and other minorities relative to the population as a whole. During the civil rights movement in the 1950s and 1960s, improved health care emerged as one of the major issues, leading Nobel Laureate and civil rights leader, the Reverend Dr. Martin Luther King, Jr., to proclaim in a 1963 speech that *"Of all forms of inequality in our society, injustice in health care is the most shocking and the most inhumane."*[16] In 1895, more than a century ago, the major *raison d'être* for the founding of the National Medical Association as the voice of black physicians and the patients they serve, was to improve the health status and outcomes of African Americans and the disadvantaged.[17]

In a specific analysis focusing on CVD, The Henry J. Kaiser Family Foundation's study, *Racial/Ethnic Differences in Cardiac Care: The Weight of the Evidence*[18] reviewed 81 studies on racial/ethnic differences in cardiac care and confirmed the IOM's findings. The study concluded that African Americans are less likely than whites to receive appropriate and necessary treatments for cardiac disease, including thrombolytics, catheterization, angioplasty, and bypass surgery, and that these racial/ethnic differences in care remained after adjustment for clinical and socioeconomic factors.

Each of the above landmark reports, in particular the IOM 2002 report, further documented and heightened awareness of a continuing national paradox in the United States—that despite the tremendous scientific achievements in terms of improvement in overall health status for the general population, significant health inequities persist among African Americans and other minorities.

Many factors contribute to health disparities, including biologic, environmental, social, cultural, behavioral, and economic. Disease burden, provider and patient factors also contribute importantly. Societal level determinants of health include poverty, unskilled job classification, lower educational attainment, and stress.[19] Patient-level potential sources of disparities in care include patient preferences, treatment refusal, different care seeking behaviors and attitudes, and clinical appropriateness of care.[14] Provider-level potential sources of disparities in care include bias, clinical uncertainty, and beliefs and stereotypes about the behavior or health of minority patients.[14]

EXCESS BURDEN OF DIABETES AND OTHER RISK FACTORS

African Americans have an excess burden of major risk factors for CVD and are more likely to have multiple risk factors than their white counterparts.[1,4,5,7,20–22] While the predictive value of most conventional risk factors appears to be similar in African Americans and whites,[23] the risk of death and other sequelae attributable to some risk factors (e.g., hypertension and diabetes) are greater for African Americans[24–26] and the risk of certain others, lipoprotein(a) (Lp(a)) are lower.[27–30] Type 2 diabetes mellitus, hypertension, left ventricular hypertrophy, obesity, cigarette smoking, and physical inactivity occur more frequently in African Americans. The increased risk factor burden plus the combination of lower screening and less effective treatment of risk factors all contribute to worse outcomes and health disparities.

Interestingly, although Hispanics in the United States have a CVD risk factor burden similarly high to that of African Americans—higher rates of diabetes, the metabolic syndrome, obesity, lower high-density lipoprotein cholesterol (HDL-C) and higher triglyceride levels, lower socioeconomic status (SES)—and barriers to health care, Hispanics have lower all-cause and cardiovascular mortality rates than non-Hispanic blacks and non-Hispanic whites (see Fig. 20-1; Table 20-1).[31–34] Some investigators refer to this observation as the "Hispanic Paradox."[33]

Diabetes Mellitus

Diabetes mellitus increases risk for CHD at least two- to fourfold.[35,36] Furthermore, vascular complications in patients with diabetes appear at a younger age, affect women as often as men, and are more often fatal than in nondiabetic patients.[35–39] African Americans and other nonwhite minorities have a greater burden of diabetes and its vascular complications are greater than in whites.[26,40,41] Compared to whites, the prevalence of type 2 diabetes

Table 20-1 **CHD Risk Factors in Hispanics and Non-Hispanic blacks Compared to Non-Hispanic whites**

More Prevalent in Non-Hispanic blacks than Non-Hispanic whites
Hypertension
Type 2 diabetes mellitus
Obesity
Metabolic syndrome (females)
Cigarette smoking
Physical inactivity

More Prevalent in Hispanics than Non-Hispanic whites
Type 2 diabetes mellitus
Obesity
Lower HDL-C (females)
Elevated triglycerides
Metabolic syndrome
Physical inactivity

Source: Adapted from Refs. 7, 28, and 31.

in African Americans is two to three times higher,[26,40,41] 2.5 times more prevalent in Hispanics (particularly those of Puerto Rican and Mexican origin), and 5 times more prevalent in Native Americans.[35] The disproportionately higher prevalence of type 2 diabetes in ethnic minorities is associated with increased morbidity and mortality.[35,36,42] Furthermore, it is projected that diabetes-related disparities will increase in the future because of the greater rate of increase for diabetes and its complications among minority groups.[42,43]

Hypertension

Both systolic hypertension and diastolic hypertension are established risk factors for CVD. Systolic blood pressure is a better predictor than diastolic blood pressure of risk for CHD, heart failure, stroke, end-stage renal disease, and overall mortality. Among African Americans, hypertension is more prevalent, develops at younger ages, and is associated with three to five times higher cardiovascular mortality rates than in whites.[20-25] African Americans also appear to experience greater cardiovascular and renal damage at any level of blood pressure than whites, although the higher mortality rates in hypertensive African Americans may reflect greater disease duration and severity.[23-25]

Obesity

Obesity, particularly abdominal obesity, increases risk for CHD, stroke, hypertension, type 2 diabetes in adults, and is also a major component of the metabolic syndrome.[44,45] The increased risk appears to be mediated chiefly through the metabolic consequences of obesity (i.e., insulin resistance, glucose intolerance, hypertriglyceridemia, reduced HDL-C, and hypertension). The prevalence of obesity among African American men is similar to that among white men. However, in African American women, obesity is twice as prevalent and the abdominal pattern of obesity is more common than in their white counterparts.[46-49]

Physical Inactivity

African Americans have a higher prevalence of physical inactivity and are less likely to get recommended amounts of exercise than their white counterparts.[5,20-22] Physical inactivity is associated with increased risk for CHD, whereas physical activity favorably modifies CHD risk.[50,51] Physical inactivity reduces caloric expenditure, contributes to obesity, other CHD risk factors, and adversely affects cardiovascular fitness and function. Physical activity decreases cardiovascular risk and favorably affects a number of CHD risk factors, including elevated blood pressure, insulin resistance, dyslipidemia, obesity, and the metabolic syndrome.

Cigarette Smoking

Cigarette smoking is a powerful CHD risk factor. More African American men smoke than white men, but African American men consume fewer cigarettes per day.[1,52] African American and white women smoke at comparable rates.[1,52] Despite the fact that African Americans tend to smoke fewer cigarettes per day and begin smoking later in life than whites, smoking-related disease morbidity and mortality are significantly higher among African Americans.[1,53,54] In one study of the smoking patterns of menthol smokers, Okuyemi et al. hypothesized that the excess smoking-related morbidity and the less successful smoking cessation rates among African Americans[54] are due to their high preference for menthol cigarettes. According to these authors, menthol cigarette smokers tend to be younger and more likely to smoke cigarettes with longer rod length, with filters, and those high in nicotine and tar. However, the mechanisms responsible for underlying differences have not been elucidated.

Risk Factor Clustering and the Metabolic Syndrome

The presence of multiple risk factors increases CHD risk synergistically. African Americans are more likely to have multiple CHD risk factors than whites.[20–22] Both genetic and environmental factors have been implicated in the etiology of risk factor clustering although the mechanisms have yet to be elucidated. The metabolic syndrome refers to a specific clustering of cardiovascular risk factors in the same individual (abdominal obesity, atherogenic dyslipidemia, elevated blood pressure, insulin resistance, a prothrombotic state, and a proinflammatory state).[55–57] Patients with the metabolic syndrome are at increased risk for the development of diabetes and CVD. African American women and Hispanic men and women have the highest prevalences of the metabolic syndrome[31] (see Chap. 14 for a more detailed discussion of the metabolic syndrome).

CORONARY HEART DISEASE

Coronary heart disease and its thrombotic complications are the major causes of morbidity and mortality in the United States. A number of differences have been reported between blacks and whites as to the extent of underlying atherosclerosis, markers of inflammation, hemostasis, endothelial dysfunction, and coronary vasospasm.[5] However, most reported differences have been modest and their clinical importance in diagnosing and treating coronary syndromes are not well documented. Nevertheless, there continues to be considerable interest in the differences in the clinical manifestations and underlying pathobiology of CHD in various ethnic groups, and whether or not these differences contribute to differences in clinical outcomes. Some of the interest exists because of an increased appreciation of the significance of CHD in ethnic minorities and some because of the apparent inconsistency with generally accepted pathophysiologic concepts. For example, among African Americans: (1) despite the greater burden of certain coronary risk factors, the incidence of angiographically significant coronary artery disease is lower than it is in whites[5,58–61] and (2) despite less severe coronary disease on angiography and fewer Q-wave (ST-elevation) myocardial infarctions, CHD events occur at younger ages and are associated with higher mortality rates than in whites.[5,7–10,62] Furthermore, and as previously noted, despite high rates of diabetes and other CHD risk factors, Hispanics in the United States have lower cardiovascular mortality rates than non-Hispanic blacks and non-Hispanic whites (see Fig. 20-1; Table 20-1)[31–34]—the *Hispanic Paradox.*[33]

Acute Coronary Syndromes

The acute coronary syndromes (ACS) refer to the spectrum of manifestations of unstable coronary artery disease, including unstable angina (UA), non-ST-segment elevation myocardial infarction (NSTEMI), ST-segment elevation myocardial infarction (STEMI), and sudden cardiac death (SCD; see Chap. 4 for a more detailed discussion of ACS). Clinical trials investigating ACS as well as clinical management guidelines often group together patients with UA and those with NSTEMI. These two entities have similar manifestations and a distinction between them can usually be made only after several hours when the results of cardiac enzymes become available.

Approximately 1.7 million individuals in the United Sates are hospitalized annually with UA and acute myocardial infarction (AMI).[1] Acute cardiac events are usually triggered by atherosclerotic plaque rupture, fissuring, or erosion with superimposed thrombosis, and coronary vasospasm.[63–67] Clinically, the risk of death and recurrent cardiac ischemic events vary among individuals and population subgroups. The heterogeneity of clinical presentations and outcomes is related to a multiplicity of factors, including: (1) the extent of underlying coronary atherosclerosis; (2) the extent and type of thrombus that forms over the ruptured plaque; (3) the degree and extent of coronary vasospasm; and (4) the underlying myocardial substrate. The degree of coronary artery luminal stenosis does not correlate well with acute cardiac events, and most myocardial infarctions occur at sites with less than 50% luminal stenosis.[68]

ACUTE CORONARY SYNDROMES IN AFRICAN AMERICANS

The clinical spectrum of African Americans presenting with ACS is the same as for white patients with ACS. However, African Americans presenting with ACS more often have non-ST-elevation syndromes (non-Q-wave myocardial infarction, UA, or sudden death) than whites, and have poorer outcomes.[69,70] The reasons for this have not been fully elucidated, but may be related to: (1) the greater prevalence and severity of certain baseline risk factors, particularly hypertension and its consequences; (2) excessive delays seeking medical care by African Americans and later presentation in the clinical evolution of the ACS; (3) delays in diagnosis of ACS in African Americans who present to emergency departments with chest pain; and (4) following confirmation of

ACS, less aggressive medical and interventional therapies (cardiac catheterization, percutaneous coronary interventions [PCI], and bypass surgery).

Prehospital delay

African Americans delay seeking medical care for ACS and present later (up to three times longer) in their clinical course than do whites.[70–74] It has now been well documented that greater benefits are achieved (infarct size reduction, mortality) when therapy is initiated earlier in the course of ACS. Delays in seeking medical care limit these benefits and contribute to increased morbidity and mortality. Many factors contribute to health care seeking behavior, including access to medical care, knowledge and beliefs concerning CHD, symptom perception and attributions, and adherence to treatment recommendations. Access to medical care is an important contributor to delays since patients without a usual care provider, patients of low SES, and patients with poor insurance coverage delay seeking care for acute events.

Emergency room evaluation

Although much of the treatment delay for African Americans with ACS can be attributed to patient delays in seeking medical care and delayed initial hospital arrival following onset of symptoms, substantial treatment delays also occur following patient arrival in the emergency department. Since African American patients present later in the clinical course of their ACS than whites and are at higher risk, there should be a greater urgency in terms of timely evaluation, diagnosis, risk assessment, and treatment. Paradoxically, the opposite is true.

Treatment delays cannot be attributed to atypical symptoms, although African Americans have been reported to more often have atypical symptoms, since most African American patients (70–85%) with myocardial ischemia and AMI present with typical chest pain.[75–80] Despite their high-risk status, in emergency departments, the index of suspicion for coronary ischemia is often lower for African Americans than it is for whites,[80] and symptoms are less often attributed to coronary disease by both patients themselves and the providers who initially evaluate them.[80] Perhaps as a consequence, first electrocardiograms are performed later than in whites, and physicians less often perform laboratory evaluation (cardiac markers), noninvasive and invasive diagnostics to evaluate for coronary disease. Even when myocardial ischemia is suspected during the initial evaluation, nonspecific (nondiagnostic) repolarization abnormalities on ECG may make diagnosis of ischemia and/or AMI difficult.

TREATMENT STRATEGIES FOR ACUTE CORONARY SYNDROMES

The optimal approach to the management of the ACS continues to evolve and in-hospital outcomes in patients with ACS continue to improve. Early, complete, and sustained reperfusion using thrombolytic therapy or PCI is the primary goal of treatment in patients with STEMI.[81] The management of patients with NSTEMI or UA is more challenging and requires careful integration of overall risk assessment, pharmacologic, and interventional/mechanical therapies.[82]

One of the guiding principles for management of patients with ACS is that the intensity of therapy should be based on the overall risk, with patients at highest risk receiving the most immediate and intensive therapy.[81-84] The goals of initial treatment in patients with ACS include relief of angina, control of the acute aspects of the pathophysiologic processes, preservation of viable myocardium, and prevention of death. Initial treatment strategies include: (1) antithrombotic and antiplatelet therapy, (2) antianginal medications, (3) mechanical revascularization, and (4) pharmacologic measures to stabilize plaques and risk factor modification. In high-risk ACS patients, an invasive strategy (early angiography and revascularization) is the preferred approach when it is available and accessible in a timely manner. However, invasive and conservative (medical) approaches should be considered complementary. Modern aggressive protocol-driven medical therapy may decrease cardiac ischemia, cardiac events, and the urgency for revascularization. Early angiography and revascularization strategies play a particularly important role in the management of patients who belong to higher risk categories.

TREATMENT OF ACUTE CORONARY SYNDROMES IN AFRICAN AMERICANS

Based on higher risk status and poorer outcomes, African Americans should be treated at least as aggressively, and perhaps more, as whites. However, this is not the case and African American patients with ACS paradoxically: (1) receive less aggressive medical therapy; and (2) are less likely to receive reperfusion therapies such as thrombolytics and coronary revascularization procedures.[14,15,18,85-91] The reasons for this are unclear but have been attributed to unmeasured confounders that may impact the process of care for black patients (such as hospital characteristics, physician and patient preferences, cultural and socioeconomic factors) and physician bias in the use of aggressive thrombolytic therapies and invasive cardiac procedures.

During the past two decades there have been considerable advances in our understanding of the pathophysiology of the ACS. The ACS (UA and NSTEMI) are heterogeneous disorders in which patients have widely varying risks. Since risk is an important driver of management decisions, accurate risk assessment is important for decision-making and optimal patient care. Physicians should employ proven strategies to assure that all patients receive appropriate and high quality of care. Use of evidence-based therapies for management of patients with ACS and better understanding of various available treatment strategies is of utmost importance. In the subset of patients who do not present with typical chest pain, yet are high risk for CAD, recognition that atypical symptoms might be due to ischemia will reduce delays in diagnosis and initiation of appropriate therapy. Thus, while typical symptoms are the strongest predictors of ACS, atypical symptoms must be recognized as well. Efforts to improve quality of care for African American patients with ACS and eliminate racial disparities must be comprehensive, and include improved strategies for: (1) decreasing patient delays in seeking medical care for ACS; (2) earlier recognition, diagnosis, and implementation of appropriate therapy in the emergency room setting; and (3) stricter adherence and implementation of evidence-based recommendations and treatment guidelines.

THE DOCTOR-PATIENT RELATIONSHIP: COMMUNICATION, CULTURAL, AND LINGUISTIC COMPETENCY

The doctor-patient relationship—the relationship between the healer and the sick person, the doctor, and the patient—has been at the heart and foundation of medicine throughout history.[92] Even in the current era in which the *doctor* and *patient* are often referred to as *provider* and *customer*, the physician-patient relationship remains a special and remarkable social contract. The recent rapid advances in cardiovascular medicine, the greater use of modern high-tech therapies and procedures, and the increased risk potential for complications, make the doctor-patient relationship and effective communication between them, more important now than ever before.

Doctor-Patient Communication and Racial/Ethnic Health Disparities

One of the major barriers to control of diabetes, prevention of CVD, and control of CHD risk factors is lack of patient compliance with recommended therapy. Important contributors to lack of compliance include poor doctor-patient communications, cost, and medication side effects.[14,93] Poor communication between physicians and patients may be the most important impediment to effective treatment adherence.[93] Good communication between physicians and patients improves patient outcomes, patient satisfaction, adherence to doctor's recommendations, and reduces the likelihood of malpractice suits.[55,93,94,96]

The lack of proper physician-patient communication is also an important contributor to health disparities[5,14,95] and worse outcomes in ethnic minorities. Although racial bias and differential patient preferences play a role, recent research suggests that the primary problem is poor communication between physician providers (most of whom are white) and their nonwhite patients.[96] When it comes to nonwhite patients, physicians' interpersonal skills are poorer, they are less supportive, provide less information, and use a decision-making style that is less participatory.[96]

Effective physician-patient communication is bidirectional and requires mutual participation and commitment. Both physician and patient must share treatment goals and mutual understandings of each other's role in managing the patient's health problem.

Physicians must convey interest in controlling the patient's risk factors, and a commitment to overcoming obstacles. This includes spending time educating patients about the importance of risk factor control, taking their medications, and achieving treatment goals. Patient responsibilities include keeping follow-up appointments, following nonpharmacologic and pharmacologic recommendations, and alerting the physician to problems with medicines.

Linguistic Barriers

Communication between physician and patient is often hindered because of linguistic barriers. The 2000 United States census estimated that more than 32 million individuals speak a language other than English at home. Persons with Limited English Proficiency (LEP) experience decreased access to hospital and medical services, decreased comprehension of diagnosis and treatment, poorer patient satisfaction, and poorer health outcomes. The care of LEP persons without proper interpreter services is also more costly, in part due to increased inefficiency and unnecessary testing. Standardization of interpreter services has been slow in coming, and national standards for interpreter services were only issued recently.[97]

Provider-Level Contributions to Disparities

Communication problems are not only issues in the care of LEP persons. The Commonwealth Fund 2001 Health Care Quality Survey[98] found that minority Americans across the board were more likely to report problems with communication and relationships with physicians. In this study, a national phone survey of 6722 adults aged 18 or older, including 3488 white Americans, 1153 Hispanics, 1037 African Americans, and 669 Asian Americans, researchers focused on: patient-physician communication, cultural competency, access and coverage, preventive care, health status, and demographics. The findings of the Commonwealth Fund study were that[98]: (1) minority patients reported more difficulty communicating with their doctors; (2) minority patients were more likely to forgo asking questions of their physicians; (3) patients of all backgrounds reported not following their doctor's advice about 20–25% of the time, but the reasons for their lack of adherence to physician advice varied by race and ethnicity; and (4) minority patients had more difficulty understanding instructions from doctor's offices.

THE ROLE OF PHYSICIAN RACE AND ETHNICITY

Cooper et al. found that African Americans rated visits with their physicians as less participatory than whites, but that racially concordant doctor visits were more likely to be participatory.[99] Minority patients of racially ethnically concordant physicians have greater patient satisfaction with and utilization of health care services.[100]

PHYSICIAN PERCEPTIONS OF MINORITY PATIENTS: BIAS AND STEREOTYPE

According to Aberegg and Terry,[101] stereotyping is common in all cultures and may have evolved as a way of simplifying decision making in complex environments. Stereotyping may also be useful in "situations characterized by time pressures, psychological stress, fatigue, or multitasking."[101] Physicians have been shown to prefer patients that are "likable," "compliant," of higher SES and physically attractive, and to find undesirable abrasive or angry patients, non-English speaking patients, and patients with varying psychosocial issues including personality disorders and suicidality."[101]

EXPLANATORY MODEL FOR DISPARITIES IN PROVIDER BEHAVIOR

Ashton et al.[93] developed a three-hypothesis explanatory model to explain differences in provider behavior by patient race. The hypotheses include:

1. *Bias hypothesis*: Unconscious bias and stereotype motivating providers
2. *Preference hypothesis*: Providers make dubious assumptions; supporting this is the reality that patient decision making is often not truly "informed" in patients of all races
3. *Communication hypothesis*: The goal of the doctor-patient interaction is for doctors and patients to reach a shared explanatory model of the illness or issue and negotiate an appropriate plan. Poor communication and negotiation interfere with reaching this goal.

These authors concluded that both doctors and patients have predisposing influences: each person has an individual communication style, self-concept (attitudes, beliefs, personality), and linguistic resources. Both parties may have different goals, different perceptions of the other person and relationship, different communication strategies, and different emotional states. All of these factors can influence both verbal and nonverbal behavior, and in turn, each person's behavior then affects the other person's behavior.

Furthermore, according to Ashton et al., the goal of each health care encounter is for the doctor to help the patient do four things: (1) provide a health narrative; (2) ask questions; (3) express concerns; and (4) to be assertive. The doctor needs to elicit their patient's explanatory model of illness and reach common understanding. In addition, patients can be empowered and educated to improve their ability to communicate with doctors. Doctors have been shown to respond to communication skills training.[93]

Patient-Level Contributions to Disparities

Patient-level potential sources of disparities in health care include patient preferences, treatment refusal, different care-seeking behaviors and attitudes, and clinical appropriateness of care. However, patient attitudes and preferences do not vary enough to explain treatment disparities.[14]

TRUST

Trust is a crucial component of the physician-patient relationship. In one national telephone survey[102] and another regional telephone survey, African American patients were found to be less trusting of their doctors and of medical research than white patients. According to Corbie-Smith et al., "Interpersonal, institutional, and societal trusts are interdependent. Trust in one's physician (interpersonal trust) is usually an iterative process. Trust in society, medical institutions, and medical research may be formed by community perceptions, public opinion, and the media."[102]

LITERACY

The Healthy People 2010 report defines literacy as "the degree to which individuals have the capacity to obtain, process, and understand basic health information and services needed to make appropriate health decisions."[103] Literacy affects health care in multiple aspects ranging from cost to compliance. In a study reported by the Institute for Health Care Advancement, the average health care cost among those with low literacy was found to be four times greater as compared to the general population.[104] In another study, poor glycemic control was found to be twice as likely in low literacy diabetics as compared to high literacy diabetics.[105] Often, physicians assume that patients understand all instructions. Frequently, due to time constraints, very little time is spent assessing the patient's comprehension of both their illness and disease process.

Patients with diabetes and chronic CVD are expected to understand, measure, monitor, and manage many variables in their daily lives that affect their disease and clinical outcomes. Literacy must be addressed and subsequent discussions should be tailored to the patient's particular literacy level.

Literacy can be addressed from the patient's perspective by building awareness about diabetes and CVD through community educational awareness programs, and improving educational information/pamphlets distributed to patients. A multidesign approach utilizing a broad range of health care workers ranging from a nurse, nurse practitioner, social worker, and case manager can facilitate and reinforce teachings initiated during the physician-patient encounter.

Steps to improve literacy should include communication that uses layman terms. The use of feedback is also an important tool that can be developed by physicians. The American Medical Association has highlighted the importance of this skill through the use of "teach back." Physicians are instructed to assess a patient's understanding of what was discussed with phrases such as "Now, to be sure we are in agreement, why don't you show me what you would do when."[106]

Enhancing the Doctor-Patient Relationship

The physician-patient relationship and in particular, communication between physicians and patients, has become increasingly challenging as health care has become more intellectually and technologically advanced. Improving patient health literacy, cultural competency among providers, and provider communication skills are keys to effective physician-patient relationships.

THE ROLE OF CULTURAL COMPETENCY

When addressing this issue of provider-patient communication, the cultural backgrounds of the patient and physician must be considered since cultural barriers between physician and patients can affect the outcome of the encounter, patient satisfaction, and patient adherence to recommendations. *Culture* refers to integrated patterns of human behavior that include the language, thoughts, communications, actions, customs, beliefs, values, and institutions of racial, ethnic, religious, or social groups.[107] *Competence* implies having the capacity to function effectively as an individual and an organization within the context of the cultural beliefs, behaviors, and needs presented by patients and their communities.[107] *Cultural and linguistic competence* has been defined as "a set of congruent behaviors, attitudes, and policies that come together in a system, agency, or among professionals that enables effective work in cross-cultural situations."[107] Cultural competence is a continuum. Cultural issues affect many patient-physician encounters, and are not unique to minority or immigrant Americans. However, enhancing culturally competent care is an important tool for addressing disparities. Cultural competence training for health care providers has focused on (1) issues of power/status of physicians; (2) language; (3) educational status and differences including the issue of health literacy; (4) the fact that socioeconomic barriers to access are greater in minority and immigrant groups; (5) diverse health and disease belief systems; (6) alternative and complementary medicine beliefs and practices versus traditional medicine; and (7) religious differences. There is some evidence that cultural competence training can address stereotyping and bias, although there has been inconsistency in methodology of implementation and evaluation.

The Office of Minority Health published the National Standards on Culturally and Linguistically Appropriate Services (CLAS) in 2001.[108] The CLAS standards are primarily directed at health care organizations; however, individual providers are also encouraged to use the standards to make their practices more culturally and linguistically accessible. The 14 standards are organized by themes: Culturally Competent Care (Standards 1–3), Language Access Services (Standards 4–7), and Organizational Supports for Cultural Competence (Standards 8–14).[108]

EFFECTIVE COMMUNICATION

Communication plays a critical role in the physician-patient relationship. The ability to know when to speak, when to listen, and what to listen for, are critical to proper communication. In one report, the average time allowed to patients to present the story of their illness before being interrupted by their clinician was found to be 18 seconds while, only 2% of those patients were ever allowed to complete their story.[109] The importance of this is seen in several studies that have shown communication to be the single most effective predictor of compliance to a treatment plan.

According to the Bayer Institute for Health Care communication model, effective communication is composed of *engagement, empathy, education, and enlistment.*[110] Serial completion of each task is required.

Engagement

Engagement requires that the physician establish a nonthreatening environment in which the clinician introduces himself or herself and begins the discussion with open-ended questions. This is a critical component in establishing a successful physician-patient relationship. If a patient does not accept the partnership, then the conversation is unilateral and authoritative. Key techniques for creating a successful engagement include acknowledging that the patient is a major player in the relationship, eliciting his or her expectations and concerns, and negotiating aspects of care if a contrary opinion is expressed by the patient. Most important is the use of layman's language instead of medical jargon.

Empathy

Empathy refers to the ability to feel and put oneself in patient's shoes. The technique that allows a physician to accomplish this includes removal of obstructions or physical barriers between the patient and physician, maintaining eye contact, and reinforcing what was stated by the patient through the use of a patient's own words. The step of engagement will facilitate a physician's empathy to be accepted and believed by the patient.

Education

Poor education and literacy on the patient's part is a by-product of poor physician communication skills. Educating a patient begins by assessing the knowledge of a patient to the issues that are presented and need to be addressed. The open-ended question model creates a nonjudgmental and multidirectional discussion. In patients not forthcoming, the skill of *empathy* allows probing of the patient to ascertain their concerns and fears. Physicians should not assume that patients understand what they are told or that they will be compliant with treatment once the examination has concluded. Educating a patient is a task that must be balanced between increasing patient knowledge and understanding while decreasing uncertainty and anxiety. The best way to increase patient awareness of their disease is to use layman terms and present the patient with questions that maintain a bidirectional discussion. The most important question before conveying a disease process is assessing the patient's understanding of "what is going on?"

In discussing the patient's condition, physicians should always try to answer the following questions which appear to be generalized concerns of patients whether they are asked directly or not[109,110]:

- What has happened to me?
- Why has this happened to me?
- What can we do about this and are there any alternatives?
- What are the side effects if this is done?
- Will it hurt?

By the end of the examination, all questions and patient's concerns should be addressed. This will increase patient compliance to treatment and follow-up.

Enlistment

The discussion should conclude with the task of *enlistment*. It is here that the clinician invites the patient to discuss the future path and treatment course that will be taken by the patient. This is another step that requires feedback from the patients to understand if they are comfortable with what was discussed and how they will move forward. Enlistment is the step that determines if an agreement will be made. This maybe a difficult task as many patients who present to the doctor's office have already made their own diagnosis with hopes of affirming it by their encounter with their physician.

All these steps are linked and moving forward to the next without being successful in the previous step will usually lead to failure.

The "LEARN" Model

Race, gender, and culture are all factors that impact effectiveness of communications. These variables must be understood and incorporated into the physician-patient relationship. A model developed by Berlin and Fowkes represents one approach to beginning the learning process of understanding and dealing with diverse groups of patients.[111] The LEARN model consists of the following:

- **L**isten with sympathy and understanding to the patient's perception of the problem.
- **E**xplain your perceptions of the problem and your strategy for treatment.
- **A**cknowledge and discuss the differences and similarities between these perceptions.
- **R**ecommend treatment while remembering the patient's cultural parameters.
- **N**egotiate agreement. It is important to understand the patient's explanatory model so that medical treatment fits into his or her cultural framework.

Using this model, physicians may begin the process of understanding folk illness among different cultures or explaining disease to patients who have no illness. Physicians must understand that being healthy requires a patient to feel a physical, cultural, moral, and social balance.

PATIENT CENTEREDNESS

Patient-centered medical encounters have been described as those that treat "patients as partners in the medical dialogue, rather than as reporters of symptoms."[112] This approach leads patients to become more willing to ask questions or express concerns, and thus, more likely to receive the kind of information about their treatment regimen that they find useful. Physicians not only try to understand the symptoms but seek to facilitate patients' expressions of their thoughts, feelings, and expectations. The patient-centered approach has been associated with better clinical outcomes. Latino patients in visits with interpreters have less patient-centered visits.[112] Physicians have been found to be more verbally dominant and engage in less patient-centered communication with African American patients compared to white patients. Interventions that increase patient centeredness and activate African American patients to enhance participation in their care would be useful strategies to address disparities in health care.[113]

ELIMINATING DISPARITIES IN CARDIOVASCULAR CARE AND OUTCOMES: THE ROADMAP TO 2010

Recent identification of some of the major contributors to observed disparities in CVD outcomes between blacks and whites—a high prevalence of diabetes and other coronary risk factors, patient delays in seeking medical care, delays in diagnosis and treatment of high-risk individuals, and limited access to cardiovascular care—present opportunities to address and reduce disparities. One of the organizations dedicated to eliminating cardiovascular disparities is the Association of Black Cardiologists, Inc. (ABC, Inc.).[114] From August 26–27, 2003, in Atlanta Georgia, the ABC, Inc. convened a special emphasis panel to develop a progressive and achievable set of recommendations to address the issue of disparities. The meeting, entitled "*Eliminating Disparities in Cardiovascular Care and Outcomes: The Roadmap to 2010,*" was cosponsored by ABC, Inc. and the NIH's National Center on Minority Health and Health Disparities, National Institute of Biomedical Imaging and Bioengineering, National Heart, Lung, and Blood Institute (NHLBI), and National Institute of Diabetes and Digestive and Kidney Diseases. The special emphasis panel summarized its findings and recommendations in a report also entitled "*Eliminating Disparities in Cardiovascular Care and Outcomes: The Roadmap to 2010.*"[114] This report identified eight essential themes for increasing capacity, evaluating impact, advancing and implementing

Table 20-2 **Recommendations of the ABC, Inc. for Eliminating Disparities in Cardiovascular Care and Outcomes by 2010**

1. Conduct additional research on access and utilization of low- and high-tech diagnostic procedures
2. Increase access and appropriate utilization of cardiac procedures and therapies
3. Enhance patient education efforts
4. Develop strategies for increasing adherence to evidence-based guidelines
5. Implement policy changes that result in fewer inequities in the health care system/infrastructure
6. Develop and evaluate strategies for optimizing physician-patient communications
7. Expand research that focuses on causes or identified practices in the delivery of care that contribute to health disparities
8. Increase awareness and monitoring of health disparities

Source: Adapted from Ref. 114.

policy, and enlisting regional and national efforts to decrease the high level of morbidity and mortality from CVDs in minority populations. These are summarized below and in Table 20-2.

Barriers and Recommendations to Eliminating Disparities in Cardiovascular Care and Outcomes

1. ACCESS AND UTILIZATION OF LOW- AND HIGH-TECH DIAGNOSTICS

There are limited data on access, utilization, and the value of low-tech diagnostic procedures such as electrocardiography (ECG) for risk assessment in African Americans. A few studies on access to ECG were completed as early as the 1960s. Since then, however, there has been little investigation of the use of ECG, echocardiography, nuclear imaging, or computerized tomography (CT) for African American patients. A better understanding is needed of differences in rates of utilization of these tests and the potential impact on risk assessment and the application of definitive therapies.

Recommendation(s):

1.1 Although some studies are underway, such as the NHLBI funded Multi-Ethnic Study of Atherosclerosis (MESA) trial, there is a need for better prognostic prospective data on the usefulness of a variety of cardiac testing procedures in identifying CVD in the early stages and improved understanding of predictive values of normal and abnormal test results in different racial/ethnic groups. This research should examine both low and high technologies used for risk stratification such as ECG, echo imaging, perfusion imaging, magnetic resonance imaging (MRI), and Computerized tomography (CT). Research should also be conducted to determine whether differences in access exist among racial groups and the potential implication for further therapies.

1.2 Physicians should apply evidence-based cardiovascular guidelines consistently. Improved strategies should be developed for more effective implementation of evidence-based treatment guidelines and the appropriate use of diagnostic studies for evaluation and risk assessment. They should also factor into care plans, the recognition that African Americans often have more aggressive diseases and may be at higher risk than suggested by commonly used risk assessment scoring algorithms.

2. ACCESS AND UTILIZATION OF CARDIAC PROCEDURES AND THERAPIES

Several recent studies have provided evidence of unequal access to cardiac procedures and therapies. In all hospitals, excluding military hospitals, African Americans are less likely than whites to undergo percutaneous transluminal coronary angioplasty (PTCA) or coronary artery bypass grafting (CABG). Since primary care physicians must often refer patients to specialists for diagnostic and therapeutic procedures, provider bias may contribute to limiting access. African American physicians, who may better understand the subtleties of clinical presentations in African American patients, are underrepresented in the cardiovascular specialties and particularly in cardiac group practices—especially in surgery and in large groups that often contract to provide interventional and surgical services to major urban hospitals. Even when African American patients are referred to a specialist, physician bias and perceptions of disease risks may inappropriately affect patients' referral for certain procedures. Furthermore, since African Americans are less likely than whites to receive preliminary diagnostic procedures, such as cardiac catheterization, the numbers of patients referred for interventions and surgery would also be fewer. In addition to increasing access and availability of providers and services, educational efforts that increase health literacy and empower African American patients regarding their therapeutic options are greatly needed.

Structural factors in health care delivery may also influence access to surgery. African Americans are more likely to have publicly funded insurance, such as Medicaid or be enrolled in health maintenance organizations among privately funded plans, two insurance options that may restrict access to and reimbursement levels for surgery. A large number of African American patients report usual care settings as a clinic, a hospital emergency room, or hospital outpatient facility, rather than a doctor's office and many of these hospitals are not equipped for endovascular procedures. These factors limit access to specialists who could provide better care and access to other resources that would support this higher level of care. The recent trends toward regionalization of cardiac surgery may have a greater impact on minority populations than whites.

Recommendation(s):

2.1 Public and private agencies should support more research on access to cardiac surgical procedures to further document disparities and more importantly, to determine why these inequities exist and practices that will lead to greater parity. The specific focus should include investigation of whether the organization of surgical units by region negatively affects access by minorities.

2.2 The Federal government, professional societies, and others should investigate ways to educate minority populations on therapeutic options and what constitutes quality care to better equip them in managing CVD and gaining better access to surgical procedures.

3. PATIENT EDUCATION

Preventing and managing CVD is a joint responsibility of physicians and patients. Among African Americans, insufficient knowledge on disease management as well as a generally lower level of educational attainment hampers effective patient participation in this process. Without a clear understanding of how CVD develops and progresses, African Americans may not seek treatment in the earlier stages or effectively contribute to the management of the disease, when it occurs.

It is generally acknowledged that health is affected by socioeconomic conditions and many of the disparities in health outcomes have roots in historical discrimination and inequities that began centuries ago and continue to have lingering effects today. Educational attainment, for example, is associated, independently of race, with major differences in mortality and may affect the quality of care because of the impact on comprehension of written health materials and numerical instructions, health beliefs, patient preferences, and compliance. African Americans are clustered at the lower end of the socioeconomic stratum, with lower levels of educational attainment. Managing diseases such as CVD that require long-term intervention and sustained behavioral changes require significant patient knowledge about lifestyle issues, as well as competence in tracking measures of improvement.

Recommendation

There is a need to raise awareness of existing educational programs and assist community groups leading these efforts in developing the grantsmanship skills required to sustain funding for effective programs. Financial support for these information dissemination efforts and widespread media campaigns should be increased, especially in the area of disease prevention. Culturally sensitive messages delivered through popular media in community settings, such as churches, worksites, beauty and barbershop may further the reach and impact of these programs. To overcome varying levels of literacy and ensure wide accessibility, an emphasis should be placed on radio and video, rather than written materials. Encouraging and supporting physicians in setting up waiting room televisions for viewing health messages, for example, may contribute to better patient education. Engaging established community organizations in educational programs creates immediate trust through recognized partners. The design of these programs should incorporate the findings of the numerous studies that have been completed on effective intervention for various racial groups and characteristics of successful programs. For example, duplicating for African Americans and other groups, the NHLBI-supported *Salud para su Corazón*, a health education program targeting Hispanics/Latinos and employing trained, lay health educators or *promoters* might be a good beginning. There should be recognition that issues of literacy and self-concept must be addressed through long-term social change.

4. ADHERENCE TO GUIDELINES FOR CARDIOVASCULAR CARE

Cardiovascular care and outcomes for African Americans would improve, if doctors consistently followed established guidelines in caring for all patients. In many instances, African American patients do not receive essential preventive services and necessary therapies. Linking compensation to compliance with accepted guidelines would encourage physicians to consistently follow these recommendations for all patients and likely lead to improvements in patient outcomes. Performance numbers on patient outcomes should also determine compensation for hospitals and other care settings.

Recommendation(s):

4.1 It is generally acknowledged that sufficient guidelines exist for cardiovascular care and more guidelines are not needed. Compensation for physicians and hospitals should reflect adherence to established guidelines. More research is needed to validate this proposition, as well as to suggest other best practices that would encourage more widespread, equitable use of evidence-based guidelines. Hospitals should monitor use of guidelines and the impact of improved compliance on disparity measures.

4.2 Research is needed to better define the barriers to effective and consistent implementation of evidence-based treatment guidelines.

4.3 Current approaches to educating physicians and other providers regarding evidence-based guidelines need to be re-evaluated and new strategies tested, especially for minorities and other difficult-to-treat patient groups.

5. Inequities in the Health Care System/Infrastructure

Structural factors and inequities in health care resources may hamper African Americans in gaining access to quality care. Large numbers of African American patients receive care in urban medical centers or community clinics. In both types of settings, resources may be lacking to deliver the high level of care required for good outcomes. Many urban hospitals are publicly funded and therefore subjected to the vagaries of politics and the government budgeting process. Inadequate or inconsistent funding often results. These institutions must absorb the cost of serving a large number of uninsured patients or patients insured by public health plans such as Medicaid that provide low levels of compensation. Without financial resources, these hospitals cannot offer the comprehensive care, including social and educational services required to address CVD.

Similar obstacles are present in community health care delivery settings where limited resources inhibit provision of preventive services and nonemergent care. These clinics, in many instances, encounter patients who have already experienced a cardiac event, but lack the resources to provide longitudinal services. Community clinics suffer from deficiencies on the most basic level, sometimes operating without data management systems to track and maintain patient data.

Some studies have suggested that the low number of cardiologists being trained, especially African American, and uneven distribution of practicing cardiologists contribute to poor cardiovascular care for African Americans. The limited numbers of practicing cardiologists seem to be concentrated in urban areas. However, both rural and urban African American communities lack the specialists required to meet their needs. Given that CVD is the number one cause of mortality for all Americans, there are not enough appropriately trained physicians to handle this demand.

Recommendation(s):

5.1 The goal of reducing disparities will not be realized unless support is generated for the types of policy changes that will result in fewer inequities in the health care system and access to quality care. Compared to many other industrialized societies, the United States has a fragmented health care delivery system that fails to provide equal care for all. Policy changes should be explored that would lead to the gradual enhancement of care for different segments of the population until universal uniform care is achieved. Recognizing that major policy changes may require a decade or more of discussion to be achieved, professional societies and others should encourage greater dialogue on this issue.

5.2 Measures must also be developed to address inconsistency in funding for large urban medical centers that serve large minority populations. Given the fluctuations in public revenues and spending, financial support from private sources should be identified to supplement and protect budgets during economic downturns.

5.3 Greater overall financial support is also needed in community care settings, but targeting patient data systems may have an immediate impact on patient care. Studies have demonstrated that the use of electronic medical records leads to better outcomes through better identification of patients at risk. Funding for computerized patient data management systems would help doctors manage patients, develop care plans, adhere to established guidelines, and potentially support more research on African American patient populations. An example would be a pilot program under development by the ABC, Inc. to use members' electronic patient records to build a database that could potentially be used for research.

5.4 More health care professionals trained to deliver cardiac care are needed. Because the training of cardiologists requires a significant number of years, consideration should be given to a two-tier system of training to most rapidly deploy cardiac professionals in a short time frame—one traditional to produce a fully trained cardiologists, and a shortened program, perhaps targeted to internists, to prepare physicians to deliver basic preventive cardiac care. Other specialists, such as gynecologists and pediatricians who serve well women and children, should also provide basic preventive care against CVD.

5.5 Given the severity of CVD in the African American community, particular emphasis should be given to training African American cardiologists who have historically provided most services for African American patients. It has been noted that if existing cardiology training programs accepted one African American each year, the number of African American cardiologists could double in 25 years. Recruitment is important, but adequate mentoring is critical to the retention of African American cardiology fellows. The diversity efforts of medical schools should aim to increase the number of African American faculty to contribute to mentoring of students and lessen the racial isolation that hampers the success of these students.

5.6 Incentives should be established to encourage greater diversity in students and faculties of medical schools. Accreditation standards for medical schools should include an assessment of diversity and the impact of diversity status on the quality of care in the local community. Federal funding for medical schools should be linked to the nation's expressed goals on diversity, perhaps becoming a criteria for research funding.

5.7 More financial support from public and private sources for individual minority medical students, including loan-forgiveness or payback programs may encourage more of these students to pursue medicine, given the very high cost of medical education. Many of the existing payback programs seem to be under subscribed. Sponsors of existing service payback programs should evaluate enrollment to determine if there are factors that limit the attractiveness of these options. Enhancement could be effected that may result in deployment of greater numbers of physicians in minority communities.

5.8 The difficulty of attracting and retaining minorities in science-based training and professions has been well documented. Significant enhancements in K-12 math and science instruction must be achieved. Increased financial support for minority undergraduates coupled with continued efforts to attract these students to science focused careers should support an increase in the pool of minority students prepared for medical training. There are some colleges that have an excellent record of medical school acceptance for graduates, such as Xavier University. Replication of the successful elements of this model is needed. Historically, Black Colleges and Universities continue to educate a very large proportion of African American science students. Programs to attract minority medical students should be national in scope, but should target these and other minority serving schools.

6. INEFFECTIVE PHYSICIAN-PATIENT COMMUNICATION

Critical to quality care, effective communication between doctor and patient may not be optimal in the interface between African American patients and their physicians. Negative historical interactions between the health care establishment and minority communities have led to a lack of trust. Racial bias and stereotyping have historically infused medical literature and continue to influence training today. In general, initial or continuing medical education (CME) does not include training on cultural diversity, producing physicians who are not equipped to overcome patient distrust or to understand the cultural nuances that may dictate different approaches in communicating with minority patients. Without exposure to health disparities in training, physicians are not prepared to incorporate issues raised in health disparities research such as differences in disease presentation and diagnostic and therapeutic evaluation when serving African American patients. Current CME lectures on health disparities and diversity do not offer the depth of training needed to produce behavioral change.

Several studies have concluded that racial concordance between physician and patient results in better care, as patients have expressed a higher level of trust in these circumstances and exhibited a greater level of compliance with treatment. Frequent achievement of this match in cardiovascular care is hampered by the continuing underrepresentation of African Americans in medical training, especially cardiology. Numerous factors feed into these low numbers as noted above, including inadequate K-12 and undergraduate science preparation, inadequate efforts to recruit, retain, and support African American medical students through initial and specialty training, and diminished support for public policies such as affirmative action that, in recent decades led to increased opportunities for African Americans in medical schools.

Language barriers contribute to poor quality care, particularly in communities with large immigrant populations. Language differences often cause patients to delay or avoid care or to misinterpret care instructions. In many health care settings, these problems may not be recognized or addressed.

Recommendation(s):

6.1 Initial medical education and CME should include training in health disparities. Using the cross-disciplinary integration of women's health into the medical curriculum as a model, medical schools should add health disparities training that include patient care considerations raised by health disparities research and cultural competency education. This training would allow physicians to potentially improve care and outcomes for minority patients and to understand general and personal biases and cultural ignorance that raise barriers to quality care. Similar training should be made available to practicing physicians through CME. As some states have done for HIV/AIDS and domestic violence training, health disparities training should be added to relicensure requirements.

6.2 As noted above, significant efforts must be put forth to increase the number of minorities completing medical training, especially in cardiology.

6.3 Support services that address language differences should be expanded, especially in the Border States and New York, where there are large immigrant populations. Professional interpretation services and culturally competent allied health professionals to assist with disease management plans are two measures that could significantly improve care for these populations.

7. HEALTH DISPARITIES RESEARCH

Despite much public discussion on health disparities over the last few decades, the Nation's biomedical research enterprise has not expanded or changed significantly to encompass an increased emphasis in these areas. While many studies have been completed that demonstrate the existence of disparities, few have pointed to causes or identified practices in the delivery of care that may lead to a reduction or elimination of these differences. Data collection to support health disparities research is inadequate. The current prevalent structure of biomedical research, including concentrated investigation in a single discipline in academic institutions, may not be optimal for addressing health disparities that call for examination from multiple perspectives. Representation of minorities in clinical research as investigators, allied health, or patients is limited, diminishing the impact and effectiveness of these studies. More research and different approaches are needed.

Recommendation(s):

7.1 Funding should be provided to support more health disparities research, particularly in the following areas:

- Cardiovascular care practices that lead to a reduction in disparities
- Differences in CABG and PTCA/PCI outcomes across ethnic groups
- The construct of race and ethnicity in novel risk factor research
- The level of contribution of traditional and novel risk factors to CVD burden
- Gene-environment interactions and risk factor clustering
- The effect of training experiences in urban hospitals on later care practices
- Differences in the effectiveness of current CVD therapies across racial and ethnic groups
- New technologies that will identify individuals at high risk for CVD
- Differences in the interpretation of diagnostic tests across racial and ethnic groups
- More longitudinal studies on CVD in African Americans

7.2 Research resources should be improved and the traditional approach to biomedical research be altered to accommodate the multidisciplinary issues involved in health disparities. Better data collection are needed at all levels—national, state, and local to monitor and track disparities. Funding agencies should support and encourage more collaborations and partnerships in research to accommodate the multifaceted nature of health disparities issues. Academic institutions should be encouraged to join with community centers to pursue multidisciplinary projects, incorporating all of the socioeconomic considerations of health disparities. As an incentive for scientists to work in these areas, NIH should establish an academic award for outstanding work in health disparities and perhaps give special consideration to institutional training grant applicants with a health disparities focus.

7.3 Measures should be taken to increase minority participation in clinical research on all levels. Much more effort should be exerted to attract minority medical students to careers in research to ensure that clinical research questions incorporate diverse perspectives and to support retention of minority patients in clinical projects. The high level of debt that minorities incur in obtaining medical training may discourage work in research when compensation for practicing physicians can be so much higher. While federal funding is available for research costs and some loan repayment, medical schools should seek private sources of discretionary funding as an incentive for minorities to pursue academic careers. Formal targeted mentoring programs should be encouraged to provide minority students greater exposure to research careers and the support network to be successful.

7.4 Allied health professionals play a major role in recruiting and retaining minority patients in clinical studies. Similar to the participation of minority researchers, the presence of a diverse group of allied health professionals encourages trust among minority patients. Success in promoting a study and gaining a commitment to participate can be more easily achieved if personnel are culturally similar to the target populations. For these reasons, investigators for projects targeting minority populations should be sensitive to the need for a diverse project team.

8. AWARENESS AND MONITORING OF HEALTH CARE DISPARITIES

Elimination of health disparities will not be achieved unless general awareness is increased. Several surveys have indicated that a large number of people in the United States are not convinced that health disparities exist, believing instead that minorities enjoy equal access to care and receive the same quality of care. Even within the medical establishment, practicing physicians often demonstrate little understanding of the severity of these problems. Many of the policy changes that must occur in the society—the processes of health care delivery and medical training—will not move forward without greater discussion of these issues on a broader level.

Recommendation(s):

8.1 Federal agencies, professional medical societies, and all concerned about disparities must work to encourage more dialogue on key policy issues on a national level. Medical professional societies can play a major role in these efforts. Greater diversity in the leadership of these groups may support elevation in priority for health disparities issues.

8.2 Efforts should be made to raise awareness of the objectives outlined in Healthy People 2010 and to track and monitor health disparity indices defined in this document.

CONCLUSION

Disparities in cardiovascular health and outcomes continue to exist. This is due to multiple factors including excessive risk factor burden, patient delays in seeking medical care, underrecognition and undertreatment of high-risk individuals, and lack of access to routine and modern cardiac medical and procedural care. Reduction and ultimate elimination of disparities in cardiovascular health and outcomes requires dedicated commitment and immediate action at the provider-patient level, from local, state, and national health agencies, from professional medical associations, and from others within and beyond the health sector.

The future of controlling diabetes and CVD is promising. However, new medications and treatments are only effective if patients understand them and are compliant in taking them. Recent scientific advances make understanding disease better today than at any other time in history. Effective communication and translation of this health information and knowledge to our patients are essential if these advances are to translate into effective reduction and ultimate elimination of health care disparities.

REFERENCES

1. American Heart Association. Heart Disease and Stroke Statistics—2006 Update. Available at: http://www.americanheart.org (accessed on May 8, 2006).

2. Anderson R, Smith B. *Deaths: Leading Causes for 2001. National Vital Statistics Reports*, Vol. 52, no. 9. Hyattsville, MD: National Center for Health Statistics, 2003.

3. Gillum RF. Coronary heart disease in black populations I, mortality and morbidity. *Am Heart J* 1982;104:839–851.

4. Gillum RF, Graham CT. Coronary heart disease in black populations II, risk factors. *Am Heart J* 1982;104:852–864.

5. Clark LT, Ferdinand KC, Flack JM, et al. Coronary heart disease in African Americans. *Heart Dis* 2001;3:97–108.

6. Centers for Disease Control and Prevention (CDC). Disparities in premature deaths from heart disease—50 states and the District of Columbia, 2001. *MMWR Morb Mortal Wkly Rep* 2004;53:121–125.

7. Clark LT. Issues in minority health: atherosclerosis and coronary heart disease in African Americans. *Med Clin North Am* 2005;89(5):977–1001.

8. Francis CK, Grant AO. Report of the Working Group on Research in Coronary Heart Disease in Blacks. National Institutes of Health, U.S. Department of Health and Human Services, 1994.

9. Traven N, Kuller L, Ives D. Coronary heart disease mortality and sudden death among the 35–44 year age group in Allegheny County, Pennsylvania. *Ann Epidemiol* 1996;6:130–136.

10. Gillium R, Mussolino M, Madans J. Coronary heart disease incidence and survival in African-American women and men. The NHANES I epidemiologic follow-up study. *Ann Intern Med* 1997;127:111–118.

11. Gillium R. Sudden cardiac death in Hispanic Americans and African Americans. *Am J Public Health* 1997;87:1461–1466.

12. Available at: http://www.cdc.gov/nchshome.htm.

13. National Institutes of Health. *Addressing Health Disparities. The NIH Program of Action. What are Health Disparities?* Available at: http://healthdisparities.nih.gov/whatare.html (accessed on May 12, 2006).

14. Smedley BD, Stith AY, Nelson AR, eds. Committee on Understanding and Eliminating Racial and Ethnic Disparities in Health Care Unequal Treatment: Confronting Racial and Ethnic Disparities in Health Care. Washington, DC: The National Academies Press, 2003.

15. U.S. Department of Health and Human Services. *Report of the Secretary's Task Force on Black and Minority Health, Volume 4: Cardiovascular and Cerebrovascular Diseases*. Washington, DC: U.S. Department of Health and Human Services, 1986.

16. Rev. Martin Luther King Jr. Speech delivered at the Second National Convention of the Medical Committee for Human Rights, Chicago, March 25, 1966.

17. NMA History. Available at: http://www.nmanet.org/History.htm (accessed on May 14, 2006).

18. The Henry J. Kaiser Family Foundation and American College of Cardiology Foundation. *Racial/Ethnic Differences in Cardiac Care: The Weight of the Evidence Summary Report*. Menlo Park, CA: The Henry J. Kaiser Family Foundation and American College of Cardiology Foundation, 2000.

19. Pincus T, Esther R, DeWalt DA, et al. Social conditions and self management are more powerful determinants of health than access to care. *Ann Intern Med* 1998;129:406–411.

20. Rowland ML, Fulwood R. Coronary heart disease risk factor trends in blacks between the First and Second National Health and Nutrition Examination Surveys, United States, 1971–1980. *Am Heart J* 1984;108:771–779.

21. Cutter GR, Burke GL, Dyer AR, et al. Cardiovascular risk factors in young adults. The CARDIA baseline monograph. *Control Clin Trials* 1991;12:1S–25S, 51S–77S.

22. Hutchinson RG, Watson RL, Davis CE, et al. Racial differences in risk factors for atherosclerosis. The ARIC study. *Angiology* 1997;48:279–290.

23. Neaton JD, Kuller LH, Wentworth D, et al. Total and cardiovascular mortality in relation to cigarette smoking, serum cholesterol concentration, and diastolic blood pressure among black and white males followed up for five years. *Am Heart J* 1984;108:759–769.

24. Cooper RS, Liao Y, Rotimi C. Is hypertension more severe among US blacks, or is severe hypertension more common? *Ann Epidemiol* 1996;6:173–180.

25. Liao Y, Cooper RS, McGee DL, et al. The relative effects of left ventricular hypertrophy, coronary artery disease, and ventricular dysfunction on survival among black adults. *JAMA* 1995;273:1592–1597.

26. Gavin JR III. Diabetes in minorities: reflections on the medical dilemma and the healthcare crisis. *Trans Am Clin Climatol Assoc* 1995;107:213–223.

27. Moliterno DJ, Jokinen EV, Miserez AR, et al. No association between plasma lipoprotein(a) concentrations and the presence or absence of coronary atherosclerosis in African-Americans. *Arterioscler Thromb Vasc Biol* 1995;15:850–855.

28. Guyton JR, Dahlen GH, Patsch W, et al. Relationship of plasma lipoprotein Lp(a) levels to race and to apolipoprotein B. *Arteriosclerosis* 1985;5:265–272.

29. Sorrentino MJ, Vielhauer C, Eisenbart JD, et al. Plasma lipoprotein(a) protein concentration and coronary artery disease in black patients compared with white patients. *Am J Med* 1992;93:658–662.

30. Schreiner PJ, Heiss G, Tyroler HA, et al. Race and gender differences in the association of Lp(a) with carotid artery wall thickness. The Atherosclerosis Risk in Communities (ARIC) study. *Arterioscler Thromb Vasc Biol* 1996;16:471–478.

31. Ford ES, Giles WH, Dietz WH. Prevalence of the metabolic syndrome among US adults: findings from the Third National Health and Nutritional Examination Survey. *JAMA* 2002;287:356–359.

32. Hunt KJ, Williams K, Resendez RG, et al. All-cause and cardiovascular mortality among diabetic participants in the San Antonio Heart Study: evidence against the "Hispanic Paradox." *Diabetes Care* 2002;25(9):1557–1563.

33. Markides KS, Coreil J. The health of Hispanics in the southwestern United States: an epidemiologic paradox. *Public Health Rep* 1986;101:253–265.

34. Liao Y, Cooper RS, Cao G, et al. Mortality from coronary heart disease and car-diovascular disease among adult U.S. Hispanics: findings from the National Health Interview Survey (1986 to 1994). *J Am Coll Cardiol* 1997;30:1200–1205.

35. Harris MI, Flegal KM, Cowie CC, et al. Prevalence of diabetes, impaired fasting glucose, and impaired glucose tolerance in US adults. The Third National Health and Nutrition Examination Survey, 1988–1994. *Diabetes Care* 1998;21:518–524.

36. Carter JS, Pugh JA, Monterrosa A. Non–insulin-dependent diabetes mellitus in minorities in the United States. *Ann Intern Med* 1996;125:221–232.

37. Folsom AR, Szklo M, Stevens J, et al. A prospective study of coronary heart dis-ease in relation to fasting insulin, glucose, and diabetes. The Atherosclerosis Risk in Communities (ARIC) study. *Diabetes Care* 1997;20:935–942.

38. Chin MH, Zhang JX, Merrell K. Diabetes in the African-American Medicare population. Morbidity, quality of care, and resource utilization. *Diabetes Care* 1998;21:1090–1095.

39. Haffner SM. Epidemiology of type 2 diabetes: risk factors. *Diabetes Care* 1998; 21(Suppl 3):C3–C6.

40. Brancati FL, Kao WHL, Folsom AR, et al. Incident type 2 diabetes mellitus in African American and white adults. The Atherosclerosis Risk in Communities study. *JAMA* 2000;283:2253–2259.

41. Bonds DE, Zaccaro DJ, Karter AJ, et al. Ethnic and racial differences in diabetes care: the Insulin Resistance Atherosclerosis Study. *Diabetes Care* 2003;26:1040–1046.

42. Dagogo-Jack S, Gavin JR III. Diabetes. In: Satcher D, Pamies RJ, eds. *Multicultural Medicine and Health Disparities*. New York: McGraw-Hill, 2005:181–196.

43. King H, Aubert RE, Herman WH. Global burden of diabetes, 1995–2025. Prevalence, numerical estimates, and projections. *Diabetes Care* 1998;21:1414–1431.

44. Brunzell JD, Hokanson JE. Dyslipidemia of central obesity and insulin resis-tance. *Diabetes Care* 1999;22:C10–C13.

45. Bjorntorp P. Body fat distribution, insulin resistance, and metabolic diseases. *Nutrition* 1997;13:795–803.

46. Bonow RO. Primary prevention of cardiovascular disease: a call to action. *Circulation* 2002;106;3140–3141.

47. Flegal KM, Carroll MD, Ogden CL, et al. Prevalence and trends in obesity among US adults, 1999–2000. *JAMA* 2002;288:1723–1727.

48. Flegal KM, Carroll MD, Kuczmarski RJ, et al. Overweight and obesity in the United States: prevalence and trends, 1960-1994. *Int J Obes Relat Metab Disord* 1998;22:39–47.

49. Perry AC, Applegate EB, Jackson ML, et al. Racial differences in visceral adipose tissue but not anthropometric markers of health-related variables. *J Appl Physiol* 2000;89:636–643.

50. Sesso HD, Paffenbarger RS, Lee I. Physical activity and coronary heart disease in men. *Circulation* 2000;102:975–980.

51. Thompson PD, Buchner D, Pina IL, et al. Exercise and physical activity in the pre-vention and treatment of atherosclerotic cardiovascular disease: a statement from the Council on Clinical Cardiology (Subcommittee on Exercise, Rehabilitation,

and Prevention) and the Council on Nutrition, Physical Activity, and Metabolism (Subcommittee on Physical Activity). *Circulation* 2003;107:3109–3116.

52. Centers for Disease Control. Prevalence of cigarette use among 14 racial/ethnic populations—United Status, 1999-2001. *MMWR Morb Mortal Wkly Rep* 2004;53: 49–52.

53. Choi WS, Okuyemi KS, Kaur H, et al. Comparison of smoking relapse curves among African-American smokers. *Addict Behav* 2004;29(8):1679–1683.

54. Okuyemi KS, Ebersole-Robinson M, Nazir N, et al. African-American menthol and nonmenthol smokers: differences in smoking and cessation experiences. *J Natl Med Assoc* 2004;96(9):1208–1211.

55. Third Report of the National Cholesterol Education Program (NCEP) Expert Panel on Detection, Evaluation, and Treatment of High Blood Cholesterol in Adults (Adult Treatment Panel III) Final Report. *Circulation* 2002;106:3146–3421.

56. Grundy SM, Cleeman JI, Daniels SR, et al. Diagnosis and management of the metabolic syndrome. An American Heart Association/National Heart, Lung, and Blood Institute Scientific Statement. *Circulation* 2005;112:2735–2752.

57. Grundy SM, Brewer HB Jr, Cleeman JI, et al. for the Conference Participants. Definition of Metabolic Syndrome: Report of the National Heart, Lung, and Blood Institute/American Heart Association Conference on Scientific Issues Related to Definition. *Circulation* 2004;109:433–438.

58. Whittle J, Kressin NR, Peterson ED, et al. Racial differences in prevalence of coronary obstructions among men with positive nuclear imaging studies. *Ann Intern Med* 2006;47:2034–2041.

59. Stone PH, Thompson B, Anderson HV, et al. for the TIMI III Registry Study Group. Influence of race, sex and age on management of unstable angina and non-Q-wave myocardial infarction. *JAMA* 1996;275:1104–1112.

60. Simmons BE, Castaner A, Campo A, et al. Coronary artery disease in blacks of lower socioeconomic status: angiographic findings from the Cook Country Hospital Heart Disease Registry. *Am Heart J* 1989;116:90–97.

61. Maynard C, Fisher LD, Passamani ER. Survival of black persons compared with white persons in the Coronary Artery Surgery Study (CASS). *Am J Cardiol* 1987;60: 513–518.

62. Thomas J, Thomas DJ, Pearson T, et al. Cardiovascular disease in African-American and white physicians: the Meharry Cohort and Meharry-Hopkins Cohort Studies. *J Health Care Poor Underserved* 1997;8:270–283.

63. Davies MJ. The role of plaque pathology in coronary thrombosis. *Clin Cardiol* 1997;20:(Suppl I):I-2–I-7.

64. Fuster V. Acute coronary syndromes: the degree and morphology of coronary stenoses. *J Am Coll Cardiol* 2000;35:52B–54B.

65. Falk E, Shah PK, Fuster V. Coronary plaque disruption. *Circulation* 1995;92: 657B–671B.

66. Selwyn AP, Kinlay S, Creager M, et al. Cell dysfunction in atherosclerosis and the ischemic manifestations of coronary artery disease. *Am J Cardiol* 1997;79: 17–23.

67. Glasser SP, Selwyn AP, Ganz P. Atherosclerosis: risk factors and the vascular endothelium. *Am Heart J* 1996;131:379–384.

68. Ambrose JA, Fuster V. The risk of coronary occlusion is not proportional to the prior severity of coronary stenosis. *Heart* 1998;79:3–4.

69. Nakamura Y, Moss AJ, Brown MW, et al. Ethnicity and long-term outcome after an acute coronary event. Multicenter Myocardial Ischemia Research Group. *Am Heart J* 1999;138:500–506.

70. Asher CR, Topol EJ, Moliterno DJ. Insights into the pathophysiology of atherosclerosis prognosis of black Americans with acute coronary syndromes. *Am Heart J* 1999;138:1073–1081.

71. Clark LT, Bellam SV, Shah AH, et al. Analysis of prehospital delay among inner-city patients with symptoms of myocardial infarction: implications for the therapeutic intervention. *J Natl Med Assoc* 1992;84:931–937.

72. Cooper RS, Simmons B, Castaner A, et al. Survival rates and prehospital delay during myocardial infarction among black persons. *Am J Cardiol* 1986;57:208–211.

73. Crawford SL, McGraw SA, Smith KW, et al. Do blacks and whites differ in their use of health care for symptoms of coronary heart disease? *Am J Public Health* 1994;84:957–964.

74. Dracup K, Moser DK, Eisenberg M, et al. Causes of delay in seeking treatment for heart attack symptoms. *Soc Sci Med* 1995;40:379–392.

75. Summers RL, Cooper GJ, Carlton FB, et al. Prevalence of atypical chest pain descriptions in a population from the southern United States. *Am J Med Sci* 1999;318:142–145.

76. Ghali JK, Cooper RS, Kowatly I, et al. Delay between onset of chest pain and arrival to the coronary care unit among minority and disadvantaged patients. *J Natl Med Assoc* 1993;85:180–184.

77. Johnson PA, Lee TH, Cook EF, et al. Effect of race on the presentation and management of patients with acute chest pain. *Ann Intern Med* 1993;118:593–601.

78. Taylor HA Jr, Canto JG, Sanderson B, et al. Management and outcomes for black patients with acute myocardial infarction in the reperfusion era. *Am J Cardiol* 1998;82:1019–1023.

79. Raczynski JM, Taylor H, Cutter G, et al. Diagnoses, symptoms, and attribution of symptoms among black and white inpatients admitted for coronary heart disease. *Am J Public Health* 1994;84:951–956.

80. Venkat A, Hoekstra J, Lindsell C, et al. The impact of race on the acute management of chest pain. *Acad Emerg Med* 2003;10:1199–1208.

81. Antman EM, Anbe DT, Armstrong PW, et al. Management of patients with STEMI: executive summary. *J Am Coll Cardiol* 2004;44:671–719.

82. Braunwald E, Antman E, Beasley J, et al. ACC/AHA 2002 guideline update for the management of patients with unstable angina and non-ST-segment elevation myocardial infarction. *J Am Coll Cardiol* 2002;40(7):1366–1374.

83. Cannon C, Weintraub W, Demopoulos L, et al. Comparison of early invasive and conservative strategies in patients with unstable coronary syndromes treated with the glycoprotein IIb/IIIa inhibitor tirofiban (TACTICS-TIMI 18). *N Engl J Med* 2001;344(25):1879–1887.

84. Fox K, Poole-Wilson P, Henderon R, et al. Interventional versus conservative treatment for patients with unstable angina or non-ST-elevation myocardial infarction: the British Heart Foundation RITA 3 randomized trial. Randomized Intervention Trial of unstable Angina. *Lancet* 2002;360:743–751.

85. Leape LL, Hilborne LH, Bell R, et al. Underuse of cardiac procedures: do women, ethnic minorities, and the uninsured fail to receive needed revascularization? *Ann Intern Med* 1999;130:183–192.

86. Scirica BM, Molitterno DJ, Every NR, et al. for the GUARANTEE Investigators. Racial differences in the management of unstable angina: results from the multicenter GUARANTEE registry. *Am Heart J* 1999;138:1065–1072.

87. Weitzman S, Cooper L, Chamblesss L, et al. Gender, racial, and geographic differences in the performance of cardiac diagnostic and therapeutic procedures for hospitalized acute myocardial infarction in four states. *Am J Cardiol* 1997;79: 722–726.

88. Gillum RF, Gillum BS, Francis CK, Coronary revascularization and cardiac catheterization in the United States: trends in racial differences. *J Am Coll Cardiol* 1997;29:1557–1562.

89. Peterson ED, Shaw LK, DeLong ER, et al. Racial variation in the use of coronary-revascularization procedures. Are the differences real? Do they matter? *N Engl J Med* 1997;336:480–486.

90. Wu AH, Parsons L, Every NR, et al. Hospital outcomes in patients presenting with congestive heart failure complicating acute myocardial infarction: a report from the Second National Registry of Myocardial Infarction (NRMI-2). *J Am Coll Cardiol* 2002;40:1389–1394.

91. Sonel AF, Good CB, Mulgund J, et al. for the CRUSADE Investigators Racial Variations in Treatment and Outcomes of Black and White Patients With High-Risk Non–ST-Elevation Acute Coronary Syndromes. Insights From CRUSADE (Can Rapid Risk Stratification of Unstable Angina Patients Suppress Adverse Outcomes With Early Implementation of the ACC/AHA Guidelines?) *Circulation* 2005;111:1225–1232.

92. Strauss EW, Straus A. *Medical Marvels: The 100 Greatest Advances in Medicine.* Amherst, New York: Prometheus Books, 2006.

93. Ashton CM, Haidet P, Paterniti DA, et al. Racial and ethnic disparities in the use of health services: bias, preferences, or poor communication? *J Gen Intern Med* 2003;18:146–152.

94. Mull JD. Cross-cultural communication in the physician's office. *West J Med* 1993;159:609–613.

95. Clark LT. Improving compliance and increasing control of hypertension: needs of the special hypertensive populations. *Am Heart J* 1991;121:664–669.

96. Aikens JE, Bingham R, Piette JD. Patient-provider communication and self-care behavior among type 2 diabetes patients. Diabetes Educ 2005;31:681–690.

97. In the Right Words: addressing language and culture in providing health care. Issues in brief #18. August 2003. Based on Grantmakers in Health Issue dialogue. Available at www.gih.org and http://www.calendow.org/reference/publications/cultural_competence.stm. Accessed Sept 28, 2006.

98. The Commonwealth Fund 2001 Health Care Quality Survey. Available at: http://www.cmwf.org/surveys/surveys_show.htm?doc_id=228171 (accessed on May 22, 2006).

99. Cooper-Patrick L, Gallo JJ, Gonzales JJ, et al. Race, gender, and partnership in the patient-physician relationship. *JAMA* 1999;282:583–589.

100. Saha S, Komaromy M, Koepsell TD, et al. Patient-physician racial concordance and the perceived quality and use of health care. *Arch Intern Med.* 1999;159: 997–1004.

101. Aberegg SK, Terry PB. Medical decision making and healthcare disparities: the physician's role. *J Lab Clin Med* 2004;144:11–17.

102. Corbie-Smith G, Thomas SB, St George DMM. Distrust, race, and research. *Arch Intern Med* 2002;162:2458–2463.

103. U.S. Department of Health & Human Services, Office of Disease Prevention & Health Promotion. Healthy People 2010, 2000.

104. Sarasohn-Kahn J. Reducing health disparities through improved communication. IhealthBeat. Available at: www.http://ihealthbeat.org/members/basecontent.asp?oldcoll=&program=1&contented=23616&collectionid=583.

105. Schillinger D, Grumbach K, Piette J, et al. Association of health literacy with diabetes outcomes. *JAMA* 2002;288:475–482.

106. American Medical Association Foundation. Facts about health literacy, 2000. Available at: www.ama-assn.org/ama/pub/article/3125-3308.html.

107. Cross T, Bazron B, Dennis K, et al. *Towards A Culturally Competent System of Care, Volume I.* Washington, DC: Georgetown University Child Development Center, CASSP Technical Assistance Center, 1989.

108. Office of Minority Health: Center for Linguistic and Cultural Competence in Health Care. Final CLAS report, policies, initiatives, and laws. Available at: http://www.omhrc.gov/clas/.

109. Mock KD. Effective clinician-patient communication. *Physicians News Digest* 2001.

110. Institute for health care communication. Available at: http://www.healthcare.org/ Accessed on September 28, 2006.

111. Berlin EA, Fowkes WC. Teaching framework for cross-cultural care: application in family practice. *West J Med* 1983;139(6):934–938.

112. Rivadeneyra R. Patient centeredness in medical encounters requiring an interpreter. *Am J Med* 2000;108:470–474.

113. Johnson RL, Roter D, Powe NR, et al. Patient race/ethnicity and quality of patient-physician communication during medical visits. *Am J Public Health* 2004;94:2084–2090.

114. Association of Black Cardiologists, Inc. Eliminating disparities in cardiovascular care and outcomes: the roadmap to 2010. *ABC Digest of Urban Cardiology* 2005;31(1): 12–25. Available at: http://www.nibib.nih.gov/nibib/File/News%20and%20Events/ABC-NIH_Final_Report-06-01-04.pdf.

BEST PRACTICES:
A CHRONIC CARE MODEL
APPROACH TO DIABETES
AND HEART FAILURE

Karen Scott Collins
Reba Williams
Luther T. Clark

INTRODUCTION

Patients with diabetes and heart disease are at high risk for acute life-threatening complications. However, both diabetes and heart disease are chronic illnesses which require ongoing long-term management and risk factor control for optimal outcomes. Recent clinical and technologic advances for diabetes and cardiovascular disease management provide great potential for increasing patient compliance, improving quality of life and health outcomes. Nevertheless, unless the health care systems in which patients receive treatment are also addressed, the disparities between the quality of health care that is delivered and the quality of health care that could be delivered will remain considerable.[1]

Health care systems and medical centers vary widely in how they manage patients with chronic illnesses. One approach to addressing some of the known deficiencies in existing health care management systems for diseases such as diabetes and heart disease is the Chronic Care Model (CCM) developed by Edward H. Wagner and colleagues at the W.A. MacColl Institute for Health Care Innovation at the Center for Health Studies Group Health Cooperative of Puget Sound in Seattle, Washington.[2-5] Wagner's CCM provides a new paradigm for improving treatment and outcomes in patients with chronic illnesses. It has specific applications in quality improvement, policy development, and research. In this chapter, we describe Wagner's CCM as a framework for treating patients with diabetes and cardiovascular diseases, and the impact of implementing this program on the treatment of diabetes and heart failure in the largest municipal hospital system in the United States, the New York City Health and Hospitals Corporation (NYCHHC).

BURDEN OF CHRONIC ILLNESSES IN THE UNITED STATES AND NEW YORK CITY

According to the U.S. Department of Health and Human Services, chronic illnesses account for 70% of deaths in the United States with associated expenditures estimated to be more than 75% of the nation's $1.5 trillion annual health care costs.[2,5] Additionally, hundreds of billions of dollars are spent annually in indirect costs, resulting from lost productivity and nonreimbursable personal costs. The Centers for Disease Control and Prevention estimates that more than 90 million Americans live with a chronic illness and that as many as 25 million Americans suffer from a disabling chronic condition.[5]

The New York City (NYC) Department of Health and Mental Hygiene's 2003 Community Health Survey reports that New York City residents are living longer than ever at a time when the city still faces significant health care challenges. Some statistics that highlight the problem include the following: more than 500,000 New Yorkers report needing care in the past 12 months, but not receiving it, suggesting a health care access issue.[6] Heart disease is still the no. 1 cause of death in NYC regardless of race, ethnicity, or sex. In 2004, 23,000 New Yorkers died from heart disease. Almost one-third of the people who died from cardiovascular disease were under the age of 75. Seventy four percent (74%) of New York residents have at least one cardiovascular risk factor. Risk factors for heart disease include diabetes, hypertension, and hyperlipidemia. Diabetes has been diagnosed in 8% of New Yorkers (454,000 people). Up to one-third of persons with cardiovascular risk factors including diabetes are not aware that they have the condition. At-risk ethnic groups in the city such as African Americans and Hispanics are more likely to die as a result of these conditions than their white or Asian counterparts. By addressing chronic illness care through an organized process, we can save thousands of New Yorker's lives. NYCHHC has a commitment to protect and serve all New Yorkers including the most vulnerable and at-risk groups. Complications due to chronic illnesses such as diabetes and heart failure disproportionately affect the most vulnerable New Yorkers served by NYCHHC. This makes developing a model health care delivery system to standardize and ensure that the highest quality care is rendered to New York residents more compelling.[6,7]

Diabetes and Heart Failure

Diabetes is a complex and increasingly common chronic disease. It requires lifelong medical and quality-of-life adjustments and frequent visits with health care providers. Diabetes increases the risk for ischemic heart disease, stroke, end-stage renal disease, peripheral vascular disease, nontraumatic lower extremity amputation, blindness, and neuropathy. Often, individuals first become aware of diabetes when confronted with one of its major complications (e.g., heart disease, blindness, stroke, or kidney problems). NYC Department of Health and Mental Hygiene reports that 454,000 New Yorkers have diabetes and another 500,000 are unaware of their disease status.[6,7] Diabetes and its complications account for approximately 10% of all health care expenses in the United States—more than $132 billion yearly.[8]

Heart failure is a major, escalating health problem in the United States. It is a chronic, long-term disease, although it can sometimes develop suddenly. It is most common in persons over the age of 65 years and the primary reason for hospitalization in this group. Heart failure is one of the top diagnostic-related groups at NYCHHC facilities. Men have a higher rate of heart failure than do women, and African Americans are at particularly increased risk.[9,10] Heart failure increases risk for death, functional decline, and hospitalization. Approximately 4.7 million Americans have symptomatic heart failure, a prevalence that is expected to increase to 10 million during the next three decades. The annual incidence of new heart failure cases is approximately 550,000 per year.[11]

Diabetes and heart failure pose an undue societal burden due to exorbitant direct and indirect cost for providing care management and delivery.[12] The extraordinarily high costs of chronic disease management, as exemplified by diabetes and heart failure, demonstrate the need for developing novel strategies to improve delivery of care to individuals with chronic conditions.

THE CHRONIC CARE MODEL

Several years ago, it became clear that changes in the approach to certain chronic illnesses were necessary in order to overcome identified deficiencies and increase the number of chronically ill patients receiving appropriate high quality medical care.[13] Numerous national and international studies have documented that chronic illnesses are often uncontrolled and that patients are unhappy with their current health care.[13] Failure to receive appropriate health care can be explained in part by reduced access and low levels of quality, particularly in underserved communities.[14]

According to a recent survey of 4000 patients conducted in five countries (Australia, Canada, New Zealand, United Kingdom, and the United States), 33–49% of respondents were not given advice on health risk behaviors and 47–67% were not asked for their opinions about treatment.[15] In the United States, estimates suggest that 40% of individuals with a chronic condition do not receive adequate health care.[4] Of the traditional care that is dispensed, 20% is deemed clinically inappropriate. New evidence has demonstrated that effective disease management systems can yield better outcomes than usual care. In essence, health care delivery needs to be transformed from a system that is basically reactive, responding mainly when a person is sick, to one that is proactive and focused on maintaining wellness.[3,4,16]

Wagner et al. developed the CCM to guide primary care providers in delivering quality chronic illness management leading to improved patient outcomes.[3,4,17] The goal is to produce improved outcomes through more productive interactions between patients and their clinical team. This evidence-based model, which first appeared in its current format in 1998,[29] identifies six elements key to improving care—community, the health system, self-management support (SMS), delivery system design, decision support, and clinical information systems. The CCM provides a template to standardized chronic care delivery and management. Health care systems that effect care delivery changes in the six areas of the CCM can expect improved clinical and process outcomes for patients as evidenced by the NYCHHC experience. Overall, the CCM focuses on the delivery of safe, effective, timely, patient-centered, efficient, and equitable health care.

In 2003, a panel of national experts, supported by the Robert Wood Johnson Foundation, further refined and revised the model.[8] The updated model was then tested nationally by the MacColl Institute, a program referred to as "Improving Chronic Illness Care (ICIC)."[19] As a result of these efforts, five new themes were incorporated into the CCM:

- Patient safety (in health system)
- Cultural competency (in delivery system design)
- Care coordination (in health system and clinical information systems)
- Community policies (in community resources and policies)
- Case management (in delivery system design)

In addition to the ICIC, several other initiatives have assessed the validity and utility of the CCM and found that it compared well relative to other leading chronic disease programs.[20,21,22] Since chronic illnesses are very prevalent in underserved communities, some investigators have wondered whether the CCM is translatable into these communities. However, the model has been demonstrated to significantly improve clinical and behavioral outcomes in patients with diabetes and in the underserved community.[23,24] Currently, the CCM is used in numerous, diverse health systems, including the NYCHHC, the Bureau of Primary Health Care hospital systems, state Medicaid agencies, and has been incorporated into work by the World Health Organization (WHO).

As noted by Wagner et al.,[3,4,21,25,26] traditional health care practices are ill-suited to address the needs of patients and families struggling with chronic

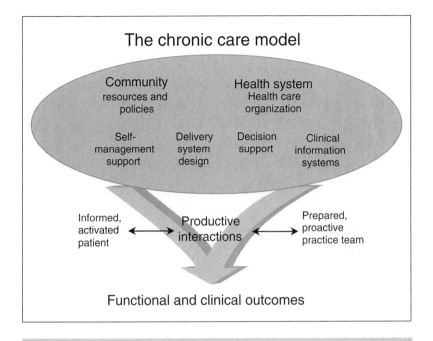

Figure 21-1 **The CCM was developed by Wagner, MD, MPH, Director of the MacColl Institute for Healthcare Innovation, Group Health Cooperative of Puget Sound.** *(Source: Adapted with permission from ICIC is a national program supported by The Robert Wood Johnson Foundation with direction and technical assistance provided by Group Health Cooperative's MacColl Institute for Healthcare Innovation and Wagner EH. Chronic disease management: What will it take to improve care for chronic illness? Effective Clinical Practice. 1998;1:2–4).*

illnesses, as these practices are mainly conceived to treat patients with acute conditions. In these conditions, the focus is on triage and patient flow, short appointments, diagnosis and treatment, reliance on prescriptions, brief patient education, and follow-up care. Relative to level of care provided to acutely ill patients, individuals with chronic illnesses require planned, regular interactions with their caretakers, while focusing on improving function and preventing exacerbations of their conditions.[19] Wagner et al. developed a model (see Fig. 21-1) for ICIC that incorporates state-of-the-art improvement initiatives and intervention strategies.[3,17] Accordingly, the model suggests that the patient-provider interactions resulting in health care that improves outcomes are found in health systems that:

- Have well-developed processes and incentives for making changes in the health care delivery system.

- Assure behaviorally sophisticated SMS that gives priority to increasing patients' confidence and skills so that they can be the ultimate manager of their illnesses.
- Reorganize team function and practice systems (e.g., appointments and follow-up) to meet the needs of chronically ill patients.
- Develop and implement evidence-based guidelines and support those guidelines through provider education, reminders, and increased interaction between generalists and specialists.
- Enhance information systems to facilitate the development of disease registries, tracking systems, and reminders and to give feedback on performance.

The CCM identifies the essential elements of a health care system that encourages high quality chronic disease care (see Fig. 21-1). These elements are the community, the health system, SMS, delivery system design, decision support, and clinical information systems. The major objectives of each element of the CCM are listed below. Each element is a principle for redesigning care and represents broad concepts that may be summarized as follows:

Self-Management Support

- Empower and prepare patients to manage their health and health care.
- Emphasize the patients' central role in managing their health.
- Use effective SMS strategies that include assessment, goal-setting, action planning, problem-solving, and follow-up care.
- Organize internal and community resources to provide ongoing SMS to patients.

Delivery System Design

- Assure the delivery of effective, efficient clinical care and SMS.
- Define roles and distribute tasks among team members.
- Use planned interactions to support evidence-based care.
- Provide clinical case management services for complex patients.
- Ensure regular follow-up by the care team.
- Give care that patients understand and that fits with their cultural background.

Decision Support

- Promote clinical care that is consistent with scientific evidence and patient preferences.
- Embed evidence-based guidelines into daily clinical practice.
- Integrate specialist expertise and primary care.
- Use proven provider education methods.
- Share evidence-based guidelines and information with patients to encourage their participation.

Clinical Information System

- Organize patient and population data to facilitate efficient and effective care.
- Provide timely reminders for providers and patients.
- Identify relevant subpopulations for proactive care.
- Facilitate individual patient care planning.
- Share information with patients and providers to coordinate care.
- Monitor performance of practice team and care system.

Health Care Organization

- Create a culture, organization, and mechanisms that promote safe, high quality care.
- Visibly support improvement at all levels of the organization, beginning with the senior leader.
- Promote effective improvement strategies aimed at comprehensive system change.
- Encourage open and systematic handling of errors and quality problems to improve care.
- Provide incentives based on quality of care.
- Develop agreements that facilitate care coordination within and across organizations.

Community

- Mobilize community resources to meet needs of patients.
- Encourage patients to participate in effective community programs.
- Form partnerships with community organizations to support and develop interventions that fill gaps in needed services.
- Advocate for policies to improve patient care.

Wagner's CCM assumes that the locus of care remains with the personal physician, anchored by an integrated practice team. Targeting and case management activities, sometimes known as carve-ins or carve-outs, do not always make this assumption. In fact, many tend to operate on four major premises:

1. Reduction in the cost of chronic illness is the major goal and is assumed to be associated with improvements in health.
2. The best way to achieve cost reduction is to focus on the highest-cost patients in the chronically ill population.
3. Primary care is not up to the task of chronic illness care.
4. Patients will do better if their chronic disease management is largely removed from primary care and is delegated to a case manager.

The CCM promotes effective change in provider groups by providing an organizational framework to support evidence-based clinical and quality improvement across a wide variety of health care settings. This model (Fig. 21-1) summarizes the basic elements for improving care in health systems at the community, organization, practice, and patient levels.

The New York City Health and Hospitals Corporation

The NYCHHC is a public benefit corporation created by legislation in 1970 and governed by a Board of Directors, to oversee the City's public health care system. NYCHHC's mission is to extend equally to all New Yorkers, regardless of their ability to pay, comprehensive health services of the highest quality in an atmosphere of humane care, dignity, and respect. The corporation promotes and protects, as innovator and advocate, the health, welfare, and safety of the people of the City of New York. We join with other health workers and with communities in a partnership that will enable each of its institutions to promote and protect health in its fullest sense, the total physical, mental, and social well-being of the people of New York. Total wellness in body, mind, and spirit is the goal of NYCHHC.

The NYCHHC consists of 11 acute care hospitals, 6 diagnostic and treatment centers, 4 long-term care facilities, a certified home health care agency, and more than 80 community health clinics, including Communicare Centers and Child Health Clinics. Through its wholly owned subsidiary, MetroPlus, NYCHHC operates a Health Plan, which enrolls members in no or low cost insurance plans such as Medicaid, Child Health Plus, and Family Health Plus. NYCHHC facilities treat 1.3 million New Yorkers annually including nearly one-fifth of all general hospital discharges in NYC and 5.5 million ambulatory care clinic visits.

NYCHHC Chronic Disease Initiatives: Diabetes and Heart Failure Collaboratives

Creation of the NYCHHC Chronic Disease Collaborative and implementation of Wagner's CCM within its corporate structure has effectuated meaningful system-wide changes leading to improved patient management in an urban, underserved, at-risk community.

NYCHHC has been particularly concerned with improving care delivery and management of chronic diseases such as diabetes and heart disease. The corporation has identified various barriers to care within the organization that must be addressed to implement and sustain comprehensive, quality health care management and delivery. Some of the specific issues targeted by the collaborative teams include:

- Wide variation in clinical practice
- Lack of care coordination among health providers
- Inadequate follow-up to ensure optimal treatment outcomes
- Inadequately trained patients to manage their own illnesses

In 2003, the NYCHHC launched Diabetes and Heart Failure Collaboratives with the goal of redesigning existing systems to improve care and outcomes for patients with diabetes and/or heart failure. Beginning with 17 teams drawn from ambulatory practices across all of NYCHHC, the *Collaborative* subsequently expanded to 28 teams, including new teams for depression and pediatric asthma, and pediatric diabetes. The *Collaborative* focuses on improving control of key clinical risk factors, using available data and information systems to support proactive care, and improving use of SMS strategies by clinicians and patients. Successful strategies for improving outcomes are being tested, implemented, and spread throughout NYCHHC facilities. The long-term goal is to maximize the length and quality of life for people with chronic diseases, such as diabetes, heart failure, depression, and asthma, and to satisfy patient and caregiver needs in a cost-effective manner. This signals an important shift in the treatment paradigm for chronic diseases, which is now being implemented in health management systems around the world.

The participating teams are supported in their work by NYCHHC and collaborative faculty in partnership with the ICIC Program of Group Health Cooperative, and the Institute for Health Care Improvement (IHI). NYCHHC collaborative faculty is comprised of internal (corporate) and external experts who are available to provide guidance and support to the teams during weekly and monthly conference calls, monthly site visits, and quarterly learning sessions or as needed. The principles adapted by NYCHHC to improve care delivery in the management of chronic diseases are based on the CCM, IHI's Breakthrough Series Collaborative and the Model for Improvement.

Collaborative Clinical Priorities

Diabetes and heart failure were the initial clinical areas of focus in the NYCHHC collaborative. Clinical priorities, or collaborative objectives, for each of these conditions were set through consensus meetings with NYCHHC clinical leadership and guidance from Dr. Wagner, ICIC, and IHI staff. Specific measures were adapted and followed throughout the collaborative work based on these priorities. For diabetes, the priorities included:

- Glycemic control
- Prevention of micro- and macrovascular complications
- Prevention of cardiovascular complications
- Self-management

For heart failure the priorities included:

- Reduction in hospitalizations
- Appropriate use of angiotensin-converting enzyme inhibitors (ACE-I) and angiotensin receptor blockers (ARBs)

- Appropriate use of beta-blockers
- Self-management

The Chronic Care Model as Used by the NYCHHC

All NYCHHC teams utilize a multifaceted, organizational approach to caring for people with chronic disease in a primary care setting as defined by the CCM. It represents a corporate shift from the reactive, acute-illness approach to a population-based system, which uses practical, supportive, evidenced-based interactions between an informed, activated patient and a prepared, proactive practice team. The NYCHHC Diabetes and Heart Failure Improvement Collaboratives utilize principles of the CCM developed by Wagner and the IHI Breakthrough Series methods for improvement collaboratives to guide primary care providers in delivering quality chronic illness care. The NYCHHC adaptation of this evidence-based model identifies six elements key to improving care: SMS, delivery system design, decision support, clinical information systems, health care organization, and community resources. Improvement teams were selected by local medical directors at NYCHHC facilities. Team members include some combination of the following staff: primary care provider, nurse, social worker, health educator, patient care associate, or clinic administrative staff. Patient (pilot) populations of focus (POF) were between 100 and 150 patients belonging to the primary care provider in the team. POF have since grown to their present size. Team members receive coaching and teaching on core elements of the CCM, how to develop and initiate change concepts at their facilities, and how to implement improvements that have proven beneficial and sustainable in the organization. Teams are supported with a core NYCHHC collaborative staff, collaborative faculty who are experts in chronic disease care and improvement, an access database registry, "change package" of practice changes and ideas to test, weekly and monthly phone calls, and quarterly learning sessions. Teams participate in weekly team meetings at the facilities, conduct small tests of change (Plan-D-Study-Act [PDSAs]), collect and report data on their population of focus, as well as on results of changes tested, meet with their local senior leadership, and participate in calls and learning sessions. A dedicated corporate intranet site houses all tools, learning session materials, and team reports. Teams share data with faculty, senior leadership, and other teams through the HHC Chronic Disease Collaborative intranet web site. The web site is also used to provide continual update to the team's recent advances in clinical care and provides access to tools.

By November 2005, more than 4600 patients were in the NYCHHC collaborative registries including 2800 persons with diabetes and 412 persons with heart failure. Also, the number of physicians using the CCM increased from 25 to 86. Clinical results for diabetes measures include patients with low-density lipoprotein cholesterol (LDL-C) <100 increased from 35 to 62%; blood pressure <130/80 increased from 30 to 54%; HgA1c <7 increased from

Table 21-1   **Results of NYCHHC Initiatives in the Management of Patients with Diabetes and Heart Failure**

Improvements in outcomes using the CCM (2003–2005)

Number of patients treated = 2800 diabetics, 412 heart failure
For diabetes patients:
   Percent with LDL <100 increased from 35 to 62%
   30% with blood pressure 130/80 at baseline increased to 54%
   Percent with self-management plans increased from 19 to 72%
   Percent with HgA1c <7 increased from 24 to 47%
For heart failure patients:
   Percent of appropriate patients on ACE-I, ARB, and beta-blockers—above
   90% in the first 2 months remain between 90 and 100%
   Percent of patients receiving follow-up within 14 days ranged from 50 to 100%

24 to 47%. The percent of patients with self-management plans increased from 19 to 72%; foot examinations from 12 to 52%. Clinical results for heart failure measures include: 30-day readmission rates 0–2%; 14-day follow-up ranged from 50 to 100% across four teams; ACE-I, ARB, and beta-blocker usage 75–100%. Self-management goals are addressed by all teams (Table 21-1).

A key message for provider teams and system leadership has been that improvements in patient outcomes, the focus of this work, do not come without working on several aspects of the overall delivery of care. Collaborative teams that realized significant improvement worked in all areas of the CCM. At NYCHHC, the collaborative teams developed and worked on several hundred (>400) specific changes that are applicable across the system. The CCM provides broad guidance on the key components of care delivery which must be addressed to improve patient outcomes; the work of the improvement teams and leadership at NYCHHC has been to use that guidance and then develop specific changes or interventions which are possible and sustainable in this system. These changes form the framework for the chronic disease delivery model at NYCHHC. Changes that have been shown to be effective in multiple NYCHHC sites and possible to incorporate into the delivery system include: using a registry to identify patients; proactively calling patients in for visits; establishing a planned visit approach; increasing access to clinic appointments; group medical visits; setting self-management goals; multiple reinforcements of the clinical goals (i.e., report cards for patients and providers) and postvisit follow-up (Table 21-2).

Impact of Implementation of NYCHHC Care Model

Using the CCM framework to guide changes in care and follow a common set of patient-based outcomes measures has shown its value in improving

Table 21-2 *The NYCHHC Adaptation of the CCM Used at All Corporate Facilities*

CRP	SMS	DSD	DS	CIS	HCO
Home care	Action plan	Redeploy staff to	Treatment	Registry on	Provide dedicated
Telehealth	Develop:	do additional or	protocols	the network server	collaborative times
Resource list	1. SMG	different duties	Reminders,	Registry uses:	Educate all staff regarding
	2. Tools	Planned visits:	ticklers, or	1. To identify outliers	the collaborative
	3. Checklist	1. Fast track	stamps	2. To identify patients	Foster collaboration
	4. Instruction sheets	2. Mini visit		lost to follow-up	between departments
	Follow-up calls and	3. Specialty visit		3. To identify patients	Redeploy staff to
	letters to patients	Open access		for planned/	appropriate functions
	Assign staff to set	sessions		group visits	Facilitate scheduling
	SMG with patient	Follow-up		4. To obtain contact	changes
		letters		information	
				5. To generate provider-	
				specific feedback	
				6. To track clinical	
				measures	
				Clinical ticklers	
				or reminders	

CRP = Community Resources and Policies; SMS = Self Management Support; DSD = Delivery System Design; DS = Decision Support; CIS = Clinical Information Systems; HCO = Health Care Organization; CCM = Chronic Care Model; NYCHHC = New York City Health and Hospitals Corporation patient outcomes in a public hospital delivery system (Table 21-1). The CCM has highlighted the importance of focusing on multiple, related aspects of delivering quality chronic disease care, and has particularly introduced self-management support and use of clinical information systems as critical to good chronic illness care. These two components were significantly underused/underdeveloped aspects of NYHHC's system.

Work on SMS required an initial focus on distinguishing this new, interactive approach to working with patients, from the more passive, provider-driven patient education approaches traditionally used. The key aspects of training staff on SMS have been to help them develop the understanding of how this differs from education, and how to work with patients on SMS in time-efficient manners. NYCHHC clinical staff have come far with helping patients set SMS goals, using simple goal setting sheets, incorporating SMS into the visit with physician, as well as follow-up from the nurse or health educator. In many clinics, standard fields for self-management goals have now been incorporated into the electronic medical record.

The CCM has also stressed the role of a registry in supporting the ability to manage a population of chronically ill patients. The development and use of registries to track our chronically ill patients, identify patients requiring specific care, and assess overall performance on key indicators has been one of the major system-wide changes of the chronic disease improvement work. The registries have progressed from stand-alone ACCESS Database registries for the pilot teams and their patients to a new corporate wide, web-based registry linked to an electronic medical record. This gives NYCHHC the ability to truly focus on entire populations receiving care from its facilities, and reduces the burdens of data collection by automating the transfer of patient data from the medical record to the registry (for review by the patient's care team). Increasingly, physicians, other clinical providers, and leadership can think in terms of the whole populations they are caring for, not just individual patients, and see how well patients are doing, or where more focus is needed. This provides a powerful tool for effecting change.

Key changes in what the CCM calls delivery system design are also becoming more standard. "Planned visits" refers to a visit in which the provider team is prepared to see the patient about their chronic illness(es)—key staff are in the clinic, key information on the patient is available, and the visit will include SMS as well as clinical management. Some NYCHHC clinics have also begun group medical visits, finding strong patient acceptance and increased efficiency with respect to physician time and ability to work on SMS. Group visits is an example where testing on a small scale has been very valuable. Many teams initially assumed patients would not want to participate, and have been surprised with the high level of participation and acceptance among patients. Nevertheless, we have also learned that an effective group visit requires excellent preparation and coordination on the part of multiple staff members.

Using the improvement models of teams working collaboratively, sharing experiences (successes and failures), sharing tools developed, "tricks" learned on how to get something done in the system has created a strong grounding and format for chronic disease improvement across this very large system. It has also contributed to a change in culture, such that exchange across NYCHHC clinics or asking colleagues at another NYCHHC facility for help are becoming more acceptable ways of interacting, rather than maintaining separate, more competitive "silos" within the system. The other powerful improvement tool has been the Model for Improvement, with a focus on both measurement and small tests of change—PDSA—cycles. Encouraging teams to test new ideas on a small scale has increased innovation, empowered more staff members to be part of change, and reduces time spent discussing why something will not work. If there's an idea someone's proposed but unsure about, we encourage him or her to do a small test and see what he or she learns.

Finally, a focus on a common set of measures has set the standard and expectations for care systemwide. These measures and goals are now incorporated into other aspects of the system, including the health plan's Pay for Performance initiative, significant reinforcement of what the collaborative started.

EXPANDING WAGNER'S CHRONIC CARE MODEL

British Columbia's Expanded Chronic Care Model

The CCM has gone through several stages of refinement and expansion. One important refinement has to do with the integration of the health system into the community framework.[27] This was necessary and reflects the realization that many resources needed to help patients manage their conditions do not exist in the health system, rather they are accessible within the community. More recently, the CCM has been studied further and as a result it has been expanded. One of the expanded models was offered by investigators from British Columbia, referred to as the British Columbia's Expanded CCM.[28] Besides the basic six elements: the community, the health system, SMS, delivery system design, decision support, and clinical information systems, they added health promotion and disease prevention. They believe that application of the expanded model can achieve better health outcomes, resulting in healthier patients, more satisfied providers, and more cost-effective expenditure of health care resources.

The Innovative Care for Chronic Conditions

The Innovative Care for Chronic Conditions (ICCC) represents an international adaptation of the CCM spearheaded by the WHO.[29] The WHO considered various programmatic options in response to the growing prevalence of chronic conditions and the ensuing need to help countries transform their health care systems. Several steps were taken to ensure the applicability of the CCM in developing countries. It was then necessary that WHO convene health leaders from several countries in Africa, Asia, Eastern Europe, and Latin America to review the CCM to ensure that it met the needs of their respective countries. Those leaders were in agreement that the adapted CCM could serve as a basis for policy development and system changes. Subsequent to this convention, the participating leaders revised the CCM. This resulted in the ICCC framework (see Fig. 21-2).[30] It should be noted that the current framework includes components at the micro (patient and family), meso (health care organization and community), and macro (policy) levels. One drawback that has been identified is that the framework does not prescribe what specific aspects must be tailored to unique needs and resources. Nonetheless, it highlights the need for comprehensive system (re)design, which is believed to be an essential requirement to foster effective care.

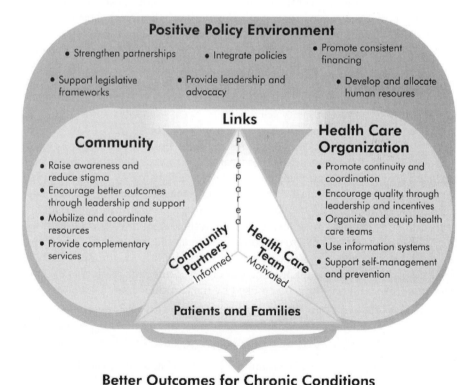

Figure 21-2 **The Innovative Care for Chronic Conditions.** (Source: Adapted with permission from Epping-Jordan JE, Pruitt,SD, Bengoa R, et al. Improving the quality of health care for chronic conditions. Qual Saf Health Care 2004;13:299–305.)

CONCLUSION

The CCM has been demonstrated to be effective in managing diabetes and heart failure in underserved communities.[24] It remains uncertain, however, how to sustain some of the innovative changes the collaborative teams have developed in the resource constrained public health systems most often providing care to underserved populations. In addition, further testing and development of model components will need to continue in order to effectively address working with different ethnic groups, cross-cultural differences, language barriers, and low health literacy—all key considerations in improving clinical outcomes in underserved communities. Presently, NYCHHC is working with its Limited English Proficiency Program to develop multilingual, culturally sensitive tools to be used by health care providers and patients in improving SMS. In many instances, these user-friendly tools have been incorporated into the electronic medical record for adaptation and use by clinical providers. In addition, several facilities use group sessions and care managers to engage patients and families in their care with much success especially with Asian, African American, and Hispanic populations. Given the diverse ethnic groups of New York Sate and other similar geographic areas, cultural differences need to be addressed to ensure the efficacy of CCMs. This is imperative as individuals have different values and expectations about the type of care they desire as they venture in differing health care venues. This constitutes one of the areas of interest of the NYCHHC.

While work continues to refine the approach to chronic illness care at NYCHHC, the system has made progress over the past 2 years with respect to some of the key challenges identified early on. Development of care teams, planned visit sessions, and use of a chronic disease registry have all contributed to improving coordination of care and a more proactive approach to management. The focus on SMS is altering the approach to working with patients, increasing engagement in their care. Finally, system-wide attention to key quality indicators in chronic illness outcomes has created an environment in which a common set of objectives is driving the work; high level attention to these indicators from senior leadership and our board of directors reinforces the clinical guidelines and protocols being used by the clinical teams.

REFERENCES

1. Bodenheimer T, Wagner EH, Grumbach K. Improving primary care for patients with chronic illness: the chronic care model, Part 2. *JAMA* 2002;288:1909–1914.

2. Kenny SJ, Smith PJ, Goldschmid MG. Survey of physician practice behaviors related to diabetes mellitus in the U.S. Physician adherence to consensus recommendations. *Diabetes Care* 1993;16:1507–1510.

3. Wagner EH, Austin BT, Von Korff M. Improving outcomes in chronic illness. *Manag Care Q* 1996;4:12–25.

4. Wagner EH, Austin BT, Von Korff M. Organizing care for patients with chronic illness. *Milbank Q* 1996;74:511–544.

5. Partnership for Solutions: Johns Hopkins University, Baltimore, MD for the Robert Wood Johnson Foundation (September 2004 Update). Chronic Conditions: Making the Case for Ongoing Care, 2004.

6. Disparities in New York City, A Report of the New York City Department of Health and Mental Hygiene. Available at: http://www.nyc.gov/html/doh/downloads/pdf/epi/disparities-2004.pdf.

7. NYC Vital Signs, A Report from the New York City Community Health Survey, Vol. 2, No. 8, 2003.

8. The Burden of Heart Disease, Stroke, Cancer, and Diabetes, United States. Available at: http://www.cdc.gov/nccdphp/burdenbook2004/Section02/diabetes.htm (accessed May 24, 2006).

9. Clark LT, Ferdinand KC, Flack JM, et al. Coronary heart disease in African Americans. *Heart Dis* 2001;3:97–108.

10. Clark LT. Issues in minority health: atherosclerosis and coronary heart disease in African Americans. *Med Clin North Am* 2005;89:977–1001.

11. American Heart Association. Heart Disease and Stroke Statistics—2004 Update. Dallas, TXx: American Heart Association, 2003.

12. American Diabetes Association. Standards of medical care in diabetes 2006. *Diabetes Care* 2006;29:S4–S42.

13. Wagner EH. Managed care and chronic illness: health services research needs. *Health Serv Res* 1997;32:702–714.

14. U.S. Department of Health and Human Services. National healthcare disparities report. Rockville, MD: Agency for Healthcare Research and Quality (AHRQ), 2003.

15. Blendon RJ, Schoen C, DesRoches CM. et al. Common concerns among diverse systems: health care experiences in five countries. *Health Aff (Millwood)* 2003;22:106–121.

16. Calkins E, Boult C, Wagner E, et al. *New Ways to Care for Older People: Building Systems Based on Evidence.* New York: Springer, 1999:1026–1031.

17. Wagner EH. Chronic disease management: what will it take to improve care for chronic illness? Available at: http://www.acponline.org/journals/ecp/augsep98/cdm.htm (accessed June 1, 2006).

18. The Chronic Disease Crisis. Robert Wood Johnson Foundation. Available at: http://www.healthyresources.com/editorials/ (accessed June 1, 2006).

19. Overview of the Chronic Care Model. Available at: http://www.improvingchroniccare.org/change/model/components.html (accessed June 1, 2006).

20. Wagner EH, Austin BT, Davis C, et al. Improving chronic illness care: translating evidence into action. *Health Aff (Millwood)* 2001;20:64–78.

21. Wagner EH. Chronic disease management: What will it take to improve care for chronic illness? *Effective Clinical Practice.* 1998;1:2–4.

22. Von Korff M, Gruman J, Schaefer J, et al. Collaborative management of chronic illness. *Ann Intern Med* 1997;127:1097–1102.

23. McCulloch DK, Price MJ, Hindmarsh M, et al. A population-based approach to diabetes management in a primary care setting: early results and lessons learned. *Eff Clin Pract* 1998;1:12–22.

24. Piatt GA, Orchard TJ, Emerson S, et al. Translating the chronic care model into the community: results from a randomized controlled trial of a multifaceted diabetes care intervention. *Diabetes Care* 2006;29:811–817.

25. Wagner EH, Bennett SM, Austin BT, et al. Finding common ground: patient-centeredness and evidence-based chronic illness care. *J Altern Complement Med* 2005;11(Suppl 1):S7–S15.

26. Strakowski SM, Stoll AL, Tohen M, et al. The Tridimensional Personality Questionnaire as a predictor of six-month outcome in first episode mania. *Psychiatry Res* 1993;48:1–8.

27. Austin B, Wagner E, Hindmarsh M, et al. Elements of effective chronic care: a model for optimizing outcomes for the chronically ill. *Epilepsy Behav* 2000;1:S15–S20.

28. British Columbia's Expanded Chronic Care Model. Available at: http://www.hlth.gov.bc.ca/cdm/cdminbc/chronic_care_model.html (accessed June 2, 2006).

29. Epping-Jordan JE, Pruitt, SD, Bengoa R, et al. Improving the quality of health care for chronic conditions. *Qual Saf Health Care* 2004;13:299–305.

30. World Health Organization. Innovative care for chronic conditions: building blocks for action. Geneva: World Health Organization, 2002.

CARDIOVASCULAR

DISEASE IN PEOPLE

WITH DIABETES:

FUTURE OUTLOOK

Luther T. Clark
Roman Royzman
Samy I. McFarlane

THE TYPE 2 DIABETES EPIDEMIC

The epidemic of diabetes mellitus continues unabated in the United States and worldwide despite the fact that diabetes is potentially preventable and its major complications treatable. The increased cardiovascular disease (CVD) morbidity and mortality associated with diabetes threaten to reverse the gains in CVD outcomes and the declining CVD mortality trend of the past several decades. The pandemic of obesity, an increasingly sedentary lifestyle, rising prevalence of other major CVD risk factors, aging population, and poor metabolic control in diabetics all contribute to this burgeoning health crisis. Obesity, in particular central obesity, is the major reason for the striking increase in type 2 diabetes—and associated complications—among adults and children. The staggering impact of diabetes and its complications—specifically, CVD—on individuals, health care costs, and health care delivery mandate (1) intensive efforts to prevent diabetes, (2) for those that have diabetes, intensive control of diabetes to prevent CVD and other complications, (3) for those that have CVD, optimal management of their CVD in addition to intensive control of diabetes and other risk factors, and (4) renewed and expanded efforts to develop more effective prevention and treatment strategies.

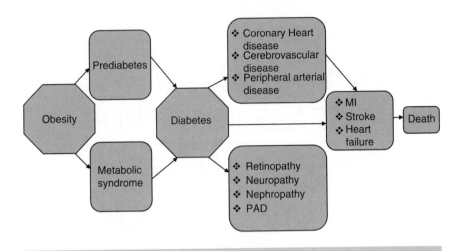

Figure 22-1 **Progression of obesity to diabetes and associated complications.**

New therapies, new technologies, and a changing clinical paradigm may provide unprecedented opportunities to unravel and control the diabetes—CVD conundrum. While the prevalence of diabetes continues to grow, concerted efforts are being made to curb this devastating epidemic and to prevent its complications.[1-14] These efforts include those aimed at prevention of diabetes in the high-risk population,[5,7,15-17] notably lifestyle interventions that have been shown in randomized-controlled trials to be even more effective than pharmacologic agents in diabetes prevention[5,7]; treatment strategies focusing on self-management; use of emerging medical informatics (information technology [IT]) and technologies (i.e., the modern closed loop monitoring).[3,4] Recent treatment advances include utilization of novel therapeutic agents that help reduce the cardiovascular risk in diabetes, the use of novel insulin delivery systems,[9,14] and other far-reaching efforts that include islet cell replacement and genetic testing (Fig. 22-1).[8,12]

PREVENTION OF DIABETES

Although the prevalence of diabetes continues to increase in the United States and worldwide, diabetes is a potentially preventable disease. Many cases of type 2 diabetes can be prevented or delayed through simple lifestyle modifications since susceptible individuals can be identified and a number of the major risk factors for diabetes (Table 22-1) are modifiable.[5,13] Prevention strategies should take full advantage of the recent clinical trial findings demonstrating that progression to type 2 diabetes can be prevented in many individuals with prediabetes and that lifestyle intervention is about twice as effective as medication.[15]

Table 22-1   **Interventions to Prevent Diabetes**

Diet and exercise	DPP
	Finnish Diabetes Prevention Study
Metformin	DPP
HMG-CoA reductase inhibitors (statins)	WOSCOPS
Acarbose	STOP-NIDDM
	Dutch Acarbose Intervention Study (DAISI)
ACE inhibitors	CAPPP, HOPE, DREAM
ARBs	LIFE, NAVIGATOR
TZD	TRIPOD, DREAM
Nateglinide	NAVIGATOR
Bezafibrate	Bezafibrate Infarction Prevention Study (BIP)
Orlistat	XENDOS

INTERVENTIONS TO PREVENT TYPE 2 DIABETES

Lifestyle Changes

Two large studies, the Diabetes Prevention Program[15] and the Finnish Diabetes Prevention Study[16] demonstrated that lifestyle changes can prevent progression of prediabetes to frank diabetes. The two studies showed that dietary modification (low-calorie and reduced fat intake), and moderate-intensity physical activity of at least 150 minutes per week, resulted in a 58% reduction in the number of participants with prediabetes (impaired fasting glucose [IFG] or impaired glucose tolerance [IGT]) who progressed to diabetes over the next 4 years.

Exercise

The protective effects of physical activity have been demonstrated in prospective cohort studies,[17,18] where the development of type 2 diabetes was significantly lower in patients who exercised regularly, even after adjustment for obesity, hypertension, and family history of diabetes. Exercise improves insulin sensitivity and peripheral glucose uptake, and leads to more efficient energy use by increasing mitochondrial enzymes, the number of slow-switch muscle fibers, and the generation of new capillaries.[5,19] Furthermore, exercise promotes translocation of insulin-responsive glucose transporters (GLUT-4) to the cell surface during exercise, enhancing glucose uptake and increasing insulin sensitivity.[20]

The Finnish Diabetes Prevention Study[16] evaluated the effects of diet and exercise on the progression from IGT to diabetes in 522 middle-aged overweight subjects followed for 3.2 years. Patients in the intervention group received individualized counseling aimed at reducing weight, total intake of fat and intake of saturated fat, and increasing intake of fiber and physical activity. After 4 years, the cumulative incidence of diabetes was 11% in the intervention group and 23% in the control group, a 58% reduction in the risk. Reduction in the incidence of diabetes was directly related to lifestyle changes.[16]

Weight Loss

Obesity, in particular central obesity,[21] is the major reason for the striking increase in type 2 diabetes among adults and children. In addition to preventive measures for overweight and obesity, effective treatment is needed for those who are already obese and those who don't respond favorably to preventive programs. In a prospective randomized-controlled study involving 154 overweight individuals with family history of diabetes (one or both parents), modest weight loss of 4.5 kg reduced the risk of type 2 diabetes by approximately 30% compared with no weight loss.[22]

In addition to dietary approaches,[22,23] some patients may benefit from pharmacologic therapy. Two of the main obesity drugs currently available include (1) sibutramine, a centrally acting inhibitor of noradrenaline and serotonin reuptake that decreases caloric intake and increases energy expenditure; and (2) orlistat, a specific lipase inhibitor that impairs fat absorption, thereby reducing fat uptake. A number of other drugs are being evaluated in clinical trials for obesity including the first in the new class of cannabinoid receptor blocking agent, rimonabant—which also appears to have favorable effects on other cardiometabolic risk factors.[24,25] For severely obese patients (>40 body mass index [BMI] or at least 100 lb over ideal weight) with medical problems such as diabetes, hypertension, and sleep apnea, surgical treatment maybe an option.

Dietary Intervention

High dietary fat intake increases risk for the development of type 2 diabetes[26,27] independent of weight gain. Decreasing fat intake improves glucose tolerance and reduces or delays development of type 2 diabetes and IGT.[28] Diet plus exercise reduces risk more than either diet or exercise alone.[15,16,29]

PHARMACOLOGIC INTERVENTIONS

In those individuals for whom lifestyle changes are not enough to normalize blood glucose, several drugs have been shown to reduce the development of diabetes (Table 22-1).

Table 22-2 **Risk Factors for Type 2 Diabetes**

Overweight (BMI ≥25 kg/m^2)

Lifestyle (physical inactivity, high-caloric, high fat intake, cigarette smoking, urbanization)

Family history of type 2 diabetes (i.e., parents or siblings with diabetes)

Race/ethnicity (e.g., African Americans, Hispanic Americans, Native Americans, Asian Americans, and Pacific Islanders)

Gestational diabetes

Impaired fasting plasma glucose (≥100 mg/dL to ≤125 mg/dL)

IGT 2 h plasma glucose (≥140 mg/dL to 199 mg/dL)

Dyslipidemia (low HDL-C, high triglycerides)

Hypertension

Polycystic ovary syndrome

Source: Adapted from Refs. 2 and 4.

Biguanides (Metformin)

Metformin is a potent insulin-sensitizing agent that acts primarily by suppressing hepatic glucose production.[30] Metformin inhibits free fatty acid (FFA) production and oxidation, thereby reducing FFA-induced insulin resistance and hepatic glucose production.[30] In the Diabetes Prevention Program (DPP) trial,[15] metformin reduced the progression of prediabetes to diabetes by 31%, compared with placebo, less risk reduction than that seen in the lifestyle-intervention group (58%). Metformin also has favorable effects in patients with the metabolic syndrome.[31]

Thiazolidinediones

Thiazolidinediones (TZDs) can delay or prevent the onset of type 2 diabetes.[14,32] The mechanism of action of TZDs involves binding to the peroxisome proliferator-activated receptor gamma (PPAR-γ), a transcription factor that regulates the expression of specific genes, especially in fat cells, but also in other tissues.[14] TZD prevention of diabetes is proportional to the reduction in plasma insulin[32]—consistent with the belief that TZDs prevent diabetes by ameliorating insulin resistance. TZDs interfere with the expression and release of mediators of insulin resistance originating in adipose tissue (e.g., FFAs, adipocytokines, such as tumor necrosis factor α, resistin, and adiponectin) in a way that result in net improvement of insulin sensitivity in muscle and liver.[33]

Alpha-Glucosidase Inhibitors

The alpha-glucosidase inhibitors such as acarbose improve glycemic control in type 2 diabetes mellitus. Acarbose decreases postprandial blood glucose, improves both insulin secretion and sensitivity,[34] and increases noninsulin reversion of IGT to normal glucose.[35]

ACE Inhibitors and ARBS

Angiotensin-converting enzyme (ACE) inhibitors and angiotensin receptor blockers (ARBs) reduce the incidence of type 2 diabetes as a secondary outcome measurement.[36–39] The mechanism by which ACE inhibition and, perhaps, ARB therapy reduce the development of type 2 diabetes in patients at risk is not clear. Several hypotheses have been proposed.[40–42] There appears to be postreceptor insulin-signaling abnormalities associated with insulin resistance that are accentuated by angiotensin II.[40,41] Thus, interruption of the renin-angiotensin system may be one mechanism for improving insulin sensitivity, and thereby preventing or delaying the onset of diabetes.[40]

Statins and Diabetes Prevention

In a subanalysis of the West of Scotland Coronary Prevention Study (WOSCOPS),[43] pravastatin therapy reduced the risk of developing diabetes by 30%. These findings, however, have not been shown in other studies, and the evidence to date for diabetes prevention with statins remains inconclusive. Additional research is necessary to clarify the role of statins alone and in combination for diabetes prevention.

CARDIOVASCULAR DISEASE PREVENTION IN TYPE 2 DIABETES

Diabetes and CVD are strongly correlated and are associated bidirectionally with increased risk. Cardiovascular risk factors in persons with diabetes include conventional risk factors, more diabetes-specific risk factors, and emerging risk factors. Most of the factors contributing to the excess risk in diabetics are modifiable and thus, opportunities for prevention and risk reduction are great. Since diabetes, hypertension, and dyslipidemia tend to cluster in patients with CVD, a multiple risk factor intervention strategy should be the primary approach to disease management.

Patients should be treated to all recommended goals using evidence-based treatment guidelines.[44–49] Patients and providers should embrace the concept of overall CVD risk and aggressively manage all coronary heart disease (CHD) risk factors. Providers and patients should commit to long-term management with special emphasis on lifestyle changes, including weight control, increased physical activity, and smoking cessation. Since diabetes is a CHD risk equivalent, all patients with type 2 diabetes should receive intensive treatment and risk modification with the same intensity as individuals with established CHD.[44–49]

Glycemic Control

Glycemic control is strongly associated with microvascular disease in individuals with diabetes, but its relation to macrovascular disease and atherosclerosis is less clear. The Diabetes Control and Complications Trial (DCCT) and the U.K. Prospective Diabetes Study (UKPDS)[50–53] demonstrated that intensive diabetes management in patients with insulin-dependent diabetes mellitus (IDDM) improves glycemic control and reduces risk of development of retinopathy, nephropathy, and neuropathy.[52] Intensive glycemic management with insulin may also reduce morbidity in patients with severe acute illness (i.e., following myocardial infarction). Epidemiologic studies and a recent meta-analysis[54–56] support the potential of aggressive intensive glycemic control to reduce CVD but this is yet to be demonstrated in randomized clinical trials.

Intensive LDL Cholesterol (LDL-C)-Lowering Therapy

Several large clinical outcomes trials of lipid lowering with 3-hydroxy-3-methylglutaryl coenzyme A reductase inhibitors (statins) have demonstrated that intensive lowering of low-density lipoprotein cholesterol (LDL-C) stabilizes atherosclerotic plaques and reduces CHD events[57–60] in both diabetic and nondiabetic patients. The PROVE IT-TIMI 22 trial (Pravastatin or Atorvastatin Evaluation and Infection Therapy-Thrombolysis in Myocardial Infarction 22)[57] evaluated the benefits of intensive LDL-C-lowering therapy to a level of approximately 70 mg/dL with atorvastatin 80 mg/day as compared to the standard LDL-C lowering to 100 mg/dL with pravastatin 40 mg/day in reducing the incidence of cardiovascular events in patients with acute coronary syndromes (ACS). At 2-years follow-up a statistically significant reduction in the primary endpoint (a composite of death, myocardial infarction, unstable angina requiring hospitalization, need for coronary revascularization, or stroke) was noted and the benefit of intensive lipid-lowering therapy was seen as early as 30 days. The results of PROVE IT-TIMI 22 demonstrated that patients presenting with ACS (unstable angina or non-ST-elevation myocardial infarction) benefit from early intensive LDL-C lowering to levels below 70 mg/dL.[45]

The REVERSAL (Reversal of Atherosclerosis with Aggressive Lipid Lowering) trial[58] was a randomized, controlled, multicenter trial comparing the effects of intensive lipid-lowering therapy with atorvastatin 80 mg/day versus the moderate LDL-C lowering with pravastatin 40 mg/day on plaque progression as measured by intravascular ultrasound (IVUS) in patients requiring coronary angiography. For the primary endpoint of percent change in total atheroma volume, a significantly lower rate of progression from baseline was observed in the intensive lipid-lowering group as compared with moderate lipid lowering. These landmark trials demonstrated that there is significant benefit from intensive lowering of LDL-C and that atherosclerosis progression could be slowed and even halted in many patients.

The ASTEROID (A Study to Evaluate the Effect of Rosuvastatin on Intravascular Ultrasound-Derived Coronary Atheroma Burden) study[60] evaluated the effect of intensive statin therapy with rosuvastatin 40 mg/day on atheroma volume as measured by IVUS. A reduction in the LDL-C level from a mean of 130 mg/dL to a mean of 60.8 mg/dL (53.2% reduction from baseline) as well as a significant increase in the high-density lipoprotein cholesterol (HDL-C) (mean increase of 14.7%) was observed on treatment. A significant reduction in total atheroma volume occurred on treatment, a statistically significant regression of atherosclerosis.

These and other clinical trials of cholesterol lowering with statins in high-risk patients demonstrate that intensive LDL-C lowering can slow progression, halt progression, and even produce regression of atherosclerotic lesions. Thus, all diabetic patients with atherosclerosis should receive intensive LDL-C lowering with a minimum goal of <70 mg/dL.[45]

HDL-Raising as a Therapeutic Target

Low HDL-C is a well recognized, strong, and independent risk factor for CHD.[44,61] Low HDL-C may be caused by insulin resistance, diabetes, elevated triglycerides, physical inactivity, cigarette smoking, and certain drugs (i.e., beta-blockers, anabolic steroids, and progesterone). Although low HDL as a CHD risk factor has been known for decades, only recently has clinical trial evidence emerged which demonstrated the benefits of raising HDL-C.[62,63] In individuals with low HDL-C levels, the primary therapeutic objective is to achieve the recommended LDL-C goal.[44] If the triglyceride level is elevated, reduction of non-HDL-C is the secondary target. Drug therapy solely for raising the HDL-C level is generally reserved for very high-risk patients. Currently available pharmacologic interventions used for low HDL levels include statins, niacin (nicotinic acid), and fibrates.[62]

The precise mechanism of HDL's protective action is not completely understood, but is thought to be multifactorial and likely includes promotion of reverse cholesterol transport from macrophages to the liver, as well as an anti-inflammatory and antioxidant activity, induction of NO synthesis, and possibly an effect on platelet aggregation. The main focus of research, however, has been the reverse cholesterol transport activity of HDL-C, whereby excess macrophage cholesterol is effluxed from endovascular sites to HDL molecules for transport to the liver. ApoA-1 (apolipoprotein A-1) is the main protein in the HDL molecule and is thought to play a crucial role in cholesterol transport. Multiple efforts are underway investigating the potential utilization of the properties of ApoA-1 for cardiovascular protection.[62]

Statins

Although statins are used primarily to lower LDL-C, they tend to increase HDL levels by 5–10%. In the ASTEROID trial, using rosuvastatin, in addition to the 53% reduction in LDL-C, there was a 14.7% increase in HDL-C.[60]

Fibrates

Fibrates, another group of lipid-modifying therapy, raise HDL-C by 5–20% while also decreasing the levels of triglycerides. In the Veteran Affairs High-density lipoprotein Intervention Trial (VA-HIT) study, HDL-C levels increased on average about 6% and was associated with a reduction in cardiovascular events.[63]

Niacin

Niacin increases HDL-C by 15–30% in some studies, making it the most potent HDL-C-raising therapy currently available.[64] Data from Coronary Drug Project demonstrated that niacin reduced the incidence of cardiovascular events. Its mechanism of action is probably multifactorial and includes slowing of HDL metabolism by the liver cells, reduction in hepatic LDL and very low-density lipoprotein (VLDL) production, inhibition of adipose tissue lipolysis, stimulation of lipoprotein lipase activity, and possibly a direct effect on the macrophages. Unfortunately, many patients have difficulties related to the drugs side effects of flushing and pruritus, which precludes its more widespread use. Therefore, there is an obvious need for development of more potent and better-tolerated HDL-raising therapies as this may turn out to be an important strategy in the treatment of coronary atherosclerosis.

ApoA-1 Milano

ApoA-1 Milano is a mutated variant of ApoA-1 lipoprotein that was identified in a small population in the Northern Italy. This variant differs from the wild-type protein by arginine for cysteine substitution at position 173, allowing for dimer formation. Patients with this mutation characteristically have very low levels of HDL-C, longevity, and low incidence of atherosclerotic heart disease. The mutation alters the protein resulting in ApoA-1 Milano being functionally much more effective than the normal ApoA-1.[65] A recombinant form of ApoA-1 Milano has been synthesized, and some early animal studies have shown very promising results for reduction of atheroma burden with infusion of this compound. To test this hypothesis, a randomized, multicenter study comparing the effects of intravenous recombinant ApoA-1 Milano-phospholipid complex on coronary atheroma volume in patients with known coronary disease and ACS was performed.[66] The study demonstrated a statistically significant reduction in the volume of coronary atheromas as measured by IVUS, following a 5-week course of ApoA-1 Milano infusion. The patients in the treatment arm of the study had an absolute reduction of 4.2% in the volume of atheroma as compared to the placebo group. These findings demonstrated atherosclerosis regression with ApoA-1 infusion therapy.

ApoA-1 Mimetic Peptides

Smaller peptide molecules that mimic the lipophilic regions of the ApoA-1 molecule, and therefore should in theory promote reverse cholesterol transport, are being developed as well. Animal studies with such compounds have shown promising results, suggesting regression of atherosclerosis with parenteral administration.[62] Most of these agents must be administered parenterally. However, an oral therapy with ApoA-1 mimetic peptide composed of D-amino acids, and thus bioavailable with oral administration is currently undergoing clinical evaluation.[61,65]

Another strategy being investigated is the use of patients' endogenous ApoA-1. Lipid-poor ApoA-1 is known to be more effective at promoting cholesterol efflux from macrophages and a technique of ex vivo delipidation with subsequent reinfusion of native HDL has been developed. However, there are currently no clinical trial data demonstrating the effectiveness of this approach.[61]

PPAR Agonists

Treatments that stimulate endogenous ApoA-1 production by turning on the genes encoding for this peptide are currently under investigation and preliminary reports are encouraging. The PPARs are ligand-activated transcription factors located in the nucleus that modulate the transcription of multiple genes.[62,64] They are active in lipid metabolism, affect vascular inflammation, and may play an important role in the rate of progression of atherosclerosis. Fibrates and TZDs—both weak agonists of PPARs—are known to upregulate ApoA-1. Therefore, an intense search for more potent PPAR agonists that may promote reverse cholesterol transport and reduce the atherosclerotic burden is underway.[62] Two compounds, dual PPAR agonists, muraglitazar and tesaglitazar, are currently being investigated.[65]

Table 22-3 **HDL-Raising Therapies**

HDL-C-Raising Therapies	Mechanism of Action on HDL-C	Available in United States
Statins	HMG-CoA reductase inhibitors	Yes
Niacin	Slows ApoA-1 catabolism	Yes
Fenofibrate, gemfibrozil	Weak PPAR-α agonists	Yes
TZDs	PPAR-γ agonists	Yes
Recombinant ApoA-1 Milano	Reverse cholesterol transport	No
Muraglitazar	PPAR-α and -γ agonist	No
Tesaglitazar	PPAR-α and -γ agonist	No
Torcetrapib	CETP inhibitor	No
Ex vivo delipidation	Reverse cholesterol transport	No
ApoA-1 mimetic peptides	Reverse cholesterol transport	No

Torcetrapib

The cholesterol ester transfer protein (CETP) is a plasma glycoprotein that facilitates the exchange of cholesterol esters for triglycerides from HDL to ApoB-containing lipoproteins.[62] Physiologically, inhibition of CETP should result in an increase of HDL-C, and clinical trials of a CETP inhibitor, torcetrapib, are currently being performed. Results of some preliminary studies have shown a significant, dose-dependant increase in HDL-C levels with torcetrapib, and are very encouraging. Larger trials of this agent, both as a monotherapy and in combination with statins are underway (Table 22-3).

FUTURE OUTLOOK FOR TREATMENT OF MYOCARDIAL ISCHEMIA

Anginal pain and its equivalents remain the most common symptoms of myocardial ischemia in patients with coronary artery disease (CAD).[67] All of these patients require medical therapy and many of them benefit from coronary revascularization procedures. Traditional pharmacotherapy for angina includes nitrates, beta-blockers, and calcium channel blockers.[67] However, despite revascularization and conventional therapy, many patients with coronary disease continue to suffer from angina with limitations of activity and reduced quality of life. Several novel pharmacologic and nonpharmacologic therapies are in development that may improve treatment for angina and patient quality of life.[67–78]

Novel Pharmacologic Therapies for Angina

RANOLAZINE

Ranolazine is a metabolic modulator as well as a late sodium channel inhibitor that has shown very promising results as an antianginal agent.[67,70,71] Similar to trimetazidine, it is believed to be a partial fatty acid oxidation inhibitor thereby improving cardiac energy metabolism and decreasing myocardial oxygen demand. The drug's action on the sodium channel may reverse action potential prolongation and suppress early after-depolarizations, which may be beneficial for patients who are at high risk for arrhythmias. The MARISA trial (Monotherapy Assessment of Ranolazine in Stable Angina)[71] showed an increase in exercise time in patients taking the drug. The CARISA trial (Combination therapy Assessment of Ranolazine in Stable Angina),[72] in which ranolazine was added to conventional therapies, demonstrated an improvement in exercise time as well as a decrease in number of anginal episodes. QT-segment prolongation was the most notable side effect, although its clinical significance was unclear.

IVABRADINE

Ivabradine is a negative chronotropic agent that acts on I(f) currents.[73] By lowering heart rate it also lowers myocardial oxygen demand, simultaneously improving oxygen supply. In a double-blind, placebo-controlled study by Borer et al.,[73] and another by Tardif et al.,[78] the drug has shown very promising results, and, was as effective as atenolol in reducing anginal symptoms.

NICORANDIL

Nicorandil is a nicotinamide ester that acts on the adenosine triphosphate-potassium channel, and also has direct vasodilatory properties.[74,75] It has activity on both arterial and venous systems, thereby reducing both preload and afterload. In the IONA trial (Impact Of Nicorandil in Angina) treatment with nicorandil resulted in reduction of the composite primary endpoint of cardiovascular death, nonfatal MI, and hospital admission for anginal symptoms.

L-ARGININE

L-Arginine may improve endothelium-dependent vasodilatation via the nitric oxide (NO) pathway, and therefore has been proposed as an alternative antianginal therapy. In a small randomized study, oral supplementation with L-arginine showed improvement in exercise time compared to placebo (Table 22-4).[76,77]

Enhanced External Counterpulsation for Refractory Angina

Enhanced external counterpulsation (EECP) represents a noninvasive non-pharmacologic outpatient therapy for anginal symptoms.[79–81] EECP consists of ECG-gated, computer-assisted sequential leg compression with three pairs of pneumatic cuffs placed on patients' lower extremities. A typical

Table 22-4 **Novel Therapies for Angina**

Antianginal Therapies	Mechanism of Action	Available in United States
Ranolazine	Late sodium channel inhibitor	No
Trimetazidine	Fatty acid oxidation inhibitor	No
Ivabradine	Acts on I(f) current (negative chronotrop)	No
Nicorandil	ATP-K+ channel, vasodilatation	No
L-Arginine	Endothelium-dependent vasodilatation	Yes
EECP	Possible hemodynamic effects	Yes
Gene therapy	Stimulation of angiogenesis in situ	No

treatment course consists of 35 treatments administered over a 7-week period. The therapy increases venous return to the heart, is postulated to augment diastolic flow, and to reduce afterload—hemodynamic effects similar to those seen with the intra-aortic balloon pump (IABP). However, the exact mechanism by which the antianginal effect is mediated is still unclear. EECP is thought to improve endothelial function and enhance vascular reactivity.[79] It also increases angiogenesis factors such as hepatocyte growth factor, vascular endothelial growth factor, and basic fibroblast growth factor.[80,81] An increase in the levels of these growth factors is thought to lead to augmentation of angiogenesis and formation of collateral circulation.[81]

The MUST-EECP (The Multicenter Study of Enhanced External Counterpulsation) study of 139 patients with chronic stable angina demonstrated an increase in exercise time and a reduction in the number of anginal episodes after 35 sessions. In another trial of EECP therapy, Masuda et al.[80] demonstrated improved myocardial perfusion, prolonged time to ECG evidence of exercise-induced ischemia, as well as increase in exercise duration. An increase in NO levels at rest, as well as a decrease in human atrial natriuretic peptide (ANP) and brain natriuretic peptide (BNP) levels were also noted after a course of EECP.[80]

In summary, EECP improves myocardial perfusion, angina symptoms, exercise tolerance, and quality of life in patients with CHD who continue to have angina despite medical therapy and coronary revascularization. It is generally well tolerated, and has been approved by the Food and Drug Administration (FDA) for use in patients with refractory angina.

CORONARY REVASCULARIZATION AND DIABETES

As the diabetes epidemic continues to grow unabated, so too does the demand for medical therapy and coronary revascularization procedures in diabetic patients. Both percutaneous coronary interventions (PCI) and coronary artery bypass graft (CABG) surgery are effective revascularization techniques in patients with diabetes. However, both PCI and CABG are associated with poorer outcomes in diabetics than nondiabetics.[82-88] The optimal revascularization strategy for diabetic patients with multivessel CAD—PCI or CABG—has not been determined and remains a matter of debate and controversy (see Chaps. 4 and 12 for a more detailed discussion).

The population of diabetic patients with coronary disease is expanding. Compared to their nondiabetic counterparts, diabetics are two to four times more likely to develop CAD, present with first myocardial infarction at younger ages, and experience greater mortality during the acute phase of myocardial infarction and during the postinfarction period.[89-93] Approximately 30% of patients hospitalized with ACS have diabetes. Despite recent advances in treatment, diabetic patients with acute myocardial infarction still have double the case fatality rate as their nondiabetic counterparts.[92]

Diabetic patients account for approximately 25% of the 1.5 million coronary revascularization procedures performed in the United States each year.[82–85] Diabetics undergoing PCI have worse survival, increased target vessel restenosis, and higher repeat revascularization rates than nondiabetics.[82,83,85] Diabetic patients undergoing CABG have increased perioperative morbidity and mortality, and poorer long-term outcomes than their nondiabetic counterparts.[82,83,85–89]

High-Risk Features of Coronary Artery Disease in Diabetes

Coronary artery disease in diabetics is characterized by several clinical, angiographic, and biologic features that confer increased risk (Table 22-5).[82–84,91] Anatomically, diabetic patients have a greater atherosclerotic burden, more diffuse and distal CAD, and smaller coronary luminal diameters. Metabolic

Table 22-5 **High-Risk Features in Diabetics with Atherosclerosis**

Metabolic Abnormalities

Hyperglycemia
Dyslipidemia
Insulin resistance
Hypertension

Coronary Angiographic Abnormalities

Greater atherosclerotic burden
Diffuse and distal CAD
Smaller coronary luminal diameters
Multivessel disease
Impaired coronary collateral development
Unfavorable coronary remodeling
High restenosis rate after PCI

Mechanistic Abnormalities

Decreased endothelial function
Inflammation
Prothrombotic state (increased thrombosis; decreased fibrinolysis)
Increased protein glycosylation
Increased intimal hyperplasia
Increased negative remodeling
Increased protein glycosylation
Increased vascular matrix deposition
Decreased collateral formation

Source: References 82–91.

and hematologic abnormalities include hyperglycemia, dyslipidemia, inflammation, and insulin resistance. Mechanistic abnormalities include a prothrombotic state, decreased endothelial function, increased protein glycosylation, decreased endothelial dysfunction, increased negative remodeling, and decreased collateral development. The clinical comorbidities in diabetics (chronic kidney disease, peripheral arterial disease [PAD]) also negatively impact outcomes following revascularization, whether PCI or CABG. All of these contribute to increased restenosis (increased hyperplasia and negative remodeling) and accelerated atherosclerosis.

Coronary Revascularization Strategies for Diabetic Patients

Coronary revascularization to restore coronary blood flow and myocardial perfusion in patients with ischemic heart disease is one of the marvels of modern medicine. However, optimizing revascularization outcomes in diabetics who require revascularization means not only selection of the most appropriate revascularization strategy (PCI, CABG, or hybrid procedures), and restoring myocardial perfusion, but also optimizing management of their ACS, as well as optimizing long-term secondary prevention and cardioprotective therapies (Table 22-6).

CORONARY ARTERY BYPASS GRAFT SURGERY

The greatest benefits from CABG surgery in terms of survival and improved quality of life have been seen in patients with left main coronary stenosis and in those with triple vessel disease and left ventricular dysfunction. Diabetes is associated with significantly greater perioperative morbidity because of wound infections, longer hospital stays, and reduced long-term survival compared to nondiabetics.[82–84,86–89]

Despite recent advances in catheter-based revascularization techniques, CABG remains the gold standard in patients with multivessel CAD. Advantages of bypass surgery for revascularization include: (1) superior long-term patency of the left internal mammary artery (LIMA) to left anterior descending (LAD) with approximately 95% patency at 15 years; (2) procedure of choice in most instances for patients with left main disease, diffuse multivessel disease, and chronic total occlusions. Disadvantages of CABG include: (1) invasiveness of the procedure (sternotomy required in many patients); (2) requirement for cardiopulmonary bypass (although some procedures can be performed off-pump); (3) high occlusion rate of bypasses if placed on hemodynamically nonsignificant stenosis; (4) patient preference for less invasive and nonsurgical procedures.

PERCUTANEOUS CORONARY INTERVENTIONS

Although the Bypass Angioplasty Revascularization Investigation (BARI) study[94,95] provided compelling evidence to some physicians that diabetic patients with multivessel CAD who need revascularization should preferably get CABG, the findings of the BARI study—fewer deaths than with PCI—have not been consistently confirmed by other registries and other studies. Furthermore, new developments in percutaneous techniques (i.e., drug coated stents) should translate to improved prognosis and may offset the advantage of CABG seen in the BARI study. Advantages of PCI include: (1) very low restenosis rates, even in long lesions and small vessels with drug-eluting stents (DES); (2) rapidly advancing technology and broadening of the spectrum of lesions that can be treated; interventionalists are increasingly tackling unprotected left main and three-vessel disease and there has been a groundswell of development in devices to cross chronic total occlusions. PCI is also associated with lower morbidity than the surgical alternatives, shorter hospital stays, potential for outpatient performance, and reduced costs. Preliminary results of complete revascularization by multivessel stenting are very encouraging. If these results are confirmed, patients in whom all lesions are amenable for PCI will probably be treated only by PCI. However, some of the advantages of PCI may be offset by newer minimally invasive surgical techniques, endarterectomy and/or transmyocardial laser revascularization in patients with diffuse coronary disease, and hybrid approaches which combine PCI and CABG.

HYBRID REVASCULARIZATION PROCEDURES

Hybrid revascularization entails performing both a PCI procedure and minimally invasive direct coronary artery bypass surgery, grafting of the LIMA to the LAD and/or a diagonal branch.[96–101] The two procedures may be performed within 1–2 days of each other (typical) or at the same time[101] in the operating room. Hybrid revascularization provides patients with a functionally complete revascularization and good outcomes with minimal surgery.[96] Patients with diabetes or other major morbidities may be particularly good candidates for this procedure where the patency advantage of the LIMA to LAD can be achieved with limited surgical intervention. This requires optimal communication and cooperation between surgeons and interventional cardiologists. The present data suggest that this hybrid strategy is a reasonable alternative that in appropriately selected patients, offers the best of both the surgical and the interventional worlds. Limitations of the hybrid strategy are: (1) requirement for antiplatelet therapy (Plavix) and bleeding; (2) many surgeons have not yet perfected the minimally invasive procedure techniques on a large enough series of patients; (3) turf wars and logistics.

However, the hybrid revascularization strategy provides a new option for treating appropriately selected patients. Although it is widely acknowledged that in some patients the hybrid approach is probably the best approach, the strategy has not yet gained much momentum (Table 22-6).

Table 22-6 **Coronary Revascularization Options in Diabetics with CHD**

CABG

Advantages:
    Superior long-term patency of the LIMA to LAD
    Procedure of choice for most patients with left main disease, diffuse
      multivessel disease, and chronic total occlusions
    More complete revascularizations
    May have mortality advantage in diabetics with multivessel disease
    Lower need for repeat revascularizations
    Procedure of choice for large atherosclerotic burden, diffuse disease, especially those
      with small vessels, left main lesions, binary stenoses, ostial lesions, severely calcified or
      thrombotic lesions, or ejection fractions below 25%
Disadvantages:
    Invasiveness of the procedure (sternotomy required in many patients)
    Requirement for cardiopulmonary bypass (although some procedures performed
      off-pump)
    High occlusion rate of bypasses if placed on hemodynamically nonsignificant stenosis
    Patient preference for less invasive procedure
    Neurocognitive dysfunction with cardiopulmonary bypass
    Vein graft attrition

PCI

Advantages:
    Very low restenosis rates with DES
    Rapidly advancing technology and broadening of spectrum of lesions that
      can be treated
    Lower morbidity than surgery
    Shorter hospital stays
    Potential for outpatient performance
    In-stent restenosis (symptomatic) <5%, similar to surgery
Disadvantages:
    Requirement for repeat procedures; greater need for repeat revascularization
    Treats only the lesion site
    In-stent restenosis (greater with bare metal stents)
    Increased restenosis risk in diabetes, long stenoses, and small vessels

Hybrid Procedures

Advantages:
    Functionally complete revascularization and good outcomes with minimal surgery
    Option for patients with major comorbidities
    Particularly good strategy where patency of LIMA to LAD and minimal surgery desired
    Offers best of both surgical and interventional worlds
Disadvantages
    Requirement for antiplatelet therapy and bleeding
    Many surgeons have not yet perfected the minimally invasive procedure techniques on
      a large enough series of patients
    Turf wars and logistics

Ongoing Clinical Trials Comparing PCI and CABG in Diabetics

Several ongoing clinical trials should help resolve the debate regarding the relative benefits of the various revascularization strategies for patients with diabetes.

The FREEDOM (Future Revascularization Evaluation in Patients with Diabetes Mellitus: Optimal Management of Multivessel Disease) is a prospective, multicenter, randomized clinical trial with the objective of evaluating whether PCI with DES is more or less effective than CABG.[102] The study will enroll 2400 adults with diabetes mellitus (type 1 or type 2) with angiographically confirmed multivessel CAD and morphology amenable to either PCI or CABG. The primary outcome measure will be the composite of all-cause mortality, nonfatal myocardial infarction, and stroke at the end of the 5-year patient accrual and follow-up with a minimum follow-up of 3 years. The main secondary endpoint will be the rate of occurrence of a major adverse cardiac or cerebrovascular event (MACCE) at the end of 1 year. MACCE is defined as the first occurrence of one of the following: death, myocardial infarction, stroke, or repeat revascularization.

The CARDia (Coronary Artery Revascularization in Diabetics) trial[103,104] is a multicenter, prospective, randomized comparison of optimal coronary angioplasty—with the use of stenting and abciximab recommended—versus CABG in patients with diabetes mellitus suitable for either intervention. The study will enroll 600 patients at 20 centers. Patients suitable for either procedure will be randomized to PCI or CABG. The PCI group will be further randomized to receive either bare stents or rapamycin-eluting stents.

Optimizing Revascularization Outcomes

Elucidation of the optimal revascularization strategy and the long-term impact of DES versus CABG in diabetics with multivessel CAD awaits the results of ongoing randomized clinical trials. Although optimizing selection of revascularization strategy—whether PCI, CABG, or hybrid—is very important for the management of diabetic patients, their ultimate survival will also depend greatly on improving management of their systemic diseases (e.g., diabetes and atherosclerosis). Coronary revascularization improves survival and quality of life for many patients. However, revascularization does not cure or reverse the underlying problem—atherosclerosis. Thus, optimally implemented secondary prevention and cardioprotective regimens are essential adjuncts to therapy and will likely have greater impact on outcomes than the specific revascularization technique.

Interventional cardiologists and cardiac surgeons have the opportunity and responsibility to provide or facilitate optimal care for their diabetic patients.

GENOMICS, DIABETES, AND CARDIOVASCULAR DISEASE

The Era of Genomics

It is well known that both genetic and environmental factors affect health, disease risk, and disease progression. We are now in the era of genomics, which can be said to have officially begun in April 2003 with completion of sequencing of the human genome and thus, ending the pregenomic era.[105,106] Whereas "genetics" refers to the study of single genes and their effects, "genomics," a term coined in 1987, refers to the study of the functions and interactions of all of the genes in the genome.[106,107] Completion of the international human genome project brings the promise of illumination of the molecular pathogenesis of many diseases—including diabetes and CVD—with new opportunities for prevention and targeted therapies. Thus, in addition to modifying environmental risk factors, an understanding and sometimes altering the genotype is emerging as a new paradigm for treatment of many diseases.[105,106,108]

According to Dr. Elias A. Zerhouni, Director of The National Institutes of Health, "We are on the brink of transforming medical treatment in the 21st Century. Our hope is to usher in an era where medicine will be *predictive, personalized and preemptive.*"[108]

PREDICTIVE

As the tools of genomic sequencing become more refined, and as we learn more about the role of various genes in the pathophysiology of CVD, we will be able to predict with a degree of certainty, which patients will be more susceptible to the disease even before the onset of symptoms or any clinical evidence of pathology.[108] The lessons learned from monogenic cardiac diseases, will help us understand genetically more complex disorders that are clearly determined by multiple genes. Identification of genes and gene polymorphisms that have high correlation with the disease processes will shed light on the molecular mechanisms involved in their pathophysiology. A current trend in biomedical science is to use new genetic strategies for screening novel genomic biomarkers that predict the risk and improve diagnosis.[108] Knowledge of underlying genetic makeup of the patient will allow prediction of disease risk and delivery of more personalized medical care.

PERSONALIZED

Even without extensive genetic work-up and knowledge of patients' genomes, important clinical differences between patients and patient populations are apparent. Certain widely used therapies have been shown to be cardioprotective, but clearly not all patients benefit.[108,109] Identification of genetic differences that affect individual patient's responses to pharmacotherapy—and other treatments—will allow the development of individualized approaches to medicine. As we gain greater knowledge of pharmacogenetics and the genetically determined effects of medications, individually customized treatments can be developed that address the specific individual needs. The strategy will be to match the appropriate therapeutic agent to the appropriate patient, and in some cases, perhaps even design individual therapies for patients according to their genotype.[109]

PREEMPTIVE

A better understanding of the genetic determinants of the disease will allow us to be preemptive[108] rather than reactive. Instead of diagnosing diseases such as diabetes or atherosclerosis only after they become clinically significant, genomics will allow preemptive treatment of high-risk patients based on their genetic makeup.

Pharmacogenomics

The pharmacologic management of CVDs is based primarily on the results of clinical trials and on guidelines developed by expert consensus panels. Since these treatment recommendations are for population groups, it is recognized and accepted that not all patients will derive the same benefits. Patients vary greatly in their responses to drugs used to treat cardiovascular disorders and diabetes. Some patients achieve the desired therapeutic responses and others do not. Furthermore, some patients will experience adverse effects, which may range from minor to life threatening. A compelling body of evidence now exists that for a number of drugs, genetic variability is an important determinant of the observed differences in responses.[105,106,108,110] It has been estimated that genetic factors may account for 20–95% of variability in drug effects.[111,112]

Pharmacogenomics is the study of genetic determinants of the body's response to drugs.[111] The promise of pharmacogenomics is that one day it will be possible to tailor-make and prescribe drugs to individual patients based on their genetic makeup. This approach has the potential for greater treatment efficacy, fewer adverse effects, and better overall disease management and outcomes.

In the fields of diabetes and cardiovascular medicine, pharmacogenomics may add to our knowledge of pharmacologic agents by: (1) identification of potentially new drug targets since it has been estimated that currently available drugs use only about 500 of the potentially 5000–10000 potential drug targets in the body[109]; and (2) provide data and new insights that elucidate the genetic or genomic contribution to variable responses to current and future drugs. However, despite the considerable data that currently exist regarding gene-drug interactions and the ongoing intensive study, translation of pharmacogenomics in clinical practice is anticipated to be a slow process that will take a decade or more before genetic/genomic information will be widely used in drug therapy decisions.[109]

Pharmacogenomics and Diabetes

Type 2 diabetes is a complex and heterogeneous metabolic disorder. Genetic factors contribute importantly to both the insulin resistance and pancreatic beta-cell failure components of type 2 diabetes although the specific responsible genes have not been identified.[113] Oral antidiabetic medications (e.g., sulfonylureas and TZDs) are very effective therapies in many patients. However, patients' responses to these agents are variable and some patients fail to respond adequately. The molecular reasons for treatment response differences to antidiabetic therapy are yet to be defined. Pharmacogenomics provides the opportunity to study and define the molecular reasons and genetic polymorphisms responsible for the variability in responses to specific drugs and for adverse effects.[114–117] This offers hope that one day pharmacogenetic principles will be translated into widespread clinical practice. The candidate genes whose polymorphisms may influence drug response belong to three main groups[113,117]: (1) genetic polymorphisms that influence drug pharmacokinetics and disposition; (2) genetic polymorphisms of drug targets and receptors; and (3) polymorphisms of genes indirectly involved in drug response.

Pharmacogenomic studies are currently underway with the goal of better understanding the genetic polymorphisms that may affect responses of patients with type 2 diabetes to antidiabetic oral treatment. For example, in a recent study by Kang et al.,[118] the investigators found that genetic variations in the adiponectin gene affects the rosiglitazone treatment response of the circulating adiponectin level and blood glucose control in type 2 diabetic patients. Specifically, these researchers found that patients with G allele homozygosity at locus 45 and locus 276 do not respond to rosiglitazone. Furthermore, variations in the adiponectin gene were found that could affect the rosiglitazone treatment response to the serum adiponectin level and blood glucose control. Such studies are potentially clinically relevant since they permit identification of patients who will respond to a specific drug—in this case rosiglitazone—and also identification of those who will not respond.

Genomics and Coronary Artery Disease

Currently there are two main areas of genetic research in patients with CAD: identification of genes or gene polymorphisms that may predispose patients to development of atherosclerotic heart disease and actual gene therapy in patients with symptomatic CAD.[108] Identification of genes important in the pathogenesis of atherosclerosis is challenging, as CAD is not inherited in a simple Mendelian fashion, has multiple genes contributing to the development of the disease, and is clearly related to environmental factors as well. However, determination of genetic risk will help, not only in improving management of CVD, but also in providing preventive tools for high-risk population such as women. For example, the identified mutation in the lipoprotein lipase gene, Asn291Ser, was associated with increased ischemic heart disease in women.[119] More recently, this mutation that is present in about 5% of the population, was also associated with increased risk for ischemic cerebrovascular disease.[119] Targeted gene therapy, as well as application of preventive measures to control CVD risk factors in susceptible patients, would help decrease the CVD burden in this vulnerable population.

Genetically determined abnormalities of lipid metabolism are likely to contribute to the pathogenesis of plaque formation. Monogenic familial hypercholesterolemia syndromes that result from mutations of genes encoding LDL receptor proteins, components of the LDL molecule, or ATP binding cassette have been described.[106,119] In most cases of dyslipidemia, however, there is no clear association with a single gene, and multiple genes are probably responsible for predisposing each particular patient to abnormal lipid metabolism. Knowing the molecular mechanisms of lipoprotein synthesis and metabolism helps researchers to identify targets for interventions as well as to screen for genetic polymorphisms that may have a meaningful predictive value for dyslipidemia or CAD.

In a similar fashion, hypertension is believed to be partially genetically induced.[106] The pathology of hypertension is complex, and in most cases there is no single identifiable gene responsible for it. Monogenic hypertensive disorders usually involve genes encoding for proteins important in synthesis of mineralocorticoid hormones, aldosterone receptor, and ENaC channel, which leads us to believe the more complex genetic disorders resulting in hypertension would involve sodium homeostasis, vascular tone, renin-angiotensin-aldosterone axis, renal function, cardiac contractility, and neurohormonal milieu.

Diabetes, clearly a very important risk factor for development of atherosclerosis, also has a significant genetic component. Identification of genetic factors predisposing patients to diabetes and metabolic syndrome will allow us to predict and prevent development of diabetes as well as its cardiovascular complications.

The HapMap Project is another way in which researchers are trying to identify genes predictive of certain diseases, including CAD and diabetes.[120] Rather than searching for specific genes, the project focuses on analyzing the haplotype patterns in different populations around the world and trying to associate them with known diseases. In this fashion, once a large enough database is built, certain genetic patterns can be identified that correlate with CAD. Even though patients identified in this manner are less likely to have a disease state that can be corrected with gene therapy, early identification of patients at risk will allow us to predict and prevent coronary disease more efficiently.

Gene Therapy

The obvious next step, after identifying a genetic abnormality or a polymorphism that increases one's chances of developing a CVD is to attempt to correct it. Even though the genetic makeup of a patient is predetermined and cannot be changed, a number of techniques have been developed and used in research in order to affect the expression of the exiting genes and to introduce new genes into the organism or sometimes to a specific tissue. The use of plasmid vectors and modified viral particles for targeted delivery of genetic material is being extensively studied. There are some limited results from human studies that may affect the future strategies for treatment of CVDs.

Collateral vessel growth induced by growth factors is a natural process and is one of the protective mechanisms to prevent ischemia.[109] Unfortunately, the angiogenesis often does not occur in a timely enough fashion to overcome the effects of atherosclerotic coronary disease, and prevent myocardial ischemia. The molecular mechanisms involved in angiogenesis and arteriogenesis are also impaired by old age, dyslipidemia states, diabetes mellitus, and endothelial dysfunction, the same factors that promote atherosclerotic disease. Therefore, the evolving paradigm of using trans-genes encoding for growth factors that are active in angiogenesis, to be delivered directly to the target areas to improve collateral circulation and to lessen the symptoms of angina by increasing oxygen supply is quite appealing.

The questions that ought to be answered by ongoing research are: "What gene targets to use?" and "Where and how to deliver it?" There are a multitude of potential gene targets,[121] as the number of proteins that play an active role in angiogenesis is large and new factors are being discovered. Some of the potential targets for genetic manipulation include HIF-1α, VEGF, Ang-1 and Ang-2, PDGF, MCP-1, FGF, PlGF, HGF, and many others.[109] The optimal target area is likely to be determined by the actual gene product, for example, stimulation of collateral circulation would be clinically beneficial in the area connecting a patent artery to hibernating myocardium. Capillary growth and improved microcirculation would probably be of greater importance in the peri-infarct area. Multiple delivery strategies exist in order to bring the trans-gene to the target area. The methods range from the delivery of soluble factors that can be introduced intravenously or via an intracoronary injection, to highly specific tissue trophic vectors that selectively target a certain tissue or cell type. The vector itself could be a plasmid, a liposome-containing genetic material, or a viral particle.

Side effects of gene therapy are not well known at this time, as it has not been studied extensively in clinical practice yet. However, in theory they may be caused by the delivery process, the vector carrying the trans-gene, or the gene product itself.

The AGENT (Angiogenic Gene Therapy)[122] trial was a study of injection of adenovirus containing basic FGF gene versus placebo in patients with refractory angina. Patients in the treatment arm of the study had a 30% improvement in their exercise time at 12-week follow-up. AGENT-2[123]—a trial of intracoronary injection of the same gene has shown a reduction in ischemic defect size as determined by single photon emission computed tomography (SPECT).

Patients in the high-dose treatment arm of the VIVA (Vascular Endothelial Growth Factor in Ischemia for Vascular Angiogenesis)[124] study had an improvement in their angina class.

At this time, gene therapy is still considered an experimental, although a very promising developing treatment of refractory angina. It may find its place in clinical practice when better gene targets as well as more reliable delivery systems become available.

GENOMICS AND CARDIOMYOPATHY

Hypertrophic cardiomyopathy is probably the best-studied genetically induced cardiomyopathy.[106] It is transmitted in an autosomal dominant pattern and is caused by the mutations of various genes encoding for the parts of the myocardial contractile apparatus. There are multiple mutations resulting in the similar phenotype of hypertrophic cardiomyopathy.[106,125]

Dilated nonischemic cardiomyopathy (DCM) is a heterogeneous diagnosis with multiple underlying pathologies that can lead to a similar clinical picture. DCMs with clearly genetic etiology, such as Duchenne's muscular dystrophy, myotonic dystrophy, and Frederick's ataxia exist, but are relatively rare. Multiple other causes exist, including alcohol, viral and autoimmune, HIV related, drug/toxicity related, tachycardia induced, hypertensive, peripartum, valvular, diabetic, or related to general systemic disease. Although identification of specific genes responsible for the disorder will only be possible in the minority of these, identification of genetic patterns that predict higher susceptibility to the environmental or iatrogenic insults will be of clinical benefit.

Ischemic cardiomyopathy is prevalent in patients with diabetes. Although not genetic in nature, the same factors—some of them genetic—that lead to the development of CAD, if not treated, may eventually result in ischemic cardiomyopathy. There is some excitement over the possibility of regenerating myocardium by the introduction of stem cells into the damaged ventricle. However, no clinically useful results are available to date. Once the ethical and scientific difficulties surrounding the issue can be resolved, it may become a valuable therapy in treatment of systolic dysfunction, ischemic cardiomyopathy.

GENOMICS AND ARRHYTHMIAS

Genetically induced arrhythmias are some of the most interesting disorders and there is a lot of interest in identifying patients and families at risk for development of malignant arrhythmias.[126] Genetic abnormalities responsible for some of the familial syndromes such as long QT syndrome, Brugada's syndrome, catecholamine-induced ventricular tachycardia (VT), and some others have been identified, creating a possibility of gene therapy development in the future to cure those disorders. At this time, patients that have been determined to be at high risk for sudden cardiac death (SCD) may benefit from automatic implantable cardioverter-defibrillator (AICD) implantation.

Although arrhythmias related to CAD are thought to be induced by ischemia or scar, and not genetically determined, there is a possibility that there is a genetic component predisposing patients to development of ventricular arrhythmias. Identifying genetic polymorphisms correlating with higher incidence of ventricular arrhythmias in CAD patients will help to determine which patients need more aggressive therapy and will allow prevention of VT and the resultant SCD.

SUMMARY AND CONCLUSION

Although preventable in many patients, the burden of diabetes and CVD in diabetics continue to increase in the United States and worldwide. The expanding epidemic of obesity, other major cardiovascular risk factors, suboptimal management of diabetes and its comorbidities account for much of the recent increased morbidity and mortality. The recent and continuing introduction of new therapies, new treatment strategies, and new technologies, as well as improved understanding of the genetics and pharmacogenomics of diabetes and CVD herald new opportunities for prevention, treatment, and stemming the tide of the diabetes-CVD conundrum.

According to the Institute of Medicine's recent report, *Crossing the Quality Chasm: A New Health System for the 21st Century*,[127] "...between the health care that we now have, and the health care we could have, lies not just a gap, but a chasm." In other words, better organization, coordination, and delivery of health care—even today—would result in improved quality and outcomes. The quality of care provided to patients with diabetes is far from optimal with <30% of diabetics achieving currently recommended treatment goals.[128,129] This is true even though optimal control and intensive management of risk factors can reduce CVD by as much as 50%.[130,131]

One of the critically important opportunities for improving the quality of care and outcomes in patients with diabetes and CVD is greater and more consistent use of recent advances in information technology (IT).[127,132] Recent advances in IT can help improve the quality of health care and improve cardiovascular outcomes[127,132] in part by (1) bringing decision support to the point of care; (2) increased automation of clinical, financial, and administrative functions that prevent errors and improve efficiency; (3) facilitation of improved implementation of evidence-based treatments through computer-assisted decision support systems; (4) enhanced communication between providers and patients; and (5) enhanced providers education.

Unraveling the diabetes-CVD conundrum and reversing the current trend of expanding diabetes and diabetes-associated complications require renewed commitment on the parts of providers, patients, and health care institutions with the primary focus on prevention and closing the chasm "between the health care that we now have, and the health care we could have."

REFERENCES

1. Engelgau MM. Trying to predict the future for people with diabetes: a tough but important task. *Ann Intern Med* 2005;143:301–302.

2. American Diabetes Association. Screening for Diabetes. Diabetes Care 2003; 26(Suppl 1):S21–S24.

3. Rohrscheib M, Robinson R, Eaton RP. Non-invasive glucose sensors and improved informatics—the future of diabetes management. *Diabetes Obes Metab* 2003;5:280–284.

4. Peeples MM. Directing the future of diabetes self-management. *Diabetes Educ* 2006;32:158–163.

5. McFarlane SI, Shin JJ, Rundek T, et al. Prevention of type 2 diabetes. *Curr Diab Rep* 2003;3:235–241.

6. Lehmann ED. Information technology in clinical diabetes care—a look to the future. *Diabetes Technol Ther* 2004;6:755–759.

7. Kriska AM, Delahanty LM, Pettee KK. Lifestyle intervention for the prevention of type 2 diabetes: translation and future recommendations. *Curr Diab Rep* 2004;4:113–118.

8. Janssens AC, Gwinn M, Khoury MJ, et al. Does genetic testing really improve the prediction of future type 2 diabetes? *PLoS Med* 2006;3:e114–e127.

9. Girish C, Manikandan S, Jayanthi M. Newer insulin analogues and inhaled insulin. *Indian J Med Sci* 2006;60:117–123.

10. Winter WE, Schatz D. Prevention strategies for type 1 diabetes mellitus: current status and future directions. *BioDrugs* 2003;17:39–64.

11. Bond MM, Yates SW. Is the future bright for diabetes? *South Med J* 2004;97: 1027–1028.

12. Adams G, Wang N, Cui Y. Future alternative therapies in a quest to halt aberrations in diabetes mellitus. *Biomed Pharmacother* 2005;59:296–301.

13. New diabetes prediction tool lets patients, providers take glimpse into the future. *Dis Manag Advis* 2005;11:103–105, 197.

14. El Atat F, Nicasio J, Clarke LT, et al. Beneficial cardiovascular effects of thiazolidinediones. *Therapy* 2005;2:113–119.

15. Knowler WC, Barrett-Connor E, Fowler SE, et al. Diabetes Prevention Program Research Group. Reduction in the incidence of type 2 diabetes with lifestyle intervention or metformin. *N Engl J Med* 2002;346:393–403.

16. Tuomilehto J, Lindstrom J, Eriksson JG, et al. Prevention of type 2 diabetes mellitus by changes in lifestyle among subjects with impaired glucose tolerance. *N Engl J Med* 2001;344:1343–1350.

17. Helmrich SP. Physical activity and reduced occurrence of non-insulin-dependent diabetes mellitus. *N Engl J Med* 1991;325:147–152.

18. Eriksson KF. Prevention of type 2 (non-insulin-dependent) diabetes mellitus by diet and physical exercise. The 6-year Malmo feasibility study. *Diabetologia* 1991;34:891–898.

19. Henriksson J. Effects of physical training on the metabolism of skeletal muscle. *Diabetes Care* 1992;15:1701–1711.

20. Devlin JT. Effects of exercise on insulin sensitivity in humans. *Diabetes Care* 1992;15:1690–1693.

21. Bjorntorp P. Abdominal obesity and the development of noninsulin-dependent diabetes mellitus. *Diabetes Metab Rev* 1988;4:615–622.

22. Wing RR, Venditti E, Jakicic JM, et al. Lifestyle intervention in overweight individuals with a family history of diabetes. *Diabetes Care* 1998;21:350–359.

23. Long SD, O'Brien K, MacDonald KG Jr, et al. Weight loss in severely obese subjects prevents the progression of impaired glucose tolerance to type II diabetes. A longitudinal interventional study. *Diabetes Care* 1994;17:372–375.

24. Després J-P, Golay A, Sjöström L. Effects of rimonabant on metabolic risk factors in overweight patients with dyslipidemia. *N Engl J Med* 2005;353:2121–2134.

25. Boyd ST, Fremming BA. Rimonabant—a selective CB1 antagonist. *Ann Pharmacother* 2005;39:684–690.

26. Feskens EJ, Virtanen SM, Rasanen L, et al. Dietary factors determining diabetes and impaired glucose tolerance. A 20-year follow-up of the Finnish and Dutch cohorts of the Seven Countries Study. *Diabetes Care* 1995;18:1104–1112.

27. Marshall JA. Dietary fat predicts conversion from impaired glucose tolerance to NIDDM. The San Luis Valley Diabetes Study. *Diabetes Care* 1994;17:50–56.

28. Swinburn BA. Long-term (5-year) effects of a reduced-fat diet intervention in individuals with glucose intolerance. *Diabetes Care* 2001;24:619–624.

29. Pan XR, Li GW, Hu YH, et al. Effects of diet and exercise in preventing NIDDM in people with impaired glucose tolerance. The Da Qing IGT and Diabetes Study. *Diabetes Care* 1997;20:537–544.

30. Kirpichnikov D. Metformin: an update. *Ann Intern Med* 2002;137:25–33.

31. Fontbonne A, Charles MA, Juhan-Vague I, et al. The effect of metformin on the metabolic abnormalities associated with upper-body fat distribution. BIGPRO Study Group. *Diabetes Care* 1996;19:920–926.

32. Buchanan TA, Xiang AH, Peters RK, et al. Preservation of pancreatic beta-cell function and prevention of type 2 diabetes by pharmacological treatment of insulin resistance in high-risk Hispanic women. *Diabetes* 2002;51:2796–2803.

33. Stumvoll M. Glitazones: clinical effects and molecular mechanisms. *Ann Med* 2002;34:217–224.

34. Delgado H, Lehmann T, Bobbioni-Harsch E, et al. Acarbose improves indirectly both insulin resistance and secretion in obese type 2 diabetic patients. *Diabetes Metab* 2002;28:195–200.

35. Chiasson JL, Josse RG, Gomis R, et al. Acarbose for prevention of type 2 diabetes mellitus: the STOP-NIDDM randomised trial. *Lancet* 2002;359:2072–2077.

36. Gerstein HC. Reduction of cardiovascular events and microvascular complications in diabetes with ACE inhibitor treatment: HOPE and MICRO-HOPE. *Diabetes Metab Res Rev* 2002;18(Suppl 3):S82–S85.

37. Hansson L, Lindholm LH, Niskanen L, et al. Effect of angiotensin-converting-enzyme inhibition compared with conventional therapy on cardiovascular morbidity and mortality in hypertension: the Captopril Prevention Project (CAPPP) randomized trial. *Lancet* 1999;353:611–616.

38. Yusuf S,Sleight P, Pogue J, et al. Effects of an angiotensin-converting-enzyme inhibitor, ramipril, on cardiovascular events in high-risk patients. The Heart Outcomes Prevention Evaluation Study Investigators. *N Engl J Med* 2000;342:145–153.

39. Lindholm LH, Ibsen H, Dahlof B, et al. Cardiovascular morbidity and mortality in patients with diabetes in the Losartan Intervention for Endpoint reduction in hypertension study (LIFE): a randomized trial against atenolol. *Lancet* 2002;359:1004–1010.

40. McFarlane SI, Kumar A, Sowers JR, et al. Mechanisms by which angiotensin-converting enzyme inhibitors prevent diabetes and cardiovascular disease. *Am J Cardiol* 2003;91(12A):30H–37H.

41. Sowers JR. Diabetes, hypertension, and cardiovascular disease: an update. *Hypertension* 2001;37:1053–1059.

42. Sharma AM, Janke J, Gorzelniak K, et al. Angiotensin blockade prevents type 2 diabetes by formation of fat cells. *Hypertension* 2002;40:609–611.

43. Freeman DJ, Norrie J, Sattar N, et al. Pravastatin and the development of diabetes mellitus: evidence for a protective treatment effect in the West of Scotland Coronary Prevention Study. *Circulation* 2001;103:357–362.

44. Third Report of the National Cholesterol Education Program (NCEP) Expert Panel on Detection, Evaluation, and Treatment of High Blood Cholesterol in Adults (Adult Treatment Panel III) Final Report. *Circulation* 2002;106:3146–3421.

45. Grundy SM, Cleeman JI, Merz CN, et al. Coordinating Committee of the National Cholesterol Education Program. Implications of recent clinical trials for the National Cholesterol Education Program Adult Treatment Panel III Guidelines. *J Am Coll Cardiol* 2004;4;44:720–732.

46. Pearson TA, Blair SN, Daniels SR, et al. AHA guidelines for primary prevention of cardiovascular disease and stroke: 2002 update. *Circulation* 2002;106:388–391.

47. Covey SS Jr, Blair SN, Bonow RO, et al. AHA/ACC guidelines for preventing heart attack and death in patients with atherosclerotic cardiovascular disease: 2001 update. *Circulation* 2001;104:1577–1579.

48. Chobanian AV, Bakris GL, Black HR, et al. The Seventh Report of the Joint National Committee on Prevention, Detection, Evaluation, and Treatment of High Blood Pressure: the JNC 7 Report. *JAMA* 2003;289:2560–2572.

49. American Diabetes Association. Standards of medical care in diabetes—2006 Diabetes Care 2006;29(Suppl 1):S4–S42.

50. U.K. Prospective Diabetes Study (UKPDS) Group: intensive blood-glucose control with sulphonylureas or insulin compared with conventional treatment and risk of complications in patients with type 2 diabetes (UKPDS 33). *Lancet* 1998;352:837–853.

51. U.K. Prospective Diabetes Study (UKPDS) Group: effect of intensive blood-glucose control with metformin on complications in overweight patients with type 2 diabetes (UKPDS 34). *Lancet* 1998;352:854–865.

52. The Diabetes Control and Complications Trial/Epidemiology of Diabetes Interventions and Complications Research Group: retinopathy and nephropathy in patients with type 1 diabetes four years after a trial of intensive therapy. *N Engl J Med* 2000;342:381–389.

53. The Diabetes Control and Complications Trial Research Group: the effect of intensive treatment of diabetes on the development and progression of long-term complications in insulin-dependent diabetes mellitus. *N Engl J Med* 1993;329:977–986.

54. Lawson ML, Gerstein HC, Tsui E, et al. Effect of intensive therapy on early macrovascular disease in young individuals with type 1 diabetes: a systematic review and meta-analysis. *Diabetes Care* 1999;22(Suppl 2):B35–B39.

55. Stratton IM, Adler AI, Neil HA, et al. Association of glycaemia with macrovascular and microvascular complications of type 2 diabetes (UKPDS 35): prospective observational study. *Br Med J* 2000;321:405–412.

56. Selvin E, Marinopoulos S, Berkenblit G, et al. Meta-analysis: glycosylated hemoglobin and cardiovascular disease in diabetes mellitus. *Ann Intern Med* 2004;141:421–431.

57. Cannon CP, Braunwald E, McCabe CH, et al. and the PROVE-IT-TIMI 22 Investigators. Comparison of intensive and moderate lipid lowering with statins after acute coronary syndromes. *N Engl J Med* 2004;350:1495–1504.

58. Nissen SE, Tsunoda T, Tuzcu EM, et al. and the REVERSAL Investigators. Effect of intensive compared with moderate lipid-lowering therapy on progression of coronary atherosclerosis. A randomized controlled trial. *JAMA* 2004;291:1071–1080.

59. La Rosa JC, Grundy SM, Waters DD, et al. Intensive lipid lowering with atorvastatin in patients with stable coronary disease. *N Engl J Med* 2005;352:1425–1435.

60. Nissen SE, Nicholls SJ, Sipahi I, et al. ASTEROID Investigators. Effect of very high-intensity statin therapy on regression of coronary atherosclerosis: the ASTEROID trial. *JAMA* 2006;295(13):1556–1565.

61. Boden WE. High-density lipoprotein cholesterol as an independent risk factor in cardiovascular disease: assessing the data from Framingham to the Veterans Affairs High-Density Lipoprotein Intervention Trial. *Am J Cardiol* 2000;86:19L–22L.

62. Duffy D, Rader DJ. Emerging therapies targeting high-density lipoprotein metabolism and reverse cholesterol transport. Circulation 2006;113:1140–1150.

63. Robins SJ, Collins D, Wittes JT, et al. VA-HIT Study Group. Veterans Affairs High-Density Lipoprotein Intervention Trial. Relation of gemfibrozil treatment

and lipid levels with major coronary events: VA-HIT: a randomized controlled trial. *JAMA* 2001;285:1585–1591.

64. Assmann G, Gotto AM Jr. HDL cholesterol and protective factors in atherosclerosis. *Circulation* 2004;109:III-8–III-14.

65. Kaul S, Shah PK. ApoA-I Milano/phospholipid complexes emerging pharmacological strategies and medications for the prevention of atherosclerotic plaque progression. *Curr Drug Targets Cardiovasc Haematol Disord* 2005;5(6): 471–479.

66. Nissen SE, Tsunoda T, Tuzcu EM, et al. Effect of recombinant ApoA-I Milano on coronary atherosclerosis in patients with acute coronary syndromes: a randomized controlled trial. *JAMA* 2003;5;290:2292–2300.

67. Abrams J. Chronic stable angina. *N Engl J Med* 2005;352:2524–2533.

68. Gaffney SM. Ranolazine, a novel agent for chronic stable angina. *Pharmacotherapy* 2006;26(1):135–142.

69. Yang EH, Barsness GW, Gersh BJ, et al. Current and future treatment strategies for refractory angina. *Mayo Clin Proc* 2004;79(10):1284–1292. Review.

70. Sulfi S, Timmis AD. Ivabradine—the first selective sinus node I(f) channel inhibitor in the treatment of stable angina. *Int J Clin Pract* 2006;60(2):222–228.

71. Chaitman BR, Skettino SL, Parker JO, et al. MARISA Investigators. Antiischemic effects and long-term survival during ranolazine monotherapy in patients with chronic severe angina. *J Am Coll Cardiol* 2004;43:1375–1382.

72. Chaitman BR, Pepine CJ, Parker JO, et al. Combination Assessment of Ranolazine In Stable Angina (CARISA) Investigators. Effects of ranolazine with atenolol, amlodipine, or diltiazem on exercise tolerance and angina frequency in patients with severe chronic angina: a randomized controlled trial. *JAMA* 2004;291: 309–316.

73. Borer JS, Fox K, Jaillon P, et al. Ivabradine Investigators Group. Antianginal and antiischemic effects of ivabradine, an I(f) inhibitor, in stable angina: a randomized, double blind, multicentered, placebo-controlled trial. *Circulation* 2003;107: 817–823.

74. Ciampricotti R, Schotborgh CE, de Kam PJ, et al. A comparison of nicorandil with isosorbide mononitrate in elderly patients with stable coronary heart disease: the SNAPE study. *Am Heart J* 2000;139:939–943.

75. IONA Study Group. Effect of nicorandil on coronary events in patients with stable angina: the Impact Of Nicorandil in Angina (IONA) randomised trial. *Lancet* 2002;359:1269–1275.

76. Egashira K, Hirooka Y, Kuga T, et al. Effects of L-arginine supplementation on endothelium-dependent coronary vasodilation in patients with angina pectoris and normal coronary arteriograms. *Circulation* 1996;94:130–134.

77. Ceremuzynski L, Chamiec T, Herbaczynska-Cedro K. Effect of supplemental oral L-arginine on exercise capacity in patients with stable angina pectoris. *Am J Cardiol* 1997;80:331–333.

78. Tardif JC, Ford I, Tendera M, et al. INITIATIVE Investigators. Efficacy of ivabradine, a new selective I(f) inhibitor, compared with atenolol in patients with chronic stable angina. *Eur Heart J* 2005;26:2529–2536.

79. Bonetti PO, Barsness GW, Keelan PC, et al. Enhanced external counter-pulsation improves endothelial function in patients with symptomatic coronary artery disease. *J Am Coll Cardiol* 2003;41:1761–1768.

80. Masuda D, Nohara R, Hirai T, et al. Enhanced external counterpulsation improved myocardial perfusion and coronary flow reserve in patients with chronic stable angina. *Eur Heart J* 2001;22:1451–1458.

81. Stys TP, Lawson WE, Hui JC, et al. Effects of enhanced external counterpulsation on stress radionuclide coronary perfusion and exercise capacity in chronic stable angina pectoris. *Am J Cardiol* 2002;89:822–824.

82. Flaherty JD, Davidson CJ. Diabetes and coronary revascularization. *JAMA* 2005;293:1501–1508.

83. Smith SC, Faxon D, Cascio W, et al. Diabetes and cardiovascular disease writing group VI: revascularization in diabetic patients. *Circulation* 2002;105:e165–e169.

84. Hammoud T, Tanguay J, Bourassa MG. Management of coronary artery disease: therapeutic options in patients with diabetes. *J Am Coll Cardiol* 2000;36:355–365.

85. Kugelmass AD, Cohen DJ, Houser F, et al. The influence of diabetes mellitus on the practice and outcomes of percutaneous coronary intervention in the community: a report from the HCA database. *J Invasive Cardiol* 2003;15:568–574.

86. Carson JL, Scholz PM, Chen AY, Peterson ED, Gold J, Schneider SH. Diabetes mellitus increases shortterm mortality and morbidity in patients undergoing coronary artery bypass graft surgery. *J Am Coll Cardiol* 2002;40:418–423.

87. Lombardero MS, Brooks MM, et al. The effects of previous coronary-artery bypass surgery on the prognosis of patients with diabetes who have acute myocardial infarction. *N Engl J Med* 2000;342:989–997.

88. Barsness GW, Peterson ED, Ohman EM, et al. Relationship between diabetes mellitus and long-term survival after coronary bypass and angioplasty. *Circulation* 1997;96:2551–2556.

89. Berger A, MacCarthy PA, Siebert U, et al. Long-term patency of internal mammary artery bypass: relationship with preoperative severity of the native coronary artery stenosis. *Circulation* 2004;100(Suppl II):II36–II40.

90. Howard BV, Rodriguez BL, Bennett PH, et al. Prevention Conference VI: diabetes and cardiovascular disease: Writing Group I: epidemiology. *Circulation* 2002;105:132–137.

91. Grundy SM, Benjamin IJ, Burke GL, et al. Diabetes and cardiovascular disease: a statement for healthcare professionals from the American Heart Association. *Circulation* 1999;100:1134–1146. [Published erratum appears in *Circulation* 2000;101:1629–1631].

92. Jacoby R. Nesto R. Acute myocardial infarction in the diabetic patient: pathophysiology, clinical course and prognosis. *J Am Coll Cardiol* 1992;20:736–744.

93. Woodfield S, Lundergan C, Reiner J, et al. Angiographic findings and outcomes in diabetic patients treated with thrombolytic therapy for acute myocardial infarction: the GUSTO-I experience. *J Am Coll Cardiol* 1996;28:1661–1669.

94. The Bypass Angioplasty Revascularization Investigation (BARI) Investigators. Comparison of coronary bypass surgery with angioplasty in patients with multivessel disease. *N Engl J Med* 1996;335:217–225.

95. The BARI Investigators. Influence of diabetes on 5-year mortality and morbidity in a randomized trial comparing CABG and PTCA in patients with multivessel disease. The Bypass Angioplasty Revascularization Investigation (BARI). *Circulation* 1997;96:1761–1769.

96. Davidavicius G, Van Praet F, Mansour S, et al. Hybrid revascularization strategy: a pilot study on the association of robotically enhanced minimally invasive direct coronary artery bypass surgery and fractional flow reserve-guided percutaneous coronary intervention. *Circulation* 2005;112:I-317–I-322.

97. Cohen HA, Zenati M, Smith AJ, et al. Feasibility of combined percutaneous transluminal angioplasty and minimally invasive direct coronary artery bypass in patients with multivessel coronary artery disease. *Circulation* 1998;98:1048–1050.

98. Lloydt CT, Calafiore AM, Wilde P, et al. Integrated left anterior small thoracotomy and angioplasty for coronary artery revascularization. *Ann Thorac Surg* 1999;68:908–912.

99. Wittwer T, Cremer J, Boonstra P, et al. Myocardial "hybrid" revascularization with minimally invasive direct coronary artery bypass grafting combined with coronary angioplasty: preliminary results of a multicentre study. *Heart* 2000;83:58–63.

100. Riess FC, Bader R, Kremer P, et al. Coronary hybrid revascularization from January 1997 to January 2001: a clinical follow-up. *Ann Thorac Surg* 2002;73:1849–1855.

101. Lewis BS, Porat E, Halon DA, et al. Same-day combined coronary angioplasty and minimally invasive coronary surgery. *Am J Cardiol* 1999;84:1246–1247.

102. Available at: *ClinicalTrials.gov* (accessed May 2, 2006).

103. Smith D. The CARDia trial protocol. *Heart* 2003;89:1125–1126.

104. Kapur A, Malik IS, Bagger JP, et al. for the CARDia Investigators. The Coronary Artery Revascularisation in Diabetes (CARDia) trial: a prospective, randomised comparison of optimal coronary angioplasty with use of stenting and abciximab recommended versus up to date coronary artery bypass grafting in patients with diabetes mellitus suitable for either intervention. *Heart* 2003;89:550.

105. Nabel EG. Genomic medicine. Cardiovascular disease. *N Engl J Med* 2003;349:60–72.

106. Guttmacher AE, Collins FS. Genomic medicine: a primer. *N Engl J Med* 2002;347: 1512–1520.

107. McKusick VA, Ruddle FH. A new discipline, a new name, a new journal. *Genomics* 1987;1:1–2.

108. Zerhouni EA. From the Desk of the NIH Director. U.S. Department of Health and Human Services, National Institute of Health. Testimony before the House Subcommittee on Labor—HHS—Education Appropriations, 2006.

109. Markkanen JE, Rissanen TT, Kivelä A, et al. Growth factor-induced therapeutic angiogenesis and arteriogenesis in the heart—gene therapy. *Cardiovasc Res* 2005;65(3):547–762.

110. Johnson JA, Cavallari LH. Cardiovascular pharmacogenomics. *Exp Physiol* 2005;90;3:283–289.

111. Evans WE, McLeod H. Pharmacogenomics. Drug disposition, drug targets, and side effects. *N Engl J Med* 2003;348:538–549.

112. Weinshilboum R. Inheritance and drug response. *N Engl J Med* 2003;348:529–537.

113. Sesti G, Hribal ML. Pharmacogenetics in type 2 diabetes: polymorphisms in candidate genes affecting responses to antidiabetic oral treatment. *Curr Pharmacogenomics* 2006;4:69–78.

114. McCarthy MI, Froguel P. Genetic approaches to the molecular understanding of type 2 diabetes. *Am J Physiol* 2002;283:E217–E225.

115. Parikh H, Groop L. Candidate genes for type 2 diabetes. *Rev Endocr Metab Disord* 2004;5:151–176.

116. Sesti G. Searching for type 2 diabetes genes: prospects in pharmacotherapy. *Pharmacogenomics J* 2002;2:25–29.

117. Goldstein DB, Take SK, Sisodiya SM. Pharmacogenetics goes genomic. *Nat Rev Genet* 2003;4:937–947.

118. Kang ES, Park SY, Kim HJ, et al. The influence of adiponectin gene polymorphism on the rosiglitazone response in patients with type 2 diabetes. *Diabetes Care* 2005;28:1139–1144.

119. Ordovas JM. Lipoprotein lipase genetic variation and gender-specific ischemic cerebrovascular disease risk. *Nutr Rev* 2000;58(10):315–318.

120. The International HapMap Project. *Nature* 2003;426:789–796.

121. Mohamed Z. The future of genetic and genomic medicine in health risk assessment and disease: a path toward individualized medicine. Annual Meeting of the International Society of Pharmacogenomics, 2004.

122. Grines CL, Watkins MW, Helmer G, et al. Angiogenic Gene Therapy (AGENT) trial in patients with stable angina pectoris. *Circulation* 2002;105:1291–1297.

123. Grines CL, Watkins MW, Mahmarian JJ, et al. Angiogene GENe Therapy (AGENT-2) Study Group. A randomized, double blind, placebo-controlled trial of Ad5FGF-4 gene therapy and its effect on myocardial perfusion in patients with stable angina. *J Am Coll Cardiol* 2003;42:1339–1347.

124. Henry TD, Annex BH, McKendall GR, et al. VIVA Investigators. The VIVA Trial: vascular endothelial growth factor in ischemia for vascular angiogenesis. *Circulation* 2003;107:1359–1365.

125. Murphy RT, Starling RC. Genetics and cardiomyopathy: where are we now. *Cleve Clin J Med* 2005;72(6):465–466, 469–470, 472–473.

126. Noble D. Unraveling the genetics and mechanisms of cardiac arrhythmia. *Proc Natl Acad Sci U S A* 2002;99(9):5755–5756.

127. The Institute of Medicine Committee on Quality of Health Care In America. *Crossing the Quality Chasm: A New Health System for the 21st Century.* Washington, DC: National Academy Press, 2001.

128. Tulloch-Reid M, Williams DE. Quality of diabetes care in the United States between 1988 and 1995. *Clin Diabetes* 2003;21:43–45.

129. McFarlane SI, Jacober SJ, Winer N, et al. Control of cardiovascular risk factors in patients with diabetes and hypertension at urban academic medical centers. *Diabetes Care* 2002;25(4):718–723.

130. Marks JB. A look back and forward. *Clin Diabetes* 2006;24:51–53.

131. Gaude P, Vedel P, Larsen N, et al. Multifactorial interventions and cardio-vascular disease in patients with type 2 diabetes. *N Engl J Med* 2003;348: 383–393.

132. Bates DW. The quality case for information technology in healthcare. BMC Medical Informatics and Decision Making 2002;2:7. Available at: http://www. biomedcentral.com/1472–6947/2/7 (accessed May 7, 2006).

NOTE: Page numbers followed by *f* or *t* indicate figures or tables, respectively.